DERMATOLOGIC
NURSING ESSENTIALS

A Core Curriculum

THIRD EDITION

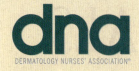

The Dermatology Nurses' Association (DNA) was established in 1981 as a not-for-profit specialty nursing organization. It serves its members through a national structure and locally through chapters. DNA also extends its services to its international members. Registered nurses, licensed practical nurses, licensed vocational nurses, and individuals involved or interested in the care of the dermatology patient are eligible for membership in the association.

PHILOSOPHY

The DNA believes that the patient is the fundamental focus of health care. We believe the quality of patient care is greatly enhanced through the promotion of education for nurses in the specialty of dermatology. We believe the advancement of dermatology nursing clinical practice is based on research, and we are committed to encouraging the testing and sharing of new ideas. We further believe that a sense of professional pride evolves with an expanded knowledge base, increased opportunity for interdisciplinary collaboration, and the recognition of superior achievement within our membership. We believe in dermatology nurse certification as a means of validating knowledge and expertise in the specialty practice of dermatology nursing.

MISSION

The Dermatology Nurses' Association is a professional nursing organization comprised of a diverse group of individuals committed to quality care through sharing knowledge and expertise. The core purpose of the DNA is to promote excellence in dermatologic care. DNA accomplishes its mission by:

- Developing and fostering the highest standards of dermatology nursing care
- Enhancing professional growth through education and research
- Facilitating communication among its members
- Providing a support system for its members
- Promoting interdisciplinary collaboration
- Providing a forum for learning and sharing
- Serving as a resource for dermatology nursing information for health care professionals

DERMATOLOGY NURSES' ASSOCIATION
435 N. Bennett Street, Southern Pines, NC 28387
Phone: 910-246-2356; 1-800-454-4DNA (4362)
Fax: 910-246-2361
Email: dna@dnanurse.org
Website: www.dnanurse.org

DERMATOLOGIC
NURSING ESSENTIALS

A Core Curriculum

THIRD EDITION

Noreen Heer Nicol, PhD, RN, FNP, NEA-BC

Associate Professor
University of Colorado College of Nursing
Denver, Colorado

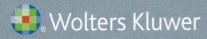

Wolters Kluwer

Philadelphia • Baltimore • New York • London
Buenos Aires • Hong Kong • Sydney • Tokyo

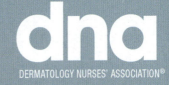

DERMATOLOGY NURSES' ASSOCIATION®

Executive Editor: Shannon W. Magee
Senior Product Development Editor: Emilie Moyer
Development Editor: Lisa Marshall
Senior Production Project Manager: Cynthia Rudy
Design Coordinator: Stephen Druding
Manufacturing Coordinator: Kathleen Brown
Prepress Vendor: SPi Global

3rd edition

Library of Congress Cataloging-in-Publication Data
Names: Nicol, Noreen, editor.
  Title: Dermatologic nursing essentials : a core curriculum / [edited by] Noreen Heer Nicol.
  Description: Third edition. | Philadelphia : Wolters Kluwer, [2016] | Includes bibliographical references and index.
  Identifiers: LCCN 2015038623 | ISBN 9781451188783
  Subjects: | MESH: Skin Diseases—nursing—Examination Questions. | Skin Diseases—nursing—Outlines. | Dermatology—Examination Questions. | Dermatology—Outlines.
  Classification: LCC RL125 | NLM WY 18.2 | DDC 616.5/0231076—dc23 LC record available at http://lccn.loc.gov/2015038623

DEDICATION

To

my husband of 33 years, Rob; our children, Erica and Brent; our large
extended family; and my parents, Lois "Chic" and Cliff Heer;

and

the nurses, physicians, and health care team at National Jewish Health in
Denver, Colorado, and the children and families with atopic dermatitis
whom they care for every day;

and

the nurses and health care professionals across the globe committed to
skin health and skin care whom I have had the pleasure of volunteering
and teaching with over the past 35 years through various professional
organizations, including the Dermatology Nurses' Association
and the International Skin Care Nursing Group.

NHN

CONTRIBUTORS TO THE THIRD EDITION

Kara Addison, FNP, MSN, DCNP, RN
Family Nurse Practitioner Dermatology Certified Nurse
    Practitioner
Associated Dermatology and Skin Cancer Clinic of Helena
Helena, Montana

Lakshi M. Aldredge, MSN, RN, ANP-BC
Dermatology Nurse Practitioner
Portland Veterans Affairs Medical Center
Portland, Oregon

Edna Atwater, BSN, RN
Director of Clinical Services
Department of Dermatology
Duke University Health System
Durham, North Carolina

Cathleen K. Case, MS, ANP-BC, DCNP
Dermatology Nurse Practitioner
Reliant Medical Group
Worcester, Massachusetts

Grace Chung, DNP, FNP-BC
Dermatology Nurse Practitioner
City of Hope National Medical Center
Duarte, California

Karen Congelio, DNP, RN, ACNP-BC
Dermatology Nurse Practitioner
Vujevich Dermatology Associates PC
Pittsburgh, Pennsylvania

Fiona Cowdell, DProf, MA, PGCE, BA(Hons), RN
Reader and Graduate Research Director
Faculty of Health and Social Care
University of Hull
East Riding, Yorkshire, United Kingdom

Theresa Coyner, MSN, ANP-BC, DCNP
Dermatology Nurse Practitioner
Randall Dermatology
West Lafayette, Indiana

Emily Croce, MSN, RN, CPNP
Pediatric Dermatology Nurse Practitioner
'Specially for Children
Dell Children's Medical Center of Central Texas
Austin, Texas

Steven J. Ersser, PhD(Lond), BSc (Hons), RN, CertTHEdb
Dame Kathleen Raven Professor of Clinical Nursing
School of Healthcare, Faculty of Medicine & Health
University of Leeds
Leeds, Yorkshire, United Kingdom

Karrie Fairbrother, BSN, RN, DNC, CDE
Nurse Educator
Prevention and Wellness, Diabetes Education
St. Peter's Hospital
Helena, Montana

Angela Hamilton, FNP-C
Family Nurse Practitioner
Department of Orthopedics
Paris Community Hospital/Family Medical Center
Paris, Illinois

Beth Haney, DNP, MSN, FNP-C
Assistant Clinical Professor
Program in Nursing Science, Nurse
    Practitioner Track
University of California, Irvine
Irvine, California

Constance L. Hayes, DNP, APRN, FNP-C
Dermatology Nurse Practitioner
Silver Falls Dermatology
Salem, Oregon

Cynthia Rena Heaton, BSN, RN
Nurse Manager
Outpatient Specialty Medicine
Veterans Administration
Iowa City, Iowa

Margaret Hirsch, BSN, RN, DNC
Staff Nurse
Dermatology Clinic
Texas Children's Hospital
Houston, Texas

**Penny S. Jones, MN, RN, CWS,
CWCN-AP, FACCWS**
Wound Management Clinical Nurse Specialist
Duke University Hospital
Durham, North Carolina

Anne Marie Ruszkowski Lord, BSN, RN, DNC
Former Director of Nursing
Department of Dermatology
Columbia University
New York, New York

Katrina Nice Masterson, DNP, RN, MS, FNP-BC, DCNP
Dermatology Nurse Practitioner
Randall Dermatology
West Lafayette, Indiana

Sarah W. Matthews, DNP, ARNP, FNP-BC
Assistant Professor
University of Washington School of Nursing
Dermatology Nurse Practitioner
Group Health Cooperative
Seattle, Washington

Noreen Heer Nicol, PhD, RN, FNP, NEA-BC
Associate Professor
University of Colorado College of Nursing
Denver, Colorado

Meghan O'Neill, BS, RN
Staff Nurse
'Specially for Children
Dell Children's Medical Center of Central Texas
Austin, Texas

Heather Onoday, MN, RN, FNP-C
Family Nurse Practitioner
Department of Dermatology
Oregon Health & Science University
Portland, Oregon

Kim B. Sanders, MPAS, PA-C
Dermatology Physician Assistant
Oregon Health & Science University
Portland, Oregon

Kelli Turgeon-Daoust, RN
Registered Nurse, Clinical Supervisor
Department of Dermatology
Reliant Medical Group
Worcester, Massachusetts

CONTRIBUTORS TO PREVIOUS EDITIONS

Lynn A. Babin, MSN, RN, CNS, AAS

Inger Christensen, BS, RN

Melissa P. Cooper, RN, CWOCN, DNC

Janice Zeigler Cuzzell, MA, RN

Bonita Drones, MSN, RN, C, CS

Maryann Forgach, BSN, RN

Janice Harris, BSN, RN

Marcia J. Hill, MSN, RN

Lauren L. Johannsen, RN

Janis S. Johnson, BSN, RN, C, DNC

Barbara Jones, BSN, RN,C

Elizabeth Bevan (Betty) Kasper, MS, ARNP-C

Glenda Killen, RN

Eileen Enny Leach, MPH, RN

Alice Liskay, BSN, RN

Sue Ann McCann, MSN, RN, DNC

Kathleen T. Moran, BSN, RN

Noreen Heer Nicol, MS, RN, FNP

Marrise M. Phillips, BS, RN, CCRC, DNC

Gwen Roof, BSN, RN

Sherrill Jantzi Rudy, MSN, RN, CRNP

Anne Marie Ruszkowski, BSN, RN, DNC

Margaret Sabatini, MS, BSN, RN

Doreen Battino Siegel, MSN, RN, C, FNP

Sharon M. Simpson, BS, RN, DNC

Dorothy Strong, BA, RN

Gerry Tetrault, BSN, RN

Nancy Vargo, RN, DNC

Robin Weber, MN, RN, FNP-C

Bonita Weyrauch, RN, CWS, CCT

Kelly N. White, MS, ARNP

REVIEWERS FOR THE THIRD EDITION

Anthony Bewley, BA(Hons), FRCP
The Royal London Hospital & Whipps Cross
    University Hospital
Barts Health NHS Trust
London, United Kingdom

Mark Boguniewicz, MD
Professor
University of Colorado School of Medicine
Division of Pediatric Allergy and Immunology,
    National Jewish Health
Denver, Colorado

Claude S. Burton III, MD
Duke Medicine, Department of Dermatology
Professor of Medicine and Dermatology
Medical Director of Dermatology Laser Facility
Medical Director of Wound Management
Durham, North Carolina

Janice T. Chussil, MSN, ANP-BC, DCNP
Dermatology Nurse Practitioner
Baker Allergy, Asthma, and Dermatology
Portland, Oregon

Vincent DeLeo, MD
Clinical Professor
Department of Dermatology, University of Southern
    California
Keck School of Medicine
Los Angeles, California

Judith Dyson, RGN, RMN, BSc(Hons), MSc, PhD, PGCHE
Senior Lecturer in Mental Health
Acting Head of Department, Psychological Health
    and Wellbeing
Faculty of Health and Science
University of Hull
East Riding, Yorkshire, United Kingdom

Benjamin D. Ehst, MD, PhD
Assistant Professor
Department of Dermatology, Oregon Health
    and Sciences University
School of Medicine
Portland, Oregon

Hilary E. Fairbrother, MD, MPH
Assistant Professor
Department of Emergency Medicine, New York University
    Langone Medical Center
New York University School of Medicine
New York, New York

Kathleen E. Dunbar Haycraft, DNP, FNP/PNP-BC, DCNP, FAANP
Nurse Practitioner
Riverside Dermatology
Hannibal, Missouri

Anjeli K. Isaac, MD
Dermatologist
Group Health Cooperative
Seattle, Washington

Sancy Leachman, MD, PhD
Professor and Chair, Department of Dermatology
Director, Melanoma Research Program,
    Knight Cancer Institute
Oregon Health & Science University
Portland, Oregon

Mandi L. Maronn, MD
Pediatric Dermatologist
Aurora Advanced Healthcare
Milwaukee, Wisconsin

Helen Page, MHP, PA-C
Dermatology Physician Assistant
Reliant Medical Group
Worcester, Massachusetts

John K. Randall, RPh, MD
Dermatologist
Randall Dermatology
West Lafayette, Indiana

Barbara Trehearne, PhD, RN
Vice President for Clinical Excellence and Nursing
Group Health Cooperative
Associate Dean for Clinical Practice
University of Washington School of Nursing
Seattle, Washington

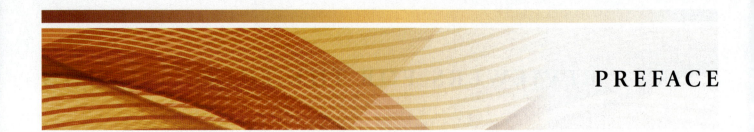

Skin, the largest and most visible organ in the body, influences everyone. Dermatology nursing focuses on the study of the skin, including its anatomic, physiologic, pathologic, psychologic, and social characteristics, as well as on the care of the patient and family with skin concerns and disorders. The Dermatology Nurses' Association (DNA) Board of Directors and I are pleased to present *Dermatologic Nursing Essentials: A Core Curriculum, third edition,* which provides the reader with core knowledge about the specialty of dermatology nursing.

Since the first edition published in 1998 and the second edition published in 2003, there has been considerable growth in the knowledge, skill, and abilities required by dermatology nurses and dermatology health care providers. As an author and reviewer in all three editions of this book, I recognize the growing scope of the audience and practice across time. This textbook is not meant to be a comprehensive review of skin or skin diseases and their treatment. The scope is intended to provide novice to expert nurses and other health care providers with essential knowledge of healthy skin and disorders of the skin to support their patient-centered care. The intention is for the book to support dermatology nursing activities as a companion piece for workshops as well as supplying the foundational information for certification and other professional needs. The content is applicable to nurses and health care providers caring for patients and families with skin disorders working in a variety of practice settings, including acute/tertiary care, outpatient, private office, schools, or community settings.

In this third edition, the 23 chapters have been expanded to reflect new trends in dermatology practice and some chapters renamed to reflect current terminology in their respective areas of skin care. Expert nurses, physicians, and health care providers from across the world authored and reviewed this book. It is through their collective generosity that this book was made possible. Almost 400 color photos have been added to enhance the learning and reading experience. Drawings, illustrations, tables, and graphs have been updated and added. The expansion of the Key Points and the addition of a Patient Education section in each chapter reflect the commitment to patient-centered care. The chapters were written or updated with the most current and factual information available to each author. In light of the dynamic and ever-changing care and treatment recommendations, readers are encouraged to always double-check information, particularly around treatment and drug therapy. This work should be used as a guide and supplemented with other references and educational formats.

My desire is for the book to serve as a reference to all nurses and health care providers to promote skin health. It is with great pride that I present the third edition of this work.

Noreen Heer Nicol, PhD, RN, FNP, NEA-BC
Editor

ACKNOWLEDGMENTS

Life is about the journey and not just the destination. Many colleagues, friends, family, and loved ones are to be acknowledged, as they supported each author in this book and my journey as editor and author. My gratitude is extended to each of them for the many tireless hours and support.

Dermatologic Nursing Essentials: A Core Curriculum, third edition could never have occurred without the original collaborative efforts of its first and second edition editor, Marcia J. Hill, the publishing staff of Anthony J. Jannetti, Inc., and the many previous contributors who are also acknowledged in this book. Marcia Hill's more than 30-year commitment to editing, authoring, mentoring dermatology nurses, and serving as one of the organization's early presidents paved the way for the growth and development of dermatology nursing.

There are many presidents, board members, and volunteers of the Dermatology Nurses' Association who have done much to mentor, educate, and influence the multitudes of dermatology health care providers; several of them are authors and reviewers in this or past editions. Individual and collective thanks for the support of the specialty and this book. My personal thanks to Edna Atwater for her mentorship years ago when I become a past president behind her. Her collegiality and support from then to now have been amazing, as well as her contributions to this third edition.

Integral to this third edition becoming a reality were the authors who spent many hours writing and rewriting and the reviewers who gave such meaningful and excellent feedback. Expert nurses, physicians, and health care providers from across the world authored and reviewed this book, often in response to my pleas for help. Words don't do justice to expressing my appreciation to the incredible panel who agreed to participate. Extra regards for those of you who took on multiple chapters or multiple roles at my request. Our physician reviewers, many of whom are recognized international experts, demonstrated ongoing professional collaboration by volunteering their time and often donating valuable clinical photos. A special thanks to Dr. Mark Boguniewicz as my colleague, copresenter, coauthor, and reviewer extraordinaire who shares my passion of working for the past 25 years with the many children and families with atopic dermatitis. Special recognition goes to Anne Marie Ruzskowski Lord for authorship in all three editions; and for choosing special life paths that hopefully allow ongoing collaborative opportunities.

The continued commitment to excellence by the staff at Wolters Kluwer was invaluable for this third edition. A special thank you goes to Lisa Marshall as Development Editor. Lisa provided her accomplished skills with formatting and writing even when it came at the end of long days and countless weeks. Appreciation also goes to Emilie Moyer, Senior Product Development Editor, and Shannon W. Magee, Executive Editor, for encouragement at the final stretch and endless review of details.

Recognition to Dr. Sue Huether and to the late Dr. Phyllis Drennan, who served as my nursing mentors. They frequently pushed me into new learning environments, which include writing and editing. Women of vision and endless energy, they gave me the opportunity to explore many dimensions of professional nursing.

Finally, appreciation and love to my husband, Rob, and our two children, Erica and Brent, along with the rest of our large extended family. Rob, Erica, and Brent, and our family endlessly changed their priorities and schedules to support mine and cared for me during my entire career; they are my anchor in life. The collective generosity of all made this book possible.

Noreen Heer Nicol, PhD, RN, FNP, NEA-BC
Editor

CONTENTS

CHAPTER 1

Anatomy and Physiology of the Integumentary System

Noreen Heer Nicol

I. OVERVIEW AND FUNCTIONS OF THE INTEGUMENTARY SYSTEM

The integumentary system is an extraordinary body system, which includes the largest and most visible organ, the skin. The skin forms the integumentary system when combined with the accessory structures of hair, nails, and glands. As the only organ of the body, which is readily available to be inspected and judged by all, the skin's very visible characteristics play a unique role in every individual's well-being. A conceptual framework for recognizing and understanding diseases of the skin relies on principles of diagnosis common to medicine and nursing, namely, historical and social factors, physical examination, and laboratory techniques. To relate these principles of diagnosis and treatment to clinicopathologic events in dermatology, it is important to start with an overview of the skin. The skin is composed of three layers: epidermis, dermis, and subcutaneous fat accounting for 15% to 20% of the body's weight (Figure 1-1). Disease may localize exclusively in one or all of these layers. There is considerable regional variation in the relative thickness of these layers. The more common skin conditions take into account a diverse spectrum of clinical pathology, which may be characterized by inflammation (noninfectious), pigmentary abnormalities, infection and infestation, benign and malignant cellular proliferations, and disease where the basic mechanisms are relatively obscure. To conceptualize skin disorders effectively, it is essential to consider the changes in the structure and function of the skin and to understand the specific clinical pathology related to the changes. The healthy integumentary system is a complex, dynamic system providing diverse functions (Table 1-1), including:

A. Protection
   1. An intact stratum corneum provides a physical barrier against foreign substances and bacteria.
   2. Mechanical strength is provided by intercellular bonding in the epidermis and collagen, elastin, and ground substance in the dermis.
   3. Subcutaneous tissue acts as a shock absorber.
   4. Melanin screens and absorbs ultraviolet radiation.

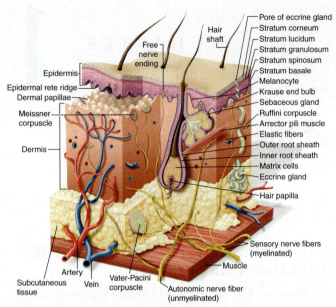

FIGURE 1-1. Anatomy of the skin. (From Anatomical Chart Co.)

B. Homeostasis
1. The skin prevents dehydration through loss of internal fluids and electrolytes.
2. The skin limits absorption of external fluids and gases.
C. Excretion
1. The glands of the skin excrete waste products, in addition to sweat, which is mostly water and electrolytes.
2. The waste products excreted can include urea, lactic acid, bile, ammonia, and even alcohol.

D. Thermoregulation
1. Body temperature is controlled by:
   a. Conduction of heat from the skin to the air or other objects
   b. Radiation of heat from the body surface
   c. Convection of heat by air currents
   d. Evaporation of perspiration
2. The cutaneous vasculature plays an important role in body temperature regulation. Blood vessels:
   a. Dilate when the external environment is warm to promote heat loss
   b. Constrict in a cold environment to conserve heat
E. Vitamin D production
1. Ultraviolet light converts 7-dehydrocholesterol to vitamin D3 in the epidermis.
2. Vitamin D3 is converted in the kidneys into the active form of vitamin D.
F. Sensory perception
1. The system contains mechanoreceptors and unmyelinated nerve fibers.
2. Touch, pressure, temperature, pain, and itch are transmitted.
G. Psychosocial
1. The skin, nails, and hair influence sexual attraction, general well-being, and self-image. Outward expressions of anxiety, fear, and anger are visible through sweating, pallor, and flushing.
2. Different societies and culture greatly influence how one accepts or rejects outward appearance of this body system.
H. Wound healing
1. The skin can repair and regenerate itself.
2. These important wound healing abilities are influenced by multiple internal and external factors.

TABLE 1-1 Function and Structure of the Healthy Integumentary System

Layer of the Skin	Function	Structure
Epidermis Pain receptors Touch receptors Keratin production Melanin production Immune system afferent limb	Water loss barrier Sensory organ Ultraviolet protection Infection barrier Excretion	**Cellular Layers** Stratum corneum Stratum lucidum (on palms and soles only) Stratum granulosum Stratum spinosum Stratum germinativum
Dermis Temperature receptors Deep pressure and touch receptors Hair shaft and follicles Lymphatic vessels Sebaceous and sweat glands Nerves Arrector pili muscles	Temperature regulation Immunoregulatory function Vitamin D production Integument strength Elastic tone	Papillary dermis Reticular dermis Connective tissue and collagen bundles
Subcutaneous Fat Layer Bulb and matrix of hair follicle Larger arteries and veins Pluripotential cells	Insulation Shock absorption Energy storage and fat metabolism Body topography	Adipose tissue Loose connective tissue

II. STRUCTURE OF THE SKIN

A. Epidermis (Figure 1-2)
  1. The epidermis is the outermost structure of the skin. It:
     a. Contains multiple layers of cells (stratified)
     b. Has considerable regional variation, depending on the site:
        (1) Thickest on palms and soles, approximately 1.5 mm
        (2) Very thin on eyelid, less than 0.4 mm
     c. Is without lymphatic and vascular channels, and connective tissue; therefore, it derives its nutritional support from the underlying dermis.
  2. Keratinization:
     a. The epidermis rejuvenates itself through the process of keratinization. Epidermal keratinization is the process of morphological and biochemical differentiation of the keratinocyte, beginning in the basal cell layer and ending in the stratum corneum as a horn or cornified cell.
  3. Keratin:
     a. Keratin, the major product of the cornified cell, is a highly resistant, insoluble, fibrous protein. It represents the end product of a differentiated epidermal keratinocyte.
     b. Keratinization also involves synthesis of several other proteins and additional substances such as keratohyalin granules, which act as glue.
  4. Layers of the epidermis:
     a. There are five layers in the epidermis.
     b. The layers are named to reflect the stage the keratinocytes are in during the process of keratinization.
     c. These layers are not independent of each other but rather are interrelated and continuous phases of the life of a keratinocyte. Keratinocytes move up as they age (Figure 1-2).

(1) Germinating or basal cell layer (stratum basale, also called stratum germinativum): the basal cell layer is the innermost layer of the epidermis. It consists of a single layer of elongated cells. Each cell divides (mitosis) into two daughter cells. One remains as "basal cell," the other migrates upward through the remainder of the epidermis.

(2) Prickle cell or spiny layer (stratum spinosum): the prickle cell layer consists of many rows of flattened polygonal cells that are held together by "prickles" or "spines." These prickles are desmosomes, which are small thickenings in an intracellular bridge.

(3) Granular cell layer (stratum granulosum): the granular cell layer is most prominent on the palms and soles. It consists of one to three layers of flattened, irregularly shaped cells that have large numbers of keratohyalin granules. Keratohyalin granules comprise particulate materials that have a high sulfur–protein content. Keratinocytes lose their nucleus in this layer, thereby becoming nonviable.

(4) Glassy layer (stratum lucidum): the stratum lucidum is made up of one or more rows of distended irregular cells. It is an even, colorless, translucent, or shiny band. The stratum lucidum is almost nonexistent except on thicker skin areas such as palms and soles.

(5) Horny cell layer (stratum corneum): the horny cell layer consists of anucleated, cornified cells. They are also known as horn cells. The nucleus and other cytoplasmic organelles have been totally degraded. The remaining material is predominantly keratin. Other substances include water, water-insoluble proteins, amino acids, sugars, urea, minerals, and lipids. These act as buffers and lubricants.
  (a) Cells of the epidermis are continuously being shed or desquamated from the stratum corneum.
  (b) It takes approximately 14 days for the keratinocyte to travel from the basal cell layer to the stratum corneum. Once in the stratum corneum, it takes another 14 days before it is shed.
  (c) New cells are formed in the basal cell layer at the same rate cells are shed in the stratum corneum.

5. Functions of the horny cell layer:
  a. The stratum corneum serves many functions for the epidermis and the skin in general:
     (1) It functions as the body's major physical barrier by being relatively impermeable to water and electrolytes.
     (2) It resists damaging chemicals, provides physical toughness, impedes passage of electrical

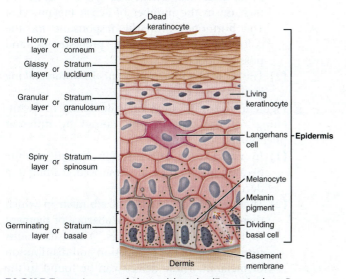

Dead keratinocyte

Horny layer or Stratum corneum
Glassy layer or Stratum lucidium
Granular layer or Stratum granulosum
Spiny layer or Stratum spinosum
Germinating layer or Stratum basale

Living keratinocyte
Langerhans cell — **Epidermis**
Melanocyte
Melanin pigment
Dividing basal cell
Basement membrane
Dermis

FIGURE 1-2. Layers of the epidermis. (From Archer, P., Nelson, L. (2012). *Applied anatomy & physiology for manual therapists*. Wolters Kluwer.)

currents, and retards the proliferation of micro-organisms through its relatively dry surface.

(3) The stratum corneum also functions as a reservoir for topical medications.

b. Although the stratum corneum is an effective barrier to most substances, some are able to pass through. Substances can be transported through the skin by three pathways:

(1) Through adnexal orifices (pilosebaceous unit) and sweat glands

(2) Through the intercellular spaces between the cornified cells

(3) Directly through the cornified cells

B. Cells in the epidermis

1. Keratinocytes account for at least 80% of the cellular components of the epidermis. They have the specialized function of producing keratin. During keratinization, the keratinocytes change shape (flatten), lose organelles, form fibrous protein (keratin), become dehydrated, and thicken their cell membrane (see discussion above).

2. Melanocyte cells:

a. Embryonic development: melanocytes are the pigment-producing cells of the epidermis. Embryonically, they are derived from the neural crest, and by the 8th week of development, melanocytes enter the epidermis. In the fetal epidermis, melanocytes are found at suprabasal levels. When the fetus is fully developed, they are located in the basal cell layer. Failure of the melanocyte to migrate to the basal cell layer results in entities such as blue nevus and mongolian spots.

b. Regional variation: melanocytes are present on all parts of the body with regional variation. There are more melanocytes on the face than on the abdomen. Ratios of melanocytes to keratinocytes vary from 1:4 to 1:10. Advancing age leads to a greater shift favoring keratinocytes.

c. Melanosome/melanin: within the cytoplasm of melanocytes are special organelles called melanosomes. Melanin is stored in the melanosome and is synthesized through the conversion of the colorless amino acid, tyrosine. There are two types of melanin. Eumelanins account for brown and black colors. Pheomelanins account for yellow to reddish brown colors.

d. Epidermal melanin unit: melanocytes are dendritic cells. Their dendrites extend for long distances in the epidermis. This allows one melanocyte to be in contact with many keratinocytes. The interaction of the melanocyte and keratinocyte forms a biologic unit called the epidermal melanin unit. Melanosomes are transferred from the dendrite of the melanocyte to keratinocytes by a process called apocopation. The keratinocyte phagocytizes the melanin-filled tips of the melanocytes. Once transferred to the keratinocyte, the fully melanized melanosomes are partially degraded by lysosomal enzymes or desquamated with cornified cells.

e. Melanin production: melanin production is controlled by genetics, hormones, and the environment. The number of melanocytes in the epidermis is the same regardless of race or sex:

(1) It is the amount of melanin in the keratinocyte that determines skin color. The difference in the skin color among individuals is the result of the differences in level of synthetic activity including degree of melanization and rate of degradation of the melanosome within the keratinocyte.

(2) There is also evidence that tyrosinase activity also plays a role in melanization. Dark-skinned people produce melanosomes that are larger than light-skinned people, resulting in more melanin synthesis. Tyrosinase activity is also increased in blacks.

(3) The size of melanosomes is the principal factor in determining how they will be distributed in the keratinocyte. The larger melanosomes of dark-skinned people are packaged individually in a membrane within the cytoplasm of the keratinocyte. In light-skinned people, smaller melanosomes are package in membrane-bound complexes in the keratinocyte.

f. Hormonal influence: hormones profoundly influence melanin pigmentation, but their precise action at the cellular level is unknown. It is presently believed that the melanocyte-stimulating hormone (MSH) causes a dispersion of melanosomes within melanocytes. Regional variations exist in the sensitivity of the epidermal melanin units to specific hormones:

(1) In pregnancy, there is increased pigmentation of the nipples and areolae, and to a lesser extent, an increased pigmentation of facial skin, midline of the abdomen, and genitalia. This is due to an increase in the number of active melanocytes. The hormones primarily responsible for the color changes are estrogen, progesterone, and possibly MSH.

(2) The same phenomenon occurs in women taking birth control pills.

g. Pigment variation: areas of leukoderma or "whitening" of the skin can be caused by different phenomena:

(1) In vitiligo, the affected skin becomes white because melanocytes are destroyed, leading to a decrease in their number.

(2) There are different types of albinism in which there is partial or complete absence of pigment in the skin, hair, and eyes. Albinism results from defects in the production and distribution of melanin. These defects can be found in the enzyme tyrosinase, melanosome development, or in the type of melanin produced.

(3) Local areas of increased pigmentation are due to a variety of causes:

(a) The typical freckle is caused by localized increased production of pigment by a normal number of melanocytes.

(b) Nevi are benign proliferations of melanocytes.

(c) Melanomas are the malignant counterparts of nevi.

h. Ultraviolet light: the most important function of melanin is to shield the skin from the sun's ultraviolet rays by absorbing its radiant energy. The absorption spectrum of melanin encompasses the entire range of ultraviolet and visible light.

(1) Melanosomes function to scatter and absorb ultraviolet light:

(a) Exposure to ultraviolet light expedites the transfer of melanosomes to keratinocytes.

(b) When the skin is tanned by ultraviolet light, an increased number of melanosomes are manufactured and available for transfer to the keratinocyte.

(c) In light-skinned people, chronic sun exposure also "tricks" the melanocyte into producing larger melanosomes.

(d) The pattern of distribution of the melanosome in the keratinocyte then resembles that of dark-skinned people.

3. Langerhans cells:

a. Langerhans cell is another dendritic cell found in the epidermis. They are found in the granular, spinous, and basal cell layers of the epidermis. Occasionally, they are seen in the normal dermis. Langerhans cells are derived from bone marrow precursor cells.

b. The Langerhans cell population is self-maintaining. There is a relatively constant number of these cells being maintained by intraepidermal mitosis and migration from the connective tissue. Langerhans cells account for approximately 4% of the epidermal cell population.

(1) Function of Langerhans cells:

(a) They are immunocompetent cells involved in the uptake, processing, and presentation of antigen to lymphocytes.

(b) It is thought that Langerhans cells are the first line of immunologic defense in the skin acting as initial receptors for the cutaneous response to external antigens.

(c) Experimental evidence shows that Langerhans cells are directly involved in allergic contact hypersensitivity.

(d) There is a decreased number of Langerhans cells in patients with skin diseases such as psoriasis and sarcoidosis.

(e) Langerhans cells are also functionally impaired by ultraviolet radiation. UVB and PUVA treatments lead to morphologic, antigenic, and enzymatic changes within the Langerhans cell. Research is under way to learn the implications of this information.

4. Merkel cells:

a. Merkel cells are also found in the basal cell layer. They are collected in specialized structures called tactile discs or touch domes. The most distal part of the Merkel cell is embedded in the dermis. Merkel cells are present in the nonhairy or smooth skin of the digits, lips, regions of the oral cavity, and outer root sheath of hair follicles.

5. Embryonic development:

a. Merkel cells originate from either the neural crest or ectoderm. They are joined to keratinocytes by "spines" or desmosomes, which project from their cytoplasm.

b. Merkel cells have characteristic organelles. They are membrane-bound granules that contain neurotransmitter substances. Distal to the granules is an unmyelinated neurite or terminal neuraxon.

c. Function:

(1) The function of Merkel cells is that of slowly adapting mechanoreceptors. The exact mechanism of action remains uncertain.

(2) The contacting membrane of the Merkel cell and the dendrite resemble pre- and postsynaptic units. It is therefore thought that the Merkel cell acts as a receptor that transmits a stimulus to the neurite via a chemical synapse.

(3) The Merkel cell may also serve a trophic (concerned with nourishment) role as well as serving as a common contact point for several associated keratinocytes.

(4) Merkel cells respond to maintained deformation of the skin surface and are involved in sensing touch and pressure.

C. Basement membrane zone (dermal–epidermal junction)

1. The basement membrane zone is found at the junction of the epidermis and dermis. It runs along the base of the epidermal rete ridges as well as the sweat glands, hair shafts, and sebaceous glands.

a. Structure:

(1) Basement membrane zone structures are formed from basal keratinocytes and dermal fibroblasts. There are several components of the basement membrane zone that are seen with the electron microscope. The plasma membrane is the most distal surface of the basal keratinocyte.

(2) Hemidesmosomes are specialized attachment plates between the basal keratinocyte and the lamina densa. The lamina densa is immediately above the dermis and comprises a collagen that provides structure and flexibility. The lamina densa also functions as a barrier/filter by the selective restriction of molecules.

(3) The lamina lucida appears as a clear zone and is found between the plasma membrane and the lamina densa.

(4) Anchoring fibrils, dermal microfibrils, and collagen fibers below the lamina densa compose the fibrous component of the basement membrane zone.

b. Function:
  (1) The basement zone serves as a porous, semipermeable filter. It:
    (a) Permits exchange of cells and fluid between the epidermis and dermis
    (b) Functions as a structural support for the epidermis and helps hold the epidermis and dermis together
c. Diseases of the basement membrane zone:
  (1) Many genetic diseases involve structural alterations in the basement membrane zone. Separation of the epidermis and dermis results in blistering. This is seen in disorders such as epidermolysis bullosa letalis, generalized atrophic benign epidermolysis bullosa, bullous pemphigoid, and recessive dystrophic epidermolysis bullosa.
D. Dermis (Figure 1-3)
  1. The dermis is the principal mass of the skin providing structural integrity and is biologically active. It is composed of collagen bundles and is 1 to 4 mm thick. It encloses the appendages of the epidermis and supports the nerve and vascular network.
    a. Function:
      (1) Functions of the dermis include preventing mechanical trauma and maintenance of homeostasis. The dermis:
        (a) Binds large amounts of water and thereby represents a water storage organ
        (b) Is also involved with thermoregulation and sensory innervation
    b. Composition:
      (1) The dermis comprises connective tissue, water, and ground substance. There are three types of connective tissue: collagen, elastic fiber, and reticulum.

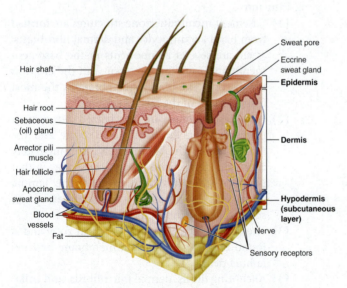

FIGURE 1-3. The dermis and its appendages. (From Archer, P., Nelson, L. (2012). *Applied anatomy & physiology for manual therapists*. Wolters Kluwer.)

        (a) Collagen constitutes the majority of fibers in the dermis:
          i. It is the major structural protein for the entire body.
          ii. Collagen is a fibrous protein synthesized by fibroblasts and degraded by the proteolytic enzyme, collagenase. Scleroderma is an example of a collagen disease that involves abnormal synthesis or degradation of collagen molecules.
          iii. Collagen is the most important stress-resistant material of the skin. It provides us with both tensile strength and the ability to resist stretching.
          iv. Individual collagen bundles become thinner in atrophic scars and thicker in keloids.
        (b) Elastic fibers represent 5% to 9% of dermal fibers. They:
          i. Differ structurally and chemically from collagen
          ii. Are made up of protein filaments and elastin
          iii. Function to restore the collagen network to a normal position following deformation, stress, or stretching. The skin's resiliency and elegant feel are attributed to the elastic fibers. There is a loss of elastic fibers in stria.
        (c) Reticular fibers are young finely formed collagen fibers:
          i. They are similar in diameter than mature collagen.
          ii. Large numbers are found in the papillary dermis where they serve as anchoring fibrils for the basal lamina.
        (d) Ground substance constitutes the interstitial component of the dermis. Ground substance:
          i. Is a viscoelastic gel
          ii. Molds to irregular objects
          iii. Is a small fraction of the dermal weight, but accounts for a substantial portion of the volume
          iv. Has a great capacity to bind water
    c. Papillary dermis:
      (1) The dermis is divided into two areas—the papillary and reticulum dermis.
      (a) The papillary dermis is the uppermost area of the dermis beginning at the basement membrane zone:
        i. The papillary dermis contains thin, haphazardly arranged collagen fibers, numerous reticular fibers, and delicate branching elastic fibers. There is abundant ground substance and numerous capillaries that extend from the superficial plexus.

       ii. The papillary dermis and the epidermis form a morphologic and functional unit. This is evident as the papillary dermis molds to the contour of the epidermal rete ridges. This relationship is seen in common inflammatory diseases when both areas show alteration.

  d. Reticular dermis:

    (1) The reticular dermis represents the bulk of the dermis. It:

      (a) Extends from the base of the papillary dermis to the subcutaneous tissue

      (b) Carries most of the physical stress of the skin

      (c) Is characterized by thick collagen bundles arranged parallel to the skin surface. Coarse elastic fibers are found around collagen bundles.

      (d) Is thicker than the capillary dermis. Proportionally, there are fewer reticular fibers, fibroblasts, and blood vessels and less ground substance in the reticular dermis, as compared to the papillary dermis.

E. Cells in the dermis

  1. Fibroblast:

    a. The principal cell of the dermis is the fibroblast. It produces collagen, elastic fibers, reticular fibers, and ground substance. Collagen fibrils are broken down and degraded by collagenase and gelatinase, both of which are also synthesized in the fibroblast.

    b. Fibroblasts have indistinct cytoplasm and spindle-shaped nuclei. They are found among and on the surface of fiber bundles.

  2. Mast cell:

    a. Mast cells are secretory cells most commonly found near the superficial plexus and in the subcutaneous fat:

      (1) The cytoplasm of mast cells contain secretory and lysosomal granules. Mediators in the granules are produced that are either vasoactive, stimulate smooth muscle contraction, or function to attract neutrophils and eosinophils.

      (2) The secretory granules contain histamine and heparin.

      (3) The lysosomal granules are nonsecretory but degrade intracellular proteoglycans and complex glycolipids.

    b. Mast cells respond to a number of physical stimuli: light, cold, heat, acute trauma, vibration, and sustained pressure, as well as chemical and immunologic stimuli:

      (1) When stimulated, the mast cell releases histamine and heparin. Once released, vasodilation and dermal edema result.

      (2) Secondly, there is an infiltration of neutrophils, eosinophils, and basophils.

      (3) Immediate hypersensitivity reactions in the skin are due to mast cells.

      (4) Subacute and chronic inflammatory disease can also be related to the mast cell.

  3. Macrophages:

    a. Originates in the bone marrow. It initially circulates as a monocyte in the blood.

    b. Macrophages in the dermis function in the immune response.

    c. Langerhans cells, along with macrophages, are capable of processing and presenting antigens to immunocompetent lymphocytes.

    d. Defend against microorganisms through phagocytosis.

    e. Important to wound healing cascade.

  4. Histiocytes:

    a. Histiocytes are cells found in the dermis, which function as scavengers. They engulf hemosiderin, melanin, lipid, and debris.

F. Dermal vasculature. The epidermis has no intrinsic blood supply so it depends on the diffusion of nutrients and oxygen from vessels in papillary dermis. The vasculature of the skin is arranged into two interconnected horizontal plexuses.

  1. Superficial plexus:

    a. The superficial plexus (subpapillary plexus) courses at the junction of the papillary and reticular dermis. It supplies capillaries, end arterioles, and venules to the dermal papillae.

  2. Deep plexus:

    a. The deep plexus is located in the base of the reticular dermis. The two plexuses are connected by blood vessels that run perpendicular to the skin surface. The communicating vessels originate from arteries and veins in the subcutaneous tissue.

  3. Functions:

    a. Thermoregulation is the most important function of the skin's vascular system. Blood flow through the dermis varies in response to changes in the core temperature of the body, as well as the temperature of the external environment.

    b. Blood pressure: the cutaneous vasculature plays a role in blood pressure regulation. Sympathetic stimulation leads to a constriction of cutaneous blood vessels, thereby, reducing blood flow to the skin. This results in increased venous return, increased cardiac output, and increased blood pressure.

    c. Nutrition is also a function of the dermal vasculature. In the capillaries and venules, oxygen, water, nutrients, and hormones are distributed from the blood to the tissues. Carbon dioxide and other products of skin metabolism are diffused for transmission to the excretory organs.

    d. Inflammation: blood vessels in the dermis also play a role in inflammation. The microcirculatory units of the papillary dermis dilate in skin diseases characterized by erythema.

G. Lymphatics
1. A lymphatic network is also found in the dermis. It parallels the vascular plexuses. The lymphatics act to filter and transport a large amount of capillary transudate or lymph and return it back to the venous system.
H. Nerves
1. Autonomic motor:
   a. Autonomic nerves are sympathetic in nature and can be divided into adrenergic and cholinergic fibers:
      (1) Adrenergic fibers regulate vasoconstriction, the apocrine gland, and arrector pili muscles.
      (2) Eccrine sweat secretion is controlled by cholinergic fibers.
2. Somatic sensory:
   a. Somatic sensory nerves are either free nerve endings or corpuscular receptors. Either together or alone, they convey touch, pressure, pain, temperature, and itch from every part of the body.
      (1) There is variation in intensity of these senses at different parts of the body. This is because the density and type of receptors are regionally variable and specific.
   b. Corpuscular receptors: Meissner and Pacini corpuscles are two mechanoreceptors in the skin conveying touch and pressure. The Meissner corpuscles are found in the papillary dermis, especially on the palms and soles. Pacini corpuscles are located in the deeper dermis of weight-bearing surfaces.
   c. Free nerve endings: temperature, pain, and itch are transmitted by unmyelinated nerve fibers, which terminate in the papillary dermis and around the hair follicles. These impulses are conveyed to the central nervous system through the dorsal root ganglion.
   d. Dermatome: the sensory nerves are arranged in dermatomal patterns. A dermatome is the cutaneous area supplied by a single spinal nerve. On the trunk, the dermatomes are horizontal; on the arms and legs, they are more vertical and irregularly distributed. Herpes zoster is an example of a disease in a dermatomal pattern.
I. Subcutaneous tissue (Also referred to as Hypodermis or Fatty Tissue) (Figure 1-3)
1. The third layer of the skin is the subcutaneous tissue. It consists of fat cells or lipocytes (adipocyte). The lobules are separated by fibrous walls (septa) of collagen and large blood vessels. Dermal collagen is continuous with the collagen found in the subcutaneous tissue.
2. The thickness of the subcutaneous tissue varies in different parts of the body. It is nearly absent in the eyelids, penis, scrotum, nipple, and overlying the tibia. It is thick in the waist, especially in middle-aged people. Distribution of subcutaneous tissue is controlled by circulating sex hormones, heredity, age, and eating habits.
3. The subcutaneous tissue has three main functions. It:
   a. Insulates the underlying tissue from extreme hot and cold
   b. Functions as a mechanical shock absorber
   c. Is a storehouse of energy (calories) used in times of nutritional deprivation

III. APPENDAGES OF THE SKIN: NAILS (SEE CHAPTER 22, HAIR AND NAILS)

A. Overview: The nail covers the upper surface of each finger and toe and acts as a protective covering to the end of each digit and aid in picking up small objects. Nails serve as scratching organs and have an increasingly important esthetic and cosmetic purpose.

IV. APPENDAGES OF THE SKIN: HAIR (SEE CHAPTER 22, HAIR AND NAILS)

A. Overview: Hair is a keratin structure of the epidermis, which serves no vital function on the human body. It does have physiologic functions including insulation, social and sexual display, camouflage, tactile perception, thermoregulation, and protection from UV light.

V. APPENDAGES OF THE SKIN: GLANDS (FIGURE 1-4)

A. Sebaceous glands
1. Sebaceous glands are found on all areas of the body except the palms, soles, and dorsum of the feet.
2. Their density varies markedly with location, being most numerous on the face, scalp, upper chest, back, and anogenital regions.
3. Most sebaceous glands are associated with hair follicles (pilosebaceous units). The pilosebaceous unit comprises the hair follicle and one or more sebaceous glands attached to it. Exceptions to this are the sebaceous glands in the following:
   a. Buccal mucosa
   b. Vermillion border of the lip
   c. Areola
   d. Prepuce
   e. Eyelids
4. Embryonic development:
   a. Embryonically, sebaceous glands are formed as an outgrowth of the upper portion of the hair follicle. They are fully developed at birth and secrete much

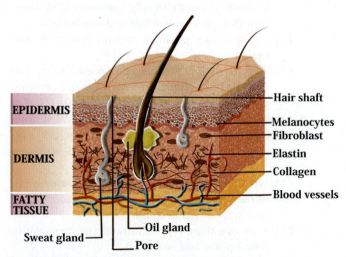

FIGURE 1-4. Vasculature and glands of the skin.

of the lipid of the vernix caseosa. Sebaceous glands are small at birth, enlarge between 8 and 10 years of age with maturation continuing through adolescence, and remain unchanged until later years. They decrease in menopause in females and after the 70th decade in males. As people age, sebum secretion decreases even though the size of sebaceous glands increases. Development of sebaceous glands and sebogenesis is hormone dependent (testosterone, androstenedione, dehydroepiandrosterone).

5. Anatomy:
   a. Germinative cells: sebaceous glands consist of one or more lobules of pale-staining cells called germinative cells. Differentiation of the germinative cells is similar to that of the keratinocyte in the epidermis. As the cells differentiate, lipid droplets accumulate, eventually filling the cytoplasm of the cell. These cells eventually rupture, discharging sebum into the sebaceous duct. Sebum is made up of cellular debris and lipids.
   b. Sebaceous duct: the sebaceous duct is the short, narrow, common excretory duct connecting several sebaceous lobules with the wider follicular infundibulum. This follicular canal is very wide throughout the entire length. It is filled not only with sebum, but keratinous materials, bacteria, and yeast.
6. Hormonal effects:
   a. There are hormonal effects on the sebaceous gland:
      (1) Sebaceous gland development is one of the earliest signs of puberty. Androgens are the principal hormonal stimulus. Testicular androgens maintain sebum production in the male and ovarian androgens in the female. Adrenal androgens also play a role.
      (2) Estrogen decreases the size of the sebaceous gland and decreases the production of sebum.
7. Sebum production:
   a. The actual production of sebum varies in relation to age and sex:
      (1) It is low in children until the time of puberty.
      (2) In adults, sebum production is higher in men than women.
      (3) In older men, production falls off slightly.
      (4) In women, production significantly decreases after 50 years of age.
8. Functions:
   a. Functions of the sebaceous gland include:
      (1) Waterproofing of the hair and skin
      (2) Promoting the absorption of fat-soluble substances
      (3) Lubrication and possibly assistance in the synthesis of vitamin D

B. Apocrine gland
1. The apocrine glands are found in the:
   a. Axilla
   b. Umbilical region
   c. Around the areolae
   d. Anogenital region
   e. External auditory canal (ceruminous gland)
   f. The eyelid (Moll gland)
2. Function:
   a. The apocrine gland has a unique scent in each individual and serves as a unique identifier.
3. Anatomy:
   a. Apocrine secretory gland:
      (1) The coiled secretory gland is located either in the lower dermis or in the subcutaneous tissue. Apocrine gland ducts usually open into the hair follicle above the entrance of the sebaceous glands, but some ducts open directly upon the surface of the skin.
      (2) It consists of secretory cells and myoepithelial cells.
      (3) Collagen and elastic fibers are found in the surrounding dermis.
   b. Apocrine duct:
      (1) The apocrine duct is the straight duct that merges with the infundibular portion of the hair follicle.
      (2) The apocrine duct consists of an inner periluminal cuticle and two to three layers of cuboidal cells. It has no myoepithelial lining.
4. Secretion composition:
   a. Apocrine gland secretions are milky in color, odorless, and sterile. The exact chemical consistency is uncertain as there is difficulty in obtaining uncontaminated specimens.
      (1) Bacteria that are present in the infundibular canal of the hair follicle, as well as bacteria on the skin surface, act upon the apocrine secretion to produce odiferous substances.
      (2) The odiferous substances contain, in part, short-chain fatty acids and ammonia.
      (3) A moist environment, conducive for bacterial proliferations, is provided by the axillary eccrine gland.
5. Stimulation:
   a. The mode of secretion of the apocrine gland is assumed to be due to the contraction of the myoepithelial cells surrounding the secretory cells.
   b. Myoepithelial contraction and the resulting emptying of the secretory coil are induced by emotional stress that leads to sympathetic nervous discharge.
   c. Like sebaceous glands, the activity of the apocrine glands is hormone dependent, but also stimulated by epinephrine and norepinephrine.
   d. Once the gland has been emptied, a refractory period ensues until the secretory gland and duct refill.

C. Eccrine sweat gland
1. Eccrine sweat glands function to help regulate the body's temperature. This is accomplished by the production of eccrine sweat that flows to the skin surface and cools by evaporation. The eccrine sweat glands are present everywhere on the body except in the ear canal,

glans penis, labia minora, prepuce, lips, and nail beds. Greatest concentration of these glands is on the palms and soles, forehead, and axilla.

    a. There are a total of two to five million eccrine sweat glands on the body.

    b. No new glands develop after birth.

    c. Each gland weighs approximately 30 to 40 mcg, the total mass equaling 100 g.

2. Anatomy:

    a. Eccrine duct: in the epidermis, the eccrine duct spirals on itself. It is lined by modified epidermal cells thought to be derived from upward migration of the dermal duct cells. There is a straight duct lying in the center of the dermis. The coiled segment of the duct is continuous with the secretary coil. It is approximately one third the length of the coil.

      (1) The eccrine duct consists of two layers of cuboidal cells:

        (a) Luminal cells: the luminal cells have a periluminal filamentous zone comprising a dense layer of tonofilaments. This adds to the rigidity of the duct.

        (b) Basal ductal cells: the basal cells have increased mitochondria and Na-K-ATPase (pump) activity.

    b. Eccrine secretory coil: the secretory coil has a larger diameter than the duct and is 2 to 5 mm in length. It makes up one half of the basal coil and lies in the lower one third of the dermis, at the dermal subcutaneous border. The secretory coil consists of three types of cells:

      (1) The mucoid or dark cells secrete a dense granule glycoprotein.

      (2) The clear or secretory cells are generally believed to be responsible for water and electrolyte secretion. The ATP-dependent NA+ pump is located within this cell. Where two or more clear cells abut, intercellular canaliculi are formed, which open into the lumen of the gland.

      (3) The myoepithelial cells lie between the secretory cells and the basement membrane. These add support to the gland. They do not expel sweat as do those in the apocrine glands.

3. Stimulation:

    a. There are three types of stimuli that promote eccrine gland secretion.

      (1) Thermal is the most important stimulus. Sweating occurs over the trunk face and sometimes the entire body. The preoptic area of the anterior hypothalamus is the heat regulating center, and it responds to changes in the core temperature. Afferent input from skin temperature also controls thermal sweating, but is not as important as core temperature.

      (2) Mental stimuli usually cause sweating on the palms, soles, and axilla, but sometimes cause generalized sweating. The frontal region of the brain is involved, but the exact pathway is unknown.

      (3) Gustatory produces sweating seen after eating hot or spicy foods. It is controlled by an unknown pathway.

4. Physiology of sweating:

    a. The physiology of sweating involves a complex process. Very basically, sweating begins in the clear secretory cells.

      (1) The intercellular canaliculi transports the solution secreted by the clear cells into the secretory coil. There is then reabsorption of sodium, chloride, and other electrolytes from the lumen of the duct.

      (2) The eccrine sweat is then secreted. It is an odorless, colorless, hypotonic solution. It has a specific gravity of approximately 1.005 and a pH between 4.5 and 5.5.

    b. Sweat contains:

      (1) Sodium
      (2) Chloride
      (3) Potassium
      (4) Urea
      (5) Lactate
      (6) Bicarbonate
      (7) Ammonia
      (8) Calcium
      (9) Phosphorus
      (10) Magnesium
      (11) Iodine
      (12) Sulfate
      (13) Iron
      (14) Zinc
      (15) Amino acids
      (16) Proteins
      (17) Immunoglobulins

    c. The sweat rate determines the concentration of the solutes.

      (1) Increased rates of sweating produce sweat with high pH, increased concentrations of sodium and chloride, and decreased concentrations of potassium, lactate, and urea.

      (2) Sweat lactate and urea may be important in controlling desquamation of the stratum corneum and may act as natural skin moisturizers.

      (3) The body may produce sweat at the rate of 2 to 4 L an hour. It may produce up to 12 L in 24 hours.

      (4) Axillary eccrine sweat glands contribute to the odor-producing secretion of the apocrine glands by providing a moist environment that is conducive to bacterial proliferation.

VI. IMMUNOLOGIC RESPONSES AND CELL TYPES

A. Humoral immunity

1. Humoral immunity is regulated by B lymphocytes that, when stimulated by antigen, form plasma cells that produce antibodies.

2. Antibodies can be divided into five classes:

    a. Immunoglobulin G (IgG)

    b. Immunoglobulin A (IgA)

c. Immunoglobulin M (IgM)

d. Immunoglobulin D (IgD)

e. Immunoglobulin E (IgE)

3. Antibodies, with varying degrees of efficiency, can:

a. Fix complement (IgG, IgM)

b. Aid macrophages in cytotoxicity or cell killing and phagocytosis (IgG)

c. Interact with antigen at mucosal surfaces (IgA)

d. Trigger release of mediators from mast cells of immunoreactive (IgE)

4. Antibodies can react to self as well as foreign antigen to cause inflammation, which in the pathogenic state can be harmful.

B. Cellular immunity

1. Cellular immunity involves T lymphocytes.

2. T lymphocytes divide into at least three subtypes:

a. T-helper cells (CD4 cells):

(1) T-helper cells activate B cells to produce antibody and activate T-cytotoxic cells.

(2) Act as killer cells against invading organisms.

(3) Can be classified as Th1 and Th2 based on cytokine profile.

(4) Secrete cytokines that increase the number of T cells, B cells, natural killer cells, and macrophages.

b. T-cytotoxic cells (CD8):

(1) T-cytotoxic cells kill target cells by binding with antigens on target cell.

(2) Cause lysis of antigen-bearing cells

c. T-memory cells (CD45RO):

(1) Play major role in inflammation seen in allergy and atopy

(2) Involved in contact and delayed hypersensitivity

3. Much T-cell function is accomplished by production of soluble proteins called lymphokines.

C. Complement system

1. A complex set of proteins that, when activated in the complement cascade, can:

a. Lyse cells

b. Aid in phagocytosis by macrophages

c. Cause mast cells to release histamines

d. Be chemotactic for neutrophils

2. Complement can be activated by:

a. Antibodies

b. Immune complexes through the classic pathway

3. Complement can also be activated by:

a. Bacteria

b. Fungi

c. Immunoglobulins and their fragments

d. Immune complexes

e. Lymphocytes

f. Endotoxins

VII. IMMUNITY AND SKIN DISEASE

A. Diseases in the skin can be caused by an immune response in three ways and in some skin diseases a combination of the three:

1. Immune response to foreign antigen

2. Response to self-antigen (autoimmunity)

3. Lack of appropriate immune response (immunodeficiency)

B. Response to an antigen (either foreign or self) is divided into four types of hypersensitivity reactions. The four hypersensitivity reactions, according to the Gel and Coombs classification are:

1. Type I—immediate allergic reaction:

a. Immediate reaction provoked by re-exposure to a specific type of antigen referred to as an allergen.

b. Exposure may be by ingestion, inhalation, injection, or direct contact.

c. An IgE-mediated response

d. Example of disease with this reaction:

(1) Urticaria (hives)

(2) Acute allergic drug reactions

2. Type II—cytotoxicity reaction:

a. Antibody is directed against antigen on cells (such as circulating red blood cells) or extracellular materials (basement membrane).

b. The resulting antigen–antibody complexes activate complement (via the classic pathway), leading to cell lysis or extracellular tissue damage.

c. Example of disease with this reaction:

(1) Transfusion reactions: incompatible RBCs or serum is transfused.

(2) Autoimmune hemolytic anemia: antibody is made against one's own RBCs.

3. Type III—immune complex-mediated reaction:

a. Mediated by circulating immune complexes

b. Often deposited in the vessel walls of the joints and kidney, initiating a local inflammatory reaction

c. Example of disease with this reaction:

(1) Serum sickness

(2) Systemic lupus erythematosus

4. Type IV—delayed-type and cell-mediated reactions:

a. Delayed hypersensitivity

b. T-cell–mediated response

c. Example of disease or testing exhibiting this reaction

(1) Allergic contact dermatitis

(2) Mantoux screening test

BIBLIOGRAPHY

Adelman, D. C., Casale, T. B., & Corren, J. (2012). *Manual of allergy and immunology* (5th ed.). Philadelphia, PA: Lippincott Williams & Wilkins.

Adkinson, N. F., Bocher, B. S., Burks, A., Busse, W. W., Holgate, S. T., Lemanske, R. F., & O'Hehir, R. E. (2014). *Middleton's allergy: Principles and practice* (8th ed.). Philadelphia, PA: Saunders-Elsevier.

Callen, J. P., Jorizzo, J. L., Zone, J. J., & Piette, W. W. (2009). *Dermatological signs of internal disease* (4th ed.). Philadelphia, PA: Saunders-Elsevier.

Chu, D. H. (2013). Development and structure of skin. In L. A. Goldsmith, S. I. Katz, B. A. Gilchrest, A. S. Paller, D. J. Leffell, & K. Wolff (Eds.), *Fitzpatrick's dermatology in general medicine* (8th ed., pp. 58–74). New York, NY: McGraw-Hill.

Garg, A., Levin, N. A., & Bernhard, J. D. (2013). Structure of skin lesions and fundamentals of clinical diagnosis. In L. A. Goldsmith, S. I. Katz, B. A. Gilchrest, A. S. Paller, D. J. Leffell, & K. Wolff (Eds.), *Fitzpatrick's dermatology in general medicine* (8th ed., pp. 26–41). New York, NY: McGraw-Hill.

Marks, J. G., & Miller, J. J. (2006). *Lookingbill and Marks' principles of dermatology* (4th ed.). Philadelphia, PA: Saunders-Elsevier.

McCann, S. E., & Huether, S. E. (2014). Structure, function, and disorders of the integument. In S. E. Huether, K. L. McCance, V. L. Brasher, & N. S. Rote (Eds.), *Pathophysiology—The biologic basics for disease in adults and children* (7th ed., pp. 1616–1652). St. Louis, MO: Mosby-Elsevier.

Nicol, N. H. (2009). Assessment of the integumentary system. In J. M. Black, & J. H. Hawks (Eds.), *Medical-surgical nursing: Clinical management for positive outcomes* (8th ed., pp. 1186–1198). Philadelphia, PA: WB Saunders Company.

Nicol, N. H., & Huether, S. E. (2012). Alterations of the integument in children. In S. E. Huether, K. L. McCance, V. L. Brasher, & N. S. Rote (Eds.), *Understanding pathophysiology* (6th ed., pp. 1070–1082). St. Louis, MO: Mosby-Elsevier.

Nicol, N. H., & Huether, S. E. (2012). Structure, function, and disorders of the integument. In S. E. Huether, K. L. McCance, V. L. Brasher, &

N. S. Rote (Eds.), *Understanding pathophysiology* (6th ed., pp. 1038–1069). St. Louis, MO: Mosby-Elsevier.

Nicol, N. H., & Huether, S. E. (2014). Alterations of the integument in children. In S. E. Huether, K. L. McCance, V. L. Brasher, & N. S. Rote (Eds.), *Pathophysiology—The biologic basics for disease in adults and children* (7th ed., pp. 1653–1667). St. Louis, MO: Mosby-Elsevier.

Penzer, R., & Ersser, S. J. (2010). *Principles of skin care*. Oxford, UK: Wiley-Blackwell.

Schalock, P. C., Hsu, J. T. S., & Arndt, K. A. (2011). *Lippincott's primary care dermatology*. Philadelphia, PA: Lippincott Williams & Wilkins.

Weinberg, S., Prose, N. S., & Kristal, L. (2008). *Color atlas of pediatric dermatology* (4th ed.). New York, NY: McGraw-Hill.

Wolff, K., Johnson, R. A., & Saavedra, A. P. (2013). *Fitzpatrick's color atlas and synopsis of clinical dermatology* (7th ed.). New York, NY: McGraw-Hill.

STUDY QUESTIONS

1. All of the following are components of the integumentary systems *except*:
   a. Skin
   b. Hair
   c. Glands
   d. Eyes
   e. Nails

2. Which of the following components of the integumentary system acts as the major barrier for the body?
   a. Dermis
   b. Epidermis
   c. Skin appendages
   d. Subcutaneous fat

3. The outermost layer of the epidermis is the:
   a. Basal cell layer
   b. Stratum lucidum
   c. Horny cell layer
   d. Granular cell layer
   e. Prickle cell layer

4. For a cell to move from the basal cell layer to the stratum corneum takes approximately:
   a. 8 to 14 days
   b. 1 to 7 days
   c. 15 to 30 days
   d. 6 weeks or more

5. Which of the following is *not* a structural component of the dermis?
   a. Collagen
   b. Elastic fibers
   c. Reticular fibers
   d. Lipocytes

6. Functions of the skin include:
   a. Temperature regulation
   b. Wound repair
   c. Vitamin D production
   d. All of the above

7. The principal cell of the epidermis is the:
   a. Keratinocyte
   b. Macrophage
   c. Mast cell
   d. Fibroblast
   e. None of the above

8. Accessory structures of the skin include the:
   a. Dermis, epidermis, and subcutaneous layers
   b. Blood vessels, macrophages, and Merkel cells
   c. Hair follicles and the sebaceous and sweat glands
   d. Cutaneous and subcutaneous layers

9. Type 1 hypersensitivity classically involves which of the following?
   a. IgM
   b. IgE
   c. Mast cells
   d. Macrophages
   e. IgD

10. Which of the following diseases displays a classic type IV hypersensitivity?
    a. Urticaria
    b. Psoriasis
    c. Allergic contact dermatitis
    d. Systemic lupus erythematosus

Answers to Study Questions: 1.d, 2.b, 3.c, 4.a, 5.d, 6.d, 7.a, 8.c, 9.b, 10.c

CHAPTER 2

Skin Assessment

Noreen Heer Nicol

OBJECTIVES

After studying this chapter, the reader will be able to:

- Define a holistic and comprehensive patient skin assessment.
- List subjective and objective data, which are necessary for a comprehensive assessment of the skin.
- Express the appropriate terminology used for primary and secondary lesions.
- Describe primary and secondary lesions of the skin and examples of dermatologic conditions exhibiting these features.
- Determine how lesion location and distribution help indicate specific diagnoses.
- Identify factors influencing professional relationship with patients and other health care professionals.

KEY POINTS

- A comprehensive, holistic skin assessment includes the history given by the patient (subjective data) and the findings of the physical exam of the skin (objective data).
- The preliminary patient history can be abbreviated to three key questions, which evaluate onset and evolution, symptoms, and treatment to date.
- Physical examination of the skin needs to be done ensuring privacy and dignity while determining whether the lesions being evaluated are primary or secondary lesions, as well as the configuration and distribution of the lesions.
- During the assessment, do not underestimate the significance of pruritus or the changes in the hair and nails.
- Specific terminology is used to describe the characteristics of skin lesions (number, color, type of lesion, configuration, distribution pattern, which can then be documented).
- Specific standardized terminology provides all care providers with a uniform description and understanding of the patient's condition. This can be especially important in completing consults with specialized providers, electronic communication, and telehealth visits.
- Documentation and communication with other health care professionals and disciplines at appropriate levels and according to identified standards are important to ensure continuity.

I. OVERVIEW

An initial assessment for patients with skin disorders should be approached as you would any patient. A comprehensive assessment of a dermatologic condition includes the history given by the patient (subjective data) and the findings of the physical examination of the integumentary system (objective data). The patient history and physical examination should also occur in an appropriately private area to ensure privacy and dignity, preferably with natural lighting. A preliminary history of a dermatologic problem can be abbreviated to three key questions, which evaluate onset and evolution, symptoms, and treatment to date (Box 2-1).

Skin provides an opportunity for visual inspection. This makes inspection the most important part of the physical examination of the skin. Physical examinations should be done in an orderly manner to insure important diagnostic clues are not missed. The initial key impression of whether the patient appears ill or not is important to note at the beginning of the physical examination.

Lesions can be defined as primary or secondary. Primary lesions are structural changes in the skin that have specific, visual characteristics and develop without any preceding skin changes (Table 2-1). Secondary lesion is one that has changed due to natural progression or due to physical factors such as rubbing or scratching (Table 2-2). Special or "other" lesions are those that occur in the skin only and in the skin most often or can be perceived most easily on the skin (Table 2-3).

Specific terminology is used to describe the characteristics of skin lesions (number, color, type of lesion, configuration, distribution pattern, which can then be documented). These descriptive clues aid in diagnosing and managing the patient by healthcare providers. It is important to use generally accepted descriptive terminology for verbal and written documentation to ensure continuity and to assist health care providers to interpret the findings. The general examination of the skin considers normal variants and general changes in the skin. A wide range of normal variations exist in the skin across the life span, which may be due to age, genetic factors, and environmental influences (Table 2-4).

II. PATIENT HISTORY (SUBJECTIVE DATA)

A. The traditional approach to assessment in general is to take the history prior to performing a physical examination. However, in dermatology, some providers prefer to do this

Box 2-1. Sample Questions for Initial Assessment or Triage

Key questions with initial history of skin problem:

Onset and Evolution: How long has the lesion been present? Has it gotten better or worse?

Symptoms: Does it itch? Or how does this bother you?

Treatment to Date: Tell me all the things that you have used to try to treat this?

Additional questions:

What did it first look like?

Has it changed, grown, bled, itched, or failed to heal?

Have you been out of the country lately?

Does it come and go?

Have you recently started any changes in your daily medicines?

Have you recently started any new medicines?

Any history of similar symptoms for you in the past?

Do any family members have the same or similar symptoms?

Have you used or done anything that seems to make it better?

is in a reverse order to expedite the process. A preliminary history helps to establish rapport and engages the patient in the process. Then, moving to physical examination allows appropriately chosen selective questions to be asked subsequently. The general history of current illness is ideally obtained by allowing patient to use their own words regarding his/her skin condition. This gives the provider a sense of direction as to which triage questions to ask. Initially, try to allow the patient to talk uninterrupted. This preliminary history can be abbreviated to three key questions, which evaluate onset and evolution, symptoms, and treatment to date (Box 2-1). Answers to these questions provide a great deal of information about how the condition has started and evolved over time. Review of systems is indicated by the acute or chronic current condition. Symptoms often drive how far one will go in looking for an etiology. Treatment is so key as oftentimes, regardless

TABLE 2-1 Primary Skin Lesions and Commonly Occurring Dermatologic Conditions

Primary Skin Lesions Description	Example of Dermatologic Condition	Example of Dermatologic Condition
Macule A circumscribed, flat discoloration, which varies widely in size, color, and shape	**Brown** Becker nevus Café au lait spot Erythrasma Fixed drug eruption Freckle Junction nevus Lentigo Lentigo maligna Melasma Photoallergic drug eruption Phototoxic drug eruption Stasis dermatitis Tinea nigra palmaris **Blue** Ink (tattoo) Maculae ceruleae (lice) Mongolian spot Ochronosis	**Red** Drug eruptions Juvenile rheumatoid arthritis Still disease Rheumatic fever Secondary syphilis Viral exanthems **Hypopigmented** Idiopathic guttate hypomelanosis Nevus anemicus Piebaldism Postinflammatory psoriasis Radiation dermatitis Tinea versicolor Tuberous sclerosis Vitiligo
Papule A solid, elevated palpable lesion on the skin <1 cm. It is round and sometimes pointed, is usually red but can be white, yellow, brown, or black, and may be associated with secondary lesions like scale and crust.	**Flesh colored, yellow, or white** Adenoma sebaceum Basal cell epithelioma Closed comedones (acne) Flat warts Granuloma annulare Lichen nitidus Lichen sclerosus et atrophicus Milium Molluscum contagiosum Nevi (dermal) Neurofibroma Pearly penile papules Sebaceous hyperplasia Skin tags Syringoma **Brown** Dermatofibroma Keratosis follicularis Melanoma Nevi Seborrheic keratosis Urticaria pigmentosa Warts	**Red** Acne vulgaris Atopic dermatitis Cholinergic urticaria Chondrodermatitis nodularis chronica helicis Eczema Folliculitis Insect bites Keratosis pilaris Leukocytoclastic vasculitis Miliaria Polymorphic light eruption Psoriasis Scabies Urticaria **Blue or violaceous** Angiokeratoma Blue nevus Lichen planus Lymphoma Kaposi sarcoma Melanoma Mycosis fungoides Venous lake

TABLE 2-1 *(Continued)*

Primary Skin Lesions Description	Example of Dermatologic Condition	Example of Dermatologic Condition
Plaque A solid lesion that covers more than 1 cm of surface skin, which is often elevated or thickened and formed by closely clustered papules	Atopic dermatitis Contact dermatitis Cutaneous T-cell lymphoma Papulosquamous (papular and scaling) lesions Discoid lupus erythematosus Lichen planus Pityriasis rosea Psoriasis Seborrheic dermatitis Syphilis (secondary) Tinea corporis Tinea versicolor	
Nodule A solid, elevated palpable mass that is usually larger than 0.5 cm. Sometimes considered a small tumor, nodules are located in the epidermis or extend deeper to the dermis or subcutaneous tissue.	Basal cell carcinoma Erythema nodosum Furuncle Hemangioma Kaposi sarcoma Keratoacanthoma Lipoma Lymphoma Melanoma	Metastatic carcinoma Mycosis fungoides Neurofibromatosis Prurigo nodularis Sporotrichosis squamous cell carcinoma Warts Xanthoma
Wheal Firm, edematous plaque resulting from infiltration of the dermis with fluid. Wheals are transient and a hypersensitivity response. Shape is often irregular. Sizes usually range from 3 mm to 12 cm.	Angioedema Dermatographism Hives Insect bites Urticaria pigmentosa (mastocytosis)	
Pustule A circumscribed elevated lesion containing whitish or yellowish elevations of the skin filled with purulent exudate, usually a collection of leukocytes and free fluid	Acne vulgaris Candidiasis Dermatophyte infection Dyshidrosis Folliculitis Gonococcemia Hidradenitis suppurativa	Herpes simplex Herpes zoster Impetigo Psoriasis Pyoderma gangrenosum Rosacea Varicella
Vesicle A round, raised lesion containing clear or purulent fluid that is up to <1 cm. They are either sparsely scattered or specifically grouped.	Herpes simplex Herpes zoster Contact dermatitis Dyshidrosis Impetigo Chickenpox	
Bulla This is a circumscribed collection of free fluid that is larger than 1 cm in diameter. It is mostly superficial in nature, and ruptures easily.	Bullous pemphigoid Pemphigus vulgaris	Bullous impetigo Bullous lichen planus

A primary lesion is a visually recognized structural change in the skin. It has specific characteristics and develops without any preceding skin change.
Adapted from Habif, T. P. (1996). *Clinical dermatology: A color guide to diagnosis and therapy* (3rd ed., pp. 3–11). St. Louis, MO: Mosby-Yearbook, Inc.

whether over-the-counter or prescription medications, it can be the very thing causing or contributing to the problem.

B. Information regarding other family members with similar symptoms, past medical history, previous and current drug therapy (including all over-the-counter preparations like herbs, vitamins, and natural supplements), occupation, and social history are all important parts of the initial interview.

1. Family history is important. Conditions such as psoriasis, eczema, skin cancer, or even keratosis pilaris have a genetic tendency. Patients may claim that another family member shares similar symptoms. For example, the diagnosis of atopic dermatitis is supported when the child presenting with chronic pruritic rash in antecubital fossa has a family history of atopic diseases (asthma, hay fever, and atopic dermatitis).

TABLE 2-2 Secondary Skin Lesions and Commonly Occurring Dermatologic Conditions

Secondary Skin Lesions Description	Commonly Occurring Dermatologic Conditions
Scales Excess dead epidermal cells that are produced by abnormal keratinization and shedding	**Fine to stratified** Erythema craquele Ichthyosis (quadrangular) Lupus erythematosus (carpet tack) Pityriasis rosea (collarette) Psoriasis (silvery) Scarlet fever (fine, on trunk) Seborrheic dermatitis Syphilis (secondary) Tinea (dermatophytes) Xerosis (dry skin) **Scaling in sheets** Scarlet fever (hands and feet) Staphylococcal scalded skin syndrome
Crusts A collection of dried serum and cellular debris; a scab	Acute eczematous inflammation Atopic dermatitis (face) Impetigo (honey colored) Pemphigus foliaceus Tinea capitis
Erosions A focal loss of epidermis; erosions do not penetrate below the dermoepidermal junction and therefore heal without scarring.	Candidiasis Dermatophyte infection Eczematous diseases Intertrigo Petechiae Senile skin Toxic epidermal necrolysis Vesiculobullous diseases
Ulcers A focal loss of epidermis and dermis; ulcers heal with scarring.	Aphthae Chancroid Decubitus Factitial Ischemic Necrobiosis lipoidica diabeticorum Neoplasms Pyoderma gangrenosum Radiodermatitis Syphilis (chancre) Stasis ulcers
Fissure A linear loss of epidermis and dermis with sharply defined, nearly vertical walls	Chapping (hands, feet) Eczema (fingertip) Intertrigo Petechiae
Atrophy A depression in the skin resulting from thinning of the epidermis or dermis	Aging Dermatomyositis Discoid lupus erythematosus Lichen sclerosus et atrophicus Morphea Necrobiosis lipoidica diabeticorum Radiodermatitis Striae Topical and intralesional steroids overuse
Scar An abnormal formation of connective tissue implying dermal damage; after injury or surgery, scars are initially thick and pink, but with time, scars become white and atrophic.	Acne Burns Herpes zoster Hidradenitis suppurativa Porphyria Varicella

A secondary lesion is a lesion that has changed due to its natural evolution or due to physical change (scratching, irritation, or secondary infection).

TABLE 2-3 Special Lesions/Other

Petechia	Hemorrhages from superficial blood vessels, <5 mm
Purpura	Hemorrhages from superficial blood vessels, 5 mm to 5 cm
Ecchymosis	Bleeding into the tissue affecting large areas
Lichenification	Thickening of the skin with exaggerated markings due to prolonged rubbing or scratching
Induration	Dermal hypertrophy causing the skin to become thicker and firmer. The skin markings remain unchanged.
Sclerosis	Circumscribed or diffuse hardening or induration of the skin resulting from dermal or subcutaneous edema, cellular infiltration, or collagen proliferation
Maceration	Thickening and whitening of the horny cell layer caused by excessive moisture
Excoriation	A linear or "dug out" traumatized area, usually self-inflicted
Cyst	A sac containing liquid or semisolid material
Furuncle	Deep form of folliculitis with pus accumulation
Abscess	Localized accumulation of purulent material deep within the dermis
Burrow	A characteristic linear lesion caused by tunneling in the stratum corneum produced by an animal parasite
Comedo	Mass of keratin and sebum within the dilated orifice of a hair follicle

2. Medical history is significant, including illnesses—particularly chronic illness, which may manifest in the skin—and surgical procedures, for example, if the patient presents with diffuse hair loss or perhaps an unusual rash that may be due to an unresolved strep infection or recent infections occupied by high fever. In another scenario, a past history of chickenpox is helpful in evaluating the patient suspected with herpes zoster.

3. Medication history and medication allergy can take time to update in a comprehensive manner. Then for example, obtaining information regarding current prescription therapy or medicines recently used, including all topicals; systemic medications including steroids; vitamins, and dietary supplements complementary or over-the-counter medications; and home remedies. Drugs or medications can cause multiple types of skin conditions.

4. Occupational history is important in skin disease when patients have occupation-associated symptoms or those which improve over a weekend or resolve while on vacation. In conditions such as occupational contact dermatitis, significant short- and long-term disability, and legal issues may coexist.

TABLE 2-4 Normal Skin Findings and Variations Across the Life Span

Areas of Concern	Normal Adult Findings	Variations in Children	Variations in Older Adults
Color and tone	Deep to light brown in blacks; whitish pink to ruddy with olive or yellow overtones in whites.	Newborn reddish first 8 to 24 h and then pale pink with transparent tone; slight jaundice starting 2nd or 3rd day of life; mottled appearance of hands and feet in newborns disappears with warming; in black newborns, melanotic pigmentation not intense with exception of nail beds and scrotum	Skin of white persons tends to look paler and more opaque.
Uniformity	Sun-darkened areas; areas of lighter pigmentation in dark-skinned persons (palms, lips, nail beds); labile pigmentation areas associated with use of hormones or pregnancy; callused areas appear yellow; crinkled skin areas darker (knees and elbows); dark-skinned (Mediterranean origin) persons may have lips with bluish hue; vascular flush areas (cheeks, neck, upper chest, or genital area) may appear red, especially with excitement or anxiety; skin color masked through use of cosmetics or tanning agents	Upper and lower extremities similar in color	More freckles; uneven tanning; pigment deposits; hypopigmented patches
Moisture	Minimum perspiration or oiliness felt; dampness in skin folds; increased perspiration associated with warm environment of activity; wet palms, scalp, forehead, and axilla associated with anxiety	Perspiration present in all children over 1 mo of age	Increased dryness, especially of extremities; decreased perspiration
Surface temperature	Cool to warm		
Texture	Smooth, even, and soft; some roughness on exposed areas (elbows and soles of feet)	Smooth, soft, flexible, dryness, and flakiness of skin in infants <1 mo of age (shedding of vernix caseosa); may appear as white cheesy skin; presence of milia; small white papules over nose and cheeks (plugged sebaceous glands) may remain for 2 mo.	Flaking and scaling associated with dry skin, especially on lower extremities
Thickness	Wide body variation; increased thickness in areas of pressure or rubbing (hands and feet)	Varying degrees of adipose tissue; dimpling of skin over joint areas	Thinner skin, especially over dorsal surface of hands and feet, forearms, lower legs, and bony prominences
Turgor	Skin moves easily when lifted and returns to place immediately when released.	Skin moves easily when lifted but falls quickly when released; skin over extremities taut.	General loss of elasticity; skin moves easily when lifted but does not return to place immediately when released; skin appears lax; increased wrinkle pattern more marked in sun-exposed areas, in fair skin, and in expressive areas of face; pendulous parts sag or droop (under chin, earlobes, breasts, and scrotum).
Hygiene	Clean, free of odor		
Alterations	Striae (stretch marks) usually silver or pinkish; freckles (prominent in sun-exposed areas); some birthmarks	Café au lait spots (light, cream-colored spots on darkened background); some nevi; stork bites (small red or pink spots on back of neck, upper lip, or upper eyelid; usually disappear by 5 y of age)	Nevi often become lighter or disappear; seborrheic keratoses (pigmented raised, warty, slightly greasy lesions most often found on trunk or face); senile (actinic) keratoses on exposed surfaces; first seen as small reddened areas and then as raised, rough, yellow to brown lesions; senile sebaceous adenomas (yellowish flat papules with central depressions); cherry adenomas (tiny, bright, ruby red, round); may become brown with age

5. Social history can be key in complex conditions. Areas to query include occupation, hobbies, sun exposure, pet exposure, alcohol consumption, recreational drugs, smoking history, travel, and sexual orientation and exposures. Long-time smokers can have physiologic changes that hinder wound healing as well as increase physical aging, particularly face.

6. Social factors including type of individual medical insurance or ability to pay for treatments also plays a particularly important role in dermatology. Over-the-counter medications or specialized topical prescriptions are frequently a part of the treatment plan. These can create financial burden to even the average patient. Providers must carefully consider these factors when delivering patient recommendations. Traditional and alternative therapies need to be explored.

7. Psychological factors in a patient's life and patient belief system may influence whether or not he/she will have a favorable or unfavorable response to treatment of a chronic skin disease. If, for example, the person prefers the added attention and sympathy the condition brings, improvement may be slow.

III. VISUAL OR PHYSICAL EXAMINATION (OBJECTIVE DATA)

A. There are many dermatologic maladies where examining the patient from head to toe is both necessary and beneficial. Whenever possible, the patient should undress and be placed in comfortable examination gown and setting. A good source of light is the best way to effectively examine the skin (and mouth). Natural lighting in the exam room improves visualization of most skin changes. Additional bright fluorescent lighting sources also are frequently used to examine the skin, mouth, and additional areas. Side lighting helps detect elevation changes.

B. Examinations should be done in an orderly manner to insure important diagnostic clues are not missed. First, note the overall impression of the patient, well or ill. Second, note weight as normal weight, obese, or cachectic. To insure the physical assessment is done in a systematic way, the general inspection of the skin should precede the lesion-specific exam. The hair, nails, mouth, and other mucous membranes should not be overlooked. All providers should strive to move to general inspections of the skin as well as any lesion-specific exams. It is unfortunate when a general physical examination of the skin is often overlooked because some lesions can be recognized at a glance. The total body examinations is completed to find lesions that may occupy the presenting complaint as well as the completely unrelated but important finding such as a skin cancer.

The general examination of the skin considers normal variants and general changes in the skin. A wide range of normal variations exist in the skin across the life span, which may be due to age, genetic factors, and environmental influences (Table 2-4). General changes can alter color (jaundice, cyanosis, pallor), turgor, thickness, temperature, and vascularity (purpura, petechiae, flushing). General findings can suggest a possible association with systemic disease. The lesion-specific examination follows the general assessment and also requires a systematic approach.

C. Gentle palpation of lesion areas, superficial and deep, should be completed to distinguish diagnostic characteristics.
1. Palpable lesions can be located in the epidermis or extend deep into the dermis or subcutaneous tissue.
2. Papules, nodules, and tumors may be smooth or rough, soft or firm, and fixed or movable.
3. Manipulation may elicit tenderness or detect localized heat.

D. Normal skin color alterations are best observed on the lips, earlobeso, oral mucous membranes, nails (fingers and toes), and extremities.
1. Natural skin color variances occur with not only the amount of melanin present in the skin but also the blood supply (from pallor to flush). Degree of pigmentation, pallor (anemia), and jaundice should be noted.
2. Abnormal conditions of hypopigmentation or hyperpigmentation may be seen in all skin colors.

E. Skin temperature depends upon the amount of vasoconstriction or vasodilation. Whereby localized inflammation causes dilatation of blood vessels and heat sensation, vasoconstriction occurs as the body tries to conserve heat.

F. When assessing for abnormality, evaluate the skin for moisture, turgor, texture, and elasticity. Note the degree of photoaging in adults.

G. The pattern, distribution, texture, and quality of hair on both the scalp and body are indicators of a person's general state of health.

H. Nails change with age and ill health. Pale nail beds can indicate circulatory impedance, whereas red inflamed nail cuticles or pitting can be a sign of psoriasis, or even bacterial or fungal infection.

IV. EVALUATION OF SPECIFIC LESIONS: PRIMARY LESIONS

Primary lesions are the physical changes caused directly by the disease process. Note the shape, morphology, distribution, and quality of the lesion(s). Also important is an accurate and precise description of the evolution of the disease condition. Some common descriptive terms follow. Table 2-1 outlines primary lesions and dermatologic conditions where they commonly occur.

A. Macule—A circumscribed, flat discoloration that varies widely in size, color, and shape, which cannot be palpated (Figure 2-1).

B. Patch—A flat discoloration that varies widely in size, color, and shape greater than 1 cm, which cannot be palpated (Figure 2-2).

C. Papule—A solid, elevated palpable lesion on the skin less than 1 cm. It is round and sometimes pointed, usually red but can be white, yellow, brown, or black and may be associated with secondary lesions like scale and crust (Figure 2-3).

D. Nodule—A solid, elevated palpable mass that is usually larger than 1 cm located in the epidermis or extend deeper to the dermis or subcutaneous tissue. Sometimes considered a small tumor, as tumors have the same features and are larger than nodules (Figure 2-4).

E. Plaque—A solid lesion that covers more than 1 cm of surface skin, which is often elevated or thickened and often formed by closely clustered papules (Figure 2-5).

F. Wheal—Firm, edematous plaque resulting from infiltration of the dermis with fluid. Wheals are transient and with an irregular shape. Sizes usually range from 3 mm to 12 cm (Figure 2-6).

G. Vesicle—A round, raised lesion containing clear or purulent fluid that is up to less than 1 cm. They are either sparsely scattered or specifically grouped (Figure 2-7).

H. Bulla—This is a circumscribed collection of free fluid that is larger than 1 cm in diameter. They are mostly superficial in nature and ruptures easily (Figure 2-8).

I. Pustule—A circumscribed elevated lesion containing whitish or yellowish elevations of the skin filled with purulent exudate, usually a collection of leukocytes and free fluid. Abscesses have the same features and are larger (Figure 2-9).

J. Telangiectasia—A permanently dilated superficial blood vessel in the skin, often seen in areas of solar damage (Figure 2-10) .

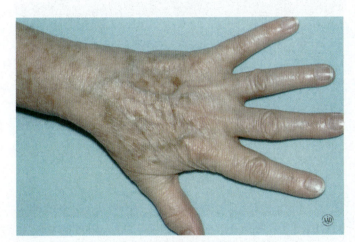

FIGURE 2-1. Macule, solar lentigines. (Provided by the American Academy of Dermatology, with permission.)

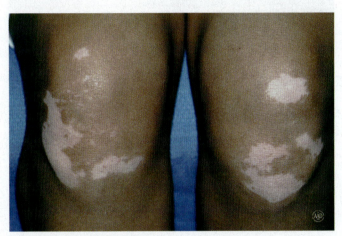

FIGURE 2-2. Patch, vitiligo. (Provided by the American Academy of Dermatology, with permission.)

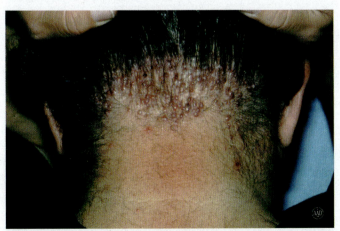

FIGURE 2-3. Papule, acne keloidalis nuchae. (Provided by the American Academy of Dermatology, with permission.)

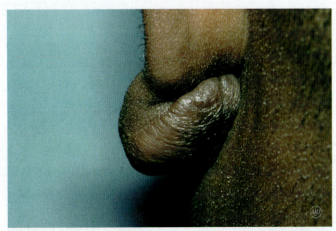

FIGURE 2-4. Nodule, keloid. (Provided by the American Academy of Dermatology, with permission.)

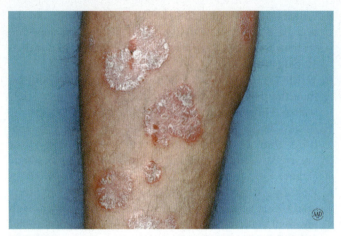

FIGURE 2-5. Plague, psoriasis. (Provided by the American Academy of Dermatology, with permission.)

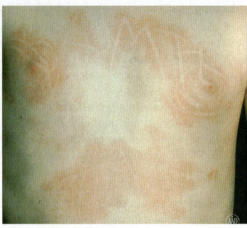

FIGURE 2-6. Wheal, dermatographism. (Provided by the American Academy of Dermatology, with permission.)

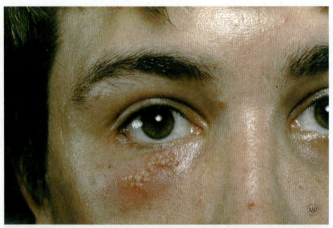

FIGURE 2-7. Vesicle, herpes simplex. (Provided by the American Academy of Dermatology, with permission.)

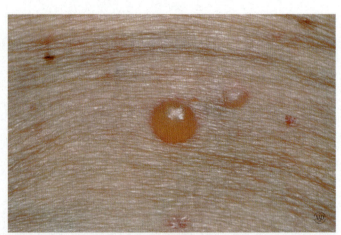

FIGURE 2-8. Bulla, bullous pemphigoid. (Provided by the American Academy of Dermatology, with permission.)

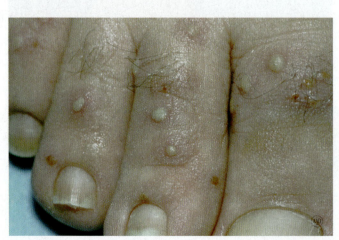

FIGURE 2-9. Pustule, insect sting, fire ant. (Provided by the American Academy of Dermatology, with permission.)

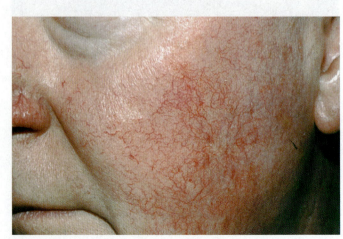

FIGURE 2-10. Telangiectasia, rosacea. (Provided by the American Academy of Dermatology, with permission.)

V. EVALUATION OF SPECIFIC LESIONS: SECONDARY LESIONS

Secondary lesions are physical changes due to natural evolution over time or environmental factors. This is the patient's response to a disease process. Secondary changes may result from scratching/rubbing, secondary infection, or therapies. Some common descriptive terms follow. Table 2-2 outlines secondary lesions and dermatologic conditions where they commonly occur.

A. Scale—Accumulated compact desquamated layers of stratum corneum, which can appear dry or greasy and range from fine and delicate as in pityriasis rosea to coarse and sheet-like as that found in exfoliative dermatitis. These are caused by abnormal keratinization and shedding (Figure 2-11).

B. Crust—Accumulated dried masses of serum, bacteria, and/or possibly blood, mixed with epithelial debris that is covering damaged skin. They vary in size, thickness, and color depending upon the cause and location (Figure 2-12, lichen simplex chronicus).

C. Fissures—Linear cracks in the epidermis, caused mainly by injury or disease. Excessive dryness of the skin may also cause this lesion. They vary in size from a tiny crack to a cleft several centimeters in length that can extend into the dermis. The hands, toes, and angles of the mouth are most commonly affected (Figure 2-13).

D. Lichenification—Areas of epidermal thickening caused by long-term rubbing or scratching. Underlying inflammation often gives a dark red appearance to the skin with exaggerated skin lines. Patient's with neurodermatitis will have lichenified areas (Figure 2-14).

E. Erosion—A temporary loss or break in the epidermis that unless secondarily infected will heal without a scar. Appearing as a slightly depressed, moist lesion, it does not extend below the epidermal junction in the skin layers. Examples of erosions are a scraped knee or elbow (Figure 2-15).

F. Ulcer—A deep erosion that extends through the epidermis down into the dermis. This type of lesion is likely to scar. The cause and location of the ulcer influence the size and type of discharge produced (Figure 2-16).

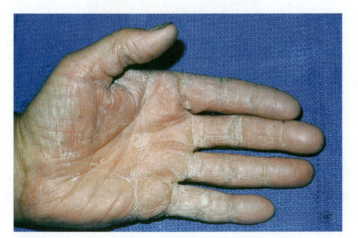

FIGURE 2-11. Scales, tinea manus. (Provided by the American Academy of Dermatology, with permission.)

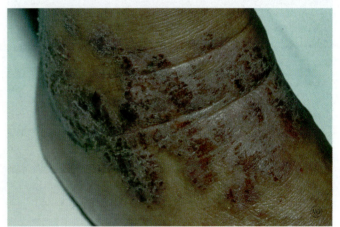

FIGURE 2-12. Crusts, lichen simplex chronicus. (Provided by the American Academy of Dermatology, with permission.)

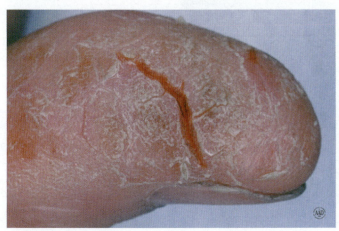

FIGURE 2-13. Fissure, hand dermatitis. (Provided by the American Academy of Dermatology, with permission.)

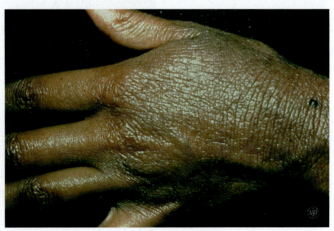

FIGURE 2-14. Lichenification, atopic dermatitis. (Provided by the American Academy of Dermatology, with permission.)

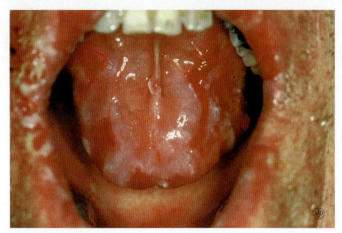

FIGURE 2-15. Erosions, oral erosions, pemphigus. (Provided by the American Academy of Dermatology, with permission.)

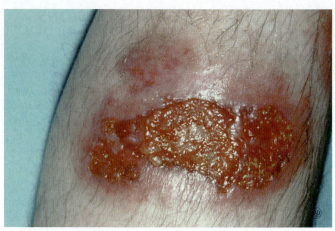

FIGURE 2-16. Ulcers, pyoderma gangrenosum. (Provided by the American Academy of Dermatology, with permission.)

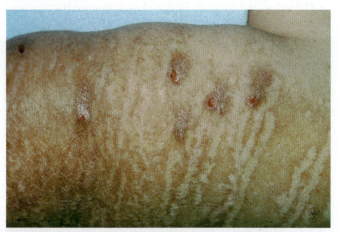

FIGURE 2-17. Excoriation with scarring, neurodermatitis. (Provided by the American Academy of Dermatology, with permission.)

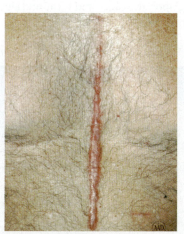

FIGURE 2-18. Scar, hypertrophic scar. (Provided by the American Academy of Dermatology, with permission.)

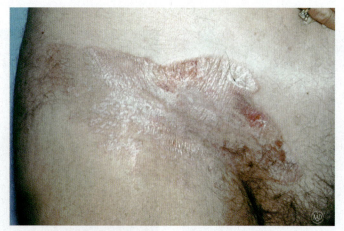

FIGURE 2-19. Atrophy, lichen sclerosus. (Provided by the American Academy of Dermatology, with permission.)

G. Excoriation—A superficial linear erosion caused by excessive scratching and other trauma. Usually self-induced and may appear linear. Commonly seen in pruritic conditions, such as patients with eczema, neurodermatitis, and scabies. Fingernails are often the source of trauma, so infection is common (Figure 2-17).

H. Scar—A normal result of skin regeneration following injury or disease. Damage to the dermis results with abnormal connective tissue patterns and frequently pigmentary changes. Scars are usually smooth and firm and appear white over time. Overproduction of collagen during the healing process produces a red, raised thickened scar known as a keloid. Burn scars are frequently keloid (Figure 2-18).

I. Atrophy—A thinning of the superficial skin layers, deeper dermal layers, and/or subcutaneous layers most commonly after injury or inflammation. The skin develops a transparent localized indentation. Some examples are post-pregnancy stretch marks or healed lesions in patients with chronic discoid lupus (Figure 2-19).

VI. EVALUATION OF LESIONS: NUMBER, COLOR, CONFIGURATION, AND DISTRIBUTION

The number, color, configuration, and distribution of the lesion(s) are often distinct enough to assist with assessment. The earliest lesion and the arrangement of the lesions in relation to each other are valuable diagnostic clues.

A. Consider the number of lesions. Are they few or numerous? Are they localized in one spot or one region? The lesions may be generalized or universal involving the hair and nails as well.
1. Some lesions affect only one side of the body and follow nerve tracts such as herpes zoster.
2. Lesion has a ringed (i.e., tinea), crescent (i.e., burn), or linear-shaped pattern (i.e., scabies).
3. Lesion location is important because some diseases only affect specific areas of the skin. For example, acne most often occurs on the face, chest, and back because of the location of sebaceous glands, whereas eczema is frequently found in the antecubital fossa and posterior knees in adolescents and adults.
   a. Lesions under a watchband, necklace, or ring might signify a nickel sensitivity.
   b. An eruption isolated where skin is exposed to direct sunlight could likely indicate a polymorphic light eruption.
   c. A rash on the "blush" areas of the face might indicate rosacea, if the history coincides.
   d. Lesions at the openings of hair follicles on the backs of upper arms likely signify keratosis pilaris.

B. Lesion color is a helpful diagnostic aid but may be confusing also since everyone's perception of color is different. A few basic shades are listed below:
1. Brown—seen with increased epidermal melanin pigmentation
2. Yellow—lipid skin lesions such as xanthomas
3. Orange—accumulated carotene in the dermis
4. Purplish red—extravasation of blood in the dermis
5. Blue-black—seen in cellular blue nevi

C. Configuration refers to the arrangement or shape of lesions in relation to other lesions. Some terms seem similar but have been common terminology for decades. The first three words below are all words for round-type lesions.
1. Annular, circinate—ring shaped with active elevated margins that spread peripherally and regress centrally, seen in granuloma annulare
2. Discoid—disk shaped seen in discoid lupus erythematosus
3. Nummular—coin shaped, found in nummular eczema
4. Linear—in a line as seen in Rhus dermatitis
5. Arciform—arc shape with an incomplete circle as found in mycosis fungoides
6. Guttate—resembling a drop as found in guttate psoriasis
7. Iris, target lesion, or "bull's-eye"—lesion which has an erythematous annular macule or papule with a purplish papular or vesicular center
8. Herpetiform—in a grouping
9. Reticulated—having a net-like appearance
10. Confluent—blending together with adjacent lesions
11. Discrete—separate lesions from each other as in varicella
12. Polymorphous or multiform—occurring in several forms
13. Punctate—marked by points or dots
14. Serpiginous—snake-like

D. Configuration refers to the arrangement or pattern of spread in relation to other lesions.
1. Dermatomal/zosteriform—band-like distributions along dermatome, which follows nerve root distribution
2. Generalized/diffuse—widely distributed
3. Localized—limited areas of involvement, which are defined clearly
4. Symmetrical—distributed in a similar way on both sides of area
5. Unilateral—affects one side of the area only
6. Truncal—prone to trunk of body, rarely affects limbs
7. Solitary—a single lesion
8. Satellite—single lesion in close proximity to a large grouping

VII. HAIR AND NAILS AS DIAGNOSTIC INDICATORS

Changes in a person's hair and nails are not necessarily indicative of a disease process. Limited to the skin, changes may be important diagnostic indicators of overall health.

A. Excessive hair (hypertrichosis) or too little hair (hypotrichosis) are findings worth noting.

B. Generalized thinning or lost patches of scalp hair or generalized hair loss in multiple body locations may be important symptoms of infections (bacterial and fungal), systemic illness, lupus erythematosus, chemicals/drugs, scarring, and many other less-common conditions.

C. Fingernails and toenails protect the digits, and changes in their appearance or color must be considered.

See Chapter 22, Hair and Nails, for more detail.

VIII. PRURITUS

A. Primary symptom found in many pathologic systemic disease processes from simple dry skin to the early symptoms of Hodgkin disease or cutaneous T-cell lymphoma.

B. The itch threshold is lower at night.

C. It is the prominent symptom in many dermatologic disorders, and in some cases, there is no apparent skin eruption.

D. To help break the itch–scratch cycle, hydration, moisturizers, sedating oral antihistamines, antipruritic lotions, and topical and injectable steroids may be used. Topical anesthetics and topical antihistamines are generally to be avoided as they may cause allergic contact dermatitis or other forms of irritation or rash. Simple cool compresses applied to the trigger point, if discernable, may help decrease symptoms.

E. Lab work such as CBC, sed rate, urinalysis, serum glucose, and/or liver/thyroid/renal function tests may be ordered. A chest x-ray, Pap smear, or stool tests for ova and parasites and occult blood might also be useful.

F. Psychologic stress and emotional well-being are considered a contributing factor in pruritus, but not solely the causing influence. Fear, tension, anxiety, stress, boredom, and depression may intensify the itch sensation.

G. Dermatologic conditions where pruritus may be a significant component are multiple. Conditions include scabies, dermatitis herpetiformis, atopic dermatitis, lichen simplex chronicus, pruritus vulvae, pruritus ani, miliaria, insect (flea or bedbug) bites, pediculosis, contact dermatitis, psoriasis (especially on scalp and genitalia), lichen planus, urticaria, and lymphoma.

IX. DOCUMENTATION

Accurate, up-to-date, and clear documentation of the patient's condition is essential to provide safe quality care. Interdisciplinary communication requires that all care providers access and contribute to the medical record in an individual and provider-unique manner. Enhanced and consistent information shared between healthcare providers promotes a continuum of care. Numerous methods and formats for documenting are available to the dermatology specialty. Many documentation specifics are now determined by the formatting established within an electronic medical record. Variations of the older S–O–A–P (subjective–objective–assessment–plan), P–I–E (problem–intervention–evaluation), D–A–R (data–action–response), freehand illustrations, body stickers, and photography have been incorporated into electronic systems. Charting by exception (CBE) while efficient still lends itself to omissions and incomplete assessment.

A. By standardizing a charting format, important patient information and details are less likely to be neglected or forgotten.

B. Body maps help indicate lesion and surgery locations. These methods work when mapping moles, too.

C. Dermatologic photography entered into the patient record is reassuring to the patient and more reliable than one's memory. A change in an acne condition, scar development, mole mapping, and hair loss or regrowth are examples of when photographic documentation are valuable.

D. Dermatologic photography is also used when teaching medical/nursing students, special courses, or relaying information to other medical associates. Written consent from the patient is necessary.

E. Photo documentation of skin surgery before, during, and after the repair is useful for the referring physician, insurance company, and dermatologist for medicolegal reasons.

BIBLIOGRAPHY

Adelman, D. C., Casale, T. B., & Corren, J. (2012). *Manual of allergy and immunology* (5th ed.). Philadelphia, PA: Lippincott Williams & Wilkins.

Adkinson, N. F., Bocher, B. S., Burks, A., Busse, W. W., Holgate, S. T., Lemanske, R. F., & O'Hehir, R. E. (2014). *Middleton's allergy: Principles and practice* (8th ed.). Philadelphia, PA: Saunders-Elsevier.

Arndt, K. A., & Hsu, J. T. S. (2007). *Manual of dermatologic therapeutics* (7th ed.). Philadelphia, PA: Lippincott Williams & Wilkins.

Callen, J. P., Jorizzo, J. L., Zone, J. J., & Piette, W. W. (2009). *Dermatological signs of internal disease* (4th ed.). Philadelphia, PA: Saunders-Elsevier.

Craven, R., Hirnle, C., & Jensen, S. (2013). *Fundamentals of nursing: Human health and function* (7th ed.). Philadelphia, PA: Lippincott Williams & Wilkins.

Desai, S., & Hsu, J. T. S. (2011). Basic definitions and differential diagnosis. In P. C. Schalock, J. T. S. Hsu, & K. A. Arndt (Eds.), *Lippincott's primary care dermatology*. Philadelphia, PA: Lippincott Williams & Wilkins.

Garg, A., Levin, N. A., & Bernhard, J. D. (2012). Structure of skin lesions and fundamentals of clinical diagnosis. In L. A. Goldsmith, S. I. Katz, B. A. Gilchrest, A. S. Paller, D. J. Leffell, & K. Wolff (Eds.), *Fitzpatrick's dermatology in general medicine* (8th ed., pp. 26–42). New York, NY: McGraw-Hill.

Garg, A., Levin, N. A., & Bernhard, J. D. (2013). Structure of skin lesions and fundamentals of clinical diagnosis. In L. A. Goldsmith, S. I. Katz, B. A. Gilchrest, A. S. Paller, D. J. Leffell, & K. Wolff (Eds.), *Fitzpatrick's dermatology in general medicine* (8th ed., pp. 26–41). New York, NY: McGraw-Hill.

Marks, J. G., & Miller, J. J. (2006). *Lookingbill and Marks' principles of dermatology* (4th ed.). Philadelphia, PA: Saunders-Elsevier.

McCann, S. E., & Huether, S. E. (2014). Structure, function, and disorders of the integument. In S. E. Huether, K. L. McCance, V. L. Brasher, & N. S. Rote (Eds.), *Pathophysiology—The biologic basics for disease in adults and children* (7th ed., pp. 1616–1652). St. Louis, MO: Mosby-Elsevier.

Nicol, N. H. (2009). Assessment of the integumentary system. In J. M. Black, & J. H. Hawks (Eds.), *Medical-surgical nursing: Clinical management for positive outcomes* (8th ed., pp. 1186–1198). Philadelphia, PA: WB Saunders Company.

Nicol, N. H., & Huether, S. E. (2012). Alterations of the integument in children. In S. E. Huether, K. L. McCance, V. L. Brasher, & N. S. Rote (Eds.), *Understanding pathophysiology* (6th ed., pp. 1070–1082). St. Louis, MO: Mosby-Elsevier.

Nicol, N. H., & Huether, S. E. (2012). Structure, function, and disorders of the integument. In S. E. Huether, K. L. McCance, V. L. Brasher, & N. S. Rote (Eds.), *Understanding pathophysiology* (6th ed., pp. 1038–1069). St. Louis, MO: Mosby-Elsevier.

Nicol, N. H., & Huether, S. E. (2014). Alterations of the integument in children. In S. E. Huether, K. L. McCance, V. L. Brasher, & N. S. Rote (Eds.), *Pathophysiology—The biologic basics for disease in adults and children* (7th ed., pp. 1653–1667). St. Louis, MO: Mosby-Elsevier.

Penzer, R., & Ersser, S.J. (2010). *Principles of skin care*. Oxford, UK: Wiley-Blackwell.

Perry, A. G., & Potter, P. A. (2002). Documenting nurses' progress notes. In A. G. Perry, & P. A. Potter (Eds.), *Clinical nursing skills & techniques* (5th ed., p. 53). St. Louis, MO: Mosby, Inc.

Weinberg, S., Prose, N. S., & Kristal, L. (2008). *Color atlas of pediatric dermatology* (4th ed.). New York, NY: McGraw-Hill.

Wolff, K., Johnson, R. A., & Saavedra, A. P. (2013). *Fitzpatrick's color atlas and synopsis of clinical dermatology* (7th ed.). New York, NY: McGraw-Hill.

STUDY QUESTIONS

1. Which of the following is *not* one of the three general questions important when taking the initial abbreviated history of a new dermatologic problem?
   a. How long have you had it?
   b. Does it itch?
   c. What blood tests have you had recently?
   d. How have you treated it?

2. Which of the following is a solid, elevated palpable mass that is usually larger than 1 cm?
   a. Plaque
   b. Nodule
   c. Patch
   d. Papule

3. The pattern, distribution, and texture of which of the following on the body is an indicator of a person's general state of health?
   a. Seborrheic keratosis
   b. Moles
   c. Hair
   d. Warts

4. A circumscribed, flat discoloration that could be brown, blue, red, or hypopigmented is a:
   a. Macule
   b. Bulla
   c. Nodule
   d. Plaque

5. Lichenification is the accumulation of dried masses of serum, bacteria, and possible blood mixed with epithelial debris that covers damaged epidermis.
   a. True
   b. False

6. Which of the following primary lesions is caused directly by a disease process?
   a. Scales
   b. Erosion
   c. Pustule
   d. Ulcer

7. A lesion that is a response to a disease process is a secondary lesion. Which of the following is an example of a secondary lesion?
   a. Wheal
   b. Crust
   c. Vesicle
   d. Plaque

8. A configuration that can be described as coin-like is:
   a. Satellite
   b. Discoid
   c. Gyrate
   d. Confluent

9. Pruritis is a major symptom of:
   a. Rosacea
   b. Keratosis pilaris
   c. Herpes zoster
   d. Atopic dermatitis

10. The itch or pruritus threshold is lower:
    a. First thing in the morning
    b. Around noontime
    c. During the evening meal
    d. In the evening during bedtime hours

Answers to Study Questions: 1.c, 2.b, 3.c, 4.a, 5.b, 6.c, 7.b, 8.b, 9.d, 10.d

CHAPTER 3

Dermatologic Diagnostic Tests and Procedures

Anne Marie Ruszkowski Lord • Noreen Heer Nicol

OBJECTIVES

After studying this chapter, the reader will be able to:

- Identify diagnostic tests and procedures commonly used on the skin, including microscopic examination, cultures, biopsy for removal and/or pathology, and patch testing.
- Describe important steps of above tests and procedures, including scrapings and swabs for microbiology, virology, and mycology.
- Describe techniques and application for patch testing in the evaluation of contact dermatitis.
- Provide effective education to patients and families to prepare them for tests and procedures.

KEY POINTS

- The skin is a highly accessible organ, making it available for several diagnostic tests that can help identify specific skin diseases.
- Diagnostic tests performed directly on the skin that are usually minimally traumatic and often highly rewarding diagnostically include microscopic examinations, cultures, biopsies, and patch testing.
- Blood, urine, and radiograph testing remain helpful when systemic disease is suspected.
- Sample selection is extremely important in obtaining the proper diagnostic specimen.
- Nursing staff is encouraged to understand each procedure and the benefit versus risk of each to teach and care for their patients more effectively.
- Patch testing is an essential tool used in diagnosing allergic contact dermatitis.
- Nursing and allied health staff are frequently key personnel participating in the preparation, interpretation, and placement of patch tests.

I. DIAGNOSTIC AIDS

As adjuncts to what is seen with the eyes or palpated with the hands, numerous diagnostic tools offer key information in making a diagnosis. Nursing staff rarely perform all steps independently in diagnostic procedures used to establish skin disorders. Therefore, this section is meant to provide an overview. Correct visualization and sample selection are critically important in obtaining the proper diagnostic specimen.

A. An alcohol wipe swept across a lesion is a method used to elucidate the small, delicate telangiectasia and translucence of that lesion, such as with a basal cell carcinoma.

B. Diascopy examination of the skin is completed by gentle pressure utilizing a translucent object, such as a glass slide, to observe the effect upon the color (erythema) of the skin.
  1. Pressure producing a reduction in erythema or pigmentation indicates blood vessel dilation.
  2. Pressure that does not produce a change in erythema or pigment indicates increased extravasation of blood, or simply an increased amount of pigment.

C. Mineral oil applied to a glass slide before using magnification helps visualize certain specimens, such as the scabies mite.

D. The microbe is stained for visibility in many microscopic examinations. In dark-field examination, the slide background is darkened to visualize the causative spirochete for syphilis. Specimens for dark-field examinations must be examined immediately.

II. DIAGNOSTIC TESTS

KOH (potassium hydroxide) preparation is a diagnostic method used to confirm the presence or absence of hyphae, spores, and pseudospores. A 10% to 20% KOH solution will digest the keratin in tissue but leave most fungal forms intact for visualization under the microscope (Figure 3-1).

A. Certain fungi have characteristic appearances.
  1. A no. 15 blade is used to scrape skin/scale from the edge of a scaling lesion onto a glass slide. The extremely thick pieces of scale should be avoided. If *Candida* infection is suspected, a pustule can be a good source of material for the exam.
  2. With the edge of the no. 15 blade, sweep scale or matter into a small pile in the center of the slide.
  3. One or two drops of 10% KOH are placed on the slide.
  4. A glass coverslip is applied over specimens. Blot out the excess KOH by firmly pressing a paper towel on top of the coverslip and slide.
  5. The slide is gently heated to dissolve the keratin, and the coverslip is gently squeezed and then examined under

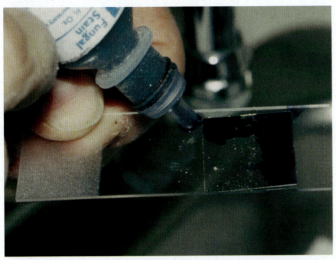

FIGURE 3-1. KOH solution and slide. (From Goodheart, H. P. (2003). *Goodheart's photoguide of common skin disorders* (2nd ed.). Philadelphia, PA: Lippincott Williams & Wilkins.)

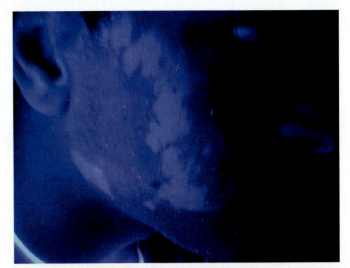

FIGURE 3-2. Vitiligo as seen with Wood's lamp. (From Goodheart, H. P. 2010. *Goodheart's same-site differential diagnosis: A rapid method of diagnosing and treating common skin disorders*. Philadelphia, PA: Wolters Kluwer.)

the microscope using low illumination. If a heat source is not available, leave the specimen set for a minimum of 30 minutes after applying the KOH prior to examination. Scan the entire coverslip first under low (X10) power and then move to higher (X45) power for confirmation.

6. Repeat the process with a new specimen if the test is negative and a high degree of suspicion remains for a fungal disorder.

B. Fungal cultures are a frequent next step when exact fungal species need to be determined to assist in treatment or the KOH test is negative in light of high suspicion of fungal disease. Scrapings obtained as above with a no. 15 blade from a dry patch of skin, intact pustule, or nail plate or from under the nail can be introduced onto a dermatophyte culture medium and aerobically incubated for a minimum of 7 to 10 days or per the specific media directions. The time required for results depends greatly on the media, lab, or process.

C. Wood's Fluoresence lamp is another simple, but less used, diagnostic tool. This handheld lamp has ultraviolet bulbs (365 nm) that cause certain microorganisms to appear colorful when illuminated. The use of this test has become limited because some common organisms do not fluoresce. This includes *T. tonsurans* which is now the most common cause of tinea capitis in the U.S. (Figure 3-2).

1. Certain fungus or ringworms glow blue-gray or yellow-green.
2. Tinea versicolor can appear gold.
3. Urine screen for porphyrins fluoresces orange.

D. Tzanck smear uses a microscope and special stain including Giemsa, methylene blue, or Wright stain. The specimen is best taken from the base of a new vesicle. The specimen slide is colored with a special dye and examined under a microscope, either at the practice office or at a pathology laboratory. The examiner looks for abnormally large cells (called giant cells) that are characteristic of herpes virus infections. This tool aids in the diagnosis of herpes simplex (which causes fever blisters) or herpes zoster (which causes chickenpox and shingles), but does not distinguish between the two.

E. Viral culture, like Tzanck smear, is ideally taken from intact vesicles and transported in a viral transport media. A vesicle is opened or crust removed and underlying serum is swabbed. The swab is placed in the viral media. Human virus types that can be identified by viral culture include adenoviruses, Cytomegalovirus, enteroviruses, herpes simplex virus, influenza viruses, parainfluenza viruses, varicella–zoster virus, measles, and mumps. Viral PCR (polymerase chain reaction) test is also frequently used.

F. Bacterial culture or microbiological culture is a method of multiplying microbial organisms by letting them reproduce in predetermined culture media under controlled laboratory conditions. The ideal specimen sources for bacterial cultures include intact pustules, bullae, and abscesses. The specimen can be obtained by a variety of methods ranging from swabbing, scrapping, aspiration, or biopsy. The cultures are used to determine the type of organism, its abundance in the sample being tested, or both.

G. Scabies scrapings are done with an oil-moistened no. 15 blade. Vigorously scrape small papules or questionable burrows, transfer to a glass slide, cover with coverslip, and examine microscopically.

H. Direct immunofluorescence of tissue is an option when trying to diagnose immunologic abnormalities in the skin. Bullous diseases and connective tissue disorders are two examples. Special tissue preparations and stains are done at a lab to microscopically visualize immunoglobulins, complement, and fibrin found in the skin or circulation.

I. Gram stain allows for identification of Gram-negative or Gram-positive organisms. Exudate from the site is smeared onto a glass slide, then stained, dried, and examined under oil immersion.

J. Hair pull (pluck) is the most accurate technique to evaluate the anagen/telogen ratio. Approximately 50 hairs of the same length are extracted using a rubber-tipped needle holder and plucked with a quick motion. Hairs are floated on a wet microscope slide or Petri dish for examination.

Dyes will be applied to determine phase of growth—anagen reacts with citrulline; telogen hairs do not stain. Hair can also be examined under a microscope to evaluate for disorders such as Netherton disease.

III. SKIN BIOPSIES

Shave, punch, and ellipse are biopsy techniques used in both diagnosis and treatment of skin diseases.

A. Shave biopsy/excision is a tangential specimen of tissue for pathology, resulting in minimal to no scarring.
1. The shave biopsy/excision is indicated for dome-shaped intradermal nevi, fibromas, warts, seborrheic keratoses, and actinic keratoses.
2. A portion of the epidermis and underlying papillary dermis is primarily involved.
3. The procedure can be both an excisional and incisional biopsy depending on whether part or all of the lesion is removed. Extremely superficial lesions are frequently removed with this method.
4. The equipment needed includes local anesthesia, gentian marker, a single-edged blade (Figure 3-3), curette (optional), hemostatic agent, pathology bottle, and appropriate dressing.
5. Postbiopsy wound care or dressings are optional depending upon the shave location and patient compliance.
6. Hypopigmentation at the shave site and localized infection are two potential complications.

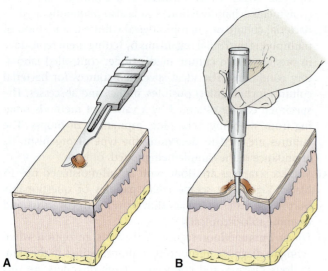

FIGURE 3-3. Straight blade and punch tools. **A:** Shave biopsy. A scalpel blade is manipulated by the operator to adjust the depth of the biopsy. Hemostasis is achieved with topical application of aqueous aluminum chloride, ferrous subsulfate, or electrocautery. **B:** Punch biopsy. The operator makes a circular incision to the level of the superficial fat, using a rotating or twisting motion of the trephine. Traction applied perpendicularly to the relaxed skin tension lines minimizes redundancy at closure. Hemostasis is commonly achieved by placement of sutures. (From DeVita, V. T., et al. 2014. *DeVita, Hellman, and Rosenberg's cancer: Principles & practice of oncology.* Philadelphia, PA: Wolters Kluwer.)

B. Punch biopsy has multiple uses: diagnosing a disease or an eruption, or simply excising a lesion. The punch instrument can be either circular or elliptical with a razor-sharp cutting edge (see Figure 3-3).
1. An early lesion is selected when an eruption needs diagnosing. If a vesicle is to be studied, a fully intact one is preferred.
2. An older lesion is needed if discoid lupus erythematosus is suspected.
3. A punch tool is advantageous in the removal of small nevi because the scar will be smaller than one from the elliptical method.
4. A punch biopsy is commonly used in diagnosing basal and squamous cell carcinomas, granuloma annulare, and other diseases that involve the deeper dermis.
5. Punch diameters are available in multiple sizes. Those most frequently used in dermatology range from 2.0 to 8.0 mm.
6. For local anesthesia, lidocaine 1%, usually with epinephrine for less bleeding depending on the site location, is administered with a 30-gauge needle by raising a wheal prior to biopsy.
7. Depth extends from the stratum corneum (outermost skin layer) to the underlying fat, providing the entire dermis for evaluation. If nonabsorbable suture is used, the patient returns for suture removal. The punch is twisted while obtaining the biopsy to sample the epidermal and deeper dermal tissue.
8. Complications to consider are infection, scarring, and nerve damage.

C. Elliptical excision/wedge biopsy is used when both normal skin and lesional skin junctions are needed for study, such as evaluating basal and squamous cell malignancies and nevi.
1. The biopsy offers greater tissue depth down to and, if necessary, into the subcutaneous fat.
2. The equipment needed includes local anesthesia, gentian marker, sterile gloves, a single-edged blade with handle, needle holder, small forceps, skin hook, small clamp, small pointed scissors, suture, curette (optional), hemostatic agent, pathology bottle, gauze, and appropriate dressing.
3. The incision length is normally 2.5 to 3 times the width of the incision.
4. Repairs require suturing, and layered closures are frequently necessary.
5. With so many different types of absorbable suture material available, patients may not need to return for suture removal, making skin surgery more convenient for their schedules. Nonabsorbable suture must be removed. The number of days until removal of nonabsorbable suture is dependent on the area of incision. For instance, facial sutures are removed earlier at 5 to 6 days versus trunk or extremity sutures, which might be left in place 1 to 2 weeks.
6. Flaps and grafts are additional options for closing large and/or inelastic skin surgery sites.

7. Scarring, possible nerve damage, and infection are the most common complications.
8. Mohs technique is a specialized procedure involving serial excisions of tissue that are systematically mapped and microscopically examined. This technique done by specially trained Mohs surgeons is used to treat basal cell and squamous cell carcinomas. It defines the extent of the cancer and ensures that the surgical margins are free of tumor .

IV. CRYOSURGERY

A. Definition. The destruction of tissue through freezing, most commonly with liquid nitrogen; it causes less scarring because of the ability to control the depth of tissue destruction. It is the simplest and least invasive method of lesion destruction, but one that yields no tissue for pathology.
B. Cryosurgery is the process of destruction by applying extreme cold to a localized site, causing ice formation at the cellular level, thermal shock to the cell, and vascular stasis, resulting in necrosis. Liquid nitrogen at −195.6°C is the standard agent used because of its availability and low cost, and because it is noncombustible (Figure 3-4).
  1. The liquid nitrogen invokes rapid cooling and slow thawing and may be applied using a direct spray or cotton-tipped applicator.
  2. Treatment causes intense stinging and burning that generally peaks 2 minutes later.
C. Indications
  1. Actinic keratoses
  2. Thin seborrheic keratosis
  3. Leukoplakia
  4. Molluscum contagiosum
  5. Common and genital warts
  6. Superficial basal cell carcinoma (BCC) and squamous cell carcinoma (SCC) in situ (rarely)
D. Nursing considerations
  1. Good cosmetic results with little anesthesia.
  2. Painful when used to treat lesions on nose, lips, ears, or eyelids; severe pain if palms, soles, or confined areas

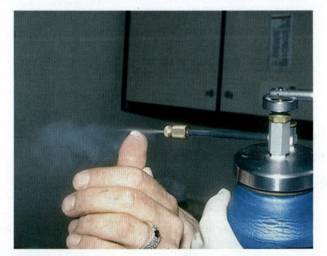

FIGURE 3-4. Liquid nitrogen as used for cryosurgery. (From Goodheart, H. P. 2010. *Goodheart's same-site differential diagnosis: A rapid method of diagnosing and treating common skin disorders*. Philadelphia: Wolters Kluwer.)

such as the area around the nails are treated; these may be better treated by another method.
3. Few side effects, but can damage vital vessels and tear ducts; hyperpigmentation in darker skin is possible.
4. Application with cotton-tipped applicator allows for more control of tissue depth.
5. Blisters form in 3 to 6 hours after application, flatten in 2 to 3 days, and peel off in approximately 2 to 3 weeks.
6. If the site is kept clean, infection is rare.

> ◉ **PATIENT EDUCATION**
> *Cryosurgery*
>
> • Understand the objective of procedures and treatment and if unclear, ask questions.
> • Acknowledge there will be some discomfort associated with the treatment.
> • Understand the sequence of skin changes associated with treatment; blistering, color changes, crusts, peeling.
> • Keep site clean and covered after wound occurs.
> • Acknowledge there will be a possible need for repeat treatments.

V. HEMOSTASIS DURING AND AFTER SURGERY

Methods frequently used to achieve hemostasis during or at the end of a surgical procedure are
A. Simple direct pressure, which is the easiest and least traumatizing to tissue.
B. Hemostatic agents such as aluminum chloride or ferric subsulfate, used after shave or curettage procedures.
C. Electrocautery or electrodesiccation using high-frequency radio current during surgical procedures. The lowest current required to achieve hemostasis is recommended.
D. Electrodesiccation and curettage is frequently used to treat selected small basal cell and squamous cell carcinomas. Selection of lesion and methodology is important to avoid reoccurrence of lesions. The practitioner needs to be sure to remove all soft cancerous tissue with curette prior to destroying the rest of the tumor with electrodesiccation and achieving hemostasis. The wound heals by secondary intention usually in 2 to 3 weeks.

VI. PATCH TESTING OVERVIEW

A. History and overview
  1. Patch testing is an essential diagnostic tool used to diagnose allergic contact dermatitis. These tests detect a type IV hypersensitivity response to contact allergens. Patients who present with dermatitis or eczema are potential candidates for patch testing.
  2. Jadassohn, a German dermatologist, is considered the father of patch testing. The first scientifically derived connection between a sensitizing substance and a

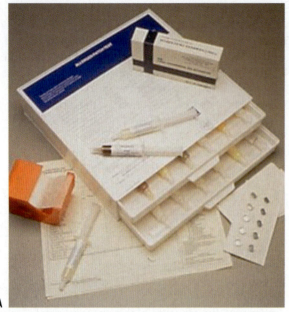
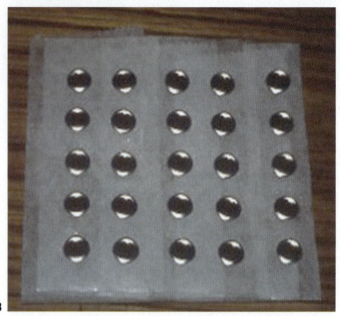

A   **B**

FIGURE 3-5. A: Finn chamber patch test supplies with Scanpor tape. **B:** Finn chambers empty to fill on Scanpor tape. (Courtesy of Noreen Heer Nicol and Anne Marie Ruskowski Lord.)

dermatologic hypersensitivity reaction was made by Jadassohn in 1895.

B. Available techniques
   1. Finn chamber/Scanpor tape is one method to test allergens. The chambers consist of shallow aluminum cups or chambers ranging from 8 to 12 mm in diameter that are affixed to a strip of Scanpor tape. Allergens, chambers, and tape are supplied separately (Figure 3-5).
   2. Al-test filament paper discs affixed to a strip of plastic-coated aluminum may also be used to test the allergens.
   3. T.R.U.E. TEST (Thin-layer Rapid Use Epicutaneous Test) is the first standardized, ready-to-use patch test system approved in the United States. This system delivers 35 common allergens and allergen mixes, which are incorporated into hydrophilic gels, printed on a water-impermeable sheet of polyester, and mounted on nonwoven cellulose tape and one negative control patch (Figure 3-6).

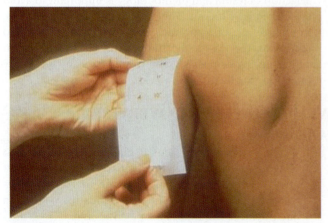

FIGURE 3-6. T.R.U.E TEST panel of 12 allergens peeled from backing. (Courtesy of Noreen Heer Nicol and Anne Marie Ruskowski Lord.)

C. Patient selection: Morphology of disease warranting patch testing
   1. Dermatitis or eczema
   2. Erythroderma
   3. Urticaria
   4. Photosensitivity
   5. Dermal inflammatory reaction
   6. Burning and itching skin with no visible pathology
D. Patient selection: Presentation that may suggest allergic contact dermatitis
   1. Highly suggestive history or distribution
   2. Suspected specific antigen or substance
   3. Other dermatitis or conditions that flare or do not respond to treatment
      a. Atopic eczema with unusual distribution
      b. Stasis dermatitis
      c. Hand dermatitis
      d. Irritant contact dermatitis
      e. Dyshidrotic eczema
      f. Seborrheic dermatitis
      g. Chronic tinea of the hands and/or feet
      h. Nummular eczema
      i. Occupationally related dermatitis

VII. PATCH TESTING APPLICATION TECHNIQUES

A. General considerations (Box 3-1)
   1. Patches should be applied to clean skin that is free of dermatitis.
   2. The preferable testing site is the upper back, avoiding midline.
   3. Patches should not be applied on hairy areas.
   4. Patients should *not* have recently taken oral steroids, had recent intramuscular injection of corticosteroid, used medium- to high-potency topical corticosteroids

to test areas, used topical calcineurin inhibitors to testing areas, or had intense sun exposure or phototherapy to testing areas. If the patient has been exposed to these in recent weeks, individual determination of appropriateness for testing must occur, as there may be a high potential for false-negative patch testing response.

5. Patch testing to unknown substances should never occur.
6. All patients should have two readings of patches.
   a. First reading must be 48 hours after initial application for the test to use the standardized parameters on which it is based.
   b. Second reading must be 24 to 96 hours after removal of patches, as the reactions are delayed and may take several days to develop.
7. Patch testing area should be kept dry during testing.
8. Patients should be instructed to remove patches if "unbearable" to wear for 48 hours. This may include severe burning, stinging, or pruritus at testing areas.

B. Finn chamber/Scanpor tape method/standard allergens
   1. Preparing patches for application
      a. Allergens are kept refrigerated before use.
      b. Anchor strips of Scanpor tape to a hard surface and then apply Finn chambers directly to tape.

c. For aqueous allergens, a filter paper disk is placed into the chamber and one drop of solution is placed on the disk immediately before application (Figure 3-7A).
   d. For allergens in an ointment vehicle, the clinician applies a 5-mm ribbon of each petroleum-base allergen directly into individual Finn chambers (Figure 3-7B).

2. Applying patches
   a. Allergen patches are placed on the patient's upper back.
   b. Patches are smoothed into place, smoothing from bottom to top (Figure 3-7C).
   c. Additional Scanpor tape may be necessary to keep patches secure.

C. T.R.U.E. TEST standard allergens (Table 3-1)
   1. Preparing patches for application
      a. Standardized, ready-to-use system consists of three panels of patches with 12 allergens per test strip. Panel one contains 11 allergens and 1 negative control.
      b. Allergens should be stored in refrigerator before application.
      c. Remove test strip from the foil outer sleeve and take off the protective plastic cover.
   2. Applying the patches
      a. Position test panel #1 on the upper part of the patient's back so that allergen #1 is in the upper left corner.
      b. Smooth the panel from the center outward toward the edges.
      c. Indicate the location on the skin by using a medical marking pen to make marks on the two notches found on the panel.
      d. Repeat the same procedure with panel #2 on the same side of the upper back so allergen #13 is in the upper left corner.
      e. Repeat the same procedure with panel #3 on the other side of the upper back so allergen #25 is in the upper left corner.
      f. Double-check that the location of all three panels on the skin is marked by using a medical marking pen to make marks on the two notches found on the panel (Figure 3-8).

D. Removing the patches: All patches must be removed 48 hours after application in standardized patch testing.
   1. Supplies needed
      a. Recording tool
      b. Surgical marking pen or permanent marker
      c. Adhesive remover
      d. Template
   2. Finn chamber method
      a. Remove test strips so that the top portion of each strip remains in place (when using template) or
      b. Remove test strips and individually mark each individual patch area (Figure 3-9).
      c. Wait 20 to 30 minutes before reading patches.
   3. T.R.U.E TEST method
      a. Check that notches on test strip are marked before removing testing panels.
      b. Position notches on template to correlate with the notch marks on the skin during application.
      c. Wait 20 to 30 minutes before reading patches.

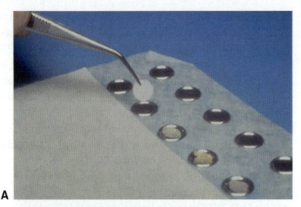

A

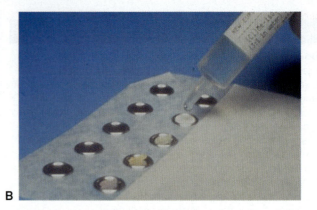

B

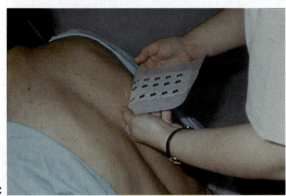

C

FIGURE 3-7. A: Finn chamber technique using filter paper disc for liquid allergen with petrolatum vehicle beside the liquid one. **B:** Finn chamber allergen preparation shows ointment and liquid with disc allergen. **C:** Finn chamber application to upper back—rolling up from bottom to top. (Courtesy of Noreen Heer Nicol and Anne Marie Ruskowski Lord.)

TABLE 3-1 Standard Allergen Tests Available in the United States

Panel	T.R.U.E TEST Allergen Panel Series
1.2	Nickel sulfate Wool alcohols Neomycin sulfate Potassium dichromate Caine mix Fragrance mix Colophony Paraben mix Negative control Balsam of Peru Ethylenediamine dihydrochloride Cobalt dichloride
2.2	p-tert-Butylphenol formaldehyde resin Epoxy resin Carba mix Black Rubber mix Cl+ Me–isothiazolinone (MCI/MI) Quaternium-15 Methyldibromo glutaronitrile p-Phenylenediamine Formaldehyde Mercapto mix Thimerosal Thiuram mix
3.2	Diazolidinyl urea Quinoline mix Tixocortol-21-pivalate Gold sodium thiosulfate Imidazolidinyl urea Budesonide Hydrocortisone-17-butyrate Mercaptobenzothiazole Bacitracin Parthenolide Disperse blue 106 2-Bromo-2-nitropropane-1,3-diol (Bronopol)

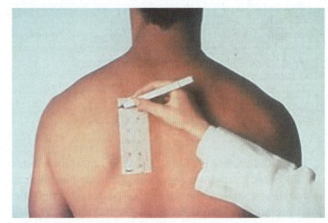

FIGURE 3-8. T.R.U.E TEST panel application and marking. (Courtesy of Noreen Heer Nicol and Anne Marie Ruskowski Lord.)

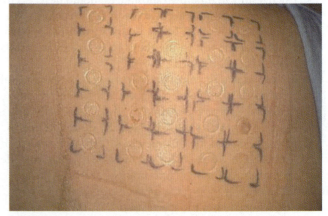

FIGURE 3-9. Finn chambers individually marked for interpretation. (Courtesy of Noreen Heer Nicol and Anne Marie Ruskowski Lord.)

TABLE 3-2 Characteristics of Positive Patch Test Reactions

Allergic Reaction	Irritant Reaction
Persists and/or worsens after patch removal or appears later	Fades rapidly after patch test removal
Spreading erythema	Glazed, scaled
Edema	Follicular
Vesicles	Pustular
	Bullous

TABLE 3-3 Morphology Codes for Patch Test Interpretation[a]

Code	Reaction
1 or +	Weak reaction: nonvesicular, but with erythema, infiltration, possibly papules
2 or ++	Strong reaction: edematous and vesicular, with erythema, edema, papules, and vesicles
3 or +++	Extreme reaction: spreading, bullous, ulcerative
4 or +/?	Doubtful reaction: macular erythema only
5	Irritant reaction
6 or −	Negative reaction
7	Excited skin
8	Not tested

Adapted From Ruszkowski, A. M., Nicol, N. H., & Moore, J. A. (1995, February). Patch testing basics: Patient selection, application techniques, and guidelines for interpretation. *Dermatology Nursing* (Suppl.)., 18.

E. Interpreting patch test results
  1. Timing
    a. All patches should be read initially at removal time (48 hours).
    b. A second reading is critical 72 to 96 hours after patch application.
  2. Irritant versus allergic reaction (Table 3-2)
  3. Morphology codes for patch test interpretation (Tables 3-3 and 3-4).
F. Patient Education (Box 3-1)
  1. Prepatch testing

    a. Explain procedure, timing of visits, and need for testing.
    b. Describe the testing materials.
    c. Explain the requirements of testing.
    d. Inform the patient about patch testing safety.

TABLE 3-4 Description of Patch Test Reactions

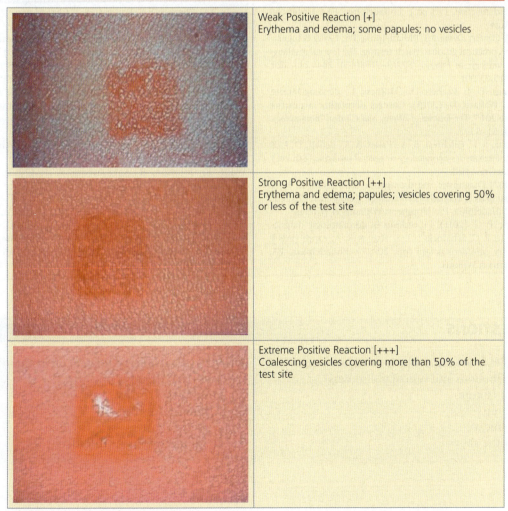

Weak Positive Reaction [+]
Erythema and edema; some papules; no vesicles

Strong Positive Reaction [++]
Erythema and edema; papules; vesicles covering 50% or less of the test site

Extreme Positive Reaction [+++]
Coalescing vesicles covering more than 50% of the test site

Images courtesy of Anne Marie Ruskowski Lord.

2. After patch testing
   a. Counsel for negative results.
   b. Counsel for positive results. The last and most important step is to determine if there is clinical relevance to a positive reaction. Clinical correlation with appropriate exposure history needs to be determined.
      1. Discuss avoidance of allergens and available alternatives.
      2. Distribute written information regarding allergens to be avoided.
      3. Be available for phone follow-up.
   c. Inform the patients that they may not have been tested to an allergen, which could have yielded a positive results due to allergen not being selected or available.

BIBLIOGRAPHY

Adelman, D. C., Casale, T. B., & Corren, J. (2012). *Manual of allergy and immunology* (5th ed.). Philadelphia, PA: Lippincott Williams & Wilkins.

Arndt, K. A. & Hsu, J. T. S. (2007). *Manual of dermatologic therapeutics* (7th ed.. Philadelphia, PA: Lippincott Williams & Wilkins.

Adkinson, N. F., Bocher, B. S., Burks, A., Busse, W. W., Holgate, S. T., Lemanske, R. F., & O'Hehir, R. E. (2014). *Middleton's allergy: Principles and practice* (8th ed.). Philadelphia, PA: Saunders-Elsevier.

Callen, J. P., Jorizzo, J. L., Zone, J. J., & Piette, W. W. (2009). *Dermatological signs of internal disease* (4th ed.). Philadelphia, PA: Saunders-Elsevier.

Craven, R., Hirnle, C., & Jensen, S. (2013). *Fundamentals of nursing: Human health and function.* (7th ed.). Philadelphia, PA.: Lippincott Williams & Wilkins.

Fisher, A. A. (1986). *Contact dermatitis.* Philadelphia, PA: Lea & Febiger.

Fonacier, L. (2015). A practical guide to patch testing. *The Journal of Allergy and Clinical Immunology: In Practice, S2213–2198*(15), 244–245. doi: 10.1016/j.jaip.2015.05.001.

Fonacier, L., Bernstein, D. I., Pacheco, K., Holness, L., Blessing-Moore, J., Khan, D., …, Wallace, D. (2015). Contact dermatitis: a practice parameter-update 2015. *The Journal of Allergy and Clinical Immunology: In Practice, 3*(3S), S1–S39.

Goldsmith, L. A., Katz, S. I., Gilchrest, B. A., Paller, A. S., Leffell, D. J., & Wolff, K. (2012). *Fitzpatrick's dermatology in general medicine* (8th ed.). New York, NY: McGraw-Hill.

Hunter-Yates, J. (2007) Diagnostic and therapeutic techniques. In K. A. Arndt & J.T.S. Hsu (Eds.), *Manual of dermatologic therapeutics,* (7th ed., pp. 255–264). Philadelphia, PA: Lippincott Williams & Wilkins.

Jarell, A. & Schalock, P. C. (2011). Procedures in dermatologic diagnosis and therapy. In P. C. Schalock, J. T. S. Hsu, & K. A. Arndt (Eds.), *Lippincott's primary care dermatology* (pp. 20–27). Philadelphia, PA: Lippincott Williams & Wilkins.

Marks, J. G., Elsner, P., & DeLeo, V. A. (2002). *Contact & occupational dermatology.* St. Louis, MO: Mosby-Year Book, Inc..

Marks, J. G. & Miller, J. J. (2006) *Lookingbill and Marks' principles of dermatology* (4th ed.). Philadelphia, PA: Saunders-Elsevier.

McCann, S. E. & Huether, S. E. (2014). Structure, function, and disorders of the integument. In S. E. Huether, K. L. McCance, V. L. Brasher, & N. S. Rote (Eds.), *Pathophysiology-the biologic basis for disease in adults and children* (7th ed., pp. 1616–1652). St. Louis, MO: Mosby-Elsevier.

Nicol, N. H. (2009). Assessment of the integumentary system. In J. M. Black & J. H. Hawks (Eds.), *Medical-surgical nursing: Clinical management for positive outcomes* (8th ed., pp. 1186–1198). Philadelphia, PA: WB Saunders Company.

Nicol, N. H., & Huether, S. E. (2014). Alterations of the integument in children. In S. E. Huether, K. L. McCance, V. L. Brasher, & N. S. Rote (Eds.), *Pathophysiology—The biologic basics for disease in adults and children* (7th ed., pp. 1653–1667). St. Louis, MO: Mosby-Elsevier.

Nicol, N. H., & Huether, S. E. (2012a). Structure, function, and disorders of the integument. In S. E. Huether, K.L. McCance, V.L. Brasher, & N.S. Rote (Eds.), *Understanding pathophysiology* (6th ed., pp. 1038–1069). St. Louis, MO: Mosby-Elsevier.

Nicol, N. H., & Huether, S. E. (2012b). Alterations of the integument in children. In S. E. Huether, K. L. McCance, V. L. Brasher, & N. S. Rote (Eds.), *Understanding pathophysiology* (6th ed., pp. 1070–1082). St. Louis, MO: Mosby-Elsevier.

Nicol, N. H., Ruszkowski, A. M., & Moore, J. A. (1995, February). Update on patch testing: Around table discussion. *Dermatology Nursing* (Suppl.), 1–30.

Penzer, R., & pages 1-30 Ersser, S. J. (2010). *Principles of skin care.* Oxford, UK: Wiley-Blackwell.

Perry, A. G., & Potter, P. A. (2002). Documenting nurses' progress notes. In A.G. Perry & P.A. Potter (Eds.), *Clinical nursing skills & techniques* (5th ed., p. 53). St. Louis, MO: Mosby, Inc.

Warshaw, E. M., Belsito, D. V., Taylor, J. S., Sasseville, D., DeKoven, J. G., Zirwas M. J., …, Maibach H. I. (2013). North American Contact Dermatitis Group patch test results: 2009 to 2010. *Dermatitis, 24*(2):50–59. doi: 10.1097/DER.0b013e3182819c51.

Warshaw, E. M., Maibach, H. I., Taylor, J. S., Sasseville, D., DeKoven, J. G., Zirwas, M. J., …, Belsito, D. V. (2015). North American contact dermatitis group patch test results: 2011–2012. *Dermatitis, 26*(1):49–59. doi: 10.1097/DER.0000000000000097.

Weinberg, S., Prose, N. S., & Kristal, L. (2008). *Color atlas of pediatric dermatology,* (4th ed.). New York, NY: McGraw-Hill.

Wolff, K., Johnson, R. A., Saavedra, A. P. (2013). *Fitzpatrick's color atlas and synopsis of clinical dermatology* (7th ed.). New York, NY: McGraw-Hill.

Zug, K. A., Pham, A. K., Belsito, D. V., DeKoven, J. G., DeLeo, V. A., Fowler, J. F. Jr, …, Zirwas, M. J. (2014). Patch testing in children from 2005 to 2012: results from the North American contact dermatitis group. *Dermatitis, 25*(6):345–55. doi:10.1097/DER.0000000000000083.

STUDY QUESTIONS

1. What of the following tools is used to aid in the diagnosis of bullous and vesicular disorders?
   a. Bacterial culture
   b. Wood lamp
   c. Tzanck smear
   d. None of the above

2. KOH (potassium hydroxide) preparation test is used to aid in the diagnosis of:
   a. Scabies
   b. Fungal disorders
   c. Herpes zoster
   d. Connective tissue disorders

3. Which of the following biopsy techniques may require the use of suturing?
   a. Shave
   b. Punch
   c. Elliptical/wedge
   d. B and C
   e. All of the above

4. Cryosurgery is frequently used to treat:
   a. Keratoses
   b. Warts
   c. Melanoma
   d. A and B.
   e. All of the above

5. Patch testing should be recommended for patients presenting with:
   a. Atopic dermatitis
   b. Dyshidrotic eczema
   c. Vitiligo
   d. A and B
   e. All of the above

6. Mr. Lyons is scheduled for patch testing. The nurse explains to him that the patches will be placed on his upper back for:
   a. 24 hours
   b. 48 hours
   c. 72 hours
   d. 96 hours

7. Mr. Lyons is instructed that during patch testing, he should:
   a. Keep patch area dry
   b. Avoid strenuous activity
   c. Wear loose clothing while patches being worn
   d. All of the above

8. Which one of the following statements is *false*?
   a. Patches should be applied to clean skin that is free of dermatitis.
   b. Patches should not be applied to the midline of the back.
   c. Patients may apply strong topical corticosteroid cream to the testing area during patch testing.
   d. Patches should not be applied on hairy areas.

9. The presentation of an extreme reaction (+3) can be characterized by:
   a. Macular erythema, only
   b. Nonvesicular reaction with erythema
   c. Spreading and bullous
   d. Edema and papules

10. Patients can be patch tested to unknown substances.
    a. True
    b. False

Answers to Study Questions: 1.c, 2.b, 3.d, 4.d, 5.d, 6.b, 7.d, 8.c, 9.c, 10.b

Therapeutic/Treatment Modalities

Beth Haney

I. OVERVIEW

The skin is the largest organ of the body; it averages 20 square feet and weighs about 9 pounds. The skin regulates body temperature, protects underlying skin cells from environmental toxins and harmful ultraviolet radiation, and acts as a barrier to prevent water loss, invasion of foreign substances, as well as immune defense. The outermost layer of the epidermis, the stratum corneum, provides these functions through a barrier that consists of fatty acids, cholesterol, and ceramides that reside between cornified cells. When the skin is intact, it also regulates percutaneous absorption. Any insult that removes lipids, water, or protein from the epidermis can severely compromise this protective function. The goal of topical and systemic preparations is to maintain and restore the functions of the skin barrier. For example, alkaline soaps affect the stratum corneum by changing the normal acidity of the skin (normal skin pH is 5.4 to 5.9). Alteration of the acid mantle can decrease bacterial resistance. Absorption rates of medications vary depending on the anatomic site, that is, eyelids, mucous membranes, palms, or soles of the feet.

II. TOPICAL AGENTS

A. Vehicles

Choice of the appropriate vehicle is paramount to successful treatment and determines the rate of the absorption of the active ingredient into the skin. Fat-soluble vehicles, especially natural emollients, are more rapidly absorbed than water-soluble vehicles.

1. Ointment: Consists primarily of greases such as petroleum jelly with little or no water and desirable for dryer lesions/conditions
   a. Increases lubrication
   b. Translucent
   c. Greater penetration of medicine than creams, which increases percutaneous absorption, thus enhancing potency of medications
   d. Usually are preservative-free
   e. Should not be used in extremely eczematous inflammation or in intertriginous areas, such as the groin due to occlusive properties
   f. May cause folliculitis when used in hairy areas
2. Creams: Mixture of organic chemicals (oil) and water emulsion and usually contains preservatives
   a. Used for lubrication and easily applied
   b. Highly versatile due to ability to use on almost any area of the body and therefore are the most prescribed
   c. Do not increase percutaneous absorption
   d. Are more cosmetically acceptable
   e. Some may cause dryness with extended use, therefore best for acute exudative inflammation
   f. White color and can be greasy in texture
   g. Can cause side effects such as burning, stinging, and/or allergy depending on components

3. Solutions and lotions: Powder suspended in liquid (may contain water and alcohol as well as other chemicals) and delivers medication as uniform film
   a. Suitable for hairy areas, frequently used for scalp due to ease of penetration, and leaves no residue
   b. Have greater content of alcohol and water
   c. May over dry the skin and wear off easily
   d. Absorb moisture, promoting drying
   e. May cause stinging and drying in intertriginous areas, such as the groin
4. Gel: Greaseless mixture of propylene glycol and water, and some contain alcohol
   a. Easily applied
   b. Drying and cooling and good for acute exudative inflammation and pruritic eruptions like poison ivy
   c. Aggravates dry, cracked lesions if it contains alcohol
   d. May cause burning on eroded skin
5. Powder: Finely ground solid particles
   a. Absorptive and promotes drying
   b. Decreases skin friction
   c. Good vehicle to deliver medication to intertriginous areas
6. Aerosols: Medications suspended in a base and delivered under pressure
   a. Similar to a lotion but more drying
   b. Useful for applying medication to hairy areas
   c. Useful on wet lesions
7. Paste: Powder in ointment and 50% or greater powder content
   a. Provides protection
   b. Decreases rate of percutaneous absorption
   c. Messy
8. Foam
   a. Useful for scalp dermatoses and spread between strands of hair until reaches the scalp where the medication is then delivered
   b. Good for acute exudative inflammation
   c. May cause stinging shortly after application
B. Application of topical agents (Tables 4-1 and 4-2): The objective of topical treatment is to lubricate or medicate, or both. Proper application technique should always be used. Hydrating the skin before application will increase percutaneous absorption. Frequency of application and amount will be dictated by severity of dermatosis and the medication chosen.
   1. Remove any "caked" topical before applying additional topical
      a. Remove creams with water.
      b. Mineral or cottonseed oil may be used to remove ointments or pastes.
      c. Always use gentle motions when removing topical medications.
   2. Applying creams and ointments
      a. The amount of cream or ointment used depends on the area to be treated.
      b. Amount can be calculated as 1 g of cream covers 100 cm^2 of skin. One fingertip unit (FTU) is the amount

TABLE 4-1 Quantity of Topical Cream to Apply and Dispense for Single or Multiple Application(s)

Area Treated	One Application (g)	BID for 10 day (g)^b	BID for 2 Weeks (g)^b	BID for 1 Month (g)^b
Face and neck	2.5 FTU^a (1.25 g)	30 g (1.07 oz.)	40 g (1.25 oz.)	75 g (2.7 oz.)
Trunk (front or back)	7 FTU (3.5 g)	75 g (2.7 oz.)	120 g (4.3 oz.)	210 g (7.5 oz.)
One arm	3 FTU (1.5 g)	30 g (1.07 oz.)	60 g (2.1 oz.)	90 g (3.2 oz.)
One hand (both sides)	1 FTU (0.5 g)	15 g (0.5 oz.)	15 g (0.5 oz.)	30 g (1.07 oz.)
One leg	6 FTU (3 g)	60 g (2.1 oz.)	90 g (3.2 oz.)	180 g (6.4 oz.)
One foot	2 FTU (1 g)	20 g (0.7 oz.)	30 g (1.07 oz.)	60 g (2.1 oz.)

^{a}FTU, fingertip unit. The amount of cream/ointment expressed from tube applied to the fingertip. FTU weighs about 0.5 g.
^{b}Weight is based on application frequency and *available tube sizing*. In some cases, the tube will have more than the prescribed amount.
Adapted from Habif, et al. (2011). *Skin disease and treatment* (3rd ed.). St. Louis, MO: Mosby.

of ointment expressed from a 5-mm nozzle applied from the distal crease of the index finger to the tip and weighs approximately 0.5 g.
   c. Apply in long downward (direction of hair growth) strokes using the palm of the hand.
   d. Only a thin film of medication is necessary.
3. Applying pastes
   a. Use tongue depressor if available.
   b. May warm container of medication in warm water to soften, thus facilitating application.
4. Applying lotions/solutions
   a. Shake well.
   b. Pour small amount in the palm of the hand.
   c. Pat onto the skin.

TABLE 4-2 Guidelines for Patient Education Regarding Application of Topical Medications

Successful topical therapy greatly depends on the patient's understanding of how to apply the topical agent as well as what product they have been prescribed. Knowledge of the drug and product and educating patients using the following guidelines will aid in achieving successful outcomes.
Review with the patient any preapplication instructions, including:
Where to apply
How much to apply How often to apply
The sequence of application for multiple products
Assess the patient's ability to comply and request at-home assistance if necessary.
Review the importance of proper application and desired outcome.
The expected results
Who and when to call with questions

Adapted from Nicol, N. H. (2005). Use of moisturizers in dermatologic disease: The role of healthcare providers in optimizing treatment outcomes. *Cutis, 76,* 32–33.

   d. A brush or gauze may be used for application; avoid use of cotton; it filters out medication and may stick to the skin.

5. Applying sprays and aerosols
   a. Shake well.
   b. Direct spray to affected area (distance as determined by package insert).
   c. Use short bursts when applying.
6. Applying powders
   a. Dry affected area thoroughly.
   b. "Dust" affected area leaving only a thin layer of powder.
   c. Gauze or powder puff facilitates application.
   d. Use caution around patients with tracheostomies or respiratory problems.
7. Applying gels
   a. Cleanse affected areas.
   b. If acne medication, wait a minimum of 30 minutes after cleansing before application to reduce incidence of irritation.

C. Occlusion: This produces a barrier usually by the use of plastic film (Figure 4-1). It enhances absorption by preventing medication evaporation and increasing hydration of stratum corneum by moisture retention. Topical medications penetrate 10 to 100 times more effectively when the stratum corneum is moist.

1. Cleanse skin of debris and other medications with soap and water.
2. Apply prescribed topical thinly while skin is damp.
3. Snugly fit plastic wrap, compress air out, and seal borders with paper tape; airtight dressing is unnecessary.
4. Leave dressing intact for prescribed time, best results are obtained if the dressing is left on for at least 2 hours, and many patients leave dressing on for 8 hours while sleeping. A reasonable schedule is twice daily occlusion for 2 hours or once daily overnight for 8 hours with simple application once or twice daily.

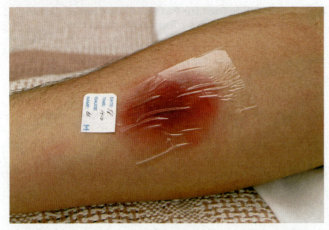

FIGURE 4-1. Occlusive dressing. (From Carter, P. J. (2011). *Lippincott textbook for nursing assistants*. Philadelphia, PA: Wolters Kluwer.)

5. Remove gently and cleanse skin.
6. Problems associated with occlusion.
   a. Sweat retention
   b. Maceration
   c. Folliculitis
   d. Atrophy
   e. Striae
   f. May increase risk for bacterial/fungal overgrowth
7. Long-term occlusion with even a low-potency topical steroid may result in temporary suppression of the hypothalamic–pituitary–adrenal (HPA) axis; this function returns after occlusion is discontinued.

III. TOPICAL MEDICATIONS

Numerous topical medications are available for treating skin disorders—corticosteroids, antifungals, antibacterials, antivirals, scabicides and pediculicides, keratolytics and caustics, and antineoplastics.

A. Topical steroids
1. Used extensively in treating skin disorders
2. Reduce inflammation through their ability to induce vasoconstriction
3. Relieve pruritus
4. Induce remission of many cutaneous disorders
5. Potency ranking—groups from 1 to 7 with 1 being the most potent; most dermatoses may be managed with low to moderately potent topical steroids (Table 4-3).

TABLE 4-3 Potency Ranking of Some Commonly Used Topical Steroids

Group	Generic Name	Brand Name
I	Clobetasol propionate	Cormax 0.05%, Olux 0.05%
	Halobetasol propionate	Ultravate 0.05%
	Betamethasone dipropionate (optimized vehicle)	Diprolene 0.05%
	Diflorasone diacetate	Psorcon 0.05%
II	Amcinonide	Cyclocort 0.1%
	Betamethasone dipropionate	Diprosone 0.05%, Elocon 0.1%
	Halcinonide	Halog 0.1%
	Fluocinonide	Lidex 0.05%
	Desoximetasone	Topicort 0.025%
III	Fluticasone propionate	Cutivate 0.005%
	Betamethasone valerate	Betatrex 0.1%
IV	Triamcinolone acetonide	Kenalog 0.1%
	Fluocinolone acetonide	Synalar 0.025%
V	Hydrocortisone butyrate	Locoid 0.1%
	Hydrocortisone valerate	Westcort 0.2%
VI	Alclometasone dipropionate	Aclovate 0.05%
	Desonide	DesOwen 0.05%
VII	Hydrocortisone	Hytone 2.5% Hytone 1.0% Many other brands

Adapted from Habif, T. P. (2016). *Clinical dermatology: A color guide to diagnosis and therapy (back inside cover)*. Philadelphia, PA: Elsevier.

6. Possible side effects
   a. Atrophy—older skin, inguinal, genital, and peri-anal areas most predisposed to atrophy and may be irreversible depending on the potency of steroid used
   b. Striae—irreversible
   c. Telangiectasia—often persists after discontinuation of steroid
   d. Acneiform eruptions—develop after months of use and reversible
   e. Interfere with epithelialization and collagen synthesis in wound healing
   f. Burning, itching, irritation, and/or dryness—usually due to the vehicle
   g. Hypo-/hyperpigmentation—reversible on discontinuation of steroid
   h. Bruising—reversible
   i. HPA axis suppression—results from application of potent (fluorinated) steroids in excess of 50 to 100 g/week in adults and 10 to 20 g in children, for 2 or more weeks, and reversible
   j. Steroid rosacea and perioral dermatitis—results from progression from weaker steroids to more potent concentrations. Strong steroids must be discontinued. Erythema and pustules eventually subside, but atrophy and telangiectasias may be permanent.
   k. Ocular hypertension, glaucoma, and cataracts when topical steroids are used around the eyes
   l. Folliculitis and milia caused from occlusive plastic dressings
   m. Hypertrichosis of the face
7. Nursing considerations
   a. Assess efficacy of medication regularly.
   b. Assess the patient for development of side effects; length of therapy increases the risk of developing side effects.
   c. Assess for tachyphylaxis, which is the tolerance to the vasoconstriction properties of topical steroids.
   d. Assess for signs of superimposed infections.
   e. Assess response related to vehicle—ointment-based preparations are generally more potent than chemically equivalent cream-based agents.
   f. Avoid use of topical steroids on the face, perineal area, or axillae unless otherwise indicated; if required, monitor closely.
   g. Hydration increases percutaneous absorption; application after soaking the skin in lukewarm water will increase absorption; in steroid-responsive generalized dermatoses, application following a bath or shower is most efficacious.
   h. Compromised skin has increased percutaneous absorption.
   i. Frequency of application depends on steroid potency and severity of dermatoses.

PATIENT EDUCATION
Topical Medications

- Understand preapplication instructions.
- Use specified and appropriate technique for application; when multiple products are to be applied, understand the order of application.
- Use the medication at specified times only.
- The medication is only to be applied to areas for which it is prescribed.
- Do not overuse or misuse medications as that can result in serious cutaneous and systemic complications.
- Monitor results of therapy.
- Do not borrow or lend medications to friends or family members.
- Use medications as directed.
- Follow up with your health care provider if any problems occur.

B. Topical calcineurin inhibitors (TCI): Tacrolimus 0.03% to 0.1% (Protopic) and pimecrolimus (Elidel)
   1. Used for treating intermittent flares of atopic dermatitis (AD) and chronic treatment of AD as alternative to topical steroids
   2. These drugs can be used as first line therapy or following treatment with topical steroids.
   3. Neither causes certain side effects, such as thinning of the skin (atrophy), or stretch marks (striae), spider veins or discoloration of the skins making them desirable when AD is on face.
   4. Side effects
      a. Burning and stinging with initial use
      b. Possible increased risk of secondary infection from bacterial, viral, and fungal infections
   5. Despite a number of epidemiological and clinical studies, no clear link between TCI use and lymphoma risk has been established.
C. Topical antifungals (antimycotic agents)
   1. Used to treat fungal or dermatophyte infections (superficial infections of the skin, hair, and nails) and also called tineas
      a. Tinea pedis (Figure 4-2)
      b. Tinea cruris (Figure 4-3)
      c. Tinea corporis (Figure 4-4)
      d. Tinea versicolor (Figure 4-5)
      e. Tinea rubrum (Figure 4-6)
      f. Tinea manuum (Figure 4-7)
   2. Antifungal–corticosteroid combinations
      a. Used to alleviate the symptoms of inflammation and pruritus secondary to certain types of fungal infection but may lead to worsening symptoms if specific type is not correctly diagnosed

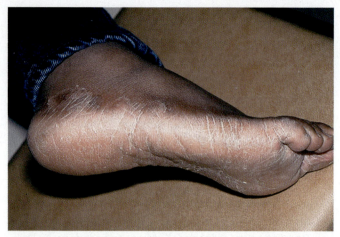

FIGURE 4-2. Tinea pedis. (From Goodheart, H. P. (2003). *Goodheart's photoguide of common skin disorders* (2nd ed.). Philadelphia, PA: Lippincott Williams & Wilkins.)

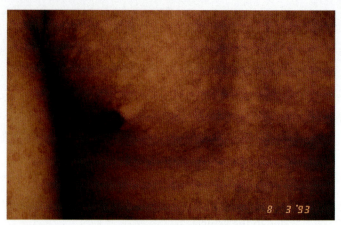

FIGURE 4-5. Tinea versicolor; note the hypopigmented areas. (From Fleisher, G. R., Ludwig, S., & Baskin, M. N. (2004). *Atlas of pediatric emergency medicine*. Philadelphia, PA: Lippincott Williams & Wilkins.)

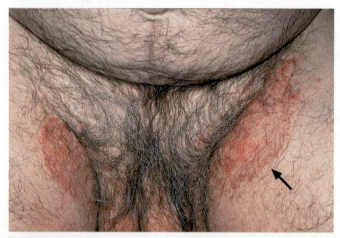

FIGURE 4-3. Tinea cruris. (From Goodheart, H. P. (2003). *Goodheart's photoguide of common skin disorders* (2nd ed.). Philadelphia, PA: Lippincott Williams & Wilkins.)

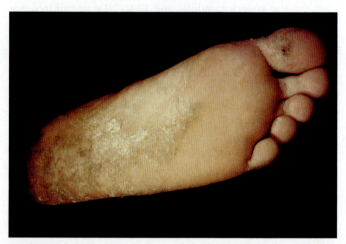

FIGURE 4-6. Tinea rubrum; chronic tinea of the sole caused by *Trichophyton rubrum*. (From Centers for Disease Control and Prevention Public Health Image Library.)

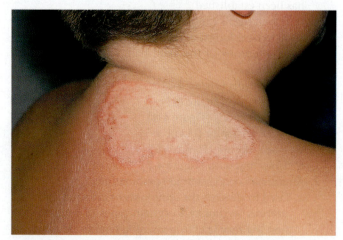

FIGURE 4-4. Tinea corporis. (From Werner, R. (2012). *Massage therapist's guide to pathology*. Philadelphia, PA: Wolters Kluwer.)

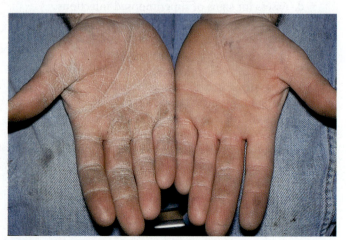

FIGURE 4-7. Tinea manuum. (From Goodheart, H. P. (2003). *Goodheart's photoguide of common skin disorders* (2nd ed.). Philadelphia, PA: Lippincott Williams & Wilkins.)

b. Produce more rapid response/alleviation of symptoms
c. May mask superimposed bacterial infections
d. Use in chronic dermatophyte-induced infections may make evaluation of response or titration of therapy difficult secondary to the topical steroid.
e. Combination medications are more expensive.
3. Antifungal chosen based on the following:
a. Species of dermatophyte
b. Body site involved
c. Severity of infection
d. Duration of infection (days, weeks, years, recurrent)
e. Patient's age and/or pregnancy status
f. Concurrent medical conditions/drug therapy
4. Possible side effects
a. Skin irritation
b. Overgrowth of fungus when occlusion is used
c. Blistering
d. Stinging
e. Peeling
f. Pruritus
5. Nursing considerations
a. Assess the patient's history for pre-existing condition that might preclude use of topical antifungal.
b. Assess for any evidence of skin irritation secondary to medication.
c. Assess patient/family/significant other's knowledge of medication and appropriate application.
d. Moist areas of the body (intertriginous and perineal areas) are particularly prone to fungal infections.
e. Ointment-based antifungal products are not desirable due to their occlusive properties.

PATIENT EDUCATION
Topical Antifungals

- Review any preapplication instructions; some products may stain fabric, skin, or hair.
- Use appropriate technique for application.
- Review frequency of applications.
- Medication is only to be used on areas for which it is prescribed; self-medication can have disastrous results.
- Need to use full course of medication unless side effects occur.
- Review expected results from therapy.
- Do not lend medication to friends/relatives.
- Keep affected areas dry; use nonocclusive, well-ventilated footwear; wash affected areas thoroughly; and change shoes and socks at least once a day.

D. Topical antipruritics
1. Usually contain camphor, menthol, phenol, or a topical anesthetic; have anesthetic and counterirritant properties that induce cooling; and indicated for the temporary relief of pruritus.

2. Examples
a. PrameGel
b. Sarna lotion and cream
c. Calamine lotion
d. Aveeno anti-itch lotion/cream
e. Pramosone
f. Benadryl cream
3. Nursing considerations
a. May be applied liberally 3 to 4 times/day
b. Underlining etiology of pruritus must be pursued and corrected.
c. Monitor for skin irritation especially with topical antipruritics.

PATIENT EDUCATION
Topical Antipruritics

- Antipruritic agents provide relief from itching.
- May be applied liberally 3 to 4 times a day.
- If no improvement, call health care provider.
- Avoid sun exposure to prevent photosensitivity reactions.
- Do not ingest.

E. Topical antibacterials
1. May be used in combination with other topical modalities
2. Suitable in treating inflammatory acne vulgaris
3. Suitable for use in open wounds and may facilitate granulation
4. Preparations chosen based on organism cultured and skin problem
5. Examples
a. Bacitracin—used for gram-positive infections and prophylaxis in minor cuts, burns, and abrasions
b. Garamycin—used for aerobic gram-negative and some gram-positive infections
c. Meclocycline sulfosalicylate—used for acne vulgaris
d. Mupirocin—greatest activity against gram-positive organisms such as *S. aureus* and streptococci. Effective treatment for impetigo and nasal colonization of methicillin-resistant *staph aureus* carrier state
e. Neomycin sulfate—used for aerobic gram-negative and some aerobic gram-positive infections, although can cause contact dermatitis for sensitive individuals
f. Nitrofurazone—used as adjunct therapy in second- and third-degree burns and in skin grafts/donor sites to prevent rejection due to bacterial contamination
g. Silver sulfadiazine—used for gram-negative and gram-positive infections
h. Erythromycin—indicated for acne vulgaris, rosacea, and folliculitis
i. Chloramphenicol—used for prophylaxis and treating superficial bacterial infections

j. Tetracycline hydrochloride—used for prophylaxis and treatment of superficial infections

k. Clindamycin—skin and soft tissue infections, impetigo, abscesses, and cellulitis

6. Nursing considerations

a. Use contraindicated in patients with a history of prior sensitization

b. Unless otherwise indicated, cleanse affected area with antibacterial soap and water before application.

c. Observe for any signs of allergic reaction—burning, swelling, redness, or worsening of condition.

d. With prolonged use, monitor for superinfections and overgrowth of nonsusceptible organisms, especially fungus.

e. Alcohol-based antibacterial solutions may cause burning upon application.

f. Nasal application of mupirocin may cause headache, cough, itching, and alterations in taste.

PATIENT EDUCATION
Topical Antibacterials

- Understand treatment objectives and if unclear, ask questions.
- Use correct application techniques, including preapplication process.
- Need to use full course of medication.
- Use medication only on affected areas.
- Call health care provider if side effects develop.
- Consult with health care provider if no improvement in 3 to 5 days.

F. Topical antivirals

1. Acyclovir and penciclovir (Denavir)—used to prevent or treat herpetic viral infections and reduce viral shedding; mode of action is interference with viral replication but is less effective than systemic therapy (Figures 4-8 and 4-9).

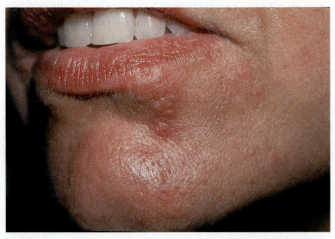

FIGURE 4-8. Herpes labialis. (From Goodheart, H. P. (2003). *Goodheart's photoguide of common skin disorders* (2nd ed.). Philadelphia, PA: Lippincott Williams & Wilkins.)

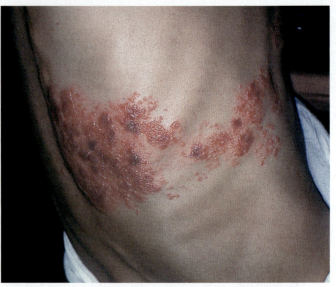

FIGURE 4-9. Herpes zoster; drying hemorrhagic crusts appear in a "zosteriform" distribution. (From Goodheart, H. P. (2003). *Goodheart's photoguide of common skin disorders* (2nd ed.). Philadelphia, PA: Lippincott Williams & Wilkins.)

2. n-docosanol (Abreva) cream—OTC and may shorten episode by hours or 1 day

3. Contraindicated with hypersensitivity to any components

4. Use cautiously during lactation, renal impairment.

5. Possible side effects: burning/stinging, pruritus, or rash

6. Nursing considerations

a. Ointment must thoroughly cover all lesions.

b. Initiate treatment as soon as possible after onset of symptoms, within 24 hours if possible.

c. Monitor for side effects and process.

PATIENT EDUCATION
Topical Antivirals

- Understand treatment objectives and if unclear, ask questions.
- Use appropriate application of topical medications.
- Important to complete therapy
- Understand possible side effects and what to do should they occur.
- The use of other creams or ointments may delay healing and may cause spreading of lesions.
- Contact health care provider if symptoms not relieved by 7 days.

G. Scabicides and pediculicides
(See Chapter 16 for further detail on infestations and the treatments indicated.)

H. Keratolytics/caustics

1. Keratolytics dissolve and separate the stratum corneum in diseases where hyperkeratosis is a manifestation; caustics have an antimitotic action.

2. Examples
   a. Coal tar (cream, shampoo, ointment, gel, lotion, soap, bath solution)
   b. Salicylic acid (cream, gel, ointment, patch, shampoo, solution)
   c. Anthralin
   d. Cantharidin
   e. Podophyllum resin
   f. Resorcinol
   g. Silver nitrate
   h. Sulfur
   i. Trichloroacetic or bichloroacetic acid
3. Possible side effects
   a. Irritation
   b. Burning
   c. Pain
   d. Inflammation
   e. Increased dryness
   f. Erosions
   g. Blistering
   h. Hyperpigmentation
   i. Hearing loss, tinnitus, dizziness, confusion, headache, and hyperventilation with salicylic acid if salicylism develops
   j. Bleeding, dizziness, hematuria, and vomiting may be seen as side effects of podophyllum resin.
4. Nursing considerations
   a. Use with caution in pregnant or lactating women.
   b. Do not apply to face, groin, axillae, mucous membranes, and broken or inflamed skin.
   c. Do not apply caustics to intertriginous areas.
   d. Do not use occlusion with caustics.
   e. Salicylic acid is contraindicated for use in children under 2 years of age, diabetics, or individuals with impaired circulation.
   f. Do not apply salicylic acid to moles, birthmarks, unusual warts with hair, genital warts, or warts on mucous membranes.
   g. Prolonged use of salicylic acid can lead to salicylate toxicity.
   h. When applying caustics, protect uninvolved skin by applying petrolatum.
   i. Apply caustics only to affected areas.

PATIENT EDUCATION
Keratolytics

- Understand treatment objectives and if unclear, ask questions.
- Use correct application of topical medications.
- Be aware of possible side effects of treatment.
- Important to complete therapy.
- Apply topicals only to affected areas and avoid surrounding skin.
- Topical is not to be applied to broken skin, wounds, or cuts.
- Do not use occlusion unless directed to do so.

I. Antineoplastics
1. Used for treating reactive and proliferative cutaneous malignancies
2. Exert action through different mechanisms.
   a. Cycle specific are more effective against proliferating cells.
   b. Phase specific are more effective against a specific phase of the cell cycle.
   c. Interfere with the synthesis of deoxyribonucleic acid (DNA) through different mechanisms
3. Categories of antineoplastics.
   a. Alkylating agents—nitrogen mustard (mechlorethamine) and BiCNU (carmustine)
   b. Disrupt the structure of DNA through nonspecific cell cycle manner
   c. Interfere with normal cell division in rapidly proliferating tissue
4. Used in treating T-cell lymphoma (mycosis fungoides)
   a. Antimetabolites—5-fluorouracil
   b. Interfere with the synthesis of nucleic acids and proteins
   c. Phase specific and inhibits RNA and DNA synthesis
5. Used in treating superficial basal cell carcinomas, multiple actinic leukoplakia, or solar keratosis
   a. Retinoid X receptors bexarotene gel (Targretin) 1% for the topical treatment of resistant T-cell lymphoma
   b. Bexarotene gel inhibits the growth of some tumor cell lines of hematopoietic and squamous cell origin.
   c. The exact mechanism of action in the treatment of T-cell lymphoma is unknown.
   d. Affects cellular differentiation and proliferation and also downregulates CCR4 and E-selectin expression, affecting malignant T-cell trafficking to the skin
6. Possible side effects
   a. Pain
   b. Pruritus
   c. Hyperpigmentation
   d. Irritation
   e. Inflammation
   f. Burning
   g. Scarring
   h. Swelling
   i. Alopecia
   j. Photosensitivity
   k. Scaling
   l. Contact dermatitis
7. Nursing considerations
   a. Apply with care near eyes, nose, and mouth.
   b. Always wear gloves when applying.
   c. Can cause photosensitivity.
   d. Avoid occlusion.
   e. Erythema, scaling, blistering, burning, and pruritus are expected results of topical treatment with 5-fluorouracil.
   f. Nitrogen mustard is applied total body with exception of the groin.
   g. Nitrogen mustard may be applied in liquid form or compounded in a petrolatum base.
   h. Inspect skin before and during treatment.

J. Vitamin A/retinoids
   1. Used in treating noninflammatory acne, photoaging, hyperpigmentation, flat warts, molluscum contagiosum, senile comedones, and actinic keratosis and to enhance percutaneous absorption of other topical agents; metabolized in the skin (Figures 4-10 through 4-12).
   2. Mechanism of action
      a. Initiates increased cell turnover in both normal follicles and comedones
      b. Reduces cohesion between keratinized cells
      c. Causes skin peeling and extrusion of comedones; new comedone formation is prevented with continued use
      d. Improves skin turgor and reduces fine wrinkling
      e. Improves circulation, which improves skin color

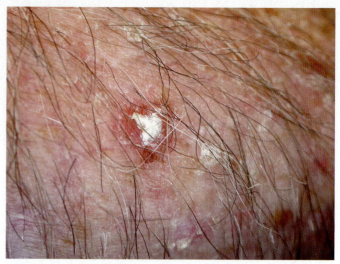

FIGURE 4-11. Actinic keratosis; keratotic papule characteristic of a hypertrophic actinic keratosis. (From Goroll, A. H., & Mulley, A. G. (2009). *Primary care medicine.* Philadelphia, PA: Wolters Kluwer.)

   3. Possible side effects
      a. Erythema
      b. Peeling
      c. Thinning of stratum corneum increasing risk of sunburn/sun damage
      d. Increased susceptibility to irritation from wind/cold
      e. Dryness
      f. Edema
      g. Blisters
      h. Stinging
   4. Nursing considerations
      a. Use with caution in pregnant or lactating women.
      b. Avoid applying around eyes, mouth, angles of the nose, and mucous membranes.
      c. Increases risk of sunburn.
      d. Astringents, alcohol-based lotions, and acne soaps may not be tolerated while using retinoids.

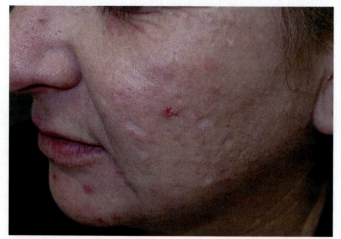

FIGURE 4-10. Acne of the face. (Image provided by Stedman's.)

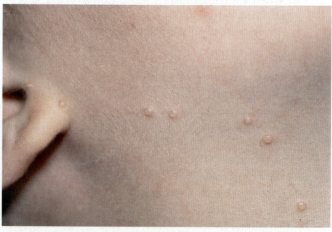

FIGURE 4-12. Molluscum contagiosum. (From Goodheart, H. P. (2003). *Goodheart's photoguide of common skin disorders* (2nd ed.). Philadelphia, PA: Lippincott Williams & Wilkins.)

IV. INTRALESIONAL THERAPY

A. Intralesional steroids
1. Injected directly into or just beneath the lesion
2. Provides a reservoir of medication that lasts for several weeks to months
3. Used to supplement other treatment modalities
4. Conditions treated
   a. Psoriasis
   b. Alopecia areata
   c. Cystic acne
   d. Hypertrophic scars/keloids
   e. Chronic eczematous inflammation and lichen simplex chronicus
   f. Discoid lupus (use lidocaine/steroid solution as for herpes zoster)
5. Most commonly used mixture: 2.5 to 10 mg/mL suspension of triamcinolone acetonide
6. Other mixtures
   a. 10 mg/mL—effective for chronic eczematous inflammation, acne, and hypertrophic scars/keloids
   b. 10 mg/mL diluted with 1% Xylocaine or physiologic saline—effective for acne and discoid lupus
   c. 2.5 to 5.0 mg/mL—effective in suppressing inflammation
7. Possible side effects
   a. Prolonged, continuous use may lead to adrenal suppression.
   b. Atrophy may result after multiple injections in same site.
8. Nursing considerations
   a. Injections may be painful.
   b. Atrophy can result from multiple treatments.
   c. Multiple treatments may be necessary in some conditions such as keloids.
   d. Vial of steroid solution must be shaken thoroughly before drawing up solution.
   e. If syringe of medication is not used immediately, syringe should be shaken immediately prior to injection.

B. Intralesional antineoplastic agents.
1. Bleomycin sulfate
   a. Useful in treating recalcitrant periungual or plantar warts and Kaposi sarcoma
   b. Solution: 1 unit/mL in physiologic saline (dissolve 15 unit vial of bleomycin in 15 mL of sterile physiologic saline)
   c. Inject 0.1 to 1.0 mL until wart blanches.
2. Vinblastine
   a. Useful in treating Kaposi sarcoma
   b. Solution: 0.1 to 0.5 mg/mL q4wk
   c. Maximum total dose to be used is 2 mg.
3. Interferon alfa-2b, recombinant, and interferon alfa-n3
   a. Treatment indications
      i. Genital warts that are unresponsive to all forms of conventional treatment, imposing significant social or physical limitations
      ii. Kaposi sarcoma
      iii. Basal/squamous cell cancers
   b. Possible side effects
      i. Injection site reactions—redness, pain, swelling, and discoloration
      ii. Flu-like symptoms
4. Nursing considerations
   a. A thorough history to determine presence of underlying medical problems (cardiac, liver, or renal)
   b. Medication must be refrigerated.
   c. Initial treatment for warts will be 3 times/week for 3 weeks.
   d. Flu-like symptoms can be managed with acetaminophen.

V. SYSTEMIC MEDICATIONS

A. Antibiotics: Act to prevent or treat infection from pathogenic microorganisms
1. Macrolides: Azithromycin and erythromycin—highly effective; one of the safest antibiotics; topical erythromycin is the drug of choice in treating acne and folliculitis.
   a. Members of macrolide group
   b. Bacteriostatic—inhibits protein synthesis
   c. Bactericidal in high concentrations
   d. Pharmacokinetics
      i. Inactivated rapidly by gastric acid
      ii. Dissolves poorly in water
      iii. Distributed well to most tissues with the exception of cerebrospinal fluid (CSF)

iv. Transported across the placenta and excreted in breast milk

v. Metabolized in the liver and excreted in the bile and small amount excreted in urine

vi. Peak serum concentration level occurs 1 to 4 hours after a single 250-mg dose of erythromycin in a fasting patient and 2.5 to 3.2 after dose of azithromycin

e. Pharmacotherapeutics

  i. Broad spectrum of antimicrobial activity, effective against the following:

    (a) *Pneumococci*

    (b) Group A *Streptococci*

    (c) *Staphylococci aureus* (not effective against methicillin-resistant *S. aureus*)

    (d) Gram-negative and gram-positive bacteria

    (e) May be used in patients with penicillin allergy who have group A beta hemolytic *streptococci* or *S. pneumoniae* infection

  ii. Dosage/indications

    (a) Erythromycin—Adults: 250 mg PO qid × 10 days, 333 mg PO q8h, or 500 mg PO q12h (base or stearate), 400 mg PO q6h or 800 mg PO q12h (ethylsuccinate); pediatric dose (base and ethylsuccinate): children greater than 1 month: 30 to 50 mg/kg/d PO in divided doses q6–8h (max. 2 g/d as base or 3.2 g/d as ethylsuccinate); 30 to 50 mg/kg/d PO divided q6h (max. 2 g/d as stearate).

    (b) Azithromycin—Adults: 500 mg PO qd on first day, then 250 mg/d PO for 4 additional days (total dose 1.5 mg): children 6 month and older: 10 mg/kg PO (not greater than 500 mg/dose) on first day, then 5 mg/kg PO (not greater than 250 mg) for four additional days.

    (c) Skin and soft tissue infections

      (i) Chlamydia trachomatis urethritis

      (ii) Erythrasma

      (iii) Gonorrhea

    (d) *Strep. pyogenes* infections

      (i) Lymphangitis

      (ii) Impetigo

      (iii) Ecthyma

    (e) *S. aureus infections*

      (i) Folliculitis

      (ii) Furunculosis

      (iii) Infected dermatitis

  iii. Adverse reactions

    (a) Commonly causes nausea and vomiting when taken on an empty stomach

    (b) Diarrhea

    (c) Cholestatic hepatitis with fever, abdominal pain, nausea, vomiting, eosinophilia, and elevated serum bilirubin

    (d) Stevens–Johnson syndrome and toxic epidermal necrolysis (azithromycin)

  iv. Drug interactions

    (a) Theophylline

    (b) Cyclosporine

    (c) Carbamazepine

    (d) Warfarin

    (e) Digitalis

    (f) Ergotamine

    (g) Methylprednisolone

    (h) Pimozide

    (i) Diltiazem

    (j) Ketoconazole

    (k) Verapamil

2. Penicillins

a. Derived from strains of *Penicillium notatum* and *Penicillium chrysogenum*, which are common molds seen on bread or fruit.

b. First generation

  i. Penicillin G and penicillin V

  ii. Newer semisynthetic penicillinase—resistant

    (a) Oxacillin

    (b) Cloxacillin

    (c) Dicloxacillin

c. Second generation

  i. Amoxicillin and clavulanate (Augmentin)

  ii. Ampicillin

  iii. Amoxicillin

  iv. Ampicillin/sulbactam (Unasyn)

d. Third generation

  i. Ticarcillin (Ticar)

  ii. Ticarcillin/potassium clavulanate (Timentin)

e. Fourth generation

  i. Piperacillin (Pipracil)

  ii. Piperacillin sodium and tazobactam sodium (Zosyn)

f. Pharmacokinetics

  i. Kills bacteria by destroying the cell walls, bactericidal

  ii. Natural penicillins (penicillin G and V) effective against the following:

    (a) Gram-positive organisms

    (b) Gram-negative organisms

    (c) Anaerobic organisms

  iii. Penicillinase-resistant penicillins (cloxacillin, dicloxacillin, nafcillin, oxacillin)

    (a) *S. aureus*

    (b) *S. epidermidis*

    (c) Some streptococci infections

  iv. Absorption

    (a) Oral absorption varies and limited by gastric acidity and binding with food. All should be taken on an empty stomach with the exception of amoxicillin.

    (b) Completely and rapidly absorbed throughout the body after parental administration.

(c) Distributed widely in fluids/tissue including liver, kidneys, bones, muscle, and placenta and enters breast milk

(d) Does not readily enter CSF

(e) Minimally metabolized in the liver

(f) Excreted unchanged and primarily through the kidneys

v. Peak serum concentrations vary from one-half hour to 24 hours depending on route of administration.

g. Pharmacotherapeutics

i. Broad spectrum of antimicrobial activity

(a) Procaine penicillin used for susceptible strains of gonorrhea

(b) Benzathine penicillin G preferred for syphilis

(c) Dicloxacillin: Treatment of osteomyelitis, suspected or proven staphylococcal infections, and most streptococci and *S. aureus* infections

(d) Aminopenicillins (ampicillin and amoxicillin): Broad spectrum, active against gram-negative bacteria, and better absorbed with less GI distress

ii. Dosage/indications

(a) Dependent on type of penicillin and route of administration

(b) Used to treat common infections, syphilis, and staph infections

iii. Adverse reactions

(a) Hypersensitivity reactions (anaphylaxis, the major adverse reaction)

(b) Neurotoxicity

(c) Nephrotoxicity

(d) Electrolyte imbalances

(e) Hematologic reactions

(f) Cardiovascular reactions

iv. Drug interactions

(a) Probenecid

(b) Methotrexate

(c) Tetracyclines

(d) Chloramphenicol

(e) Aminoglycosides (penicillin G, azlocillin, carbenicillin, mezlocillin, piperacillin, ticarcillin)

(f) Neomycin (penicillin V)

(g) Allopurinol

3. Cephalosporins

a. Pharmacokinetics

i. Properties and mechanisms of action resemble penicillins.

ii. Semisynthetic derivation of cephalosporin C (produced by fungus *Acremonium chrysogenum*); classified by generation, which is determined by spectra of activity. As progression is made from the first generation to the fourth generation, the activity against gram-negative bacteria increases, the ability to penetrate CSF increases, and there is greater resistance to beta lactamases.

iii. Rapidly absorbed by the GI tract

iv. May take with or without food

v. Distributed widely through soft tissue and bodily fluids except CSF

vi. Excreted essentially unchanged by the kidneys except for cefoperazone, which is excreted in bile, and ceftriaxone, which is partly metabolized and partly excreted in urine, and are excreted in the feces

vii. Oral cephalosporins reach a peak serum concentration level within 1 to 6 hours after administration; IV administration levels achieved within 30 minutes; IM administration in 15 minutes to 3 hours

b. First generation

i. Parenteral

(a) Cefazolin

ii. Oral

(a) Cephalexin

(b) Cefadroxil

iii. Treatment of gram-positive and gram-negative organisms (most staphylococci, groups A and B hemolytic streptococci, most streptococci)

c. Second generation

i. Parenteral

(a) Cefoxitin

(b) Cefotetan

(c) Cefuroxime

ii. Oral

(a) Cefaclor

(b) Cefprozil

(c) Cefuroxime

iii. Treatment of gram-negative, gram-positive, and anaerobic organisms (same as first generation as well as *Escherichia coli, Neisseria gonorrhoeae, Neisseria meningitidis, Enterobacter, Citrobacter, Clostridium, Bacteroides*)

d. Third generation

i. Parenteral

(a) Cefotaxime

(b) Ceftriaxone

(c) Ceftazidime

(d) Cefoperazone

ii. Oral

(a) Cefixime

(b) Cefdinir

(c) Cefditoren

(d) Cefpodoxime

(e) Ceftibuten

iii. Treatment of gram-negative, gram-positive, and anaerobic organisms (same as first and second generation as well as *Pseudomonas aeruginosa, Enterobacter*)

e. Fourth generation

i. Parenteral

(a) Cefepime

ii. Treatment of gram-negative, gram-positive, and anaerobic organisms (same as third generation but also effective against *P. aeruginosa*)

f. Fifth generation
  i. Parenteral
    (a) Ceftaroline
  ii. Treatment of gram-negative, gram-positive, and anaerobic organisms (same as third generation but also effective against *P. aeruginosa* and with improved gram-positive activity, in particular MRSA)
g. Pharmacotherapeutics—ineffective against enterococci (*Streptococcus faecalis*), methicillin-resistant staphylococci, and beta hemolytic streptococci
h. Dosage/indications
  i. Based on drug and condition being treated and route of administration
  ii. Treatment of skin infections due to *S. aureus* and group A and B beta hemolytic strep
  iii. Cellulitis due to *H. influenzae*
i. Adverse reactions (considered to be very safe)
  i. Hypersensitivity reactions (most common)
  ii. Cross-reactivity in patients who are sensitive to penicillins
  iii. Pain, induration, and tenderness at site of injection
  iv. In patients with impaired renal function, confusion, and seizures
  v. In orally administered drug: nausea, vomiting, and diarrhea
  vi. Cephalosporins may produce nephrotoxicity.
  vii. Possibility of superinfection
j. Drug interactions
  i. Disulfiram-like reaction with cefoperazone and cefotetan
    (a) Headache
    (b) Flushing
    (c) Dizziness
    (d) Nausea, vomiting, and abdominal cramping
  ii. Concomitant use of cephalosporins and imipenem/cilastatin
    (a) Antagonizes antibacterial activity of beta lactam cephalosporins

4. Tetracyclines
a. Pharmacokinetics
  i. Absorbed from the duodenum
  ii. Distributed widely into the body tissues, fluids with some penetration into CSF, placenta, and breast milk
  iii. Excreted primarily unchanged by the kidneys (except for doxycycline and minocycline; bile and feces)
  iv. Onset, peak, and duration of action vary among tetracyclines; ranges from 30 minutes to 4 hours.
b. Pharmacotherapeutics
  i. Provide broad-spectrum coverage against gram-positive, gram-negative, aerobic, and anaerobic bacteria, spirochetes, mycoplasmas, rickettsieae, chlamydiae, and some protozoa
  ii. Doxycycline and minocycline provide more action against various organisms.
c. Dosage/indications
  i. Minocycline hydrochloride (Minocin)
    (a) Treatment of severe acne: 50 mg qid or 100 mg bid
    (b) Not recommended in children under 8 years old
  ii. Tetracycline hydrochloride
    (a) Treatment of acne, Lyme disease, and syphilis in penicillin-allergic patients
      (i) 250 to 500 mg PO q6h for gram-positive and gram-negative organisms
      (ii) 500 mg PO qid for 10 to 30 days for Lyme disease
      (iii) 250 to 500 PO mg qid for acne
    (b) Pediatric dose (>8 years old): 25 to 50 mg/kg/d PO in divided doses every 6 hours
  iii. Doxycycline (Vibramycin, Doryx)
    (a) Treatment of acne, anthrax, malaria prophylaxis, as well as other infections treated with tetracyclines
      (i) Most infections: 100 mg PO q12h
      (ii) Malaria prophylaxis: 100 mg PO qd
      (iii) Lyme disease: 100 mg PO q12h
      (iv) Anthrax: 100 mg PO q12h × 60 days
    (b) Pediatric dose (>8 years old): Oral: 25 to 50 mg/kg/d in divided doses every 6 hours
d. Adverse reactions
  i. GI disturbances—nausea, vomiting, and diarrhea (Tetracycline must be taken on an empty stomach with either juice or water for proper absorption.)
  ii. Risk of superinfection
  iii. Significantly affects tooth enamel, therefore not recommended in children under age of 8 or pregnant patients
  iv. Photosensitivity reactions
  v. Nephrotoxicity in patients with renal failure
  vi. Hepatotoxic reactions in patients with an excessive serum concentration due to renal failure
  vii. Light-headedness, loss of balance, dizziness, and tinnitus (most common with minocycline)
  viii. Yeast infections
  ix. Hypersensitivity reactions, though uncommon
e. Drug interactions
  i. Antacids with calcium, aluminum, and magnesium—chlortetracycline, doxycycline, minocycline, and tetracycline
  ii. Iron salts, bismuth, subsalicylate, and zinc sulfate—tetracycline and doxycycline
  iii. Barbiturates, carbamazepine, and phenytoin—decrease effects of doxycycline
  iv. Decreases effect of penicillin—all tetracyclines
  v. Decreases effect of warfarin—all tetracyclines

B. Antifungals (antimycotics): Used to treat superficial (topical) and systemic infections

1. Nystatin
   a. Pharmacokinetics
      i. Little or no absorption, distribution, or metabolism
      ii. Excretion negligible with local application
   b. Pharmacotherapeutics
      i. Primarily treat superficial skin infections
      ii. Effective against *Candida albicans, Candida guilliermondii,* and other Candida species
      iii. Oral nystatin is used to prevent fungal infection in neutropenic patients
   c. Dosage
      i. For oral candidiasis: 400,000 to 600,000 units swish and swallow (retain in the mouth as long as possible) qid, or 500,000 to 1,000,000 units oral tablets dissolved in the mouth q8h
   d. Adverse reactions
      i. Hypersensitivity reactions (uncommon)
      ii. Bitter taste
      iii. High doses may cause diarrhea, nausea, vomiting, and abdominal pain
   e. Drug interactions
      i. None
2. Amphotericin B intravenous (IV)
   a. Pharmacokinetics
      i. Distributed throughout the body tissues and fluids and poor CSF penetration
      ii. Very prolonged and excreted by the kidneys
   b. Pharmacotherapeutics
      i. Indicated for treating severe, potentially fatal systemic fungal infections
      ii. Extremely toxic; therefore, risk/benefit must be weighed carefully
      iii. Used to treat aspergillosis, coccidiomycosis, cryptococcus, candidiasis, and phycomycosis infections
   c. Dosage
      i. Test dose: 1 mg in 250 mL of dextrose 5% over 20 to 30 minutes
      ii. Systemic fungal infections: 0.25 mg to 1.5 mg/kg/d based on organism present and patient's tolerance and infused over 4 to 6 hours
      iii. Pediatric dosage: Infants and children: 0.1 mg/kg/dose to a maximum of 1 mg; infuse over 30 to 60 minutes. Maintenance dose: 0.25 to 1 mg/kg/d given once daily; infuse over 2 to 6 hours. Once therapy has been established, amphotericin B can be administered on an every-other-day basis at 1 to 1.5 mg/kg/dose; cumulative dose: 1.5 to 2 g over 6 to 10 weeks
   d. Adverse reactions
      i. Nephrotoxicity
      ii. Hypokalemia
      iii. Chills and fever
      iv. Nausea, vomiting, and anorexia
      v. Muscle and joint pain
      vi. Headache and chest pain
      vii. Abdominal pain
      viii. Normochromic or normocytic anemia
      ix. Phlebitis/thrombophlebitis
      x. Hypotension/hypertension
      xi. Flushing
      xii. Hypersensitivity reactions, chills, and fever
      xiii. Leukocytosis
   e. Drug interactions
      i. Aminoglycosides
      ii. Cyclosporine
      iii. Azole antifungals
      iv. Corticosteroids
      v. Extended-spectrum penicillins
      vi. Pancuronium bromide
      vii. Electrolyte solutions
3. Fluconazole (Diflucan)
   a. Pharmacokinetics
      i. Synthetic, broad-spectrum agent
      ii. Well absorbed after oral administration
      iii. Distributed in all body fluids, including CSF and breast milk
      iv. Excreted unchanged in the urine
      v. Peak plasma concentration 2 to 4 hours after administration
   b. Pharmacotherapeutics: Indicated for treating candidal and cryptococcal infections and used in neonates and children
   c. Dosage
      i. Oropharyngeal candidiasis: 200 mg PO first day, then 100 mg PO daily for 2 weeks
   d. Adverse reactions: All reactions are more common in HIV patients.
      i. Transient elevations in serum glutamic oxaloacetic transaminase (SGOT)/serum glutamic pyruvic transaminase (SGPT) alkaline phosphatase, and bilirubin, hepatotoxicity
      ii. Dizziness
      iii. Nausea, vomiting, diarrhea, and abdominal pain
      iv. Skin rash, Stevens–Johnson syndrome, and anaphylaxis
      v. Headache
   e. Drug interactions
      i. Warfarin
      ii. Levels of phenytoin, theophylline, tacrolimus, and cyclosporine may increase with fluconazole.
      iii. Patients taking rifampin, rifabutin, and isoniazid may require higher doses of fluconazole to get therapeutic results.
4. Terbinafine (Lamisil)
   a. Pharmacokinetics
      i. Disrupts the cell wall of fungal hyphae (fungicidal). Metabolized in the liver and excreted in the feces
   b. Pharmacotherapeutics
      i. Indicated for treating widespread tinea infections of the skin and onychomycosis
   c. Dosage: 250 mg PO qd × 1 to 2 weeks for tinea corporis, 2 weeks for tinea pedis, 6 weeks for fingernail involvement, and 12 weeks for toenails
   d. Adverse reactions
      i. Elevated liver enzymes (rare)

ii. Leukocytopenia (rare)

iii. Stevens–Johnson-type reaction (rare)

iv. Taste disruption

v. Indigestion, anorexia, diarrhea, nausea, and vomiting

vi. Headache

e. Drug interactions

  i. Rifampin

  ii. Cyclosporine

  iii. Tagamet (oral antacid may decrease absorption)

5. Ketoconazole (Nizoral). Oral ketoconazole is less often prescribed now than in the past years because newer azole drugs such as itraconazole and fluconazole are less likely to cause liver dysfunction.

a. Pharmacokinetics

  i. Varied absorption and distribution and pH dependent

  ii. Metabolized in the liver and excreted through bile and feces

  iii. Peak plasma concentration reached in 1 to 4 hours.

b. Pharmacotherapeutics

  i. Treatment of superficial and systemic infections with susceptible fungal organisms

    (a) Active against certain dermatophytes (tinea corporis, tinea cruris, tinea versicolor)

    (b) Yeasts such as candida and malassezia

  ii. Response to treatment

    (a) Mucosal infections—respond in days

    (b) Skin infections—respond in weeks

    (c) Nail infections—respond in months

c. Dosage

  i. 200 mg PO daily; may increase to 400 mg if unresponsive

  ii. Duration varies with organism/site.

    (a) 2 weeks for oral candidiasis

    (b) 2 to 6 weeks for dermatophyte infections

    (c) 6 to 12 months for chronic mucocutaneous candidiasis and tinea unguium

d. Adverse reactions

  i. Nausea/vomiting and diarrhea

  ii. Pruritus, skin rash, dermatitis, and urticaria

  iii. Headache

  iv. Insomnia and lethargy

  v. Dizziness

  vi. Interference with adrenal and corticosteroid synthesis leading to decreased circulatory testosterone

  vii. Disulfiram-like reaction if alcohol is ingested

e. Drug interactions

  i. Warfarin

  ii. Methylprednisolone

  iii. Cyclosporine

  iv. Some hypoglycemic medications

  v. Quinidine

  vi. Corticosteroids

6. Itraconazole (Sporanox)

a. Pharmacokinetics

  i. Bioavailability maximal when taken with food

  ii. Metabolized in the liver and excreted in feces

b. Pharmacotherapeutics: Indicated in treating onychomycosis of the nails and deep fungal infections (blastomycosis, aspergillosis, and histoplasmosis)

c. Dosage

  i. Toenails with or without fingernail involvement: 200 mg qd for 12 consecutive weeks

  ii. Fingernails only: 200 mg bid for 1 week; 3-week period without therapy, then 200 mg bid for an additional week to 6 months

d. Adverse reactions

  i. Elevated liver enzymes

  ii. GI disorders

  iii. Rash/pruritus

  iv. Hypertension/orthostatic hypotension

  v. Headache

  vi. Malaise

  vii. Myalgia

  viii. Nausea

  ix. Vertigo

e. Drug interactions

  i. Warfarin

  ii. Antihistamines

  iii. Ritonavir and indinavir

  iv. Benzodiazepines: Midazolam, triazolam, and diazepam

  v. Calcium channel blockers

  vi. Cyclosporine

  vii. Methylprednisolone

  viii. Digoxin and quinidine

  ix. Phenobarbital, carbamazepine, and phenytoin

  x. Isoniazid, rifampin, and rifabutin

Note: Sporanox increases plasma concentrations of drugs from 1 through 8 and decreases plasma concentrations of drugs from 9 through 10.

7. Griseofulvin

a. Pharmacokinetics: Disrupts mitosis of fungal cells

  i. Metabolized by the liver and excreted through urine, feces, and perspiration

b. Pharmacotherapeutics

  i. Indicated for treating fungal infections of the skin except tinea versicolor and not effective for nails

  ii. Duration of therapy varies with site of infection.

c. Dosage

  i. Gris-PEG: 125 to 250 mg PO in single or divided doses for 2 to 8 weeks

  ii. Grifulvin V : 500 to 1,000 mg in single or divided doses for 2 to 8 weeks

  iii. Pediatric: Gris-PEG and grifulvin V 125 mg/5 cc suspension; 10 to 25 mg/kg/d

d. Adverse reactions

  i. Nausea, vomiting, and diarrhea

  ii. Fatigue

  iii. Confusion

iv. Headaches

v. Rare: Proteinuria, urticaria, rash, serum sickness, photosensitivity, hearing loss, paresthesia, dizziness, insomnia, leukopenia, and oral candidiasis

e. Drug interactions

i. Alcohol

ii. Barbiturates

iii. Warfarin

C. Antivirals

1. Acyclovir, famciclovir, and valacyclovir—used in the management of herpes simplex viruses.

a. Pharmacokinetics

i. Absorbed in the GI tract

ii. Distributed throughout the body

iii. Crosses the placenta and enters breast milk

iv. Metabolized in the liver

v. Excreted in the urine

vi. Peak concentration levels reached within 1.5 to 2.5 hours after oral administration; immediately after IV administration.

b. Pharmacotherapeutics

i. Effectiveness limited to herpes viruses (HSV 1 and 2; varicella-zoster virus)

ii. Initial and recurrent genital herpes treated with oral acyclovir, valacyclovir, or famciclovir; all are effective for suppressive therapy

iii. Recurrences may be reduced with long-term use

iv. Severe initial and recurrent mucocutaneous HSV infections and varicella-zoster, particularly in immunocompromised patients, require parenteral administration

v. Decreases severity, pain, and viral shedding

vi. Decreases duration of lesions

c. Dosage depends on disease and type of episode (must be adjusted in patients with renal dysfunction).

i. Acyclovir: 200 to 800 mg 5/day for 7 to 10 days

ii. Famvir: 125 to 1,000 mg bid to tid for 1 to 10 days

iii. Valacyclovir: 500 to 1,000 mg 1 to 2 times a day for 3 to 10 days

iv. Medication must be started within 72 hours for optimal reduction in shedding.

v. All three medications are indicated to help prevent postherpetic neuralgia.

d. Adverse reactions

i. Headache and dizziness

ii. Nausea, vomiting, and diarrhea

iii. Pruritus

iv. Fatigue

v. Insomnia

vi. Irritability

vii. Depression

viii. Hypotension

ix. Rare: Thrombocytosis, thrombocytopenia, transient lymphopenia, transient leukopenia, and bone marrow hypoplasia

e. Drug interactions

i. Probenecid (and other drugs that inhibit tubular secretion or absorption)

ii. Cimetidine

iii. Phenytoin

iv. Theophylline

D. Antineoplastics

1. Methotrexate

a. Pharmacokinetics

i. Well absorbed and distributed throughout the body

ii. Undergoes minimal metabolism and mostly excreted by the kidneys

iii. Peak plasma concentration reached 1 hour after oral dosing

iv. Crosses placenta and enters breast milk and very little concentration in CSF

b. Pharmacotherapeutics

i. Used for treating recalcitrant, severe psoriasis, mycosis fungoides, and psoriatic/rheumatoid arthritis

ii. May be used as steroid-sparing drug in immunobullous diseases

(a) A folic acid antagonist and inhibits cell division

(b) Has some activity as an immunosuppressive agent

c. Dosage: Varies from 10 mg to 30 mg/week

d. Adverse reactions

i. Hepatic fibrosis and cirrhosis with long-term use

(a) Liver function may be abnormal despite frequently normal blood tests.

(b) Liver biopsy should be done periodically with long-term use.

ii. Bone marrow suppression is usually dose dependent; white blood cell (WBC) must be monitored carefully.

iii. Nausea

iv. Malaise

v. Headaches

vi. Teratogenic in females, harmful to male sperm, and birth control indicated during course of medication

e. Drug interactions

i. Probenecid

ii. Salicylates and non-steroidal anti-inflammatory drugs (NSAIDS)

iii. Alcohol

iv. Cholestyramine

v. Live vaccines

vi. Penicillins

vii. Oral hypoglycemic agents

2. Cyclophosphamide (Cytoxan)

a. Pharmacokinetics

i. Synthesized derivation of nitrogen mustard

ii. Alkylating agent—disrupt the structure of DNA

iii. Absorbed well

iv. Peak plasma concentration reached 1 hour after oral dosing.

v. Hepatic metabolism

vi. Excreted in the urine

b. Pharmacotherapeutics
   i. Used for steroid-sparing therapy of immunobullous diseases and leukocytoclastic vasculitis
   ii. Used in advanced mycosis fungoides and in connective tissue diseases
   iii. Activity and effectiveness depend on type of cancer, the extent of disease, and patient's overall condition.
c. Dosage
   i. 1 to 5 mg/kg up to 100 mg/kg PO
   ii. Dosage must be adjusted in patient with impaired liver or renal function
d. Adverse reactions
   i. Bone marrow suppression
   ii. Late lymphoreticular malignancies
   iii. Hemorrhagic cystitis
   iv. Anorexia, nausea, and vomiting
   v. Secondary neoplasms
   vi. Pulmonary fibrosis
e. Drug interactions
   i. Succinylcholine
   ii. Allopurinol
   iii. Warfarin
   iv. Live virus vaccines (decreases antibody response)

E. Retinoid (vitamin A)
  1. Isotretinoin (Accutane)
   a. Pharmacokinetics
      i. Isomer of retinoic acid, a metabolite of vitamin A
      ii. Inhibits sebaceous gland function
      iii. Prevents abnormal keratinization
      iv. Peak plasma concentrations reached 3 to 5 hours after dosing
      v. Metabolized in the liver and excreted in urine and feces
   b. Pharmacotherapeutics
      i. Indicated in treating recalcitrant cystic and nodular acne
      ii. May be used in ichthyosis, pityriasis rubra pilaris, and Darier disease
      iii. May affect basal cell carcinoma (BCC), squamous cell carcinoma (SCC), cutaneous T-cell lymphoma (CTCL), keratoacanthoma, verruca vulgaris, discoid lupus erythemetosus (DLE), and pustular/erythrodermic psoriasis
      iv. Females must have a negative pregnancy test before initiation of treatment and must use birth control for the duration of treatment. Women should continue contraception for one month and be reassured they may safely become pregnant one month after stopping isotretinoin treatment
      v. iPLEDGE program: Computer-based risk management program designed to eliminate fetal exposure to isotretinoin. All prescribers, pharmacists, men, and women must be registered with the iPLEDGE program
   c. Dosage
      i. 0.5 to 2 mg/kg PO daily in two divided doses for 15 to 20 weeks

      ii. Contraindicated if patient is sensitive to any ingredients or sensitivity to parabens, glycerin, or soybean oil
      iii. Use with caution in diabetics and patients with hepatic disease and hypertriglyceridemia
   d. Adverse reactions
      i. Cheilitis
      ii. Conjunctivitis
      iii. Skin fragility
      iv. Dry skin and mucous membranes
      v. Epistaxis
      vi. Dry nose and mouth
      vii. Corneal opacities
      viii. Inflammatory bowel disease
      ix. Hypertriglyceridemia
      x. Arthralgia
      xi. Hepatotoxicity
      xii. Photosensitivity
      xiii. Pseudotumor cerebri
   e. Drug interactions
      i. Vitamin A or vitamin A supplements, may result in hypervitaminosis
      ii. Minocycline
      iii. Tetracycline
      iv. Drugs with anticholinergic properties
      v. Alcohol-containing acne preparations or cosmetics
      vi. Alcohol

  2. Acitretin (Soriatane)
   a. Pharmacokinetics—binds to and activates retinoid X receptors; results in anti-inflammatory, antiproliferative, and normalization of keratinocyte differentiation
   b. Pharmacotherapeutics
      i. Treatment of ichthyosis, pityriasis rubra pilaris, and pustular and erythrodermic psoriasis; monotherapy is less effective for plaque psoriasis (Figure 4-13)
      ii. Contraindicated in pregnant patients or women who may become pregnant within 3 years
      iii. Complete blood count (CBC), baseline liver function, pregnancy test, lipid profile, and renal function tests must be checked before beginning treatment and 1- to 2-week intervals for the first 2 months decreasing to 1 to 3 months if values are within normal limits
      iv. Pregnancy tests monthly during treatment and every 3 months for 3 years after treatment
   c. Dosage
      i. 10 to 50 mg/d qd. Doses of about 25 mg/d decrease side effects.
      ii. Maintenance dose: 25 to 50 mg/d
   d. Adverse reactions
      i. Cheilitis (>75%)
      ii. Pseudotumor cerebri
      iii. Headache
      iv. Dizziness
      v. Alopecia (50% to 75%)

Scales

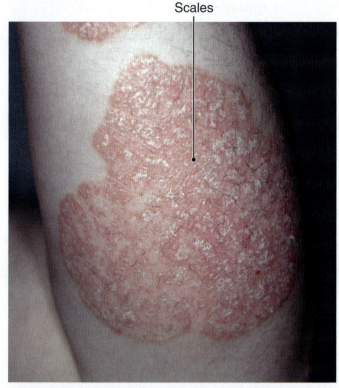

FIGURE 4-13. Plaque psoriasis showing erythematous plaques with secondary scaling.

    vi. Dryness of skin and mucous membranes
    vii. Elevated liver enzymes
   viii. Hypo- or hyperkalemia and hyperlipidemia
    ix. Bone pain
    x. Photosensitivity
    xi. Xerostomia
  e. Drug interactions
    i. Alcohol
    ii. Hepatotoxic medications
   iii. Vitamins/minerals with A, D, E, K, folate, and iron
    iv. Tetracyclines
    v. Vitamin A/vitamin A supplements
F. Corticosteroids
  1. Pharmacokinetics
    a. Absorbed well through the gastrointestinal (GI) tract and intra muscular (IM) absorption slower
    b. Metabolized in the liver
    c. Excreted by the kidneys
    d. Cross the placenta and are distributed in breast milk
    e. Rapid onset of action, usually within 1 hour after oral dosing
  2. Pharmacotherapeutics
    a. Anti-inflammatory
    b. Immunosuppressive
    c. Indicated for a wide variety of conditions and diseases including recalcitrant cases of acne, dermatomyositis, and cutaneous lichen planus
  3. Dosage: Based on disease process and severity
  4. Adverse reactions: Usually seen with long-term treatment
    a. Adrenocortical insufficiency

    b. Muscle wasting
    c. Cataracts
    d. Cushingoid signs and symptoms
    e. Skin atrophy, striae, and hirsutism
    f. Petechiae and ecchymoses
    g. Polycythemia and enhanced coagulability
    h. Fluid/electrolyte imbalance
    i. Weight gain
    j. Immunosuppression
    k. Mood changes
    l. Psychosis, depression, and euphoria
    m. Osteoporosis
    n. Hypertension
  5. Drug interactions
    a. Barbiturates
    b. Phenytoin
    c. Rifampin
    d. Amphotericin B
    e. Furosemide
    f. Thiazide diuretics
    g. Erythromycin
    h. Salicylates
    i. NSAIDs
    j. Vaccines and toxoids
    k. Estrogen, oral contraceptives that contain estrogen
    l. Hypoglycemic agents
    m. Isoniazid
    n. Fluoroquinolones
G. Psoralens (methoxsalen, oxsoralen, oxsoralen ultra, methoxypsoralen (8-MOP))
  1. Pharmacokinetics
    a. Increase melanization of the epidermis and thickening of the stratum corneum
    b. Photosensitizer
    c. Bonds with cellular DNA and causes cell damage when exposed to ultraviolet A (UVA) light, decreasing cell turnover rate
    d. 95% absorbed from the GI tract
    e. Peak serum concentration increased when taken with food
      i. Oxsoralen-Ultra reaches peak serum concentration 30 minutes to 1 hour after ingestion
      ii. Oxsoralen reaches peak level in 1.5 to 6 hours after ingestion, with half-life being 2 hours
    f. Metabolized in the liver and excreted in urine
  2. Pharmacotherapeutics
    a. Used in treating psoriasis, CTCL, and vitiligo
    b. Contraindicated if patient has increased risk for developing melanoma and SCC
    c. Contraindicated if patient is aphakic, has disorder associated with photosensitivity, is an albino, or has documented cataracts
  3. Dosage
    a. Psoriasis: Individualized according to weight
    b. Vitiligo: 20 mg with food or milk 2 to 4 hours prior to treatment
    c. CTCL: Individualized according to stage, overall prognosis, and quality of life

4. Adverse reactions
   a. Severe burns (must avoid sun exposure for 24-hour postingestion)
   b. Rash and pruritus
   c. Erythema and peeling
   d. Nausea
   e. Nervousness
   f. Insomnia
   g. Dizziness
   h. Headache
   i. Depression
   j. Malaise
   k. Cataract
   l. Infection
5. Drug interactions
   a. Photosensitizing drugs
      i. Phenothiazines
      ii. Thiazides
      iii. Sulfonamides
      iv. Tetracyclines
      v. Griseofulvin
      vi. Coal tar derivatives
      vii. Nalidixic acid
      viii. Halogenated salicylamides

H. Immunosuppressants
1. Cyclosporine (Neoral)
   a. Pharmacokinetics
      i. Distributed widely throughout the body; skin shows high concentrations.
      ii. Crosses the placenta and enters breast milk
      iii. Metabolized in the liver
      iv. Excreted primarily in bile
      v. Peak serum concentration reached within 2 to 6 hours after oral dosing.
      vi. Variable absorption through GI tract
   b. Pharmacotherapeutics
      i. Prevention of graft rejection without destruction of bone marrow
      ii. Used for treating psoriasis, alopecia areata, pyoderma gangrenosum, Behcet disease, AD, and lichen planus
      iii. Limited to treating moderately severe to severe recalcitrant psoriasis
      iv. Contraindicated in patients with renal impairment, severe hepatic impairment, uncontrolled hypertension, other infections, prone to infection or malignancy, and vaccination with live viruses
   c. Dosage
      i. Determined on body weight
      ii. Psoriasis: 2.5 to 5 mg/kg/d in one or two divided doses
      iii. Initial dosing may be at maximum level (5 mg/kg/d) for rapid response with adjustment of 0.5 to 1 mg/kg/d each week as needed
   d. Adverse reactions
      i. Tremor

      ii. Hypertension
      iii. Hepatotoxicity
      iv. Diarrhea, nausea, vomiting, and anorexia
      v. Nephrotoxicity
      vi. Hirsutism and acne
   e. Drug interactions
      i. Many drugs in many classes including antibiotics, antifungals, retinoids, antiepileptics, NSAIDs, and antihypertensives
2. Azathioprine (Imuran)
   a. Pharmacokinetics—see cyclosporine
   b. Pharmacotherapeutics
      i. Immunosuppressive effect and steroid sparing
      ii. Used in immunobullous diseases, leukoplastic vasculitis, and connective tissue disease
   c. Dosage
      i. 1 to 3 mg/kg/d PO, based on severity of disease
      ii. If no response after 6 to 8 weeks, dose may be increased by 0.5 mg/kg/d.
   d. Adverse reactions
      i. Leukopenia, anemia, pancytopenia, and thrombocytopenia
      ii. Bone marrow suppression
      iii. Nausea, vomiting, and anorexia
      iv. Pancreatitis
      v. Malaise
      vi. Hepatotoxicity
      vii. Rash
      viii. Alopecia
      ix. Increased risk of SCC and infections
   e. Drug interactions
      i. Allopurinol
      ii. Nondepolarizing neuromuscular blocking agents
      iii. Antineoplastics, cyclosporine, live virus vaccines, Echinacea, and melatonin

I. Antihistamines
1. Nonsedating (Claritin, Zyrtec, Allegra)
   a. Pharmacokinetics
      i. Peak plasma levels reached in 2 to 12 hours.
      ii. Metabolized in the liver and excreted in feces
      iii. H1-receptor antagonist
   b. Pharmacotherapeutics
      i. Relief of allergic rhinitis
      ii. Chronic idiopathic urticaria
   c. Dosage
      i. Loratadine (Claritin): one 10-mg tablet daily
      ii. Cetirizine HCL (Zyrtec): Adults and children over 6 years old 5 mg to 10 mg PO qd
      iii. Fexofenadine (Allegra): Adults and children 12 or older 60 mg PO bid or 180 mg qd
   d. Adverse reactions
      i. Confusion
      ii. Blurred vision
      iii. Pharyngitis
      iv. Increased appetite
      v. Nausea

vi. Nervousness
vii. Dry mouth
viii. Fatigue
ix. Photosensitivity
x. Rash
  e. Drug interactions
    i. Central nervous system (CNS) depressants and alcohol
    ii. Grapefruit, apple, and orange juice.
    iii. Tricyclic antidepressants
    iv. Monoamine oxidase (MAO) inhibitors
    v. Phenothiazines
    vi. Norepinephrine/phenylephrine
    vii. Amiodarone
  2. Benadryl, Atarax, Tavist, and Periactin: H1 antagonists have the same pharmacokinetics/pharmacotherapeutics as the nonsedating drugs except they cause drowsiness.

VI. LOCAL ANESTHETICS

A. Local anesthetics are drugs that slow or stop nerve conduction when applied close to nerve tissue. Local anesthetics block the flow of sodium ions, thereby preventing transmission of the impulse. Both temporary sensory and motor nerve paralyses occur in the affected nerve distribution with complete recovery in the normal course of events.
B. Injectable anesthetics
  1. Ester linked—cocaine, procaine (Novocain), and tetracaine (Pontocaine)
    a. Metabolized in plasma or local tissue by the enzyme pseudocholinesterase
    b. Metabolized to para-aminobenzoic acid (PABA) among other metabolites to which patients may already have been sensitized and may lead to severe allergic reactions
    c. Metabolized by the liver and excreted through the kidneys
  2. Amide linked
    a. Metabolized in the liver and excreted by the kidneys.
    b. Allergies to the amide group of anesthetics are rare.
    c. Common amide anesthetics include the following:
      i. Lidocaine (Xylocaine)—rapid onset, low toxicity and allergic potential, water soluble, and compatible with vasoconstrictors and tissue fluid. Intermediate acting and duration of 30 to 60 minutes
      ii. Mepivacaine (Carbocaine)—less toxic than lidocaine or procaine but slower onset of action. Intermediate acting and duration of 45 to 90 minutes
      iii. Bupivacaine (Marcaine)—more potent and toxic than lidocaine and mepivacaine. Longer duration of action, onset of action delayed. Long acting and duration of 2 to 4 hours
      iv. Etidocaine (Duranest)—four times more potent than lidocaine and lasts two times longer; useful for nerve blocks. Long acting and duration of 5 to 10 hours

3. Other agents
  a. Antihistamines (Benadryl)
    i. May be combined with epinephrine
    ii. Benadryl produces sedative effect if over 50 mg given. One suggested formula: 2 mL Benadryl (25 mg/mL), 8 mL normal saline, and 0.1 mL epinephrine (1:1,000)
    iii. Normal saline (to be effective must be injected to produce wheal; is inadequate for large procedures)
C. Vasoconstrictors (epinephrine premixed 1:100,000 to 1:200,000)
  1. Shortens time of onset, prolongs durations, and increases the depth of anesthesia
  2. Reduces systemic absorption and toxicity by reducing rate of clearance, gaining more effective anesthesia with less drug volume
  3. Reduces bleeding during procedure (plain lidocaine is a vasodilator)
  4. Useful with shorter-acting anesthetics and of little benefit with Marcaine or Duranest, although may provide hemostatic benefit
D. Untoward effects of systemic absorption of epinephrine
  1. Normal reaction to epinephrine includes restlessness, increased heart rate, palpitations, pounding in the head, and chest pain. These symptoms alert the provider of pending CNS toxicity with further absorption.
  2. Avoid vasoconstrictors.
    a. Digits with compromised digital circulation
    b. Patients with catecholamine sensitivity and patients taking ergot alkaloids or lurasidone
    c. For patients with normal circulation, it is safe to use epinephrine in areas including tip of the nose, fingers, toes, ears, and penis although not recommended for field or ring blocks in these areas.
  3. Dilute concentration of epinephrine.
    a. Hypertensive patients or those with cardiovascular disease
    b. Anxious or nervous patients
    c. When patient is taking phenothiazines, MAO inhibitors, beta blockers, and tricyclic antidepressants (raises blood pressure)
E. Adverse reactions to local anesthesia
  1. Usually related to vasoconstrictors and may result in anxiety, tremor, tachycardia, and diaphoresis when absorbed.
  2. Vasovagal reactions include hyperventilation, apprehension, and syncope.
  3. Local reactions such as delayed swelling, erythema, and blistering.
  4. True allergic reaction includes pruritus, hypotension, hives, urticaria, and angioedema with bronchospasm manifested by wheezing and coughing.
F. Systemic toxicity depends on concentration of local anesthesia in blood.
  1. Maximum safe doses:
    a. Adult: Repeated doses at 2-hour intervals
      i. 1% lidocaine with epinephrine 50 mL
      ii. 1% lidocaine without epinephrine 30 mL

iii. Suggest 0.5% lidocaine when large amounts required.
iv. Mepivacaine without epinephrine 30 mL
v. Mepivacaine with epinephrine 50 mL
vi. Bupivacaine 0.25% with epinephrine 90 mL
vii. Bupivacaine 0.25% without epinephrine 70 mL
viii. Etidocaine 0.5% with epinephrine 400 mg
ix. Etidocaine 0.5% without epinephrine 300 mg
b. Children less than 8 years old: 80% of the maximum allowable dose
2. Plasma concentration is the result of a balance between the rate of absorption and its rate of elimination dependent upon the following:
a. Inadvertent intravascular injection (into an artery or vein)
i. May occur with nerve blocks
ii. Inadvertent injection into scalp artery may more easily reach cerebral circulation and produce CNS response
b. Total dosage (see above)
c. Speed of injection
d. Vascularity of injection site
e. Presence of vasoconstrictors in solution
f. Physiologic characteristics of local anesthetics
g. Decreased metabolism of local anesthesia
h. Health status of patient (be cautious in elderly, sick, and patient with renal or hepatic disease)
G. Systemic toxicity mainly involves CNS and cardiovascular system.
1. Toxic blood levels of 1% lidocaine
a. Concentrations of 1% lidocaine—10 mg/mL
b. Depending on site, peak blood level of between 0.5 and 2.0 µg/mL is reached for every 100 mg lidocaine given; therapeutic range—1.5 to 5 µg/mL.
c. 50 mg IV results in blood level of about 1 µg/mL.
d. Avoid in patients with Wolf–Parkinson–White syndrome
2. CNS toxicity (mirrors blood concentration of local anesthetic)
a. 1 to 5 µg/mL
i. Ringing in ears
ii. Perioral numbness and tingling
iii. Metallic taste in mouth
iv. Light-headedness and talkativeness
v. Nausea and vomiting
vi. Double vision
b. 5 to 7.5 µg/mL may precede seizure activity.
i. Nystagmus
ii. Slurred speech
iii. Hallucinations
iv. Localized muscle twitching
v. Fine tremors of face and hands
c. 7.5 to 10 µg/mL: Focal seizure activity may increase to culminate in grand mal seizures (may be life threatening).
i. Seizure is usually self-limiting.
(a) Protect from injury and lie patient flat and maintain open airway

(b) Oxygen delivery with mask
(c) IV diazepam if necessary
d. 20 to 25 µg/mL: Cardiac toxicity, hypertension, arrhythmias, CNS depression, CV collapse, bronchospasm, and coma
3. Cardiovascular effects (heart and peripheral arteries)
a. All anesthetics except cocaine are vasodilators and can result in hypotension; patient may become pale, nauseated, with cold sweating.
b. Inject with patient lying flat.
c. Trendelenburg position if reactions appear. Apply cool wet washcloth to forehead, monitor vital signs, and physician may order oxygen.
H. Preventing CNS and cardiovascular reactions
1. Use minimum effective dose, especially on head and neck.
2. Aspirate before injection.
3. Use nerve block whenever possible.
4. Allow sufficient time for anesthesia before reinjecting.
5. Avoid injection of inflamed tissue, which results in unsatisfactory anesthesia due to lower tissue pH.
6. Use vasoconstrictors when indicated.
7. Some providers consider preoperative diazepam when large amounts of local anesthetics must be used; this raises seizure threshold but may induce respiratory depression.
8. Consider pre-existing renal, hepatic, and cardiac failure that may decrease clearance and increase risk of toxic dose.
9. Reduce dose in elderly, pts. weighing less than 50 kg, and children.
I. Allergy
1. More common in patients with underlying atopic or immunologic problems and multiple drug allergies (especially procaine penicillin)
2. Ester groups primarily responsible for allergic reactions and less incidence (rare) in amide groups
3. Topical sensitization to lidocaine has been substantiated leading to anaphylaxis
4. Allergy symptoms
a. Skin: Pruritus, urticaria, erythema, and facial swelling
b. GI: Nausea, vomiting, abdominal cramps, and diarrhea
c. Respiratory: Bronchospasm and hypoxia
5. Treatment of allergy to local anesthetic
a. SQ epinephrine (may need IV epinephrine)
b. Maintain airway
c. Oxygen and IV fluids
d. Transport to acute care facility (needs observation for 6 hours)
J. Effects on fetus/newborns
1. Avoid during first trimester while organogenesis has begun.
2. Postpone large procedures if possible until after delivery (hepatic system of fetus is immature).
3. Small procedures require minimal anesthetic and may be performed if necessary. Dilute epinephrine 1:300,000; fetal heart monitoring is recommended.

4. All local anesthetics are excreted into breast milk, and toxicity to infant is possible.

K. Topical anesthetics: The epidermis offers an effective barrier to diffusion of anesthetic agents while absorption through mucous membranes occurs quickly.

1. Cocaine (4% solution): A vasoconstrictor useful for anesthesia of nasal mucosa
   a. Maximum safe dose: 5 mL (200 mg) in adult
   b. Soak cotton ball in solution and apply topically to nasal mucosa with forceps.
   c. Peak effect is 2 to 5 minutes lasting 30 to 40 minutes.
   d. Absorption in mucosa is slow; increased cocaine blood level may occur 4 to 6 hours after nasal application.
   e. Renders superficial (not deep) anesthesia only.

2. Benzocaine available as 20% gel or aerosol, gel 7.5% to 20%, 20% solution, 2% to 20% ointment, or liquid 10% to 20%
   a. Useful in oral mucosa
   b. Associated with increased risk of contact allergy
   c. Cetacaine, used by otolaryngologists, is:
      i. 14% benzocaine
      ii. 2% tetracaine
      iii. 2% butamben
      iv. Spray of 1 second with 0.1 cc solution produces 30 seconds mucosal anesthesia.

3. 2% lidocaine jelly
   a. Contains parabens
   b. Maximum dose: 30 mL (600 mg) in 12-hour period

4. EMLA, cream (lidocaine 2.5% and prilocaine 2.5%), is an emulsion in which the oil phase is an eutectic mixture of lidocaine and prilocaine in a ratio of 1:1 by weight.
   a. Applied to intact skin under occlusive dressing at least 1 to 2 hours before procedure
   b. May cause a transient local blanching followed by temporary local erythema
   c. Application of EMLA cream to larger areas or for longer times than those recommended could result in overabsorption of anesthetic resulting in serious side effects

5. 0.5% proparacaine (Alcaine, Parcaine)—1 to 2 gtts on conjunctival surface prior to administering local anesthesia will prevent sting of lidocaine in eye and help eliminate blink reflex.

6. Viscous lidocaine for oral mucosa.

7. Oraqix gel is used orally.

L. Injection technique: Patient comfort and safety
1. Discuss procedure, goals, and expectations with patient.
2. Consider need for preoperative sedation.
3. Comfort measures
   a. Positioning, distraction (conversation, music), and ice prior to injection
   b. Eliminate preservatives that are acidic and contribute to the "sting" of local anesthesia infiltration by:
      i. Mix fresh solution of 0.1 mL epinephrine (1:1,000) to each 10-mL plain lidocaine. pH 6.5 to 6.8. Tissue fluid pH is 7.3 to 7.4.

      ii. Buffer stock lidocaine with epinephrine 1:100,000 with 1 cc sodium bicarb (8.4% solution) to every 10-mL lidocaine. Results in pH of 7.0 to 7.3.
         (a) Decreased duration may be due to more rapid absorption of less-charged buffered agents.
         (b) Epinephrine concentration reduced to 1:200,000.
         (c) Do not buffer bupivacaine (Marcaine) with epinephrine—may result in prolonged numbness of injection site.
         (d) Some providers keep buffered solution up to 1 week. Loss of 25% epinephrine effect occurs by that time.

4. Infiltration of anesthesia
   a. Equipment includes gloves, goggles, 18- to 20-gauge needle for drawing up solutions, 30 gauge 1" needles for injection, Luer-Lock syringes, alcohol prep, preloaded syringes may save time.
   b. Pain is caused by inevitable expansion of tissue on injection and the speed with which it occurs.
      i. SQ injection is less painful since tissue is more distensible but onset is delayed (and duration of reaction is longer).
      ii. Intradermal injection produces immediate anesthesia with prolonged effect due to placement but is more painful.
      iii. Whenever dermis is bound tightly to underlying tissue and there is little fat (e.g., nose), there is more resistance to instillation of local anesthetic and increased pain.
      iv. Use careful approach to bone.
   c. Proper technique includes the following:
      i. Rapid needle penetration into tense skin
      ii. SLOW INJECTION to lessen burning sensation
      iii. Limit number of punctures by trailing the needle; inject proximal to distal. Injecting from within the laceration or wound is less painful than into intact skin
      iv. Proper placement of anesthesia (not too deep)
      v. Allow time for vasoconstrictors to take effect, at least 10 to 15 minutes
      vi. Carefully test injected areas by "light" touch with needle—not dart-like jabs. Make sure patients are well anesthetized prior to procedure

M. Field block: Circumferential injections in superficial and deep planes
1. Avoids distortion of surgical field
2. Prevents possible implantation of cancer cells beyond surgical margins
3. Limits amount of anesthesia required to anesthetize area
4. Paralysis due to anesthesia of motor nerves; prepare patient in advance

N. Nerve block
1. Requires less anesthetic volume and higher concentration such as 2% lidocaine useful

a. Duration of action may be prolonged with use of long-acting agent such as Duranest.

b. Use of vasoconstrictors in blocks does not decrease bleeding at operative site, but does increase duration of anesthetic.

2. Requires greater skill and knowledge of anatomy

3. Allow time for block to take effect—10 minutes minimum

4. Complications of nerve blocks

  a. Laceration of nerve—long-term or permanent anesthesia in area supplied by nerve.

  b. Intravascular injection may lead to acute toxicity.

  c. Nurse should maintain observation of patient following nerve blocks.

  d. Hematoma formation—apply firm pressure for 5 minutes to injection site to avoid hematoma formation resulting from vessel laceration.

  e. Needle breakage usually resulting from attempt to change needle position while in contact with bone.

  f. Infection or abscess—nerve blocks are considered an invasive procedure, maintain sterile technique.

VII. TOPICAL TREATMENTS

A. Balneotherapy

  1. Objectives

    a. Cleansing

    b. Hydration

    c. Enhance delivery of medication

    d. Pain relief

  2. Types of baths

    a. Antibacterial: Potassium permanganate (1:32,000; 1:64,000)

      i. Used for infected eczema, dirty ulcerations, and furunculosis

      ii. Lowers bacterial load

    b. Colloidal: Starch/baking soda and Aveeno colloidal or oilated colloidal

      i. Used for red, pruritic, or oozing conditions

      ii. Soothing; helps relieve pruritus

    c. Emollient: Bath oils

      i. Dry skin conditions

      ii. Cleanse and hydrate

d. Tar: Oils with tar and coal tar concentrate (liquor carbonis detergens)

  i. Scaly dermatoses (psoriasis)

  ii. Relieve pruritus

  iii. Loosen scale

  iv. Potentiate UVB/UVA

e. Paraffin dips

  i. Wax is melted.

  ii. Usually used for hands, arms, and feet

3. Nursing considerations

  a. Average home tub holds 150 to 200 L of water.

  b. Hot water and soap are drying, increasing pruritus; use tepid water and limit soap use.

  c. Pat dry leaving some moisture on the skin.

  d. Apply medication or emollient immediately after patting skin dry.

PATIENT EDUCATION
Balneotherapy

- Use appropriate bath preparation.
- Hot water increases drying and itching; use tepid water to decrease pruritus.
- Bath additives can cause slippery conditions; use rubber mats.

B. Soaks

  1. Objectives

    a. Loosen eschar/crusts

    b. Decrease/prevent infection

    c. Relieve pruritus

    d. Promote drying in moist dermatoses

    e. Enhance re-epithelialization

    f. Decrease pain

  2. Types of soaks (see Table 4-4 for wet dressings)

    a. Tap water

      i. Cooling

      ii. Relieve pruritus

      iii. Loosen eschar/crust

TABLE 4-4 Examples of Wet Dressings

Agent	Strength	Preparation	Germicidal Activity	Astringent Activity	Comments
Normal saline	0.9%	1 tsp to a pint of water	–	–	Inexpensive, easy to prepare
Burow solution (aluminum acetate) Domeboro packets/tablets	5%	Dilute to 1:10–1:40 One packet/table to a pint of water yields a 1:40 solution; two yields a 1:20 solution.	Mild Mild	+ +	
			–		
Silver nitrate	0.1%–0.5%	1 tsp or a 50% stock solution to 1,000 cc yields a 0.25% solution.	Good	+	Stains, can cause pain
Acetic acid (vinegar is 5% acetic acid)	1%–2.5%	Dilute 1:5 with standard 5% household vinegar	Good	+	Odiferous, can be irritating

Adapted from Habif, T. P. (2010). *Clinical dermatology: A color guide to diagnosis and therapy (back inside cover)*. St. Louis, MO: Mosby.

b. Aluminum acetate (Domeboro, Aluwets, Burow solution); one tablet in one quart of water
 i. Cooling
 ii. Relieve pruritus
 iii. Loosen eschar/crust
 iv. Promote drying in moist dermatoses
 v. Provides mild antiseptic effect (mix 1 tablet with 1 pint water)

c. Potassium permanganate ($KMNO_4$): 0.25% to 0.5%
 i. Cooling
 ii. Relieve pruritus
 iii. Loosen eschar/crust
 iv. Provide astringent effect
 v. Provide antimicrobial effect (especially *P. aeruginosa*)

d. Normal saline: 0.9%
 i. Cooling
 ii. Relieve pruritus
 iii. Loosen eschar/crust

e. Silver nitrate ($AgNO_3$): 0.5% to 50% solution
 i. Astringent
 ii. Antibacterial

3. Nursing considerations
 a. Soaks must be kept wet.
 b. Gauze pads with fillers should not be used for soaks (retain too much solution/fibers may be left in wounds).

PATIENT EDUCATION
Soaks

- Understand objective of soak, and if unclear, ask questions.
- Demonstrate mixing of solution (if applicable) and appropriate application technique.

C. Therapeutic shampoos
 1. Objective
  a. Cleansing
  b. Remove accumulated scales, crusts, or medications
  c. Deliver medication
 2. Types of shampoos
  a. Salicylic acid/sulfur
  b. Zinc pyrithione (Denorex, Head and Shoulders)
  c. Surfactants
  d. Tar
  e. Selenium sulfide
  f. Nizoral
 3. Nursing considerations
  a. Avoid scrubbing scalp with fingernails to remove scale.
  b. Allow shampoo to stay on scalp to enhance penetration.
  c. Dryers may increase scaling and pruritus.
  d. Rinsing with a solution of two tablespoons of white vinegar in one gallon of water will help prevent hair from becoming dry.

PATIENT EDUCATION
Therapeutic Shampoos

- Understand the objective of therapy, and if unclear, ask questions.
- Use appropriate technique for therapeutic shampoo.
- Tar shampoos may cause discoloration.

VIII. LASER

A. Definition: Laser is an acronym for light amplification by stimulated emission of radiation. The energy from the laser is directed at the skin, and the majority will be absorbed by chromophores. Lasers produce measurable, repeatable, consistent zones of tissue damage. They can cut, coagulate, and vaporize tissue to some degree.
B. Types: See Tables 4-5, 4-6 through 4-7 for types and indications for use.
C. Nursing considerations
 1. Must have thorough knowledge of laser safety for both patient and health care providers
 2. Written policy and procedures addressing laser safety must be in place, and a laser safety course is highly recommended.
 3. Pre- and posttreatment education is essential.
 4. Photosensitivity may occur after photodynamic therapy, lasting 4 to 6 weeks.
 5. Laser light is damaging to structures of the eye; therefore, safety glasses or goggles that protect against the specific wavelengths used must be worn by both operator and patient.

PATIENT EDUCATION
Laser Treatment

- Understand objective of treatment, risks, side effects, and benefits.
- Understand pre- and posttreatment interventions.
- There is an increased vulnerability of skin; need to avoid environmental stresses including UV radiation.
- Possible need for multiple treatments when indicated.

IX. DERMATOLOGIC SURGERY

A. Shave biopsy: See Diagnostic Options, Chapter 3.
B. Punch biopsy: See Diagnostic Options, Chapter 3.
C. Excisional biopsy: See Diagnostic Options, Chapter 3.
D. Wedge biopsy: See Diagnostic Options, Chapter 3.
E. Mohs: See Chapter 3.
F. Dermabrasion
 1. Definition: The process of planing the superficial layer of epidermis and dermis. The area to be treated may be

TABLE 4-5 Lasers Used to Treat Cutaneous Lesions

Laser Type	Wavelength (nm)	Mode of Output	Clinical Use
Argon (blue–green)	488; 514	Continuous	Vascular and pigmented lesions
Argon-pumped tunable dye (green–yellow–red)	504–690	Continuous	Vascular and pigmented lesions; photodynamic therapy
Flashlamp-pumped pigmented lesion dye (green)	510	Short pulsed	Pigmented lesions; tattoos—epidermal
Copper vapor/bromide (green)	511	Pseudocontinuous	Pigmented lesions—epidermal
Krypton (green)	521; 531	Continuous	Pigmented lesions—epidermal
KTP-potassium titanyl phosphate (green)	532	Pseudocontinuous	Vascular and pigmented lesions
KTP-potassium titanyl phosphate (green)	532	Long pulsed	Vascular and pigmented lesions
Frequency-doubled Q-switched Nd:YAG (green)	532	Pulsed	Vascular and pigmented lesions; tattoos
Krypton (yellow)	568	Continuous	Vascular lesions
Copper vapor/bromide (yellow)	578	Pseudocontinuous	Vascular lesions
Flashlamp-pumped dye (yellow)	585–600	Long pulsed	Vascular lesions, warts, hypertrophic scars, striae
Q-switched ruby (red)	694	Pulsed	Pigmented lesions; tattoos
Q-switched ruby (red)	694	Long pulsed	Hair reduction, pigmented lesions—dermal
Q-switched alexandrite (infrared)	755	Pulsed	Pigmented lesions—epidermal and dermal; tattoos
Alexandrite (infrared)	755	Long	Hair reduction
Diode (infrared)	810	Long pulsed	Hair reduction
Q-switched Nd:YAG (infrared)	1,064	Pulsed	Pigmented lesions—dermal; tattoos
Nd:YAG (infrared)	1,064	Continuous	Deep coagulation of tissue
Nd:YAG (infrared)	1,064	Long pulsed	Hair reduction
Nd:YAG (infrared)	1,320	Pulsed	Nonablative skin resurfacing
Er:YAG (infrared)	2,940	Pulsed	Skin resurfacing
Carbon dioxide (infrared)	10,600	Continuous/pulsed	Tissue cutting; coagulation; vaporization/skin resurfacing

Adapted from Habif, T. P. (2010). *Clinical dermatology: A color guide to diagnosis and therapy (back inside cover)*. St. Louis, MO: Mosby.

anesthetized by injecting local anesthesia or freezing the area with fluoroethyl spray.

2. Indications
   a. Removal of superficial scars, that is, acne scarring
   b. Removal of hyperplastic tissue
   c. Tattoo removal
   d. Rhinophyma
   e. Sun-damaged skin
3. Nursing considerations
   a. Patient expectations may be unrealistic; be clear and direct when informing patient of outcome.
   b. Results are seen slowly.
   c. Discomfort may increase as lesions dry and heal.
   d. Risk of infection due to loss of protective barrier.
   e. Photosensitivity postprocedure.
   f. Edema is common postprocedure; keep head elevated at least 45 degrees during first 24 to 48 hours.
   g. Analgesics may be indicated for postprocedure discomfort.

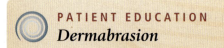

PATIENT EDUCATION
Dermabrasion

- Understand procedure process.
- A thorough understanding of the treatment effects will be paramount to satisfaction; understand the need for follow-up treatments or therapies.
- May use petrolatum to relieve tightness after treatment.
- Keep head elevated for 24 to 48 hours postprocedure to reduce edema.
- Use saline solution for wound cleansing to help reduce edema.
- Monitor for signs of infection, that is, increasing pain, pus, and unusual swelling.
- Use sun protection at all times when outside.
- Take analgesics as directed for discomfort.
- Expect oozing for at least 24 hours.
- Crust will form and will last approximately 1 week.
- Skin may remain red for approximately 2 to 3 months.

TABLE 4-6 Vascular Lesions Treated with Lasers

Laser Type	Clinical Use	Other Considerations
KTP	Telangiectases; thick PWS in adults	Increased risk of scarring
Frequency-doubled Q-switched Nd:YAG	Telangiectases, cherry angioma, capillary hemangioma	Temporary unsightly purpura
Krypton	Telangiectases; thick PWS in adults	Better for large-caliber vascular lesions; increased risk of scarring
Copper vapor	Telangiectases; thick PWS in adults	Better for large-caliber vascular lesions; increased risk of scarring
Flashlamp-pumped dye	Flat PWS and PWS in children; telangiectases	Least risk of scarring; temporary unsightly purpura
Nd:YAG	Deep coagulation of tissue; cavernous hemangioma	Better for deep, large-caliber vascular lesions; increased risk of scarring
	PWS	Angiokeratoma
	Capillary (cutaneous) hemangioma	Adenoma sebaceum
	Cavernous (subcutaneous) hemangioma	Angiolymphoid hyperplasia
	Cherry angioma	Rosacea
	Nevus araneus (spider nevi)	Poikiloderma of Civatte
	Venous lake	Telangiectases
	Glomus tumor	Verrucae
	Kaposi sarcoma	Hypertrophic scars
	Pyogenic granuloma	Striae Some scars

PWS, port-wine stain.
Adapted from Habif, T. P. (2010). *Clinical dermatology: A color guide to diagnosis and therapy (back inside cover)*. St. Louis, MO: Mosby.

TABLE 4-7 Pigmented Lesions Treated with Lasers

Laser Type	Clinical Use		Other Considerations
Argon	Epidermal pigmented lesions		Scarring
Argon	Epidermal pigmented lesions		Scarring
Flashlamp-pumped pigmented lesion dye	Epidermal pigmented lesions; tattoos (red, orange, purple, yellow, tan)		
Copper vapor	Epidermal pigmented lesions		
Krypton	Epidermal pigmented lesions		
KTP	Epidermal pigmented lesions		
Frequency-doubled Q-switched Nd:YAG	Epidermal pigmented lesions; tattoos (red, orange, purple, tan)		
Q-switched ruby	Dermal and epidermal pigmented lesions; tattoos (black, blue, green)		
Q-switched alexandrite	Dermal and epidermal pigmented lesions; tattoos (black, blue, green)		
Q-switched Nd:YAG	Dermal pigmented lesions; tattoos (black, blue)		
Nd:YAG	Dermal pigmented lesions; tattoos (black, blue)		
	Tattoos		
	Dermal pigmented lesions	Nevus of Ota, Becker nevus, Melasma	
	Epidermal pigmented lesions	Solar lentigo, ephilides, epidermal nevus, Café au lait	

Cafe au lait, melasma, and Becker's nevi have variable responses to laser treatment.
Adapted from Habif, T.P. (2016). *Clinical dermatology: A color guide to diagnosis and treatment (6th ed.)*. Philadelphia, PA. Elsevier.
Adapted from Marcus, J., & Goldberg, D. J. (1996). Lasers in dermatology: A nursing perspective. *Dermatology Nursing, 8*(3), 181–195.

X. UNNA'S BOOT

A. Definition: A dressing for venous ulcers consisting of 3- to 4-inch bandage impregnated with calamine–gelatin–zinc oxide paste. It is applied to the leg and produces a semirigid boot.

B. Indications

1. To reduce edema
2. Decrease healing time in stasis ulcers
3. Give support to surgical wounds
4. Protect lesions from manipulation
5. Excellent alternative to elastic wraps particularly for patients who are not self-sufficient
6. Reduction of pain
7. Soothing and antipruritic
8. Acute and chronic tendonitis
9. Ankle sprain, with or without fracture

C. Application

1. Can be applied to legs before arising in the morning to prevent edema.
2. Applied with graduated pressure with greatest pressure at ankle and gradually lessening as wrapped up the leg.
3. Use Unna paste boot gauze.
4. Wash leg with warm water and dry thoroughly.
5. Apply a thin layer of topical medication, when indicated (bacitracin zinc/polymyxin B sulfate ointment).
6. Apply hydrocolloid or hydrogel dressing over ulcer.
7. Begin wrap behind first metatarsal prominence.
8. Wrap, enclosing the heel and being certain there are no wrinkles to cause discomfort, and keep ankle at a right angle.
9. Use only one layer of Kling or Kerlix as an underlayer if desired.
10. When passing over the ulcer, do not allow edge of gauze to lie directly on ulcer; this will cause pain.
11. Continue wrapping proximally, with a 50% overlap with each wrap (Figure 4-14).
12. Be sure that pressure of wrap is greater at ankle, decreasing to knee.

13. Wrap the leg with three layers and stop wrap just below popliteal space.
14. Gently mold the wrap by gently rubbing.
15. Place about 2.5 yards of tube gauze, Kling, Coban, or a stockinette over the form.
16. Have patient secure the gauze at the knee and then begin stretching while rotating the tube gauze form.
17. Relax tension when at the foot, rotating the form once.
18. Push back over the foot rotating toward the knee.
19. Pull tension on loose ends of tube gauze and secure with 2-inch Elastoplast (see Figure 4-15).
20. Fold down and trim loose edges and secure with tape.
21. Unna's boot should remain comfortably in place for 3 to 11 days.

Note: It may be helpful to apply a bland emollient to the unaffected areas of the legs to decrease dryness and pruritus during time boot is in place.

XI. PHOTOPHERESIS

A. Indications

Photopheresis is indicated for the palliative treatment of the skin manifestations of CTCL (Figure 4-16).

B. Overview

1. Photopheresis, or extracorporeal photochemotherapy (ECP), is an FDA-approved therapy for CTCL (see Chapter 6). CTCL is a malignancy of human T lymphocytes (helper T cells). These malignant lymphocytes often target the skin and spend part of their life cycle residing there. This infiltration of malignant cells into the skin can be seen in several variations and ranges. Manifesting various lesions including patch-plaque–type disease, fissures and ulcerations, tumors, and/or a universal erythrodermic scaly version that may cover the entire skin surface.
2. Treatment is determined primarily by the extent of disease, quality of life, age, and comorbidities.
   a. The photopheresis UVAR XTS instrument integrates three main subsystems designed to collect and separate a portion of the patient's blood and to photoactivate the collected WBCs.
   b. In photopheresis, the injectable drug, methoxsalen (UVADEX), is given directly into the reservoir

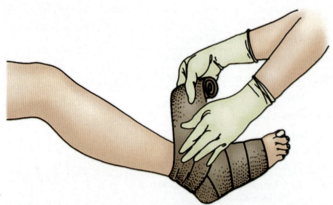

FIGURE 4-14. Unna's boot application. Begin behind first metatarsal prominence and continue wrapping proximally, with a 50% overlap. Be sure that pressure of wrap is greater at ankle, decreasing to knee. Wrap the leg with three layers and stop wrap just below popliteal space. (From Lippincott's Nursing Procedures and Skills, 2007.)

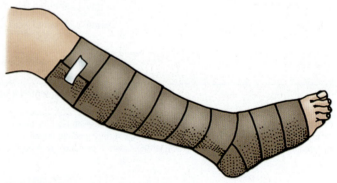

FIGURE 4-15. Completed Unna's boot. (From Lippincott's Nursing Procedures and Skills, 2007.)

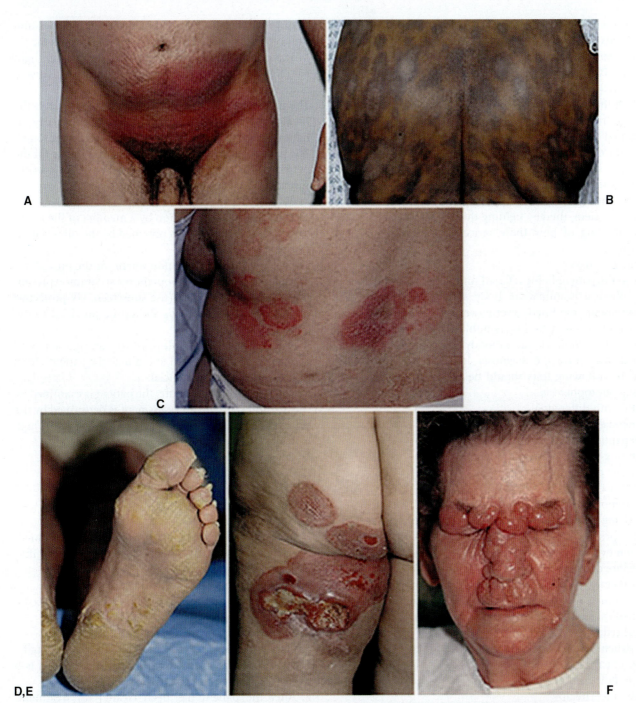

FIGURE 4-16. The cutaneous phases of mycosis fungoides. **A:** Early patch-stage lesions in a sun-protected region. **B:** Hyperpigmented diffuse patches on the back of a dark-skinned patient. **C:** Scattered thin and thick plaques on the back. **D:** Early keratoderma of the sole. **E:** Ulcerated tumor within a plaque on the posterior leg. **F:** Coalescing nodules and tumors with dermal thickening forming "leonine facies" in this patient with transformed cutaneous T-cell lymphoma (CTCL). (From Greer, J. P., et al. (2013). *Wintrobe's clinical hematology.* Philadelphia, PA: Wolters Kluwer.)

collection bag (collected WBCs) just prior to the photoactivation phase.

c. Using a 16- to 17-gauge butterfly needle inserted in the antecubital vein, a portion of blood is removed (300 to 400 mL) and then processed through a centrifuge where the individual components of the blood are separated. Some of the plasma and as many of the white blood cells as can be collected are stored in a reservoir bag.

d. The red blood cells are returned to the patient immediately. The plasma and the white blood cells are then circulated through an ultraviolet light field where the UV light activates the methoxsalen that is now attached to the lymphocytes.

3. How the UVA-activated methoxsalen affects the white blood cells and primarily the malignant T cells found in CTCL is still not completely understood. We do know that the UVA light activates the methoxsalen inside the cell. This leads to cross-linking of the DNA and the death of the cell.

4. Ongoing research also suggests that the methoxsalen combined with UVA may somehow affect the presentation of endogenous antigens on the cell surface. When these treated white blood cells are returned to the patient, it appears that they are now capable of stimulating the patient's previously unresponsive immune system, thereby fighting the disease. The total understanding of how these processes take place is unknown.

C. Pretreatment Workup
1. Prior to the patient being referred for treatment, a complete physical examination, body surface area (BSA) measurement, modified severity-weighted assessment tool (mSWAT), skin biopsy, lymph node biopsy, flow cytometry, or monoclonal antibody test must be performed to confirm the diagnosis. In addition, results from the following tests should be evaluated prior to starting photopheresis.
   a. CBC with differential
   b. Chemistry panel
   c. Hepatitis and HIV screening
   d. Chest x-ray and electrocardiogram
   e. Lactate dehydrogenase
   f. PET or CT scan
2. It is important that the patient is screened for any underlying renal, hepatic, cardiovascular, or infectious disease prior to starting the photopheresis procedure. The removal of close to a unit of blood during the procedure can put the patient at risk for a hypotensive/hypovolemic episode. Therefore, the above tests should be performed and the results evaluated very carefully by the medical staff to ensure that the patient can tolerate the procedure.
3. The patient's disease should be staged by an experienced practitioner, usually a specialized dermatologist or hematologist–oncologist.

D. Orientation to Therapy
1. Prior to starting the actual treatment, the patient should be introduced to the photopheresis nursing staff and undergo an orientation to the unit and its procedures. One of the nurses' most important roles is to be an advocate for the patient.
2. Any interested relatives should be invited to participate with the patient to establish as much support as possible. The Cutaneous Lymphoma Foundation (CLF) was formed in 1998 and is dedicated to supporting people with cutaneous lymphomas. The website is www.clfoundation.org
3. Written material regarding the disease and the procedure should be offered to the patient and copies given to relatives.

4. Additional written instructions regarding policies and unit procedures should be provided for the patient.
5. Written information regarding the ultraviolet light should be presented; precautions should be discussed and provided.
6. The patient should be instructed in how to contact the medical/nursing staff in case of potential emergency situations (fever, pain, bleeding, or other acute symptoms).
7. The primary nurse in charge should also arrange for the patient to meet with the office staff to review health insurance coverage for the procedure.

E. Procedure Information
1. After a thorough explanation by a member of the medical staff, a consent form is obtained by the physician in charge.
2. The patient is given an appointment for the procedure.
3. The patient is reminded about the most common precautions that must be taken (use sunscreen, UV-protective glasses). These instructions should be provided to the patient in writing.
4. A follow-up telephone call prior to starting therapy to review all instructions and to evaluate the patient's level of understanding is beneficial.
5. Prior to the actual procedure, the patient is examined by the medical staff and an assessment is performed by the primary nurse. This assessment includes the following:
   a. Recent medical history
   b. Review of allergies
   c. Review of medications currently being used
   d. Vital signs
   e. Physical exam
   f. A brief review of the recent social history
6. If the patient is cleared, the procedure is performed. After the procedure, the patient may be discharged if:
   a. Vital signs are normal
   b. He/she has no new complaints
   c. He/she has a secured pressure dressing on the needle site
   d. He/she uses appropriate sun protection
   e. He/she is cleared for discharge by the medical staff
7. The photopheresis procedure in most institutions is a 3- to 4-hour outpatient procedure.
   a. After the patient has been cleared for treatment, venous access is obtained using a 16- to 17-gauge intravenous needle.
   b. The preferred access site is one of the large antecubital veins.
   c. In some patients, it can be very difficult to obtain a sufficient access. It might be necessary to insert some type of a central line, similar to those used for chemotherapy or hyperalimentation. This increases the risk for infections in this high-risk group of patients and should be avoided if possible.
   d. The photopheresis UVAR XTS system automatically sets the photoactivation time (light exposure time) based upon the total treatment volume, hematocrit of the treatment volume, and remaining UVA lamp life.

e. During the procedure, the patient will also receive between 500 to 650 mL of 0.9% saline, some mixed with heparin to prevent the blood from clotting as it goes through the instrument. It is also given to maintain the patient's blood volume and to prevent any hypovolemia. Patients who are susceptible to fluid shifts may experience an exacerbation of congestive heart failure symptoms if they cannot tolerate this fluid during treatment.

F. Post-treatment Precautions
  1. Prior to leaving, the patient is instructed as to the following precautions:
    a. Bleeding tendency
      i. Due to the use of heparin as an anticoagulant during the procedure, the patient should be instructed to watch for bleeding immediately after the treatment primarily from the needle site. The amount of heparin used during the treatment is fairly low (between 6,000 and 10,000 units of heparin) and will rarely cause such complications.
      ii. The pressure dressing that is applied to the needle insertion site should remain in place for at least 4 hours. When it is removed, the patient may place an adhesive bandage over the site.
      iii. If any bleeding occurs from the needle site, the patient should be instructed to apply pressure to the site. If the bleeding does not stop within a reasonable period of time, the patient should be instructed to either seek help from his/her local health care provider and emergency room or call 9-1-1 and request help.
    b. Methoxsalen
      i. When using methoxsalen, a drug that causes sensitivity when activated by ultraviolet light, the patient should be instructed in specific precautions (as recommended by the manufacturer).
        a. Sun exposure should be avoided for 24 hours after treatment, and sunscreen should be applied to the skin areas that may be exposed to sunlight.
        b. Protective UV wraparound sunglasses should be worn during daylight for the next 24 hours.
        c. It is recommended by the drug manufacturer that all patients should have an annual eye exam to monitor the effects of the methoxsalen (cataracts).
    c. Additional information
      i. Patient should be instructed that a small fever spike may occur 4 to 6 hours after the treatment. This is a common reaction and there is no cause for alarm. This usually will subside without any need for treatment. If it does persist for longer than 24 hours, patient should notify their provider.
      ii. Patient should be instructed how to avoid potential light-sensitive medications that might interfere with the photopheresis treatment. A list of light-sensitive drugs should be provided and reviewed with the patient and/or significant other.
      iii. Patient and significant others should be informed how to contact the unit staff and/or provider for any emergencies or concerns.

G. Scheduling
  1. The photopheresis treatments are always given on 2 consecutive days every 2 to 4 weeks for 6 months. The physician in charge determines the actual treatment schedule depending on the severity of the patient's condition. As the patient's condition improves, the interval between the treatments may be extended.

H. Adjunctive Therapy
  1. Patients with a partial response to photopheresis can often gain additional improvement if an adjunctive therapy is selected. The physician, together with the patient, will determine when and if any additional therapy is needed. Some of the adjunctive therapies used are the following:
    a. Total skin electron beam therapy (TSEBT) is given to selected skin areas or to the total skin surface and is best used for patients with extensive skin involvement.
    b. Chemotherapeutic agents such as methotrexate, nitrogen mustard, and carmustine
    c. The different interferons can also be used.
    d. Psoralen and ultraviolet A radiation (PUVA) PUVA
    e. Bexarotene (Targretin) (oral or topical)
    f. Noncytotoxic and biologic agents: Corticosteroids (oral or topical), denileukin diftitox, alemtuzumab, and histone deacetylase inhibitors
    g. Allogeneic stem cell transplantation

I. Complications
  1. Photopheresis has been used worldwide since 1987 and was FDA approved in 1988. Presently, no major side effects have been identified. The photopheresis treatment does not appear to suppress the immune system or expose the patient to an increased risk of opportunistic infections or other malignant diseases.
    a. Minor side effects that can occasionally occur:
      i. Hematoma and bleeding from needle site that can be easily treated with pressure dressings and ice packs
      ii. Slight fever spike 4 to 8 hours after reinfusion of the treated cells that usually does not require treatment
      iii. Increased erythema and itching immediately after the treatment. This will most often respond to oral antihistamines
      iv. Hypovolemia/hypotension caused by volume shifts during treatment. In most situations, this can be corrected by infusion of intravenous fluids and positioning the patient in a Trendelenburg position
      v. Nausea from ingestion of 8-MOP
      vi. Catheter-related infection, headache, and chills

J. Response

1. During the initial clinical trials that led to the FDA approval of photopheresis (1984 to 1987), the data showed that approximately 30% of patients treated with photopheresis had an excellent response to the therapy. Thirty percent had some response but might benefit from adjunctive treatments, and 30% showed no response. Recent clinical publications have reported 33% to 88% response rates.

K. Nursing Considerations

1. Evaluation and teaching

   a. It is very important that the patient receives a general medical evaluation prior to starting therapy to exclude any significant medical problems that might be a contraindication to photopheresis (cardiac, renal, hepatic disease, or any infectious disease).

   b. Both the patient and significant others should receive a detailed orientation to the procedure, the unit, and its policies.

      i. The unit coordinator or the primary nurse should meet with the patient and significant others and provide additional verbal information as needed. Make sure that the patient has plenty of opportunities to ask questions.

      ii. If possible, have the patient observe an actual treatment and meet other patients who are receiving therapy.

   c. Allow the patient time to absorb the information given. Do not start treatment on the same day patient is being oriented to the procedure.

   d. Give the patient detailed instructions regarding possible side effects, expectations, and information regarding other forms of therapy that may be needed.

   e. Communicate all test data and results to the patient directly, if the patient has requested this information.

   f. Provide a multidisciplinary approach using all disciplines within the system (medicine, nursing, social work, psychiatry, dietary, and other resources from within the institution as they are needed).

PATIENT EDUCATION

Photopheresis

- Understand the objectives, outcomes, and side effects of treatment, and if unclear, ask questions.
- Expect a fever for a couple of hours after treatment; this is common and usually does not require treatment.
- If you experience increased redness or itching post-treatment, antihistamines help relieve these symptoms.
- Contact your health care provider if you have any vision changes or other unexpected side effects.

BIBLIOGRAPHY

Beckmann, C. R. B., Ling, F. W., Herbert, W. N. P., Laube, D. W., Smith, R. P., Casanova, R., ..., Weiss, P. M. (2014). *Obstetrics and gynecology* (2nd ed.). Philadelphia, PA: Lippincott Williams & Wilkins.

Calderwood, S. B. (2014). Cephalosporins. *UptoDate.* Retrieved from http://www.uptodate.com/contents/cephalosporins?source=preview&language=en-US&anchor=H12&selectedTitle=1~150#H2999961

De Lima, E. L., Salome, G. M., De Brito Rocha, M. J. A., & Ferreira, L. M. (2013). The impact of compression therapy with Unna's boot on the functional status of VLU patients. *Journal of Wound Care*, 22(10), 558–561.

Domino, F. J., Baldor, R. A., Golding, J., Grimes, J. A., & Scott-Taylor, J. (Eds.) (2013). *The 5-minute clinical consult 2013* (21st ed.). Philadelphia, PA: Lippincott Williams & Wilkins.

Edmunds, M. W., & Mayhew, M. S. (2009). *Pharmacology for the primary care provider* (3rd ed.). St. Louis, MO: Mosby.

Ersser, S. J., Maguire, S., Nicol, N., Penzer, R., & Peters, J. (2009). Best practice in emollient therapy: A statement for health care professionals (2nd ed.). *Dermatological Nursing (Supplement)*, 8(3), 1–22.

Frye, R., Myers, M., Axelrod, K. C., Ness, E. A., Piekarz, R. L., Bates, S. E., & Booher, S. (2012). Romidepsin: A new drug for the treatment of cutaneous T-cell lymphoma. *Clinical Journal of Oncology Nursing*, 16(2), 195–204.

Goldstein, A. O., & Goldstein, B. G. (2014a). Cutaneous warts. Retrieved from: http://www.uptodate.com/contents/cutaneous-warts?source=search_result&search=warts&selectedTitle=1%7E21

Goldstein, A. O., & Goldstein, B. G. (2014b). Dermatophyte (tinea) infections. *UptoDate.* Retrieved from: http://www.uptodate.com/contents/dermatophyte-tinea-infections?source=search_result&search=tinea&selectedTitle=1%7E109#H1

Habif, T. P. (2010). *Clinical dermatology: A color guide to diagnosis and therapy.* St. Louis, MO: Mosby

Habif, T. P. (2016). *Clinical dermatology: a Color guide to diagnosis and therapy* (6th ed.). Philadelphia, PA: Elsevier

Habif, T. P., Campbell, J. L., Chapman, M. S., Dinulos, J. G., & Zug, K. A. (2011). *Skin disease and treatment* (3rd ed.). St. Louis, MO: Mosby.

Herhert-Ashton, M., & Clarkson, N. (2008). *Quick look nursing: Pharmacology* (2nd ed.). Burlington, MA: Jones and Bartlett.

Hsu, D. C. (2014). Infiltration of local anesthetics. *UptoDate.* Retrieved from: http://www.uptodate.com/contents/infiltration-of-local-anesthetics?source=search_result&search=anesthetics&selectedTitle=4%7E150#H2694370

Jablonski, N. (2006). *Skin: A natural history.* Los Angeles, CA: UC Press.

Jawed, S. I., Mykowski, P. L., Horowitz, S., Moskowitz, A., & Querfeld, C. (2014a). Primary cutaneous T-cell lymphoma (mycosis fungoides and Sezary syndrome): Part I. Clinical and histopathologic features and new molecular and biologic markers. *Journal of the American Academy of Dermatology*, 70(2), 205-e1–205-e16.

Jawed, S. I., Mykowski, P. L., Horowitz, S., Moskowitz, A., & Querfeld, C. (2014b). Primary cutaneous T-cell lymphoma (mycosis fungoides and Sezary syndrome): Part II. Prognosis, management, and future directions. *Journal of the American Academy of Dermatology*, 70(2), 223-e1–223-e17.

Katsambas, A., & Dessinioti, C. D. (2014). Pityriasis rubra pilaris. Retrieved from: http://www.uptodate.com/contents/pityriasis-rubra-pilaris?source=search_result&search=retinoids&selectedTitle=13%7E150#H427352231

Klein, M. J. (2013). Superficial heat and cold. *Medscape.* Retrieved from: http://emedicine.medscape.com/article/1833084-overview#a01

Kolarsick, P. A., Kolarsick, M. A., & Goodwin, C. (2011). Anatomy and physiology of the skin. *Journal of the Dermatology Nurses Association*, 3(4), 203–213.

Lapolla, W., Yentzer, B.a., Bagel, J., Halvorson, C. R., & Feldman, S., R. (2011). A review of phototherapy protocols for psoriasis treatment. *Journal of the American academy of dermatology*, vol. 64(5), 936–949.

Lansigan, F., & Foss, F. (2010). Current and emerging treatment strategies for cutaneous T-cell lymphoma. *Drugs*, 70(3), 273–286 .

Lee, M., & Kalb, R. E. (2008). Systemic therapy for psoriasis. *Dermatology Nursing, 20*(2), 105–111.

Macksey, L. F. (2011). *Surgical procedures and anesthetic implications: A handbook for nurse anesthesia practice.* Burlington, MA: Jones and Bartlett.

Malamed, S. F. (2013). *Handbook of local anesthesia* (6th ed.). Missouri, MO: Mosby.

McCann, S. A. (2007). Cutaneous T-cell lymphoma: Overview and nursing perspectives. *Nursing Clinics of North America, 42,* 421–455.

Medscape (no author, 2014). Coal tar shampoo. Retrieved from: http://reference.medscape.com/drug/neutrogena-t-gel-original-dhs-tar-coal-tar-shampoo-999365#4

Menter, A.,…Bhushan, R. (2010) Guidelines of care for the management of psoriasis and psoriatic arthritis: Section five. Guidelines of care for the treatment of psoriasis with phototherapy and photochemotherapy. *Journal of the American academy of dermatology,* vol *62*(1), 114–135.

Nicol, N. H. (2005). Use of moisturizers in dermatologic disease: The role of healthcare providers in optimizing treatment outcomes. *Cutis, 76,* 32–33.

Nicol, N. H. (2011). Efficacy and safety considerations in topical treatments for atopic dermatitis. *Pediatric Nursing, 37*(6), 295–302.

Phenniger, J. L., & Fowler, G. C. (2011). *Procedures for primary care* (3rd ed.). St. Louis, MO: Elsevier.

Richards, E.G. & Morison, W. (2014). Psoralen plus ultraviolet A (PUVA) photochemotherapy. Retrieved from: www.uptodate.com/contents/psoralen-plus-ultraviolet-a-puva-photochemotherapy

Schreml, S., Szeimies, R. M., Karrer, S., Heinlin, J., Landthaler, M., & Babilos, P. (2010). The impact of the pH value on skin integrity and cutaneous wound healing. *Journal of the European Academy of Dermatology and Venereology, 24*(4), 373–378.

Talpur, R., Demierre, M. F., Geskin, L., Baron, E., Pugliese, S., Eubank, K., …, Duvic, M. (2011). Multicenter photopheresis intervention trial in early stage mycosis fungoides. *Clinical Lymphoma, Myeloma, & Leukemia, 11*(2), 219–227.

Travers, N. (2013). Overview of laser therapy for common vascular lesion. *Journal of Dermatology Nurses' Association, 5*(5), 280–285.

Ustine, R. P., & Pfenniger, J. L. (2012). *Dermatologic and cosmetic procedures in office practice.* Philadelphia, PA: Saunders.

Vallerand, A. H., Sanoski, C. A., & Deglin, J. H. (2013). *Davis's drug guide for nurses* (13th ed.). Philadelphia, PA: F.A. Davis.

Wheeler, T. (2010). Psoriasis: Impact and management of moderate to severe disease. *British Journal of Nursing, 19*(1), 10–17.

STUDY QUESTIONS

1. Intralesional steroids can be appropriate for patients with:
   a. Psoriasis.
   b. Alopecia areata.
   c. Cystic acne.
   d. Hypertrophic scars.
   e. All of the above.

2. There is a higher risk of burning and blistering with systemic psoralen than with topical application.
   a. True
   b. False

3. Properties of antimetabolites (e.g., 5-fluorouracil) include all of the following *except:*
   a. Interferes with the synthesis of nucleic acids and proteins.
   b. Phase specific; inhibits RNA and DNA synthesis.
   c. Used in treating superficial basal cell carcinomas, multiple actinic leukoplakia, or solar keratosis.
   d. Affects cellular differentiation and proliferation and also down-regulates CCR4 and E-selectin expression, affecting malignant T-cell trafficking to the skin.

4. Side effects of retinoid therapy include:
   a. Erythema and dryness of skin.
   b. Blisters and stinging.
   c. Peeling and edema.
   d. All of the above.

5. Side effects of steroid therapy include all of the following *except:*
   a. Mood changes.
   b. Muscle wasting.
   c. Hypopigmentation/hyperpigmentation.
   d. Alopecia.

6. Local anesthetics block the flow of sodium ions, thereby preventing transmission of the impulse.
   a. True
   b. False

7. Epinephrine has all of the following properties *except:*
   a. Shortens time of onset, prolongs durations, and increases the depth of anesthesia.
   b. Reduces systemic absorption and toxicity by reducing rate of clearance, gaining more effective anesthesia with less drug volume.
   c. Useful with longer-acting anesthetics.
   d. Reduces bleeding during procedure (plain lidocaine is a vasodilator).

8. CNS and cardiovascular reactions with local anesthetics can be managed by injecting quickly to avoid prolonged burning at the injection site.
   a. True
   b. False

9. Cryosurgery is indicated for which of the following conditions?
   a. Thickened seborrheic keratosis.
   b. Molluscum contagiosum.
   c. Psoriasis.
   d. Cutaneous melanoma.

10. Salicylic acid should not be applied to any of the following *except:*
    a. Warts.
    b. Moles.
    c. Birthmarks.
    d. Mucous membranes.

11. Possible side effects of antifungals include:
   a. Overgrowth of fungus when occlusion is used.
   b. Blistering.
   c. Skin irritation.
   d. Overgrowth of fungus when occlusion is used.
   e. All of the above.

12. Antimicrobial activity of the macrolide class of antibiotics includes all of the following *except*:
   a. Pneumococci.
   b. Group A Streptococci.
   c. *Staphylococci aureus* (not methicillin-resistant *S. aureus*).
   d. Gram-positive bacteria only.

13. Isotretinoin is an effective drug for cystic acne, but the following must be considered:
   a. May impair ability to drive.
   b. Must be prescribed and used by providers and patients who have successfully registered in the iPLEDGE program.
   c. Should be taken with caution because it inhibits adrenal gland function.
   d. Patients should increase their intake of vitamin A supplements.

14. Properties of cephalosporins include all of the following *except*:
   a. Rapidly absorbed by the GI tract.
   b. Must be taken with food.
   c. Distributed widely through soft tissue and bodily fluids except CSF.
   d. Oral cephalosporins reach a peak serum concentration level within 1 to 6 hours after administration.

Answers to Study Questions: 1.e, 2.b, 3.d, 4.d, 5.d, 6.a, 7.c, 8.b, 9.b, 10.a, 11.d, 12.d, 13.b, 14.b

CHAPTER 5

Biologic Therapies for Dermatology Conditions

Lakshi M. Aldredge

LEARNING OBJECTIVES

After studying this chapter, the reader will be able to:

- Identify common biologic agents used in the treatment of dermatologic conditions.
- Understand clinical criteria, side effects, and monitoring parameters of biologic agents.
- Counsel patients and other health care providers regarding proper use and side effect monitoring of biologic agents.

KEY POINTS

- Appropriate identification of patients who are candidates for biologic therapy is important. A thorough knowledge of their medical history, current medication profile, and family history of medical conditions must be ensured.
- Patients must be aware of the risks and benefits of biologic therapy including their side effect profile, the need for close monitoring, and consistent follow-up with their dermatology provider.
- Patients need to be appropriately counseled regarding healthy lifestyle modifications in order to ensure successful outcomes with their biologics, including smoking cessation, appropriate immunization practices, and diet and weight control.

I. OVERVIEW

Biologic agents (biologic response modifiers) are protein-based drugs targeting specific inflammatory immune mediators that contribute to the development of cutaneous and systemic disorders. They are the newest therapeutic modalities used to treat dermatologic and other conditions. These agents are derived from biologic synthesis using living cells rather than a chemical process.

Because they are large protein molecules, there are no oral biologic agents and they must, therefore, be administered either subcutaneously or intravenously. Biologics tend to initiate a significant therapeutic response within a relatively short time period and are highly efficacious, often providing 50% to 75% improvement in most patients. Because they

target specific immune markers, such as cytokines, enzymes, and growth factors, they are considered less likely to cause end-organ toxicity as compared to traditional systemic agents, such as methotrexate and cyclosporine. However, due to their immune-modifying ability, some agents may be associated with increased risk of infection and malignancy as well as other side effects. Biologic agents have also been associated with the development of antidrug antibodies, which may inhibit long-term use. Patients should be carefully screened in order to determine if they are an appropriate candidate for biologic therapy because of the aforementioned risks.

Most patients find biologic agents convenient to use and well tolerated compared with other therapies, such as conventional systemics and phototherapy. They are an expensive alternate to conventional systemic agents and most insurance carriers require failure of one or more traditional therapies prior to authorization of a biologic. Traditionally approved for use in psoriatic disease, biologics are now being studied in other challenging dermatology conditions. As researchers and scientists continue to discover new immune-mediated therapeutic targets for dermatologic conditions, newer biologic agents are being developed that will continue to significantly impact the way in which dermatologic conditions are managed in the near future.

II. BIOLOGICS IN TREATMENT OF PSORIASIS

A. Overview
1. Psoriasis is a common autoimmune inflammatory disorder characterized by hyperproliferation of keratinocytes resulting in thickened, scaling plaques and may be accompanied by inflammation and destruction of joints and enthesis (areas where tendons/ligaments bind to bone). It is associated with numerous comorbidities including cardiovascular disease, metabolic disorders, and psychosocial conditions. In addition to the physical symptoms associated with psoriasis, this complex condition can result in significant impairment in patients' quality of life (see Chapter 8).
2. The pathogenesis of psoriasis is highly complex, and while the exact cause is unknown, it is thought to be

a T-cell–mediated disease involving the production of inflammatory cytokines such as tumor necrosis factor (TNF), interleukins (IL-23, IL-17), and other mediators. There is no cure for psoriasis, although research in the past two decades has helped to identify immunological pathways that lead to psoriatic disease development and progression. The therapies focusing on these immunological pathways are known as biologics.

3. The first biologic agent approved for psoriasis by the U.S. Food and Drug Administration (FDA) was alefacept in 2003. The company took it off the market in 2011. In the United States, there are currently four biologic agents approved for psoriasis: adalimumab,

etanercept, infliximab, and ustekinumab. These four biologic agents used in the treatment of psoriasis are summarized in Table 5-1. Adalimumab, etanercept, and infliximab are TNF-alpha inhibitors, and ustekinumab is an IL-12/IL-23 blocker.

4. Patient education for patients with psoriasis considering the use of these biologic agents is essential. Important points to emphasize are noted in Box 5-1.

B. TNF-alpha (TNF-α) blockers
  1. Overview
    a. TNF-α blockers are the most common biologics used in the treatment of psoriasis and psoriatic arthritis worldwide.

TABLE 5-1 Biologic Agents for Psoriasis

Agent	Mechanism of Action	Dosing	Screening	Efficacy	Side Effects
Adalimumab (Humira)	TNF-α inhibitor	80 mg SC week 0, then 40 mg 7 days later, then 40 mg every other week	Baseline: Hepatitis B, TB, CBC, LFTs, and chemistry panel Annual: TB Periodic CBC, LFTs, and chemistry panels as warranted	53%–80% of patients achieved PASI 75 with doses of 40 mg every other week and 40 mg every week, respectively	Common: Injection site reactions, URI, headache, and fatigue. Rare: Serious infection including TB, malignancy, hepatitis B reactivation, development of positive antinuclear antibodies, development of lupus-like syndrome anaphylaxis, and new-onset demyelinating disease
Etanercept (Enbrel)	TNF-α inhibitor	50 mg SC twice a week × 3 months, then 50 mg every week	Baseline: Hepatitis B, TB, CBC, LFTs, and chemistry panel Annual: TB Periodic CBC, LFTs, and chemistry panels as warranted	Approximately 30% of patients treated with 25 mg BIW achieved PASI 75 after 12 weeks. 50% of patients treated with 50 mg BIW achieved PASI 75	Common: Injection site reactions, URI, headache, and fatigue. Rare: Serious infection including TB, malignancy, hepatitis B reactivation, new-onset or worsening CHF, pancytopenia, development of positive antinuclear antibodies, development of lupus-like syndrome anaphylaxis, and new-onset demyelinating disease
Infliximab (Remicade)	TNF-α inhibitor	5 mg/kg IV infusion weeks 0, 2, and 6 and then every 8 weeks	Baseline: Hepatitis B, TB, CBC, LFTs, and chemistry panel Annual: TB Periodic CBC, LFTs, and chemistry panels as warranted	75% of patients receiving 5 mg/kg achieved a PASI 75 at week 10	Common: URI, headache, and fatigue Rare: Acute infusion site reactions, delayed hypersensitivity reaction (myalgia, arthralgia, fever, rash, pruritus, edema, dysphagia, urticaria, sore throat, headache), serious infection including TB, malignancy, hepatitis B reactivation, new-onset or worsening CHF, pancytopenia, development of positive antinuclear antibodies, development of lupus-like syndrome anaphylaxis, and new-onset demyelinating disease
Ustekinumab (Stelara)	Blocks the p40 subunit of IL-12/IL-23	45 mg (patients <100 kg) and 90 mg (patients over 100 kg) weeks 0 and 4 and then every 12 weeks thereafter	Baseline: TB Can consider CBC, LFTs, and chemistry panel Annual: TB Periodic CBC, LFTs, and chemistry panels as warranted	45 mg dosing: 65% of patients achieved PASI 75. 90 mg dosing: 76% of patients achieved PASI 75	No clear side effect patterns emerged in clinical trials. However, there is a risk for injection site reactions, and because it targets the immune system, there is a theoretical risk of serious infection and malignancy. There is one reported case of posterior leukoencephalopathy syndrome
Secukinumab (Cosentyx)	IL-17A agonist	150 or 300 mg SC Week 0, 1, 2, 3, 4 and then every 4 weeks thereafter	Baseline: TB Can consider CBC, LFTs, chemistry panel Annual: TB Periodic CBC, LFTs, chemistry panels as warranted	150 mg dosing: 71.6% of patients achieved PASI 75 at week 12 300 mg dosing: 81.6% of patients achieved PASI 75 at week 12	No clear side effect patterns emerged in clinical trials. There was an increase in Crohn disease exacerbations during clinical trials, and as such, secukinumab should be used cautiously in this population. Because it targets the immune system, there is a *theoretical* risk of increased risk of infection and malignancy.

TNF-α, tumor necrosis factor alpha; CBC, complete blood count; TB, tuberculosis.

BOX 5-1. Use of Biologic Agents in Psoriasis: Patient Screening, Education, and Monitoring

Patients should be advised that as there is no cure for psoriasis, treatment with biologic agents must be consistent and ongoing.

Biologics used for psoriasis seem to be well tolerated with minimal side effects, but they should still be considered immunosuppressive and therefore used cautiously.

All patients should be carefully screened for history of serious infections and malignancies prior to initiating any biologic therapy. If considering a TNF-α blocker, patients should also be screened for history of hepatitis B, CHF, and demyelinating conditions.

Patients undergoing biologic therapy require baseline and annual TB screening.

Adherence with the prescribed dosing regimen is essential and patients should be advised to avoid skipping doses or "stockpiling" medications.

Etanercept, adalimumab, and ustekinumab may be self-administered and should be stored appropriately. After injection, pens or syringes should be disposed in approved sharps containers.

Patients should refrain from taking their biologic agent should they develop any significant health changes, specifically signs and symptoms of infection (fevers, chills, nausea, vomiting, abdominal pain, diarrhea, wounds that fail to heal) or other health changes including weight loss, loss of appetite, significant fatigue, persistent headache, vision changes, and loss of large muscle strength.

No live vaccinations should be given during biologic therapy. Live vaccinations should be given at least 4 weeks prior to starting a biologic drug. If a live vaccine is warranted after biologic therapy is initiated (for travel or for age-specific conditions), patients should be advised to hold dosing for at least 4 weeks prior to administration of vaccine and resume therapy 4 weeks postvaccination.

If patients have injection site reactions, they can apply ice to the injection site prior to injection, as well as postinjection. Anti-inflammatory medications can be taken as needed for mild symptoms.

Injection sites should be rotated and monitored for signs and symptoms of infection.

b. Infliximab and adalimumab are anti-TNF monoclonal antibodies, whereas etanercept is a human TNF receptor fusion protein. These agents bind to soluble and transmembrane forms of TNF, disrupting inflammatory cascade resulting in skin and joint disease, in the case of psoriasis.

c. Adalimumab and etanercept are subcutaneous injections that can be administered by the patient. Infliximab is an intravenous infusion that is usually administered in an infusion center.

2. FDA-approved indications in dermatology
  a. Adalimumab, etanercept, and infliximab are approved for adult patients with moderate-to-severe plaque psoriasis and should be considered first-line therapy according to psoriasis treatment guidelines recommended by the American Academy of Dermatology (AAD).

3. Screening
  a. Patients should be thoroughly screened for current or past history of serious infection (including tuberculosis [TB]), malignancy, history of heart failure, personal or family history of demyelinating conditions, and hepatitis B.
  b. While there are no standardized guidelines for laboratory monitoring of any biologic agents, most experts recommend baseline labs to include complete blood count (CBC), metabolic panel including liver function tests, screening for hepatitis B core antibody, hepatitis B surface antibody, and hepatitis B surface antigen. TB screening can be done with either PPD skin testing or QuantiFERON Gold serum testing. Ongoing labs should be done every 3 to 6 months in the first 2 years of treatment and at least annually thereafter as indicated by the patient's health status.

C. IL-12 and IL-23 blockers
  1. Overview
    a. Ustekinumab is a fully human monoclonal antibody, which binds with high affinity and specificity to the subunit p40, which is common to both IL-12 and IL-23. Increased levels of IL-23 have been detected in psoriasis plaques and have also been shown to induce psoriasis-like disease in mice.
    b. Ustekinumab is highly efficacious providing significant clearance in most patients, and 5-year trial data have indicated a favorable safety profile.
    c. The dosing schedule of a single injection at week 0, week 4, and every 12 weeks following is highly appealing to patients.
  2. FDA-approved indications in dermatology
    a. Infliximab is approved for adult patients with moderate-to-severe plaque psoriasis and should be considered first-line therapy according to psoriasis treatment guidelines recommended by the AAD. Unfortunately, many insurance companies require patients to have failed at least one TNF-α blocker prior to approval of ustekinumab, despite its more convenient dosing schedule (Table 5-1) and long-term favorable safety data.
  3. Screening
    a. Patients should be thoroughly screened for current or past history of serious infection (including TB), malignancy, and any immunosuppressive conditions.
    b. While there are no standardized guidelines for laboratory monitoring of any biologic agents including ustekinumab, most experts recommend baseline labs to include CBC and TB screening with either PPD skin testing or QuantiFERON Gold serum testing. Repeat CBC should be considered every 3 to 6 months in the first 2 years of treatment and annually thereafter as indicated by the patient's health status.

D. IL-17 Agonist
  1. Overview
    a. IL-17A is considered to be a central target in the pathogenesis of psoriasis as it stimulates keratinocytes, and other cells, to secrete numerous

proinflammatory mediators that play a role in the development of psoriatic disease. IL-17A is a primary effector of Th17 cells that is believed to be a central pathway of numerous inflammatory disorders, including psoriasis.

b. Secukinumab is the first FDA-approved IL-17A agonist indicated for the treatment of moderate-to-severe plaque psoriasis. Clinical trials of secukinumab in psoriasis demonstrated high efficacy with a favorable safety profile.

c. The recommended dosing for secukinumab is 300 mg; however, 150 mg can be used although clinical trials demonstrated slightly inferior efficacy (81.6% vs. 71.6%, respectively). The subcutaneous injection is given at weeks 0, 1, 2, 3, and 4 and every 4 weeks thereafter.

2. FDA-approved indications in dermatology
   a. Secukinumab is approved for adult patients with moderate-to-severe plaque psoriasis and psoriatic arthritis. Because it is the newest biologic agent approved for psoriasis, most insurance companies require failure of conventional systemic therapy or other biologic agents.

3. Screening
   a. Patients should be thoroughly screened for current or past history of serious infection (including TB), malignancy, and any immunosuppressive conditions. Patients with a history of Crohn disease should receive consideration prior to secukinumab therapy as these patients were noted to have an increase in Crohn's exacerbations while undergoing treatment in secukinumab clinical trials.
   b. While there are no standardized guidelines for laboratory monitoring of any biologic agents including secukinumab, most experts recommend baseline labs to include complete blood count (CBC), and TB screening with either PPD skin testing or QuantiFERON gold serum testing should also occur annually. Repeat CBC should be considered every 3 to 6 months in the first 2 years of treatment and annually thereafter as indicated by the patient's health status.

E. Biologics and pregnancy
   1. Pregnancy category
      a. All biologic agents are Pregnancy Category B, meaning animal studies have failed to demonstrate a risk to the fetus, and there are no adequate and well-controlled studies in pregnant women.
   2. Safety considerations
      a. Psoriasis can confer independent risks during pregnancy including increased risk of spontaneous abortion, placenta previa, ectopic pregnancy, and preeclampsia.
      b. Patients should be counseled regarding the risks and benefits of initiating or continuing biologic therapy during pregnancy. Consultation with the patient's obstetrician is strongly recommended in order to arrive upon a mutually agreeable treatment plan during pregnancy.

c. The National Psoriasis Foundation (NPF) recommends that biologic agents should only be used if there is a clear medical need. TNF-α inhibitors may be used with caution in the second and third trimesters.

III. RITUXIMAB

A. Overview
   1. Rituximab is a monoclonal antibody and an antineoplastic agent whose primary mode of action is through the depletion of CD20+ B cells.
   2. FDA-approved indications in dermatology
      a. Rituximab is approved for non-Hodgkin lymphoma (B cell, follicular, CD20 positive) in combination with first-line chemotherapy and can be used as a single agent for disease maintenance.
      b. Wegener granulomatosis, in combination with glucocorticoids.
   3. Screening
      a. Rituximab is contraindicated in patients with known anaphylaxis or IgE hypersensitivity to murine proteins or other components of the rituximab. It is also contraindicated in patients with hypotension, bronchospasm, and angioedema. It should be used cautiously in patients with active infections.
      b. Patient's should be screened for underlying cardiac disorders, particularly hypertension, angina, or arrhythmias. Health care providers should consider withholding scheduled antihypertensive medications for 12 hours before infusing rituximab in order to avoid enhanced hypotensive effects. Frequent blood pressure monitoring is critical during the first dose of rituximab.
      c. Rituximab is Pregnancy Category C, and there are no human or animal studies including pregnant women. It should only be used if the risks outweigh the benefits and if there is a clear clinical need.

IV. NON–FDA-APPROVED USES OF BIOLOGIC AGENTS

A. Eczematous disorders
   1. Atopic dermatitis is a common inflammatory skin disease whose pathogenesis involves both immune dysregulation and disruption in the epidermal barrier. Numerous biologic agents have been tested in this disease state including TNF-α blockers (etanercept and infliximab), and while clinical improvement has been demonstrated, sustained clinical response has been lacking, although there are two cases in which etanercept maintained disease clearance.
   2. Inflammatory dermal diseases
      a. TNF-α has been identified as playing a definitive role in the pathogenesis of sarcoid. Subsequently, TNF-α blockers have been used in the treatment of this disease state with some success (adalimumab and infliximab had greater efficacy than etanercept). It is important to note, however, that numerous case reports identify TNF-α as a trigger for sarcoid as well.
      b. TNF-α has also been identified as playing a definitive role in the pathogenesis of granuloma annulare

(GA) being treated with TNF-α blockers successfully. Adalimumab and infliximab have demonstrated efficacy in treating GA (in its disseminated form, primarily), while etanercept has shown both success and failure, although there have been no randomized controlled trials for this condition with TNF-α inhibitors.

c. Necrobiosis lipoidica has also shown responsiveness to TNF-α blockers, although the case reports are sparse.

3. Neutrophilic dermatoses

a. Biologics have been used in the treatment of pyoderma gangrenosum, with a small study of 30 patients showing significant improvement with infliximab as well as other reported cases. Other studies have shown variable treatment success with adalimumab and etanercept in this difficult, ulcerating disease. IL-23 has been demonstrated to be elevated in PG lesions, and one case report demonstrated complete ulcer healing with ustekinumab.

b. TNF-α levels have been shown to be increased in Sweet syndrome; however, due to the concern of underlying malignancy in this disease state, there have been concerns about utilizing this class of drugs for treatment. There have been at least two case reports demonstrating efficacy in treating Sweet syndrome.

4. Autoimmune bullous skin diseases

a. Bullous pemphigoid and pemphigus vulgaris (along with other pemphigus-related disorders) have demonstrated responsiveness to both TNF-α blockers and ustekinumab. As with the inflammatory and neutrophilic dermatoses, numerous cytokines, including TNF-α, have been shown to play a role in disease activity. In the unfortunate patients having concomitant psoriatic disease and bullous disease, case reports have demonstrated resolution of both conditions with etanercept, and in one case, ustekinumab. Etanercept has been the most often used biologic agent in patients with these disorders; however, there have also been reports of the development of pemphigoid and pemphigus in patients being treated with TNF-α blockers for other conditions, such as psoriasis.

b. Rituximab has been used in both pemphigoid and pemphigus, with greater success in pemphigus-related diseases. In fact, it should be considered as a steroid-sparing agent in the treatment of pemphigus vulgaris.

5. Connective tissue disorders

a. Systemic lupus erythematosus can be a treatment challenge. Both TNF-α blockers and rituximab have been shown to be successful in the management of this complex disease.

b. Some case reports of generalized morphea (scleroderma) treated with infliximab have been hopeful. There is a study which failed to show clinically significant improvement with infliximab. Many patients in the same study also experienced significant side effects.

c. Dermatomyositis has been successfully treated with infliximab, although the case reports are few. In contrast, there is a report of a dermatomyositis patient who developed sepsis and then lymphoma after an infliximab infusion.

6. Disorders of follicular occlusion

a. Hidradenitis suppurativa (HS) is an incredibly difficult condition to treat and can be both physically and psychologically debilitating. TNF-α levels have been demonstrated to be elevated in HS, and there are numerous case reports and small studies demonstrating efficacy in the treatment of HS with all the biologic agents. The earliest case reports utilized infliximab, while the most recent phase 2 clinical trials (with the largest number of HS patients) showed significant improvement with adalimumab. Etanercept has also been shown to be efficacious, but the studies were with smaller numbers of patients. While all agents are useful in treating this challenging disease, infliximab may demonstrate earlier onset of symptom and disease improvement.

7. Other disorders

a. There are numerous other dermatologic conditions in which biologics have been used, including pityriasis rubra pilaris, graft versus host disease, urticaria, and others.

b. While it is beyond the scope of this chapter to review all of these conditions, it is important to understand the role of biologic agents in the treatment paradigm of all dermatoses and the promise they hold for disease management.

BIBLIOGRAPHY

Castelo-Soccio, L., & van Vorhees, A. S. (2009). Long-term efficacy of biologics in dermatology. *Dermatologic Therapy, 22,* 22–33.

Graves, J. E., Nunley, K., & Heffernan, M. P. (2007). Off-label uses of biologics in dermatology: Rituximab, omalizumab, infliximab, etanercept, adalimumab, efalizumab and alefacept (Part 2 of 2). *Journal of the American Academy of Dermatology, 56*(1), e55–e79.

Guttman-Yassky, E., Dhingra, N., & Leung, D. Y. (2013). New era of biologic therapeutics in atopic dermatitis. *Expert Opinion on Biological Therapy, 13*(4), 549–561. Retrieved from http://informahealthcare.com/doi/abs/10.1517/14712598.2013.758708?journalCode=ebt

Han, G. (2014). Biologics in dermatology and beyond. *Cutis, 93.* Retrieved from www.cutis.com

Kimball, A. B., Gladman, D., Gelfand, J. M., Gordon, K., Horn, E. J., Korman, N. J., …, National Psoriasis Foundation. (2008). National Psoriasis Foundation clinical consensus on psoriasis co morbidities and recommendations for screening. *Journal of the American Academy of Dermatology, 58*(6), 1031–1042.

Langley, R. G., Elewski, B. E., Lebwohl, M., et al. (2014). Secukinumab in plaque psoriasis: results of two phase 3 trials. *The New England Journal of Medicine, 371,* 326–338. DOI: 10.1056/NEJMoa1314258.

Lima, S. T., Seidler, E. M., Lima, H. C., & Kimball, A. B. (2009). Long-term safety of biologics in dermatology. *Dermatologic Therapy, 22,* 2–21.

Menter, A., Gottlieb, A., Feldman, S. R., et al. (2008). Guidelines of care for the management of psoriasis and psoriatic arthritis. *Journal of the American Academy of Dermatology, 58*(5), 826–850.

Narahari, B. S., & Feldman, S. R. (2012). Biologics 101. *The Dermatologist, 20*(2). Retrieved from http://www.the-dermatologist.com/content/biologics-101

National Psoriasis Foundation. Moderate to severe psoriasis and psoriatic arthritis: Biologic drugs. Retrieved from http://www.psoriasis.org/about-psoriasis/treatments/biologics

Prussick, R., & Prussick, L. (2013). Biologic therapies for 2013: Do we use them enough? *Practical Dermatology*. Retrieved from http://practicaldermatology.com/2013/02/biologic-therapies-for-2013-do-we-use-them-enough

Santoro, F. A., Rothe, M. J., & Strober, B. E. (2012). Ethical considerations when prescribing biologics in dermatology. *Clinics in Dermatology, 30*, 492–495.

Van de Kerkhof, P. C. M., & Schalkwijk, J. (2008). Psoriasis. In J. L. Bolognia, J. L. Jorizzo, R. P. Rapini (Eds.), *Dermatology* (2nd ed., pp. 115–135). Spain: Mosby Elsevier.

STUDY QUESTIONS

1. Which of the following biologic therapies is *not* considered a TNF-α inhibitor?
   a. Infliximab
   b. Etanercept
   c. Ustekinumab
   d. Adalimumab

2. Baseline screening for *all* patients prior to initiating a biologic agent must include:
   a. Chest x-ray
   b. C-reactive protein
   c. TB screening
   d. Hepatitis B screening

3. Women of childbearing age and pregnant women should be counseled regarding the risks and benefits of biologic therapy for the treatment of psoriasis. The biologics approved for the treatment of plaque psoriasis are FDA Pregnancy Category:
   a. C
   b. A
   c. D
   d. B

4. Rituximab is a biologic agent whose primary mechanism of action is:
   a. Blocking of IL-12 and IL-23
   b. Depletion of CD20+ B cells
   c. Depletion of CD4+ T cells
   d. Targeted blocking of TNF-α

5. Long-term use of biologic therapy has been associated with:
   a. Serious infection and serum sickness
   b. Weight loss and loss of appetite
   c. Recurrent minor infections
   d. Development of antinuclear antibodies to drug

Answers to Study Questions: 1.c, 2.c, 3.d, 4.b, 5.a

CHAPTER 6

Phototherapy

Cynthia Rena Heaton • Margaret Hirsch • Angela Hamilton

LEARNING OBJECTIVES

After studying this chapter, the reader will be able to:

- Identify skin disorders that would be appropriate for phototherapy and desired outcomes.
- Describe the differences between ultraviolet radiation A (UVA) and ultraviolet radiation B (UVB) light.
- Identify the different types of lights and metering equipment.
- Describe the different protocols for UVA and UVB therapy.
- Identify the appropriate patients for the different therapies.
- Describe the different ways to manage side effects of phototherapy.
- Understand the purpose of shielding and ways to shield.
- Understand the importance of proper use of topical therapy in combination with phototherapy.
- Counsel patients that each individual responds differently to phototherapy.
- Counsel patients regarding proper and safe care during phototherapy.

KEY POINTS

- Phototherapy is an important health care intervention and should be administered with the same precautions as a drug using specialized equipment. A prescription is needed before a treatment is given.
- Patient education regarding the importance of home care, protecting against extra ultraviolet light, and consistency of treatments are the keys to success.
- The maximum amount of ultraviolet light a patient can receive is measured by risk versus benefit and quality of life.
- Documentation of patient education, treatments, and missed treatments is required, as well as patient concerns.
- Multiple regulations and guidelines must be considered including state and federal guidelines, Centers for Disease Control, Food and Drug Administration, Joint Commission, and manufacturer recommendations and guidelines.
- Treatments are determined by the prescriber, previous dose given, patient response to previous dose, and unit lamp output.
- Understand that when switching from UVA to UVB, there is no crossover protection.

I. OVERVIEW

Phototherapy is the exposure of nonionizing radiation for therapeutic benefit; ultraviolet light (UVL) is not visible and is classified by wavelength—UVC, UVB, and UVA; UVB and UVA are used in treating dermatologic diseases. Phototherapy is the use of UVL to clear skin diseases. This is also referred to as *photomedicine*. Phototherapy is prescribed by dermatologists and other physicians, nurse practitioners, and/or physician assistants.

A. Evolution of phototherapy
1. Broadband (BB) UVB—first used in the 1920s (290 to 320 nm).
2. Full-body cabinets—first used in the 1970s.
3. Narrowband (NB) UVB—first used in the 1980s (311 to 313 nm).
4. Psoralen plus UVA (PUVA) gets Food and Drug Administration (FDA) approval in 1982 (320 to 400 nm).
5. Ultraviolet A1 (UA1), the long-wavelength band of UVA—first used in the 2000s (340 to 400 nm).

B. Ultraviolet light (Figure 6-1)
1. Phototherapy terms
   a. Wavelength—the distance measured along the wave from any given point to the next similar point, as from crest to crest (peaks).
   b. Nanometer (nm)—the unit of measurement used to describe the distance between wavelengths. One billion nanometers equals 1 m or 39.37 inches.
   c. Photons—the energy emitted from the UVL wavelength.
   d. Joules (J)—the dosing unit for UVA. One joule equals 1,000 millijoules.
   e. Millijoules (mJ)—the dosing unit for UVB.

C. Facts about UVL
1. Longer wavelengths produce fewer photons, resulting in less energy.
2. Shorter wavelengths produce more photons, resulting in more energy.
3. UVL can do one of three things. It can be reflected, transmitted, or absorbed. When UVL is absorbed, photons activate specific cells in the dermis and epidermis called chromophores, resulting in a biological response.
4. Most natural sunlight exposure occurs in the first 18 to 20 years of life, and phototherapy adds to total lifetime accumulation. Overexposure to UVL increases the risk of skin damage. Therefore, risks versus benefits of therapy must be considered.

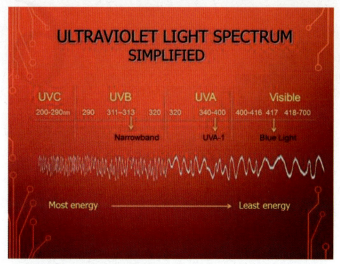

FIGURE 6-1. UVL spectrum.

5. UVL's therapeutic physiological effects are immune function manipulation, decreased DNA synthesis, and selective cytotoxicity.

D. Common diseases treated with phototherapy

The most common dermatological diseases treated with phototherapy are psoriasis, vitiligo, various types of dermatitis, and cutaneous T-cell lymphoma (CTCL). The goals of phototherapy are different depending on the disease being treated (Table 6-1).

1. Psoriasis: goal is to depress the immune system and slow down T-cell activity, which will then result in thinning of plaques, decreased pruritus, decreased scaling, and induction of remission.

TABLE 6-1 Photoresponsive Diseases

Photoresponsive Diseases	BB-UVB	NB-UVB	UVA	UVA-1	PUVA
Alopecia					X
Atopic dermatitis/other eczemas	X	X	X	X	X
Folliculitis	X	X	X		X
Graft vs. host disease				X	X
Granuloma annulare		X		X	X
IRBD ("itchy red bump disease")	X	X	X		X
Lichen planus		X			X
Localized scleroderma				X	
Mycosis fungoides (CTCL)	X	X		X	X
Parapsoriasis	X	X	X		X
Photosensitivity	X	X	X		X
Pityriasis rosea	X	X			
Prurigo, pruritus				X	
Psoriasis	X	X	X		X
Uremic pruritus	X	X	X		
Urticaria pigmentosa				X	
Vitiligo		X			X

BB, broadband; NB, narrowband; UVA, ultraviolet A; UVB, ultraviolet B; PUVA, methoxsalen + ultraviolet A.

2. Vitiligo: goal is repigmentation, which will occur in 50% to 80% of patients.
3. Dermatitis: goal is to depress the immune system resulting in elimination or reduction of pruritus. Improvement of the rash is secondary. This group includes atopic dermatitis, eczema, folliculitis, IRBD or papular dermatitis, and lichen planus.
4. CTCL: goal is to slow the systemic progression of the disease as evidenced by flattening of plaques and normalization of skin pigmentation.

II. PHOTOTHERAPY

UVL waves found in sunlight have a therapeutic effect. The types of UVL used to treat skin diseases are UVB and UVA (Figure 6-2).

A. UVB

UVB is referred to as the sunburn ray. It is 1,000 times more capable of producing erythema than UVA and is dosed in millijoules (mJ). It has shallow penetration into the epidermis, takes a short time to develop erythema (4 to 6 hours), and the erythema resolves quickly (18 to 24 hours). Skin protection against UVB is referred to as hyperplasia, thickening of the top layer of skin.

1. Broadband UVB (BB-UVB) wavelength 290 to 320 nm
   a. Must wear goggles, as corneal burns can occur (Figure 6-3).
   b. Sunburning spectrum of light, therefore potentially the most damaging.
   c. Potential carcinogenesis following long-term exposure.
   d. No medications needed as epidermis has sufficient chromophores to absorb UVB. When phototherapy truly indicated in pregnant women, UVB is frequently the type chosen because no additional medications are used with this treatment.
2. Excimer laser UVB–wave length of 308 nm.
   a. Treatment twice a week.
   b. Emits light that is monochromatic and coherent.
   c. Handheld device with a fiber-optic arm allows for targeted application of light while avoiding unaffected skin.
   d. Uses a spot diameter of 14 to 30 mm.

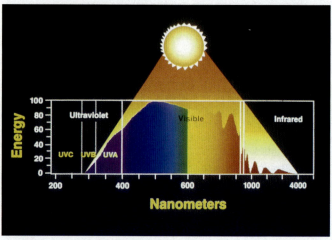

FIGURE 6-2. Energy of UVL.

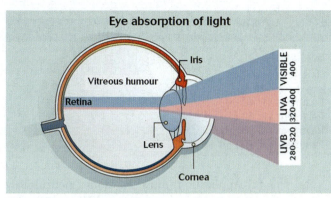

FIGURE 6-3. Eye light absorption.

TABLE 6-3 Comparison of Ultraviolet B Narrowband and Broadband Protocols

Skin Type	Broadband	Narrowband (NBC protocol)
I	10 mJ	120 mJ
II	20 mJ	220 mJ
III	30 mJ	260 mJ
IV	40 mJ	330 mJ
V	50 mJ	350 mJ
VI	60 mJ	400 mJ

3. Narrowband UVB (NB-UVB) wavelength of 311 to 313 nm.
   a. Clears lesions faster than BB-UVB.
   b. Fewer treatments necessary.
   c. Treatment Schedule.
      (1) Clearing phase: three to five treatments per week until disease clears.
      (2) Maintenance phase: every 9 to 11 days to maintain clearance.
4. Indications (BB-UVB and NB-UVB).
   a. Treatment of photosensitive dermatoses.
   b. Pregnant women and children may be treated since there are no drugs needed for UVB to be effective.
   c. Used for patients with UVA contraindications, such as previous arsenic or x-ray therapy.
5. Absolute contraindications (BB-UVB and NB-UVB).
   a. Xeroderma pigmentosum
   b. Albinism
   c. Porphyria
6. Relative contraindications (BB-UVB and NB-UVB).
   a. Can exacerbate photodermatoses.
   b. Previous nonmelanoma skin cancers or family history of melanoma.
   c. Inability of patient to stand due to physical limitations.

   d. Noncompliance with regular treatment schedule.
   e. Physically or mentally unstable, debilitated, or intoxicated patients.
7. Dosing (BB-UVB and NB-UVB).
   a. Skin type—estimate of patient's ability to tolerate UVL (Table 6-2).
   b. Intensity and dosage length are increased as tolerated per a specific protocol designated by the prescribing provider (Tables 6-3 through 6-5; Boxes 6-1 through 6-2).
   c. Minimal erythema dose (MED)—smallest amount of UVL needed to produce mild erythema.
      (1) Small sections of the patient's skin are exposed to increasing doses of UVB.
      (2) Results are read within 18 to 24 hours.
8. Nursing considerations (BB-UVB and NB-UVB).
   a. Always evaluate extent of erythema prior to each treatment.
   b. Arms and legs may require extra dosing; if so, all other areas must be shielded.
   c. Always question the patient regarding new medications as they may be photosensitizing.
   d. Protective goggles must be worn during treatment, genital shields for males.
   e. Do not increase dose if it has been 7 days since last treatment (or per facility protocol).

B. UVA

UVA is referred to as the suntanning ray. It is 1,000 times less effective in producing erythema than UVB and is dosed in joules (J). UVA penetrates deep into the dermis, takes a longer time for erythema to develop (12 to 36 hours) and can take days to resolve. Skin protection against UVA is referred to as melanogenesis, which leads to hyperpigmentation (tanning).

TABLE 6-2 Skin Typing

Type*	Characteristic	Example
I	Always burns, never tans	Celtic or Irish, often blue eyes, red hair, freckles
II	Burns easily, tans slightly	Fair skin, often blonde hair; many whites
III	Sometimes burns, then tans gradually, and moderately	Mediterranean's and some Hispanics
IV	Burns minimally, always tans well	Asians and darker Hispanics
V	Burns rarely, tans deeply	Middle Easterners, Asians, dark brown-black skin, African American
VI	Almost never burns, deeply pigmented	Black skin, African American

*Reflects color of unexposed buttock skin. Skin types I to III are white, type IV is white or faint brown, type V is brown, and type VI have dark brown or black buttock skin.

TABLE 6-4 Narrowband Treatment Protocol

Skin Type	Initial Dose	Subsequent Dose
I	120 mJ	15–25 mJ
II	220 mJ	25–40 mJ
III	260 mJ	40–45 mJ
IV	330 mJ	45–60 mJ
V	350 mJ	60–65 mJ
VI	400 mJ	65–100 mJ

TABLE 6-5 Broadband Treatment Protocol

Skin Type	Initial Dose	Subsequent Dose
I	10 mJ	5–10 mJ
II	20 mJ	5–20 mJ
III	30 mJ	5–30 mJ
IV	40 mJ	5–40 mJ
V	50 mJ	5–50 mJ
VI	60 mJ	5–60 mJ

BOX 6-2. Broadband Treatment Flow Sheet

Skin Type IV
Starting dose: 40 mJ
Increase by: 20 mJ
Treatment #1: 40 mJ
Treatment #2: 60 mJ
Treatment #3: 80 mJ
Treatment #4: 100 mJ

1. UVA
   a. Wavelength 320 to 400 nm; to be effective, must be given with UVB or a photosensitizing medication.
   b. UVA at this wavelength may enhance the photobiologic effects of UVB.
   c. May cause retinal and lens damage leading to cataracts, so goggles are required.
2. UVA-1
   a. Wavelength 340 to 400 nm.
   b. Long wavelength penetrates deep into the reticular layer of the dermis.
   c. Induces T-cell apoptosis and activates fibroblasts, which lead to the breakdown of excess collagen.
   d. See immediate hyperpigmentation, but the patient is at lower risk for burning.
   e. Dosing regimen is one of three protocols: low, medium, and high.
   f. Treatment times are longer, ranging from 10 to 40 minutes per visit.
   g. A course of therapy can range from 10 to 40 treatments.
   h. Continued improvement can be noted for up to several months after completion of therapy.
3. Psoralen/UVA (PUVA). This is the interaction and absorption of the drug psoralen (methoxsalen) and UVA by specific chromophores in the dermis to produce a therapeutic effect.
   a. Methoxsalen, a photosensitizing drug from the psoralen family, is administered topically or systemically to be effective. PUVA can be more effective than UVB, but it also has more potential side effects. Patients are at increased risk for malignant melanoma, squamous cell carcinoma, skin aging, actinic keratosis, and lentigines.
      (1) Topical methoxsalen (paint PUVA)
         (a) Useful for localized lesions and is very potent.
         (b) Higher risk of burning or blistering than with systemic methoxsalen.

BOX 6-1. Narrowband Treatment Flow Sheet

Skin Type IV
Starting dose: 330 mJ
Increase by: 45 mJ
Treatment #1: 330 mJ
Treatment #2: 375 mJ
Treatment #3: 420 mJ
Treatment #4: 465 mJ

         (c) Application must be done meticulously 15 to 90 minutes prior to UVA exposure (or per facility protocol).
         (d) After treatment with topical methoxsalen, site must be washed with soapless cleanser; moisturizing sunscreen and/or appropriate clothing must be worn over site for 8 hours.
      (2) Systemic methoxsalen
         (a) Methoxsalen is available in 10-mg capsules, and dosing is weight based. Patients ingest a prescribed dose of methoxsalen approximately 1½ to 2 hours before being treated with UVA.
   b. Dosage.
      (1) MED or skin type dosing is done to establish the baseline dose.
      (2) Intensity and dosage length are increased as tolerated per a specific protocol designated by the prescribing provider (Table 6-6 and Box 6-3).
   c. Treatment schedule.
      (1) Clearing phase: three times per week on alternate days until clearing of disease is noted.
      (2) Maintenance phase: usually once every 2 to 3 weeks. This is individualized, but should be often enough to prevent flare-ups.
   d. Indications.
      (1) Failure of topical steroids, tar, anthralin, or UVB
      (2) Extensive skin involvement
      (3) Nail disease
      (4) Geographic, social, or occupational factors that necessitate keeping treatments to a minimum
      (5) Photosensitivity to UVB
   e. Absolute contraindications.
      (1) Xeroderma pigmentosum
      (2) Lupus
      (3) Lactation

TABLE 6-6 Ultraviolet Radiation A Protocol

Skin Type	Initial Joules	Joule Increments
I	0.5 jl	0.5 jl
II	1.0 jl	0.5 jl
III	1.5 jl	0.5–1.0 jl
IV	2.0 jl	0.5–1.0 jl
V	2.5 jl	1.0–1.5 jl
VI	3.0 jl	1.0–1.5 jl

Skin Type II

Starting dose: 2 joule
Increase by: 5.1 joule
Treatment #1: 2.0 jl
Treatment #2: 2.5 jl
Treatment #3: 3.0 jl
Treatment #4: 4.0 jl

    (4) Porphyria cutanea tarda, erythropoietic porphyria, variegate porphyria
    (5) Albinism
    (6) Pregnancy/lactation
    (7) No longer approved by the American Academy of Pediatrics for use in children
  f. Relative contraindications.
    (1) Age and infirmity
    (2) Pemphigus and pemphigoid exacerbated by UVA/UVB
    (3) Uremia or severe hepatic failure
    (4) History or family history of melanoma
    (5) Past history of nonmelanoma skin cancer
    (6) Extensive solar damage
    (7) Previous treatment with ionizing radiation or arsenic
    (8) Patients with cataracts or who are aphakic
    (9) Dysplastic nevus syndrome
    (10) Photosensitizing medications
    (11) Severe cardiac disease
    (12) Immunosuppression
  g. Complete an individualized patient assessment prior to making a therapy decision (Box 6-4).

Subjective Data

1. Motivation to adhere to regimen
2. Ability to alter work and personal schedule to adhere to therapy schedule
3. Financial needs/concerns regarding prescribed drug and treatment, physicians' fees, and transportation

Objective Data

1. Determine skin type.
2. Perform thorough assessment of skin area to be treated.
3. Obtain results of patient's initial ophthalmology exam.
4. Obtain complete history of other medications patient is taking—prescription and over the counter. Pay particular attention to any that may cause photosensitivity.
5. Obtain complete health history—particularly in regard to liver problems, skin cancer, heart problems, hypertension, and lupus erythematosus.

The nurse will notify physician of inability to initiate therapy if a problem exists with the patient's ability to begin PUVA therapy.

From Galloway, G. A., & Lawson, G. B. (1995). Photochemotherapy (PUVA) protocol. *Dermatology Nursing, 7*(6), 348–351.

  h. Nursing considerations.
    (1) Review prescription and over-the-counter medications every treatment.
    (2) Review time methoxsalen was ingested or applied.
    (3) Review response to last treatment.

III. PHOTOTHERAPY EQUIPMENT

A. Phototherapy units
  1. There are many manufacturers and a variety of models available (Figure 6-4).
    a. Full-body cabinets.
    b. Panels.
    c. Hand and foot units.
    d. Handheld units for treating the scalp and selective treatment of body lesions.
    e. Models for professional use.
    f. Models for home use.
    g. Models are designated for a single UVL wavelength or for a combination of UVL wavelengths.
B. Safety
  1. Equipment should be maintained and operated following manufacturer guidelines and facility policy.
  2. All state and federal applicable regulations should be adhered to including the FDA.
  3. Phototherapy units are considered radiology devices. Standards set by the Joint Commission, OSHA, and other agencies must be followed. Only authorized staff should operate the equipment.
  4. Each phototherapy unit should have an individual breaker box in the event of fire.
  5. Routine cleaning should be done to keep unit functioning at maximum level and for infection control purposes.
C. UVL lamps (Figure 6-5)
  1. New lamps contain maximum energy and cannot be recharged.
    a. Lamps will only lose power when illuminated.
    b. Unused lamps do not have expiration dates or a limited shelf-life.
  2. Power is gradually lost with use resulting in less energy.
    a. Longer treatments occur as time to complete session increases to compensate for lower energy. Long treatments may:
     (1) Increase patient fatigue
     (2) Result in reduction of patient scheduling
  3. Lamps should be changed when burnt out or damaged.
    a. Replace lamps in an even distribution pattern to avoid "hot spots"—uneven energy output that could result in patient injury.
    b. Ensure the correct UVL lamp is placed in the corresponding socket, that is, NB-UVB lamps should not

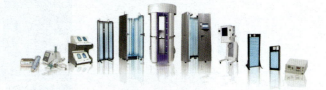

FIGURE 6-4. Phototherapy equipment.

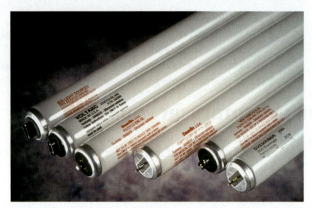

FIGURE 6-5. Phototherapy lamps.

be placed in sockets made for UVA lamps. Doing so may lead to treatment error and harm the patient.

   c. Keep a record of lamp installation, lamp removal, lamp life (per manufacturer), and energy output.

4. Lamps are designated by wave length and are either fluorescent or metal halide.

   a. Broadband UVB (290 to 320 nm)
     (1) Low-pressure mercury vapor fluorescent lamp.
     (2) Red lettering is a visual indicator of this wavelength.

   b. Narrowband UVB (311 to 313 nm)
     (1) Low-pressure mercury vapor fluorescent lamp.
     (2) Gold lettering is a visual indicator of this wavelength.

   c. UVA (320 to 400 nm)
     (1) Low-pressure mercury vapor fluorescent lamp.
     (2) Black lettering is a visual indicator of this wavelength.

   d. UVA-1 (340 to 400 nm)
     (1) Metal halide high-pressure lamp.
     (2) Special optical filters are required for use with these lamps.
     (3) A heat removal system is required for UVA-1 units as metal halide lamps generate more heat than fluorescent lamps.

D. Metering

Metering determines the lamp energy/power as output declines over time. Treatments are determined by the energy/power output and past treatment dose (Figures 6-6 and 6-7).

1. There are no FDA standards for metering.
2. Phototherapy units have either integrated dosimetry or require external dosimetry.
   a. Integrated dosimetry is a term used to describe phototherapy units with a built-in meter or sensor.
     (1) The meter located inside the cabinet internally monitors the lamp energy.
     (2) Unit will self-adjust the treatment time resulting in automatic shut off when the desired dose is reached.
   b. Nondosimetry equipment refers to phototherapy units without a built-in meter or sensor.
     (1) An external meter is a portable device used to measure the lamp energy.
     (2) Meter reading is used along with desired dose to determine treatment time.
3. External metering.
   a. Meter new lamps daily until readings stabilize (approximately 2 weeks).
   b. Metering once a week is standard after readings are stable.
   c. Cold lamps emit less energy.
     (1) A warm-up of 5 to 10 minutes prior to metering allows for lamps to reach maximum output.
       (a) Refer to manufacturer recommendation for specific warm-up time.
   d. Consistency is critical for accurate results.
     (1) Only use the meter that is recommended by the unit's manufacturer.
     (2) Use the same warm-up time prior to each meter reading.

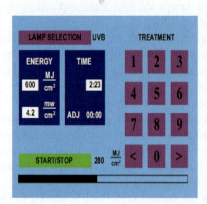

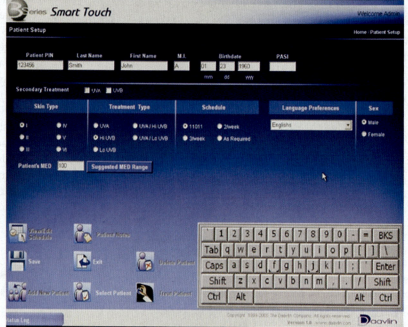

FIGURE 6-6. Phototherapy control panels.

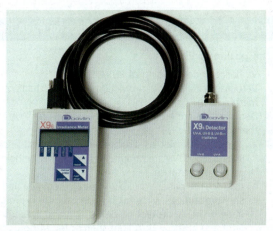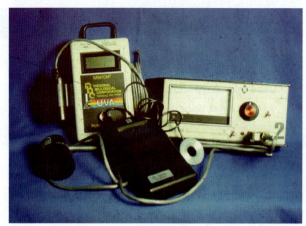

FIGURE 6-7. Phototherapy meters.

(3) Place the meter sensor at the same location and distance from the lamps per manufacturer recommendation.
4. Care of portable meters.
   a. Clean and protect the sensor lens on the meter.
   b. Send meter to manufacturer annually for recalibration.
   c. Investigate sudden or rapid changes in readings. Send to manufacturer if meter is dropped or damaged in any way.

IV. ADVERSE EFFECTS OF PHOTOTHERAPY

A. Side effects
1. Erythema (Table 6-7)
   a. BB-UVB: mild erythema is expected and acceptable; pale pink is optimal if no pain and not lasting over 24 hours.
   b. NB-UVB: erythema is more intense in color, less painful, and longer lasting.
   c. UVB erythema lasting more than 24 hours is a concern. Localized erythema should be shielded. If the patient has generalized erythema, consider holding treatment. Onset of erythema is 2 to 6 hours peaking at 12 to 24 hours, with a normal duration of 24 to 48 hours.
   d. PUVA: erythema is not required or desirable with exception of vitiligo and alopecia treatment. Hold treatment until erythema is resolved. Shield localized areas until healed. Onset of erythema is 12 to 36 hours peaking at 48 to 96 hours, with a normal duration of 7 days. Erythema lasting over 48 hours is concerning.
   e. UVA-1: Low risk of erythema in UVA-1 compared to other light. Pink is not desirable and would require

further evaluation. Immediate hyperpigmentation (tanning) is expected.
   f. Nursing considerations:
      (1) Document any erythema onset, grade, location, duration, discomfort, itching, and inability to sleep.
      (2) Document any changes in prescription and over-the-counter medications.
      (3) Document environmental changes, such as golfing, vacation, and outdoor activities.
      (4) Treatment—corticosteroids, systemic or topical, aspirin, and cool compresses.
2. Pruritus and xerosis
   a. Recommend use of an itch scale (0 to 10, 0 being no itch and 10 being severe itch). Ask if the itch has changed intensity, and if constant or intermittent.
   b. Treatment: emollients, antipruritics, cool compresses, and antihistamines.
3. Koebnerization
   a. Process where injury to the skin causes further formation of psoriasis.
   b. Treatment: avoid injury, scratching, picking, or aggressive removal of plaques.
4. Lentigines and skin aging
   a. Lentigines are blemishes of the skin associated with aging and exposure to UVL.
   b. Treatment: sunscreens and shielding.
5. Skin cancers and precancers
   a. Most common types: actinic keratosis or precancers, basal cell carcinoma, squamous cell carcinoma, and melanoma.
   b. Treatment: early detection and prevention, topical medications, cryotherapy, and biopsies with follow-up removal.
6. Eye damage
   a. Cataracts and keratitis (corneal burns)
   b. Treatment: surgical removal of cataracts
7. Exacerbation of other medical conditions
   a. Lupus, herpes simplex, rosacea, and polymorphous light eruption.
   b. Treatment: usual course of treatment for the exacerbated condition may be needed.

TABLE 6-7 Erythema Grading

Grade	Description of Erythema
0	No erythema or pinkness
1+	Slightly pink
2+	Marked erythema, no edema
3+	Fiery erythema with edema
4+	Fiery erythema with edema/blisters

TABLE 6-8 Shielding

Areas	Items Used for Shielding
Eyes	UVA/UVB goggles, glasses
Face/head	Face shields, bags, sunscreens, glasses, and towels
Body	Gowns, towels, bathing suits, sunscreens or sunblocks
Hands	Sunscreens or sunblocks, gloves
Male genitals	Shorts, jockstraps, socks

B. Protection from adverse effects: shielding (Table 6-8)
1. Methods, materials, and devices used to shield can vary depending on unit resources.
   a. Shielding is the protection of unaffected skin or eyes from UVL.
   b. The goal of shielding is to protect the unaffected skin and prevent skin/eye damage from UVL.
   c. Material used for shielding should be thick enough to block all UVA. Meter these items to ensure protection. UVB is easily blocked, and shielding material does not require metering.
   d. Eyewear is a must for the patient during treatment and the staff during metering of the phototherapy unit. Sunscreen, broad-spectrum UVA/UVB lip protection, and face and genital shielding are strongly recommended if not affected by disease.

V. PHOTOTHERAPY PEARLS

Phototherapy can be the last resort for the treatment of some skin diseases. Two primary goals of phototherapy are to provide safe treatment and to ensure the patient is well educated (Box 6-5). Explanation of the procedure, desired effects, and possible complications should be discussed and documented. See Patient Education Points Related To Phototherapy.

A. Set realistic expectations by discussing the following with each patient prior to the onset of phototherapy:
1. Response to phototherapy is not immediate.
2. Individuals respond differently to phototherapy, and some may not respond at all.
3. 100% clearing is usually not attainable.
4. Patient must continue with home care of skin to get the best benefit from phototherapy.

B. The phototherapist's role in treatment
1. Know and follow the facilities policies and procedures for:
   a. Safe operation of the phototherapy unit(s)
   b. Treatment documentation/charting
   c. Treatment protocols
   d. Missed treatment protocols
   e. Treatment adjustment for potential photosensitizing medications
   f. Erythema protocols
   g. Reporting of treatment errors or adverse events
   h. Management of noncompliant patients

BOX 6-5. Patient Education Objectives for PUVA Treatment

The patient will:
1. Verbalize understanding of PUVA therapy.
2. Verbalize understanding of action and side effects of oral methoxsalen.
3. Demonstrate adherence to correct regimen for PUVA therapy.
   a. Take methoxsalen as directed—1.5 to 2 hours prior to scheduled PUVA treatment. Treatment will be held if medication is not taken.
   b. Instruct the patient on PUVA therapy regimen and necessary precautions while taking photosensitizing medication. Patient should protect his or her skin and eyes from sunlight and artificial UVA light sources for 24 hours following ingestion of psoralens and following the light treatment.
4. Demonstrate physical signs of therapeutic response to PUVA without side effects as evidenced by:
   a. Light-to-medium pink erythemal response 24 to 48 hours following each treatment.
   b. Tolerance of methoxsalen by no complaints of nausea and vomiting.
   c. Lab values maintained within normal limits.
   d. Ophthalmologic exams saw no evidence of cataract formation.

From Galloway, G. A., & Lawson, G. B. (1995). Photochemotherapy (PUVA) protocol. *Dermatology Nursing, 7*(6), 348–351.

2. Administer phototherapy as one would a medication.
   a. There should be an order which includes:
      (1) Condition being treated
      (2) Type of UVL to be given
      (3) Skin type
      (4) Number of treatments prescribed

PATIENT EDUCATION
Phototherapy

- Explain objective of treatment.
- Stress that individuals respond differently to phototherapy and that some may not respond at all; 100% clearing is usually not attainable.
- Explain possible side effects of treatment.
- Emphasize the importance of patient reporting any new medications—prescription or OTC—to avoid potential photosensitization.
- Reinforce the importance of compliance with treatment regimen including any topical medications prescribed or recommended prior to therapy.
- Instruct patient to use emollients frequently, but especially after treatment, to prevent dryness and pruritus.
- Patients with psoriasis should prepare skin at home prior to treatment by soaking and then gently debriding plaques.
- Instruct patients about interventions for erythema or other common side effects.
- Emphasize the need for regular sunscreen use and avoidance of additional UVL exposure.

b. Follow the "five rights" of phototherapy. These are very similar to the rights emphasized in proper medication administration.

   (1) Right patient

   (2) Right chart

   (3) Right UVL and dose

   (4) Right phototherapy unit

   (5) Right shielding

3. Assess the patient prior to every treatment and document his or her condition.

  a. Assess response to previous treatment including:

   (1) New erythema

   (2) Irritation

   (3) Pruritus

   (4) Pain

  b. Assess if condition has improved, has stayed the same, or is worse.

  c. Ask if the patient has taken or used new oral or topical medications, including prescription, over-the-counter, and herbal products.

  d. Assess if the patient appears physically unwell or mentally unstable.

  e. Assess if the patient appears intoxicated or under the influence of drugs.

4. Patient instructions

  a. Tell the patient how long the treatment will take.

  b. Eye protection must be in place before unit is started and is to remain in place the entire treatment.

  c. Shielding should be appropriate, consistently placed, and secured.

  d. Direct patient to stand in center of the phototherapy unit.

  e. Discuss appropriate posturing to expose all affected areas.

  f. Instruct the patient to call out or exit unit if any problems.

5. There is a professional obligation to ensure patient safety during treatments.

  a. One of the primary staff responsibilities in phototherapy is to ensure the safe entry into and exit from all phototherapy equipment.

  b. Many potential issues may occur during treatment:

   (1) Removal of goggles

   (2) Removal of shielding

   (3) Position change so patient is standing too close to the lamps

   (4) Fainting

   (5) Claustrophobia

   (6) Seizure

   (7) Cardiac arrest

  c. Booth timers can fail. It is recommended to have a backup timer as a precautionary measure.

C. Treatment failures

1. Disorder is simply nonresponsive.

2. Monotherapy is often less effective. At each visit, reinforce continued use of topical or oral medications as prescribed.

3. Wrong type of UVL used.

4. Side effects too troublesome.

  a. Pruritus

  b. Persistent erythema

  c. Nausea

5. Patient is noncompliant.

D. Important points to remember

1. Recognize that patient outcomes will vary.

2. Aggressive treatment is sometimes required to achieve desired outcome.

3. The number one fear in phototherapy is overtreatment.

4. The number one error in phototherapy is undertreatment.

5. The ultimate goal of phototherapy is to provide safe and effective treatment.

BIBLIOGRAPHY

Abdulla, F., Breneman, C., Adams, B., & Breneman, D. (2010). Standards for genital protections in phototherapy units. *Journal of the American Academy of Dermatology, 62*(2), 223–226.

Dahl, M. V. (2012). UVA1 is often A1. *Journal Watch Dermatology.* doi: 10.1056/JD201204270000001

Galloway, G. A., & Lawson, G. B. (1995). Photochemotherapy (PUVA) protocol. *Dermatology Nursing, 7*(6), 348–351.

Habif, T. P. (2010). *Clinical dermatology: A color guide to diagnosis and therapy.* Mosby Elsevier.

Hearn, R. M. R., Kerr, A. C., Rahim, K. F., Ferguson, J., & Dawe, R. S. (2008). Incidence of skin cancers in 3867 patients treated with narrow-band ultraviolet B phototherapy. *British Journal of Dermatology, 159*(4), 931–935. doi: 10.1111/j.1365-2133.2008.08776.x

Herr, H., Cho, H. J., & Yu, S. (2007). Burns caused by accidental overdose of photochemotherapy (PUVA). *Burns, 33*(3), 372–375. doi: 10.1016/j.burns.2006.07.005

Kerr, A. C., Ferguson, J., Attili, S. K., Beattie, P. E., Coleman, A. J., Dawe, R. S., …, Sarkany, R. P. E. (2012). Ultraviolet A1 phototherapy: A British photodermatology group workshop report. *Clinical and Experimental Dermatology, 37*(3), 219–226. doi: 10.1111/j.1365-2230.2011.04256.x

Koh, M. J., & Chong, W. (2014). Narrow-band ultraviolet B phototherapy for mycosis fungoides in children. *Clinical and Experimental Dermatology, 39*(4), 474–478. doi: 10.1111/ced.12364

Krutmann, J., & Moriat, A. (2012). UVA1 phototherapy. http://www.uptodate.com/contents/uva1-phototherapy?source=search_result&search=UVA1&selectedTitle=1~19

Lapolla, W., Yentzer, B. A., Bagel, J., Halvorson, C. R., & Feldman, S. R. (2011). A review of phototherapy protocols for psoriasis treatment. *Journal of the American Academy of Dermatology, 64*(5), 936–949.

Leach, E. E., McClelland, P. B., Morgan, P., & Shelk, J. (1996). Basic principles of photobiology and photochemistry for nurse phototherapists and phototechnicians. *Dermatology Nursing, 8*(4), 235–241, 258.

Majid, I. (2014). Efficacy of targeted narrowband ultraviolet B therapy in vitiligo. *Indian Journal of Dermatology, 59*(5), 485. doi: 10.4103/0019-5154.139892

Martin, J. A., Laube, S., Edwards, C., Gambles, B., & Anstey, A. V. (2007). Rate of acute adverse events for narrow-band UVB and Psoralen-UVA phototherapy. *Photodermatology, Photoimmunology & Photomedicine, 23*(2–3), 68–72. doi: 10.1111/j.1600-0781.2007.00278.x

Menter, A., & Bhushan, R. (2010). Guidelines of care for the management of psoriasis and psoriatic arthritis: Section 5. Guidelines of care for the treatment of psoriasis with phototherapy and photochemotherapy. *Journal of the American Academy of Dermatology, 62*(1), 114–135.

Morita, A. (2010). *Ultraviolet (UV) A and (UV) B phototherapy* (pp. 87–91). Berlin/Heidelberg: Springer. doi: 10.1007/978-3-540-78814-0_9

Mysore, V. (2009). Targeted phototherapy. *Indian Journal of Dermatology, Venereology and Leprology, 75*(2), 119–125. doi: 10.4103/0378-6323.48655

Osorio, F., & Magina, S. (2011). *Phototherapy and photopheresis: Old and new indications.* London, UK: Expert Reviews, Ltd. doi: 10.1586/edm.11.71

Percivalle, S., Piccinno, R., Caccialanza, M., & Forti, S. (2012). Narrowband ultraviolet B phototherapy in childhood vitiligo: Evaluation of results in 28 patients. *Pediatric Dermatology, 29*(2), 160–165. doi: 10.1111/j.1525-1470.2011.01683.x

Syed, Z. U., & Hamzavi, I. H. (2011). Photomedicine and phototherapy considerations for patients with skin of color. *Photodermatology, Photoimmunology & Photomedicine, 27*(1), 10–16. doi: 10.1111/j.1600-0781.2010.00554.x

Tartar, D., Bhutani, T., Huynh, M., Berger, T., & Koo, J. (2014). Update on the immunological mechanism of action behind phototherapy. *Journal of Drugs in Dermatology, 13*(5), 564.

The Joan Shelk Fundamentals of Phototherapy Workshop, Dermatology Nurses' Association. Copyright 2011.

Tilkorn, D. J., Schaffran, A., Al-Benna, S., Benna, S. A., Hauser, J., Steinau, H. U., & Ring, A. (2013/2012). Severe burn injuries induced by PUVA chemotherapy. *Journal of Burn Care & Research, 34*(3), e195. doi: 10.1097/BCR.0b013e318257d932

Verhaeghe, E., Lodewick, E., van Geel, N., & Lambert, J. (2011). Intrapatient comparison of 308-nm monochromatic excimer light and localized narrow-band UVB phototherapy in the treatment of vitiligo: A randomized controlled trial. *Dermatology, 223*(4), 343–348. doi: 10.1159/000335272

Wallengren, J. (2010). *Ultraviolet phototherapy of pruritus* (pp. 325–334). London, UK: Springer. doi: 10.1007/978-1-84882-322-8_51

Weichenthal, M., & Schwarz, T. (2005). Phototherapy: How does UV work?. *Photodermatology, Photoimmunology & Photomedicine, 21*(5), 260–266. doi: 10.1111/j.1600-0781.2005.00173.x

York, N. R., & Jacobe, H. T. (2010). UVA1 phototherapy: A review of mechanism and therapeutic application. *International Journal of Dermatology, 49*(6), 623–630. doi: 10.1111/j.1365-4632.2009.04427x

Zandi, S., Kalia, S., & Lui, H. (2012). UVA1 phototherapy: A concise and practical review. *Skin Therapy Letter, 17*(1), 1.

Zhang, A. Y. (2014). Drug-induced photosensitivity. http://emedicine.medscape.com/article/1049648

STUDY QUESTIONS

1. Which of the following statements about metering is *false*?
   a. Metering determines the power/energy output of the phototherapy equipment.
   b. Metering is done to adjust the amount of energy being emitted from UVL lamps.
   c. There are no FDA standards for metering.
   d. Metering should be done consistently and according to manufacturer recommendations.

2. Both old and new lamps can provide effective phototherapy treatment; however, treatment times with older lamps may be longer.
   a. True
   b. False

3. Which of the following is *not* a side effect of phototherapy?
   a. Erythema
   b. Pruritus
   c. Nail peeling
   d. Skin damage

4. Sunscreens can be used for shielding of unaffected areas.
   a. True
   b. False

5. Which of the following light spectra is also referred to as the burning ray?
   a. UVC
   b. UVA
   c. UVB
   d. Both A and C

6. Which of the following is *not* a question to ask a patient before administering PUVA?
   a. Have you started any new medications?
   b. Have you used artificial hair dye since the last treatment?
   c. Is there any possibility you could be pregnant?
   d. Did you develop erythema with the last dose?

7. Erythema lasting more than 24 hours after narrowband UVB is concerning.
   a. True
   b. False

8. Diseases such as lupus can be exacerbated by UVL use.
   a. True
   b. False

9. Phototherapy is always effective as a monotherapy, replacing the need for the patient to use topical or oral medications for the condition.
   a. True
   b. False

10. All of the following statements about phototherapy are true *except*:
    a. Staff members are responsible for ensuring safe entry into and exit out of the phototherapy unit.
    b. A backup timer should always be employed as a precautionary safety measure with each treatment.
    c. Patient observation during treatment is only necessary for pediatric and elderly patients.
    d. Persistent pruritus, erythema, and nausea can result in treatment failure.

Answers to Study Questions: 1.b, 2.a, 3.c, 4.a, 5.c, 6.b, 7.a, 8.a, 9.b, 10.c

Psychosocial Effects and Nursing Interventions for Dermatological Disease and Psychodermatoses

Fiona Cowdell • *Steven J. Ersser*

OBJECTIVES

After studying this chapter, the reader will be able to:

- Identify the functions of the skin that are related to psychosocial well-being.
- Describe the psychosocial effects of dermatological disease.
- Describe the classification of psychodermatological disorders.
- Identify holistic approaches to consultation that support recognition of psychodermatoses and enhance the therapeutic nature of dermatological consultations.
- Select appropriate measures that assess skin-related psychological status accurately and measure learning and support needs.
- Assess when patients have psychodermatological conditions that are amenable to nursing intervention and when specialist psychodermatology referral is required.
- Explain the principles of three evidence-based behavioral interventions that may be used by nurses to support patients with psychodermatological conditions with a focus on promoting effective self-management.

KEY POINTS

- The skin is the largest and most visible organ of the body, and changes to the skin can have a major impact on psychosocial well-being.
- Skin diseases cause alterations in appearance and thereby affect body image.
- Psychodermatoses or psychocutaneous diseases are skin diseases with a psychological origin.
- People with skin conditions may suffer physical and psychosocial discomfort as well as being stigmatized by others because of their appearance.
- It is important to integrate psychosocial assessment into dermatological consultations.
- Patients presenting with dermatological symptoms should be assessed for dermatological and systemic disease before a psychological or psychiatric cause is diagnosed.

- A long-term skin condition can be very challenging for patients to cope with, and poor self-management can increase psychodermatological suffering and the quality-of-life impact.
- Many psychodermatological issues are amenable to nursing intervention, while others need specialist referral.

INTRODUCTION

This chapter is divided into four sections. The first section examines the effects of dermatological disease on health and well-being. The second provides a summary of psychodermatological disease classification. The third examines how assessment of psychodermatological health and well-being can be integrated into nursing consultation and offers some measurement tools for assessment and evaluation. Recognition of conditions that are responsive to nursing intervention and those that require specialist referral is also considered in Section 2. The final section outlines three evidence-based approaches for psychodermatological disorders that are amenable to nursing intervention through promotion of health and well-being and effective self-management.

EFFECTS OF DERMATOLOGICAL DISEASE ON HEALTH AND WELL-BEING

I. PSYCHOSOCIAL FUNCTIONS AND IMPACTS OF THE SKIN

A. The skin is the largest and most visible organ of the body that serves as the barrier between the individual and the external environment, including the interpersonal and social environment.

   1. As a society, we tend to place a high value on flawless skin and can be quick to judge people on their appearance.

   2. The visual appearance of skin disease may lead to the development of disruption of normal interpersonal relationships.

3. Rejection by others frequently occurs.
4. Interpretation of outside stimuli is adversely affected.
5. Expression of enjoyment from outside stimulation is adversely affected.
6. Sensory pleasure is adversely affected.

B. The skin affects the mind.
   1. The skin acts as a sense organ for touch, cold, heat, and pain and is an erogenous organ.
   2. The skin separates us from the outside world but provides an interface with the psychosocial environment.
   3. The skin may be a source of anxiety and stress.
   4. Early experiences of skin contact may have far-reaching impact on physical and emotional development.
   5. The skin's condition is influenced by the "look good–feel good" factor. If the skin has imperfections, this can have a detrimental effect on psychosocial well-being and body image, depending on the individual reaction.

C. The mind affects the skin.
   1. The skin acts as a facade that displays us and serves as a means of nonverbal communication with the outside world.
   2. The skin involuntarily communicates to others some of our emotional states.
   3. The skin acts as an intermediary between the individual's inner self and the external environment.
   4. The skin is an organ of emotional expression.
   5. The skin conveys varied external stimuli, including temperature differences, pain, affection, tenderness, and sexual identity and stimulation.
   6. There is complex interplay between stress, anxiety, and depression in the skin; these factors can precipitate or worsen skin conditions. Living with skin conditions can cause or exacerbate stress, anxiety, and/or depression.

D. The skin is one of the most important psychosomatic organs.
   1. The impression an individual makes on another person depends partly on their skin condition/health.
   2. Unsightly skin typically provokes negative feelings in the observer.
   3. Unsightly the skin may trigger feelings of revulsion, shame, and inferiority.

CLASSIFICATION OF PSYCHODERMATOLOGICAL DISORDERS

I. OVERVIEW

A. The skin has multiple functions and plays a crucial role in psychological and social well-being.
B. The concepts of psychological and social well-being are two distinct but related states but are often unhelpfully merged.
C. Psychological well-being refers to issues related to the mind, how the person copes with their experiences and surroundings.
D. Social well-being is concerned with how effectively the person interacts with others in society.

E. Several factors can precipitate psychodermatological disorders including stress, the impact of mood and anxiety, the presence or absence of social support, and, in some cases, mental ill health.
F. The visibility of the skin conditions can have a negative impact on body image, that is, the mental picture of how individuals view their bodies including their perception of how their body looks and the feelings, attitudes, and their emotions toward it.
G. If body image becomes very negative, the person may become obsessional about the appearance of their skin; this may lead to misperceptions of delusional proportion. People with dermatological conditions and those undergoing dermatological treatments often experience uncomfortable and unsightly skin.
H. Treatment for skin conditions may be time consuming and require expensive and unpleasant topical medications.
I. Dermatological treatments may be slow to show an effect, and their use may be required over prolonged periods of time; this may impact on motivation and thus well-being.
J. There is often a high self-management burden when living with chronic dermatoses.
K. While skin conditions present physical problems, they elicit emotional reactions as well, both for the person living with the disease and their significant others.
L. Significant others and the public often do not understand skin diseases and are typically repulsed at the site of their appearance.
M. A common fear is that the diseases are contagious and communicate their thoughts and feelings, both verbally and nonverbally, to the individuals with the diseases. The public may also misinterpret skin lesions as a sign of poor personal hygiene.

II. CLASSIFICATION

A. Primary psychiatric disease presenting to dermatology health care professionals
   1. Delusional disorders
      a. Olfactory syndromes
      b. Dysmorphic syndromes
      c. Others
   2. Obsessive–compulsive disorders (OCD)
      a. Body dysmorphic disorders
      b. Other obsessive–compulsive disorders, for example, excessive hand washing
      c. Health anxieties
      d. Skin picking disorders
      e. Trichotillomania
   3. Dysesthesias, for example, burning syndrome, vulvodynia, and scrotal dysesthesias
   4. Anxiety disorders
      a. General anxiety disorder
      b. Specific anxieties
         i. Syphilis phobia
         ii. Cancer phobia
         iii. Others

5. Chronic pruritus
    a. Psychogenic pruritus
    b. Nodular prurigo
6. Factitious disorders
    a. Dermatitis artefacta
    b. Factitious and induced illness
    c. Malingering
    d. Abuse (sexual/emotional)
B. Dermatological disorders with potential psychosocial comorbid conditions: for example, acne, eczema, psoriasis, vitiligo, and others with psychiatric disorders such as anxiety, depression, suicidal ideation, and social phobia
C. Suicidal ideation associated with skin disorders
D. Psychopharmacologically related disorders
    1. Medication which dermatologists use that may lead to psychiatric disorders (e.g., isotretinoin and depression)
    2. Psychiatric medication that may lead to skin disorder (e.g., lithium and psoriasis)
E. Skin disorders that may be induced by stress (e.g., psoriasis)
F. Site-specific skin disorder that may have a site-specific psychosocial comorbid condition, such as the following:
    1. Alopecia areata and hair appearance–related comorbid condition
    2. Genital dysesthesias and psychosexual comorbid condition

III. CLINICAL FEATURES OF FREQUENTLY SEEN DERMATOLOGICAL DISORDERS

A. The clinical features, etiology, and treatment of the most frequently seen dermatology-related primary psychiatric conditions are summarized in Table 7-1.
B. These psychiatric disorders require more specialized care and are beyond the scope of this chapter.

IV. DERMATOLOGY-RELATED PSYCHOSOCIAL COMORBIDITIES

A. Psychological and social experiences in dermatological disease
    1. Patients with dermatology-related psychosocial comorbid conditions may encounter one or more of the psychological and/or social experiences listed in Box 7-1.
    2. Any of these experiences and feelings can hinder people's ability to self-manage effectively; this can lead to a downward spiral, as self-care diminishes skin condition and quality of life deteriorates.
    3. This may result in impaired ability to self-care and ever-worsening skin condition; this in turn can impact on psychosocial well-being and self-care ability.
    4. Experiences listed in Box 7-1 may be considered within the realms of "normal" reactions and are likely to be amenable to nursing intervention.

HOLISTIC APPROACHES TO NURSING CONSULTATION AND ASSESSMENT

I. OVERVIEW

A. Dermatology-related psychosocial comorbid conditions are amenable to nursing care through effective assessment, consultation, and psychological interventions.
B. Accurate, holistic patient assessment is essential in identifying and understanding psychosocial health in patients with skin conditions in planning appropriate care and referral.
C. Most nurses will already have an extensive skill set that will inform consultations. There are additional techniques that may be integrated into consultations to enhance communication, develop therapeutic effectiveness, and ensure that psychosocial issues are identified and addressed.

TABLE 7-1 Clinical Features and Treatment of Common Dermatology-Related Primary Psychiatric Conditions

Condition	Etiology	Treatment
Delusional parasitosis (DP) Also known as Ekbom syndrome	Currently unknown Can be associated with dementia in older people, drug and alcohol misuse and rarely neurological disease can mimic DP	Can be difficult as patients often lack insight. Exclusion of organic cause is essential. Patients should not be accused of false claims as this will breakdown the therapeutic relationship and may trigger the patient seeking alternative medical care. Conventional antipsychotics are sometimes effective.
Body dysmorphic disorder (BDD) Characterized by imagined or exaggerated defect in physical appearance	May be familial and may be related to obsessive–compulsive disorder	Patients may lack insight and decline psychological or psychiatric treatment. High doses over long periods of seronergic antidepressants may be effective.
Trichotillomania Hair pulling May occur alone or as part of another disorder, for example, schizophrenia, borderline personality disorder, or depression	Unknown at present	Comorbid psychiatric disorders should be excluded. Patient support groups and general supportive psychotherapy may be helpful in helping patients cope with their condition. Antidepressant and behavioral therapy have been used with some success.
Dermatitis artefacta Patient-created skin lesions, may be produced to satisfy a personal psychological need. May include linear tears and bruising	Many patients have personality disorders and may have experienced physical or sexual abuse	Dermatological diseases must be excluded. Skin lesions must be treated. Patients should be reviewed regularly in the dermatology clinic to prevent escalations of help-seeking behaviors. Psychiatric treatment may include antidepressants or atypical antipsychotics.

BOX 7-1.   Experiences of People with Dermatology-
            Related Psychosocial Comorbid Conditions

Anger
Anxiety
Avoidance
Bullying
Concealment
Depression
Embarrassment
Exhaustion
Frustration
Guilt
Helplessness
Increased alcohol intake
Irritability
Low confidence
Low self-esteem
Performance issues
Poor body image
Relationship issues
Resentment
Secretiveness
Self-consciousness
Sexual problems
Sleep deprivation/sleeplessness
Social isolation
Social phobia
Stigmatization
Stress
Suicidal thoughts
Suicide
Teasing
Unemployment
Withdrawal

II. NURSING CONSULTATION

In any nursing consultation, the patient must have the opportunity to express their thoughts and feelings. The consultation should take place in a quiet, comfortable environment
in which there are no disturbances. This information below
is not intended to be a checklist but rather a number of ideas
that may be introduced in the course of consultations using a
mixture of open and closed questions as appropriate.

A. Objectives of the nursing consultation:
   1. To provide support and education to patients with skin
      disease to aid their adaptation and promote well-being
      and quality of life.
   2. To enhance their mental health and well-being and so
      enable patients to manage their condition as effectively
      as possible.
   3. To identify patients with psychiatric conditions or com-
      plex clinical psychological needs who require specialist
      care and so referral to psychological or psychiatric services.

B. The four-stage therapeutic consultation
   A four-stage therapeutic consultation approach allows the
   person to be examined holistically and provides a basis for
   effective care planning:
   1. The clinical observation: global evaluation
      a. How does the patient behave?—for example, do they
         appear worried, relaxed, and defensive?

b. How are they talking?—for example, do they provide
   a concise or a long and complex history?
c. What about nonverbal language?—for example, do
   they exhibit signs of stress?
d. How do they look?—how are they dressed; what is
   the first impression of their skin condition?
e. How are they interacting with others?—For example,
   are they accompanied by a friend or relative, who
   talks first, and are they able to listen to and understand information?

   2. The clinician's thoughts:
      a. What is the overall impression of the patient (physi-
         cal and psychosocial presentation)?
      b. Is the initial impression of the patient and what they
         are saying is congruent? For example, does the patient
         given nonverbal cues that they are distressed but try
         to discuss their condition in purely physical terms?
      c. Is there a sense of reality in what the patient is tell-
         ing you?
   3. Questions—it is always useful to discuss sleep distur-
      bance, appetite, weight change, their quality of life, and
      how they manage stress.
   4. Validated questionnaires can help to more accurately
      assess problems with psychosocial well-being and con-
      sequence of disease. (See section below on assessment of
      psychological health and disease-related quality of life.)

C. Communication
   1. Communication is central in any consultation, and
      there are three core conditions that need to be met by
      the nurse within a therapeutic consultation:
      a. Congruence (genuineness)
      b. Empathy
      c. Unconditional positive regard (acceptance and sup-
         port of a person)
   2. Critical elements of consultation include the following:
      a. Establishing rapport
      b. Agenda setting (what does each person expect from
         the consultation)
      c. Asking open-ended questions to elicit a fuller picture
         of how the patient is feeling:
         Are you happy with your skin?
         What are your feelings about your skin?
         Help me to understand how you feel about your skin?
         Talk me through ....

      d. Using reflective listening—a communication tech-
         nique with two steps: firstly understanding what the
         patient is trying to convey and then offering the idea
         back to the patient to ensure that they have been cor-
         rectly understood.
         Simply paraphrasing what you think they have said
         Stating "It sounds like you are feeling ...."
         Stating "It sounds like you are having trouble
         with ...."
         Or the more sophisticated approach of tentatively
         interpreting the emotion of what they have said
         Stating "You're not able to ...."
         Stating "You're having a problem with ..."
         Stating "You're feeling that ...."

e. Adopting a nonjudgmental, nonconfrontational, and nonadversarial position and try to understand what the patient is experiencing.

f. Establishing some of the following on the nature and potential impact of their condition:

  i. What patients know about the disease.
  ii. How they feel it affects their appearance.
  iii. How it impacts on their body image.
  iv. How they feel if it affects the texture of their skin.
  v. How they feel if it affects their personal odor.
  vi. How the condition is affecting their daily lives.
  vii. If they are anxious or depressed.
  viii. If they can do the things they want to do.
  ix. If they obtain and use treatments as agreed.
  x. If they feel supported by family and friends.
  xi. How it is affecting their interaction and relationships with others.
  xii. The impact the condition is having on their work or education.
  xiii. How others are reacting to their skin condition and how they are responding to others.
  xiv. If they have developed effective coping mechanisms.
  xv. What their expectations are for the outcomes of treatment.

In addition to talking with patients, it may be useful to invite them to complete questionnaires about their well-being and disease-related quality of life. These can be completed prior to the consultation and provide a basis for discussion, which should include considering physical and psychological health, their interrelationship, and self-management strategies. They can also provide a basis for evaluating the impact of support and treatment.

ASSESSMENT TOOLS USED IN DERMATOLOGY SELF-MANAGEMENT

I. OVERVIEW

A. There are many validated measures of quality of life, defined as the differences between the person's hopes and expectations and their current experience.

B. Tools may be generic, applying to diseases affecting one system (e.g., skin) or be disease specific.

C. There are also tools that measure self-management ability (e.g., the Person-Centered Dermatology Self-Management Index, Cowdell et al., 2012).

D. Assessment tools can be used as a guide for discussion and when repeated allow the patient and the nurse to see change over time.

II. ASSESSMENT TOOLS

A. Generic and disease-specific quality-of-life tools

There are many generic and disease-specific quality-of-life impact tools (Table 7-2).

TABLE 7-2 Quality-of-Life Measures Used in Dermatology

Tool	Components	Authors
Dermatology Life Quality Index (DLQI)	10 items Score range 0–30 Completed by the patient	Finlay and Khan (1994)
Family Dermatology Life Quality Index (FDLQI)	10 items Score range 0–30 Completed by the parent	Basra et al. (2007)
Children's Dermatology Life Quality Index (CDLQI)	10 items Score range 0–30 Completed by children aged 5–16 y assisted by parents if needed Word or cartoon versions available	Lewis-Jones and Finlay (1995)
Infants Dermatology Quality of Life Index (IDQOL)	1-item dermatitis severity 10-items quality of life Score range 0–30 Completed by parents or carers of children from birth to 4 y The severity of eczema is scored separately and can be correlated with the IDQOL	Lewis-Jones et al. (2001)
Dermatitis Family Impact Questionnaire (DFI)	10 items Score range 0–30 Completed by the parent	Lawson et al. (1998)
Skindex-16	16 items Score range 0–96 Completed by the patient	Chren et al. (2001)
Cardiff Acne Disability Index (CADI)	5 items Score range 0–15 Completed by the patient	Motley and Finlay (1992)
Psoriasis Disability Index	15 items Score range 0–45 Completed by the patient Visual analogue or tick box version available	Finlay and Kelly (1987)

Name: Condition: Topical treatment(s):

Please score each area of ability in discussion with the person using treatment(s) by ticking the relevant boxes.

PeDeSI number:	Degree of independence				
Ability	0 = No ability	1 = Some ability	2 = Sufficient ability	3 = Full ability	**Agreed Action Plan**
1. Do you have an understanding of your skin condition?					
2. Do you know what things make your skin condition better and worse?					
3. What is this treatment(s) used for?					
4. Are you aware of how long initial treatment will take to be effective?					
5. Do you know what the common side-effects of your treatment(s) are?					
6. Do you know how much cream / ointment / lotion should be applied each time and at what time(s)?					
7. Can you apply the treatment(s) to the affected areas? (demonstrate)					
8. Do you know how and when to adapt treatment / seek help if condition gets worse?					
9. Do you know how to obtain a repeat prescription?					
10. Do you feel confident to use treatment(s) at home yourself?					

Total Score   / 30 (maximum total score)
Total scores in range: 0–10 needs intensive education and support to develop knowledge, ability and confidence
Total scores in range: 11–20 needs some education and support to develop knowledge, ability and confidence
Total scores in range 21–29 needs limited education and support to develop knowledge, ability and confidence
Total score of 30 has sufficient knowledge, ability and confidence to manage on their own

Signature   Date

FIGURE 7-1. Person-Centered Dermatology Self-care Index (PeDeSI). (© Ersser, Cowdell, Gradwell & Langford December 2011.)

B. The Person-Centered Dermatology Self-Care Index (PeDeSI)

PeDeSI (Figure 7-1) is a validated, behaviorally based tool; the theoretical underpinnings are the self-efficacy construct (the belief that a person has that they are able to successfully undertake a specific behavior) and the concordance model (the process of prescribing and using medications based on a partnership approach between the patient and health professional). This simple, evidence-based questionnaire, which is completed collaboratively between the patient and nurse, identifies education and support needs that, if met, will enhance self-management and concordance with the treatment regimen.

While none of these tools is a panacea, they can help to understand the impact of the psychosocial state of the patient, which may have a bearing on their ability to cope and engage in their own self-management. In combination with the consultation and clinical judgment, they will help you to identify when referral to specialist psychodermatology care is required.

III. SPECIALIST REFERRAL

The need for psychological or psychiatric referral is always a matter for clinical judgment; however, there are some specific factors that should alert the nurse to this requirement (Box 7-2).

BOX 7-2. Indicators that Psychological or Psychiatric Referral May Be Required

High scores in the quality-of-life indices (but not in isolation)

Anxiety and profound preoccupation with a delusional belief (e.g., of parasitical infestation)

Difficult-to-engage patients who recount in minute detail their medical history and treatment failures

Adults exhibiting personality disordered behavior characterized by infantile, dependent, manipulative behavior and poor impulse control

Unusual skin appearance, for example, single or multiple, bilateral or symmetrical, or within easy reach of the dominant hand, which may be self-inflicted

There is a sense of unreality in what the patient is telling you.

Serious deterioration in their condition and self-care ability, which is primarily related to their psychosocial state

There are a range of treatment options for patients who need care that is beyond purely nursing intervention. Complex psychological or psychiatric care and counseling are the major treatments. Medication can be helpful and may include, according to condition, antidepressants and occasionally atypical antipsychotics.

If a higher level of specialized psychological or psychiatric care is required, this idea should be put to the patient sensitively as some may resist referral, partly due to perceived stigma. One of the major advantages of having psychological support within or via a dermatology department is that such care may be "normalized" if provided in "normal" health care settings.

Conducting a systematic and thorough consultation with the patient, careful examination of the skin, and completion of measurement tools will help the nurse determine key aspects of the psychosocial health and well-being and care needs of the patient.

EVIDENCE-BASED NURSING INTERVENTIONS FOR PSYCHODERMATOLOGICAL DISORDERS

I. OVERVIEW

1. There is overwhelming evidence that changing people's health-related behavior can have a major favorable impact on physical and psychosocial well-being.
2. It is essential that behavioral change interventions are built on a strong theoretical base to strengthen their effectiveness and are appropriate for the individual patient.
3. Following consultation, the nurse will have built up a picture of the patient, their support and education needs, and whether onward referral for psychological or psychiatric care is necessary.
4. If the patient's condition is amenable to nursing intervention, it may be helpful to use elements from the following psychological techniques as an adjunct to conventional dermatology treatments during regular consultations. These techniques are particularly useful for people with chronic dermatoses, which they are finding difficult to self-manage and which is having a detrimental impact on their quality of life.

5. The patient should be assured that behavioral therapies are complementary to other dermatological treatment and that use of a psychological intervention does not imply that they have a mental illness as this can be a common misunderstanding.

The intention here is to give an illustrative flavor of these techniques rather than an exhaustive account. Readers will not become experts; however, they will have an understanding of key concepts and how these may practically be applied and provides a basis to guide further more specialist reading.

A. Cognitive–Behavioral Therapy
1. Cognitive–behavioral therapy (CBT) is a form of therapy that aims to change thoughts and behavior to improve mental and emotional health and well-being.
2. CBT originates from the work of Aaron Beck in the 1970s and has been developed over time.
3. It is based on the concept that the way we think about things affects how we feel emotionally and physically and how we behave.
4. The aim of CBT is to help patients focus on changing their unhelpful thinking patterns in order to change their behavior and emotional state. It is categorized as a "talking therapy" but can be delivered face to face or electronically.
5. CBT concentrates on the present rather than trying to make links with the individual's past.
6. Therapy requires a collaborative relationship between the patient and nurse. The patient needs to be motivated to want to change as they are very involved in the process, which takes significant effort, active participation, and willingness to do "homework."
7. If the fundamental principles are used skillfully, CBT can help the patient to make sense of problems that may seem insurmountable at the time.
8. There is a sound evidence base for CBT. It is recommended by NICE for mental ill health such as anxiety and depression and has also been used successfully in a range of long-term conditions including, to a limited extent, in dermatology.
9. There are several models of CBT; one suggests a six-phase approach. These are outlined and allied activities summarized in Table 7-3.

B. Habit Reversal
1. Habit reversal (HR) therapy is a brief intervention with a strong theoretical underpinning, which is historically linked to behavioral theory.
2. It was originally developed by Azrin and Nunn as a multicomponent treatment and based on the premise that an old habit can be broken by replacing it with a new more desirable habit.
3. A habit is defined as a recurrent, often subconscious, or automatic pattern of behavior that is acquired through frequent repetition.
4. HR has been used successfully in dermatology primarily to manage the itch–scratch cycle for use in conditions such as eczema but also for trichotillomania and skin picking. A clinical intervention model for use with chronic scratching has been developed (Table 7-4).

TABLE 7-3 Six Phases in the Cognitive–Behavioral Therapy Process and Allied Activities

Phase	Activity
1. Assessment	Conversation with patients and their families, series of self-reported measures to identify degree of psychosocial impairment and determine appropriate course of action. The patient is helped to appraise the personal meaning and significance of events and consider his or her capacity to cope with the situation. For each situation, there are helpful and unhelpful ways of responding.
2. Reconceptualization	The nurse assists the patient to reframe his or her experiences; this may simply require the nurse to draw the negative response to the attention of the patient. For example, "I am a failure in life because I have bad skin." Alternatively could involve: Asking the patient to complete a thought diary to identify antecedents to negative thoughts.
3. Skills acquisition	Teach patients how to deal with day-to-day obstacles in their everyday life and how to avoid falling into a pattern of automatic thought. The patient needs to understand the direct connection between thoughts and feelings (having more positive thoughts is likely to lead to more positive feelings) and that physical/bodily feelings can be changed. Techniques may be used to support this: Square breathing (in for a count of two, hold for two, out for two, hold for two) Progressive muscle relaxation Challenging negative automatic thoughts Behavioral strategies (e.g., building up social contact one step at a time)
4. Skills consolidation	Patients given "homework" to help them reinforce newly acquired skills. Changing habitual responses takes time and effort, and for those with skin disease, there is the added challenge of coping with the discomfort and complexity of treatment regimes. Example of this are as follows: Activity scheduling (planning achievable and rewarding daily tasks) Replacing maladaptive coping behaviors (e.g., avoidance of situations) with adaptive mechanisms (e.g., challenging negative automatic thoughts) Mindfulness practice (exercises that focus on awareness of the present moment)
5. Generalization and maintenance	The patient and the nurse discuss and agree how the patient is going to maintain his or her skills, for example: Diary Support groups
6. Posttreatment assessment follow-up	The nurse and the patient monitor and evaluate how CBT skills have been incorporated into everyday life.

CBT, cognitive–behavioral therapy.

TABLE 7-4 Habit Reversal Clinical Intervention Model for Use in Chronic Scratching

Stage of Habit Reversal	Actions
Habit concept education	Provide the patient with a straightforward explanation of what a habit is and why HR may be a useful technique for he or she to learn.
Itch–scratch cycle education	Patient's own itch–scratch cycle should be defined and represented diagrammatically; this requires a conversation with the patient and detailed behavioral profile.
Situation awareness training	The person needs to become aware of their scratching behavior; this can be achieved by the following: Asking the patient to keep a scratch diary for a fixed time period Learning to recognize early moves to scratch
Behavioral assessment	Patients need to learn the difference between itch and scratch (as some use these terms interchangeably). Assessment should include the following: How the patient actually scratches (with what, where, when, frequency, intensity, duration, and bouts of scratching triggers) must be identified (temperature, friction, atmosphere, etc.). Define thoughts after the itch. Define the scratching behavior. Consider the consequences. What makes the problem better and worse? What does the problem prevent the patient from doing? List the goals that the patient wishes to achieve (stop scratching, allow the skin to heal, etc.).
Design brief	Based on assessment, a design brief for the competing response exercise can be developed; this may include factors such as the following: Can be done in bed or in public Incompatible with scratching Lasts for at least 1 min Anatomically opposite of scratching compatible with normal activity
Competing response practice	The exercise needs to be practiced to teach the patient a competing nondestructive behavior to replace scratching (e.g., patting or stroking the skin) or a proxy (e.g., a chamois leather pad attached to a belt loop). This should be used for at least 10 min per day and also when trigger or to scratch is experienced.
Symbolic rehearsal	The patient is asked to describe the itching and scratching in detail while performing the competing response.

TABLE 7-5 Elements and Application of Self-efficacy[a]

Element of Self-efficacy	Description	Application to Practice
Mastery experience	Most effective way of creating a strong sense of self-efficacy Enables people to master tasks Tasks must be pitched at the right level for the individual If too easy, people will expect instant success and will be discouraged by failure Essential to avoid early failure as this undermines self-efficacy To develop resilient self-efficacy, it is important that people learn to overcome obstacles and persevere	Break tasks down into component parts, for example, if a person needs to learn to apply a range of topical treatments to different areas of the body, they might first be taught how/when to use emollients and then their suitable quantities The person needs to practice this task repeatedly in different environments with the required support, encouragement, and feedback When person is confident in this element of the task, further actions may be added
Vicarious experience	Particularly useful in people with little experience or confidence. Watching someone similar to oneself successfully achieving a specific task (modeling) can be a powerful way of convincing individuals that they can master the skills needed to be successful	Demonstrate the application of medication In a group learning situation, more experienced members may be able to demonstrate a particular skill such as applying a topical treatment to a plaque while avoiding healthy skin Social learning supports the development for self-efficacy
Social persuasion	People can be persuaded verbally that they are able to master tasks and succeed Through effective communication and social persuasion, the patient may begin to understand and accept how seemingly difficult treatments can be incorporated into his or her lives	Expose patients to situations where they can succeed and avoid situations too early in which they are likely to fail Emphasize success as a personal gain during consultations Agree on achievable personalized goals Those goals developed through a true partnership interaction style and that are written and reviewed are most likely to be achieved Encourage patients to consider carefully what they really want to achieve; goals may often be quite different to those anticipated by nurses
Emotional regulation	Teach patients how to interpret their physical and psychological states that may impact on their self-management accurately They may see physiological and emotional reactions such as those of stress as signs of inability to complete certain tasks Positive mood enhances perceived self-efficacy; despondent mood diminishes it It is not the degree of emotional and physical reactions that are important but how these are perceived and interpreted	Identify where responses to stress are maladaptive, for example, the use of alcohol Advise on stress management and relaxation techniques

[a]These techniques may be a valuable adjunct to other dermatologic therapies. Although they will only work for some patients and under variable conditions, this does not mean that they are not successful. Reinforcement, perseverance, and practice are essential.

5. Prior to attempting HR, it is important that the nurse acknowledges the patient's affect and feelings about health care professionals and treatments including adherence. There should be a review of chronic illness factors and current medications.

C. Social Cognitive Theory (SCT) and its relationship to self-management support

1. SCT and in particular the self-efficacy construct underpin many behavioral interventions to enhance self-management of long-term conditions.

2. Developed by Albert Bandura, the central concept is the development of self-efficacy, that is, the belief that a person has in their ability to successfully initiate and complete the actions required in specific situations to achieve particular outcomes.

3. Enhanced self-efficacy in self-management ability will help the person to self-manage their skin condition more effectively.

4. To help people develop a robust sense of self-efficacy, we need to ensure that they acquire sufficient knowledge, skills, and confidence to self-manage their skin condition as effectively as possible.

5. Self-efficacy is measured using the PeDeSI referred to above.

6. Self-efficacy is acquired through mastery experience, vicarious experience, social persuasion, and emotional regulation. These elements are explained in detail in Table 7-5.

BIBLIOGRAPHY

Azrin, N. H., & Nunn, R. G. (1973). Habit-reversal—Method of eliminating nervous habits and tics. *Behaviour Research and Therapy, 11*(4), 619–628.

Bandura, A. (1997). *Self-efficacy: The exercise of control.* New York, NY: W.H. Freeman.

Basra, M. K. A., Sue-Ho, R., & Finlay, A. Y. (2007). The Family Dermatology Life Quality Index: Measuring the secondary impact of skin disease. *British Journal of Dermatology, 156*, 528–538. Erratum: *British Journal of Dermatology* 2007;156:791.

Bewley, A., Taylor, R., Reichenberg, J., & Magid, M. (2014). *Practical psychodermatology.* Chichester, UK: John Wiley & Sons, Ltd.

Cowdell, F., Ersser, S., Gradwell, C., & Thomas, P. (2012). The Person-Centred Dermatology Self-Care Index: A tool to measure education and support needs of patients with long-term skin conditions. *Archives of Dermatology, 148*(11), 1251–1256. doi: 10.1001/archdermatol.2012.1892

Cowdell, F., & Ersser, S. J. (2014). Nursing interventions in psychodermatology. In A. Bewley, R. Taylor, J. Reichenberg, & M. Magid (Eds.), *Practical psychodermatology (Chapter 9).* Chichester, UK: John Wiley & Sons, Ltd.

Chren, M. M., Lasek, R. J., Sahay, A. P., Sands, & L. P. (2001). Measurement properties of Skindex-16: A brief quality-of-life measure for patients with skin diseases. *Journal of Cutaneous Medicine and Surgery, 5*(2), 105–110.

Dryden, W., & Branch, R. (2012). *The CBT handbook*. London, UK: Sage.

Ersser, S. J., & Nicol, N. H. (2012). Chapter 3: Educational interventions for the management of children with dry skin. In M. Lodén, & H. Maibach (Eds.), *Treatment of dry skin syndrome—The art and science of moisturizers*. Berlin/Heidelberg: Springer.

Finlay, A. Y., & Kelly, S. E. (1987). Psoriasis—An index of disability. *Clinical and Experimental Dermatology, 12*, 8–11.

Finlay, A. Y., & Khan, G. K. (1994). Dermatology Life Quality Index (DLQI): A simple practical measure for routine clinical use. *Clinical and Experimental Dermatology, 19*, 210–216.

Lawson, V., Lewis-Jones, M. S., Finlay, A. Y., Reid, P., Owens, R. G. (1998). The family impact of childhood atopic dermatitis: The Dermatitis Family Impact Questionnaire. *British Journal of Dermatology, 138*, 107–113.

Lewis-Jones, M. S., & Finlay, A. Y. (1995). The children's dermatology life quality index (CDLQI): Initial validation and practical use. *British Journal of Dermatology, 132*, 942–949.

Lewis-Jones, M. S., Finlay, A. Y., & Dykes, P. J. (2001). The infants' dermatitis quality of life index. *British Journal of Dermatology, 144*, 104–110.

Motley, R. J., & Finlay, A. Y. (1992). Practical use of a disability index in the routine management of acne. *Clinical and Experimental Dermatology, 17*, 1–3.

Nicol, N. H., & Ersser, S. J. (2010). The role of the nurse educator in atopic dermatitis. (Issue Ed: Prof. M. Boguniewicz-University of Colorado.) *Immunology and Allergy Clinics of North America, 30*, 369–385.

Penzer, R., & Ersser, S. J. (Eds.) (2010). *Principles of skin care: A guide for nurses and other health care professionals*. Chichester, UK: Wiley Blackwell.

Walker, C., & Papadopoulos, L. (2005). *Psychodermatology: The psychological impact of skin disorders*. Cambridge, UK: Cambridge University Press.

STUDY QUESTIONS

1. Which of the following is one of the most important psychosomatic organs?
   a. Heart
   b. Brain
   c. Lungs
   d. Skin

2. Which of the following *best* describes a dermatological disorder with a psychosocial comorbid condition?
   a. Skin condition precipitated by exposure to allergens
   b. Psychiatric disease that presents as a skin disorder
   c. Skin condition that precipitated by exposure to irritants
   d. Psychological distress due to skin disease

3. John, a 13-year-old male, presents in the dermatology clinic for evaluation of an obvious skin problem. His mother reports difficulties in school, difficulties making friends, and that her son is generally rebellious and uncooperative. John is exhibiting:
   a. Typical teenage behavior
   b. Schizophrenic behavior
   c. An emotional reaction to a dermatological condition
   d. A neurotic reaction to a dermatological condition

4. Dermatological conditions often heal:
   a. Readily and easily
   b. Slowly with careful treatment
   c. Rapidly with the correct treatment
   d. Completely without relapse

5. The public often interprets skin lesions as a sign of which of the following:
   a. Poor personal hygiene
   b. Good personal hygiene
   c. A neurotic condition
   d. A psychotic condition

6. Body image is defined as how individuals:
   a. View bodies of others
   b. View their own bodies
   c. Display their bodies in pictures
   d. Present their bodies to the public

7. Psychodermatoses are conditions that primarily have which of the following origins:
   a. Physiological
   b. Sociological
   c. Psychological
   d. Biological

8. Therapeutic consultations are characterized by:
   a. Compliant patient engagement and sympathy
   b. Concordant patient engagement and empathy
   c. Unconditional positive regard
   d. Conditional positive regard

9. Habit reversal has several key stages, some of which include:
   a. Situation awareness training and scratching gently.
   b. Itch–scratch education only.
   c. Competing response practice and distraction.
   d. Situation awareness training, itch–scratch education, and competing response practice.

10. Self-efficacy is mastered in part through:
    a. Trying to be self-confident
    b. Support from a nurse
    c. Vicarious experience and social persuasion
    d. Deep breathing

Answers to Study Questions: 1.d, 2.d, 3.c, 4.b, 5.a, 6.b, 7.c, 8.b, 9.d, 10.c

CHAPTER 8

Papulosquamous Diseases

Sarah W. Matthews

OBJECTIVES

After studying this chapter, the reader will be able to:

- Describe the prevalence and epidemiology of psoriasis, lichen planus, pityriasis rosea, keratosis pilaris, and lichen simplex chronicus.
- Identify the most common areas of the body affected by each condition.
- Discuss the current understanding of the pathophysiology of each condition.
- Explain the various challenges in treating them.
- Classify the most common treatment modalities.
- Utilize teaching points in the education and engagement of patients with these conditions (etiology, triggers, self-care, optimizing treatment modalities, and follow-up).

KEY POINTS

- Understanding the common clinical features and the distinguishing etiologies of these papulosquamous diseases are essential to appropriate assessment and treatment.
- Assessing and supporting the patient's knowledge of his/her disease and his/her engagement in self-care is key to achieving successful management.
- Psoriasis is a chronic, lifelong disease with natural exacerbations and remissions that require long-term treatment affecting about 1% to 3% of the population worldwide. Multiple internal and external factors can trigger psoriasis in genetically susceptible people.
- Psoriasis is a T-lymphocyte–mediated autoimmune disease, and a variety of topical and systemic treatments exist for the management of psoriasis.
- Lichen planus can be either an acute or a chronic inflammatory disease of the skin, mucous membranes, hair, and nails. It may be idiopathic or caused by a drug, contact allergen, or viral infection (hepatitis B or C).
- Classic cutaneous lichen planus is often described using the five Ps—purple, polygonal, pruritic, planar, and papules.
- Pityriasis rosea is a mild acute, self-limiting exanthematous eruption characterized by a distinctive morphology of oval-shaped salmon-colored papules and macules with a collarette of scaling seen on the trunk and proximal extremities.

- Pityriasis rosea typically begins with a solitary patch on the trunk called the "herald patch."
- Keratosis pilaris is a very common chronic condition, which affects nearly 50% to 80% of all adolescents and approximately 40% of adults. It can be very difficult to treat but may resolve in the fourth or fifth decade.
- Lichen simplex chronicus is a disorder characterized by skin thickening (lichenification) secondary to excessive scratching and rubbing of the skin. Treatment is aimed at reducing pruritus to break the itch–scratch cycle.

INTRODUCTION

Papulosquamous diseases are varied. They have some shared morphologic features, which can lead to challenges in diagnosis. Interestingly though, their etiologies are different. Some of the common diseases in this group are psoriasis, pityriasis rosea (PR), lichen planus (LP), and lichen simplex chronicus (LSC).

I. PSORIASIS

Psoriasis is a chronic skin condition that presents in a variety of ways among individuals. It is a genetic condition triggered by environmental factors such as infection, medications, and trauma. It is characterized by exaggerated and disordered epidermal cell proliferation and keratinization. Typical lesions are well-defined erythematous, indurated papules, and plaques with white or silvery scale. It may also involve the nails and joints (Figure 8-1).

A. Definition

1. Psoriasis is thought to be a T-lymphocyte–mediated autoimmune disease. The skin lesions of psoriasis are characterized by cells multiplying much more quickly than normal (epidermal hyperproliferation), cells that do not mature normally (abnormal keratinocyte differentiation), and the presence of proinflammatory cells (a lymphocyte inflammatory infiltrate).

B. Background and etiology

1. Affects about 1% to 3% of the population worldwide depending on the study reviewed. It is seen equally in men and women, and people of all races are affected. Prevalence estimates vary in relation to age and geographic region, being more frequent in countries farther from the equator.

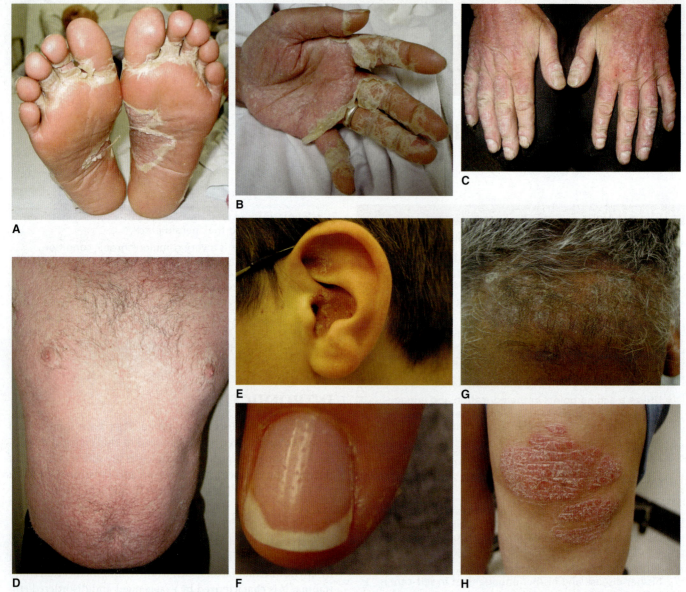

FIGURE 8-1. Psoriasis. **A:** Desquamating erythrodermic. **B:** Desquamating erythrodermic, hand. **C:** Hands. **D:** Abdomen and chest. **E:** Ear. **F:** Nail pitting. **G:** Forehead. **H:** Knee, plaque form. (From Stedman's Medical Dictionary for the Health Professions and Nursing.)

2. US prevalence in Caucasians is 3.6%, in African Americans is 1.9%, in Hispanics is 1.6%, and in other groups is 1.4%.

3. Prevalence varies throughout the world. The highest rates are in Norway of 8.5%, and the lowest rates in Asia of less than 0.5%.

4. Age at onset ranges from infancy to the end of life. The incidence of psoriasis commonly peaks at two different times across the life span (the early peak is between 20 and 30 years and the late peak is 50 and 60 years). Early onset usually leads to a more severe course of the disease.

5. Multifactorial and polygenetically inherited disease. The role of hereditary transmission is supported by familial association, twin studies, and correlation with human leukocyte antigens (HLA). Numerous studies have proven that certain antigens are positively associated with psoriasis and that Cw6 antigen has been shown to be the most significant marker for the risk prediction of the disease.

6. On the basis of epidemiological studies, the theory of two distinct disease patterns of psoriasis has been suggested. In type I psoriasis, the disease has an early onset and familial inheritance. Type II psoriasis has a late onset and sporadic familial occurrence.

7. If one parent is affected, 8% of children will develop psoriasis. If both parents are affected, then 41% of children develop psoriasis. Twin studies by Farber et al. showed that monozygotic twin pairs tend to be similar with respect to age of onset and pattern of disease. This was not the case in concordant dizygotic twins. The fact that not all monozygotic twins exhibited the same

disease characteristics indicates the influence of environmental triggering factors.

8. Trigger factors. Multiple internal and external factors can trigger psoriasis in genetically susceptible people.

a. Infections: In some cases, bacterial infections are the initial trigger for psoriasis. A correlation between streptococcal infection and psoriasis has been identified using both clinical and epidemiological data. Acute streptococcal infections, often associated with pharyngitis, are the most common and are specifically associated with the guttate form of psoriasis (Figure 8-2). Children and adolescents are the most susceptible, but it may also precipitate pustular psoriasis or exacerbations of plaque psoriasis. HIV and other immune-suppressing infections can significantly worsen psoriasis. Other infections, such as respiratory, gastrointestinal, and genitourinary, may also trigger psoriasis, although less often.

b. Psychological stress: Stress is a well-known trigger for psoriasis. Zachariae et al. found that 66% of patients reported exacerbations of their psoriasis related to stress and 35% reported that the onset of their psoriasis occurred during a time of stress. Those who were the most stressed reported greater disease severity, psoriasis-related stress, and quality-of-life (QOL) impairment. Depression can be a significant barrier to improving the patient's condition. When severe psoriasis is present or the patient expresses distress related to the psoriasis, depression screening should be considered at the initial visit, as well as follow-up visits. The PHQ-2 depression scale can be used as an initial screening tool for undiagnosed depression. It consists of the first two questions on the PHQ-9 depression questionnaire (PHQ-9 Depression Scale. AIMS Center: Advancing Integrated Mental Health Solutions). If the patient answers affirmatively to either question, the other seven questions should be asked. If depression is identified, the nurse or provider should connect the patient to his/her primary care provider or to behavioral health for follow-up. See Chapter 7 for additional information on psychosocial effects and nursing interventions for psoriasis.

c. Drugs: Multiple medications have been implicated as inducers of psoriasis including beta-blockers, lithium, antimalarials, interferon, NSAIDs, and tetracyclines. The degree of impact from each of these medications varies. Rapid discontinuation of corticosteroids can lead to exacerbations of plaque and pustular psoriasis. This is why oral prednisone is generally advised to be avoided, and topical steroids should be tapered instead of abruptly stopped.

d. Smoking and alcohol: Smoking and alcohol both have effects on psoriasis. Smoking seems to be a more significant trigger in women, while alcohol may have more impact on the evolution of the disease, particularly in men. Smoking is also strongly associated with pustular psoriasis. Helping patients understand the impact of alcohol and smoking on psoriasis has the potential to significantly impact the course of the disease.

e. Trauma: The Koebner phenomenon (Figure 8-3), a condition induced by trauma to the skin, is common in patients with psoriasis. It was first described by Heinrich Koebner in 1876 as the formation of psoriatic lesions in uninvolved skin of patients after cutaneous trauma. It can be triggered by virtually any form of trauma, such as scratching, picking, rubbing, sunburn, drug eruptions, and tattoos. Patient education is important in the prevention of this type of trigger.

C. Immunopathogenesis

1. Studies indicate that psoriasis is a T-lymphocyte–mediated autoimmune disease. Its pathophysiology is complex, involving parts of the innate and adaptive immune systems, genetics, and the environment. This

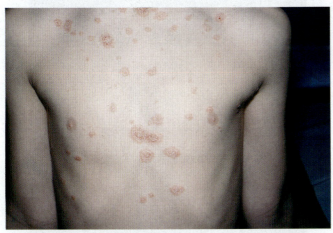

FIGURE 8-2. Guttate psoriasis associated with a recent group A beta-hemolytic streptococcal infection. (From Goodheart, H. P. (2003). *Goodheart's photoguide of common skin disorders* (2nd ed.). Philadelphia, PA: Lippincott Williams & Wilkins.)

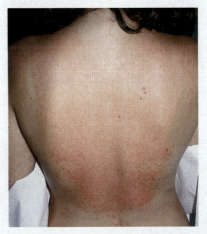

FIGURE 8-3. The Koebner phenomenon is localized to the area of sunburn. The region that had been covered by the patient's bathing suit is almost free of lesions. (From Goodheart, H. P. (2003). *Goodheart's photoguide of common skin disorders* (2nd ed.). Philadelphia, PA: Lippincott Williams & Wilkins.)

interaction of multiple systemic factors results in an increase in antigen presentation and the activation of T-helper cell type 1 (TH1) and T-helper cell type 17 (TH17), resulting in what we recognize as typical cutaneous plaques of psoriasis.

2. The skin lesions of psoriasis are characterized by cells multiplying much more quickly than normal (epidermal hyperproliferation), cells that do not mature normally (abnormal keratinocyte differentiation), and the presence of proinflammatory cells (a lymphocyte inflammatory infiltrate).

3. The T-lymphocyte subsets seen in the early phase of psoriasis and the response to T-lymphocyte targeting therapies strongly suggest that the T lymphocytes are the main players in the pathogenesis of psoriasis. Activated T cells in psoriasis secrete cytokines, which can account for many characteristics of the psoriasis lesions. See Chapter 5 to learn more about immunology and its influence on psoriasis treatment decisions.

D. Comorbidities

1. Since psoriasis and psoriatic arthritis are immune-mediated inflammatory disorders, they are associated with multiple comorbidities and cardiovascular risk factors. Patients with psoriasis have an increased risk of atherosclerosis, myocardial infarction, stroke, and cardiovascular death. It has been suggested that overlapping mechanisms of systemic inflammation contribute to the connection between psoriasis and cardiovascular disease.

2. An association with metabolic dysfunction, including obesity and metabolic syndrome (ischemic heart disease, hypertension, nonalcoholic fatty liver disease, diabetes, and obesity), with subsequent effects on morbidity and mortality, has been documented in psoriasis. It is also associated with inflammatory bowel disease (Crohn disease).

3. Psychiatric/psychological comorbidities that are associated with psoriasis include depression, anxiety, suicidal ideation, and poor QOL. Psoriasis often causes significant psychosocial burden affecting all aspects of a person's life—relationships, social activities, work, and emotional well-being. The collective effect may be self-perpetuating social withdrawal. Health-related QOL studies have measured the burden of psoriasis, and some new studies have attempted to assess the significant cumulative disability over a person's lifetime. Psoriasis is known to affect QOL and emotional well-being in a way that is comparable with other major conditions, including diabetes, arthritis, and cancer. It is imperative to support patients to discuss their feelings and how the condition affects their lives.

E. Assessment

1. Clinical manifestations and therapeutic modalities: Psoriasis can be classified by its different phenotypes, which include the following:

a. Chronic plaque psoriasis: About 90% of psoriasis is the plaque type and is characterized by well-defined red or salmon-colored, scaly plaques that are usually fairly symmetrically distributed (Figure 8-4). The degree of body surface involvement varies from limited to extensive. The scalp, elbows, knees, and low back/sacral area are the most common sites (Figure 8-5). Hands and feet are also frequently involved. In about 30% of people, the genitals are affected. Treatments range from topical medications (e.g., corticosteroids, vitamin D preparations, coal tar, calcineurin inhibitors) to systemic medications (e.g., methotrexate, acitretin, biologics) and phototherapy for widespread and recalcitrant cases. Depending on the location and severity of the disease, the treatment will need to be individualized to meet the patient's needs. In clinical trials, a method call Psoriasis Area and Severity Index (PASI) is used to evaluate the

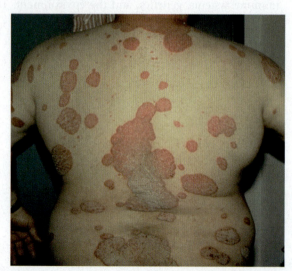

FIGURE 8-4. Moderately severe case of psoriasis characterized by sharply defined, erythematous plaques on the trunk. (From Rubin, E., & Farber, J. L. (1999). *Pathology* (3rd ed.). Philadelphia, PA: Lippincott Williams & Wilkins.)

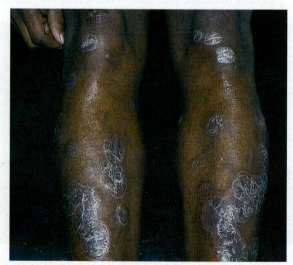

FIGURE 8-5. Well-defined plaques with silvery scale on the lower extremities. (From Goodheart, H. P. (2003). *Goodheart's photoguide of common skin disorders* (2nd ed.). Philadelphia, PA: Lippincott Williams & Wilkins.)

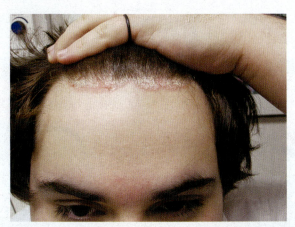

FIGURE 8-6. Scalp psoriasis. (From Goodheart, H. P. (2010). *Goodheart's same-site differential diagnosis: A rapid method of diagnosing and treating common skin disorders.* Philadelphia, PA: Wolters Kluwer.)

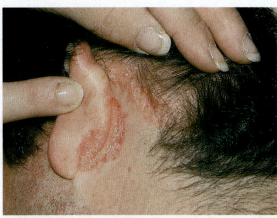

FIGURE 8-7. Psoriasis of the scalp and ears. (From Goodheart, H. P. (2003). *Goodheart's photoguide of common skin disorders* (2nd ed.). Philadelphia, PA: Lippincott Williams & Wilkins.)

percentage of body involvement and plaque severity evident on the day of the exam. The PASI scores are then evaluated over time. A PASI score is determined based on the amount of erythema, scaling, and thickness of an "average" plaque on the patient and the percentage of body areas affected. The evaluator must be well trained in how to determine the PASI score in order for the assessment to be accurate and consistent throughout the clinic trial. Because of the complexity and tediousness of PASI scoring, it is not typically used in most dermatology clinics.

b. Scalp: Well-demarcated red, scaly plaques on the scalp are usually classic for psoriasis, but it can sometimes be difficult to differentiate from seborrheic dermatitis (Figure 8-6). Posterior or temporal scalp involvement is often suggestive of psoriasis versus a frontal or diffuse scalp flaking that may be more suggestive of seborrheic dermatitis. There is certainly overlap between the two conditions. Scalp psoriasis can be especially distressing to patients due to itching, its visibility, and difficulty in treatment (Figure 8-7). The presence of hair can make application of topical medications very challenging. Solutions and gels are frequently utilized, but if the person has more course or very curly short hair, then oils, creams, or ointments may be appropriate. Very recalcitrant scalp psoriasis may require phototherapy or another systemic treatment such as methotrexate. When there are thick adherent scales, a keratolytic preparation such as salicylic acid and coal tar may be needed.

c. Guttate: Widespread erythematous papules with scale, which may be preceded by streptococcal infection. For this reason, underlying infection should be suspected and treated if present. Often, a throat culture is done in new cases whether or not patient complains of sore throat. Regardless of culture results, many patients are treated empirically for streptococcal infections in new cases of guttate pso-

riasis with a course of amoxicillin. Guttate lesions are often too widespread for topical therapy, so most patients are started on phototherapy (narrowband ultraviolet B [UVB]). It usually responds well so it is only occasionally necessary to use a more aggressive second-line therapy (Figure 8-8).

d. Inverse psoriasis: Characterized by plaques in the intertriginous areas (axillae, inframammary area, gluteal cleft, umbilicus, abdominal folds, and genital area). These plaques tend to be red, thinner, and without scale (Figure 8-9). The intertriginous areas are usually treated with mild topical steroids. Because they are more at risk for steroid atrophy and striae long term, continuous use of even mild steroids should be avoided, though short courses are appro-

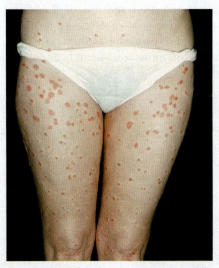

FIGURE 8-8. Papules of various sizes, with small guttate lesions on the abdomen. Scale is not obvious, and there is a perilesional ring of blanching that may be seen in psoriasis before treatment that is common in the late stages of treatment. (From Craft, N., et al. (2010). *VisualDx: Essential adult dermatology.* Philadelphia, PA: Wolters Kluwer.)

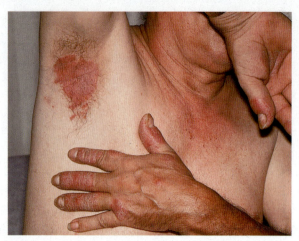

FIGURE 8-9. Inverse psoriasis. Close inspection of this patient reveals typical psoriasis on the hands. (From Goodheart, H. P. (2003). *Goodheart's photoguide of common skin disorders* (2nd ed.). Philadelphia, PA: Lippincott Williams & Wilkins.)

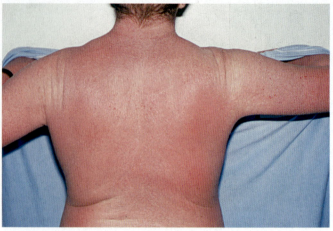

FIGURE 8-10. Psoriasis, erythrodermic variant. (From Goodheart, H. P. (2003). *Goodheart's photoguide of common skin disorders* (2nd ed.). Philadelphia, PA: Lippincott Williams & Wilkins.)

priate. Therefore, nonsteroid treatment is often appropriate, such as tacrolimus or pimecrolimus.

e. Erythrodermic: An uncommon but severe and disabling variant of psoriasis occurring in 1.5% of cases characterized by widespread deep erythema and scaling affecting the entire cutaneous surface (Figure 8-10). Withdrawal of systemic steroid therapy, infections, and drugs are frequent causes in erythrodermic exacerbations. Thus, use of systemic steroids in patients with psoriasis should be avoided. Punch biopsies are important to obtain in any erythrodermic patient to rule out erythrodermic T-cell lymphoma and other conditions that can mimic erythrodermic psoriasis. The protective functions of the skin are lost so these patients are susceptible to infection and loss of fluids and nutrients. Cyclosporine is often necessary for rapid control of this form of psoriasis. Methotrexate or biologics are useful for more long-term treatment, but caution

is essential given the risk for complications due to immunosuppression and infection.

f. Pustular psoriasis: Localized or generalized noninfectious pustules. It is characterized by pustules, not papules, found on normal or erythematous skin. There are two types, palmoplantar (Figure 8-11) and generalized (Figure 8-12) acute pustular psoriasis. Incidence of palmoplantar is low compared to psoriasis vulgaris and is seen more frequently in smokers. It tends to be chronic with intermittent exacerbations that are limited to the palms and soles. The lesions are sterile, yellow, deep-seated pustules. It is known to be refractory to many therapeutic approaches. Generalized acute pustular psoriasis is rare and life threatening. It is characterized by burning erythema with widespread sterile pustules, fever, malaise, and leukocytosis. These patients are often admitted to the hospital or should be monitored very closely, and a dermatologist

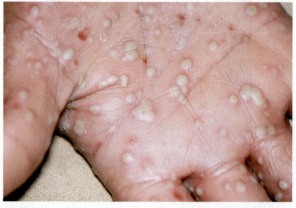

FIGURE 8-11. Psoriasis, pustular variant. (From Goodheart, H. P. (2003). *Goodheart's photoguide of common skin disorders* (2nd ed.). Philadelphia, PA: Lippincott Williams & Wilkins.)

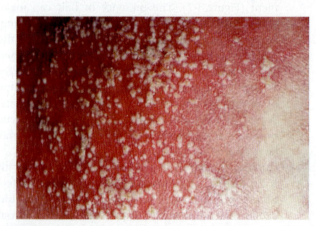

FIGURE 8-12. Pustular psoriasis. Rapid development of sterile pustules complicated a case of erythroderma. (From Elder, D. E., et al. (2012). *Atlas and synopsis of Lever's histopathology of the skin*. Philadelphia, PA: Wolters Kluwer.)

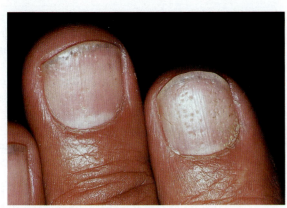

FIGURE 8-13. In confusing diagnostic cases, the identification of typical psoriasis on other skin surfaces such as the scalp, elbows, or nail pits, such as these, can be very useful. (From Edwards, L., & Lynch, P. J. (2010). *Genital dermatology atlas*. Philadelphia, PA: Wolters Kluwer.)

should be called to distinguish this entity from a pustular drug eruption.

g. Nail disease: Occurs in about 50% of people with psoriasis and is more common in those with associated psoriatic arthritis. There are a variety of nail abnormalities associated with psoriasis. The most common change is pitting (Figure 8-13). Loosening of the nail plate from the underlying nail bed, onycholysis, is also fairly common (Figure 8-14). Oil spots may also be seen in the nail bed.

h. Psoriatic arthritis: Psoriatic arthritis is associated with cutaneous psoriasis in 7% to 26% of cases. It is a seronegative inflammatory arthritis that is usually asymmetric (60% to 70% of the time) and involves the proximal and distal joints of the fingers or toes (Figure 8-15). It may also manifest as sausage fingers (dactylitis). The axial form involves the vertebra and sacral joints and occurs approximately 5% of the time. It is a destructive arthritis; therefore, early

diagnosis and treatment is critical for optimal control and averting joint destruction, functional disability, and reduced QOL.
2. Diagnostic tests
   a. Diagnosis is most often based on clinical findings.
   b. Punch biopsy may be considered if diagnosis is unclear.
F. Nursing considerations
   1. Medical intervention overview
      a. A variety of topical and systemic treatments exist for the management of psoriasis. It is a chronic, lifelong disease with natural exacerbations and remissions that require long-term treatment. There is a range of treatments available to manage the condition, but the response to treatment is unique to each individual. For that reason, finding an effective treatment plan can be a process of trial and error.
      b. Eighty percent of psoriasis patients have mild-to-moderate disease, so topical therapies play a central role in the treatment of their psoriasis. Patients usually start with a single type of therapy; however, in more severe cases (>10% body surface area, severely impaired QOL, or recalcitrant psoriatic lesions), multiple treatment approaches may be used as part of combination, successive, or rotational therapeutic regimen.
      c. The main treatment options include topical steroids, topical vitamin D, retinoids, phototherapy, oral systemic therapies (methotrexate, acitretin, cyclosporine), and biologic therapies. Recently, laser has been developed as another modality to treat psoriasis.
      d. Other topical therapies include the following steroid-sparing agents: coal tar, anthralin, calcineurin inhibitors, keratolytics, and emollients.
      e. Therapeutic approaches should take into consideration the main goal of improving the patient's QOL, the individual patient's likelihood of adherence, and promoting a therapeutic relationship with the patient (Table 8-1).

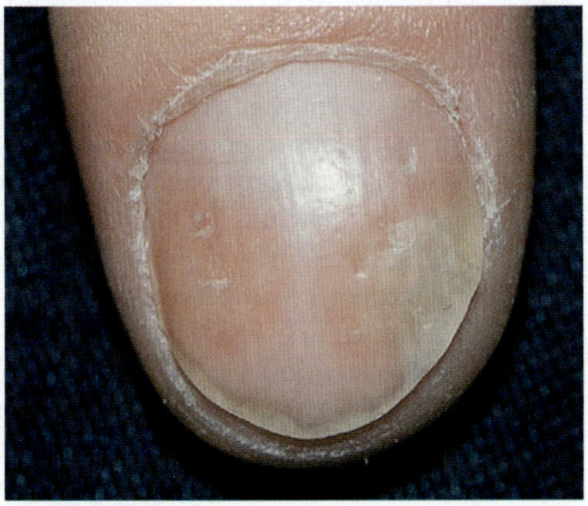

FIGURE 8-14. Orange-brown coloration appears under the nail plate, presumably the result of psoriasis of the nail bed. (From Goodheart, H. P. (2003). *Goodheart's photoguide of common skin disorders* (2nd ed.). Philadelphia, PA: Lippincott Williams & Wilkins.)

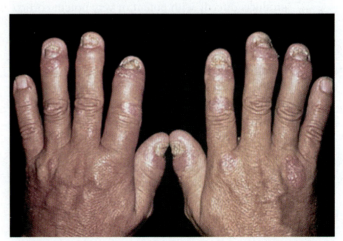

FIGURE 8-15. Pitting and onycholysis of nails of a patient with psoriatic arthritis. (From Huang, J. J., & Gaudio, P. A. (2010). *Ocular inflammatory disease and uveitis manual*. Philadelphia, PA: Wolters Kluwer.)

TABLE 8-1 Factors to Consider When Choosing Psoriasis Therapies

Age	Associated medical disorders HIV Liver disease Cardiovascular disease Skin cancer
Type of psoriasis and severity Guttate Plaque Palmoplantar Generalized pustular Erythrodermic	Psychosocial factors Engagement in self-care Perceived impact on quality of life Depression Financial challenges Proximity to clinic
Sites and extent of involvement Localized vs. widespread Localized but on the palms and soles (very debilitating) Scalp (difficult to treat due to hair-impeding topicals) Anogenital area (psychosocial impact) Scattered plaques but <5% involvement Generalized and >30% involvement	Previous treatments and response to therapy Systemic glucocorticoids (may exacerbate psoriasis) Narrowband UVB phototherapy (did it work well previously?) PUVA (increased skin cancer risk) Cyclosporine (blood pressure and nephrotoxicity issues) Methotrexate (potential liver toxicity) Biologics

HIV, human immunodeficiency virus; PUVA, ; UVB, ultraviolet B.
Adapted from Wolff, K., Johnson, R. A., & Saavedra, A. P. (2013). *Fitzpatrick's color atlas* (7th ed., pp. 49–57). United States: The McGraw-Hill Companies.

2. Medications
   a. Topical corticosteroids were first introduced in the early 1950s and have been the most common treatment for psoriasis. They are often the first-line therapy in mild-to-moderate psoriasis but are also used as adjunct therapy in more severe psoriasis. For plaque psoriasis, medium- to high-potency steroids used one to two times a day can lead to significant improvements. Itching, scale, and inflammation improve quickly. Potent topical corticosteroids (e.g., betamethasone dipropionate) and very high-potency (e.g., clobetasol propionate) topical corticosteroids are most effective. Some studies compared vitamin D products directly with potent or very potent corticosteroids and found that they have comparable effects when applied to the body, but corticosteroids were more effective than vitamin D for scalp psoriasis. Combination therapy with a topical vitamin D with topical corticosteroid is more powerful than either alone. On both the body and the scalp, potent corticosteroids were less likely than vitamin D to cause local adverse events, such as skin irritation or burning, so people were consequently more likely to stop using vitamin D products.
      (1) Factors that increase the risk of side effects from corticosteroids include the following:
         (a) Potency.
         (b) Length of treatment: the longer the topical corticosteroid is applied, especially on a daily basis, the greater the risk.
         (c) Surface area of skin being treated: the larger the area treated with a topical corticosteroid, the greater the risk.
         (d) Location being treated: more sensitive skin locations such as the face, axillae, and groin are at higher risk than thicker-skinned areas such as the palms and soles.
         (e) Patient's age—young children and people aged over 70 have a greater risk because of thinner skin.
      (2) Side effects include the following:
         (a) Burning or stinging of the skin: usually occurs when first started; improves as skin gets used to the medication.
         (b) Atrophy (thinning of the skin): skin may bruise or tear more easily than normal. May cause visible telangiectasias.
         (c) Worsening of a preexisting skin infection.
         (d) Acne with over use (especially on the face) or worsening of existing acne.
         (e) Rosacea: face becomes red and flushed with acne-form lesions.
         (f) Hypopigmentation: more common in skin types with more natural pigment.
         (g) Contact dermatitis related to allergic reaction to the substances in the topical corticosteroid, which can manifest as worsening or persistent psoriasis.
         (h) Striae (stretch marks): due to prolonged application or excessive potency. The highest risk areas are the axilla, groin, and inner thighs.
         (i) Tachyphylaxis: steroids work less well over time if they are overused or breaks are not taken (often, "a 2-week on, 2-week off" regimen is recommended for psoriasis).
      (3) Prevention of side effects
         (a) Prudent use of topical steroids includes using the minimal strength needed to get results, attention to the area of application (e.g., weaker topical steroids should be used on the face and intertriginous areas), duration (usually a maximum 2 weeks then taking a break or rotating with nonsteroids), and vehicle (e.g., ointments are more potent than creams).
         (b) In general, use a potent preparation for short term and weaker preparation for maintenance between flare-ups or nonsteroidal topicals such as tacrolimus or pimecrolimus. Even the application of weaker or safer steroids should be limited to 2 weeks on those sites.
   b. Systemic corticosteroids
      (1) Can rapidly clear psoriasis, but the psoriasis eventually worsens again requiring higher and higher doses and can lead to a severe rebounding or more severe disease, even erythrodermic or widespread pustular psoriasis.
   c. Calcipotriene
      (1) Vitamin D products (calcipotriene) affect keratinocyte differentiation. Treatment with calcipotriene (Dovonex) in ointment, cream, or solution is

steroid sparing and has been shown to be very effective in the treatment of plaque and scalp psoriasis.

(2) Combination therapy with calcipotriene and high-potency steroids appears to provide greater improvement rates and fewer adverse effects.

(3) Calcipotriene degrades in the presence of UV light, so it should not be used prior to sun exposure or phototherapy. Calcipotriene plus betamethasone dipropionate is more effective than either agent alone. Calcipotriene performs better than tar products.

d. Other topicals: salicylic acid, tar, anthralin, tazarotene, and calcineurin inhibitors

(1) Salicylic acid is used as a keratolytic agent in shampoos, creams, and gels. It helps to chemically exfoliate scale and promote the absorption of other topical agents. Widespread application should be avoided due to potential for salicylate toxicity.

(2) Coal tar is frequently used in over-the-counter shampoos. Oil of cade (pine tar) or birch tar can be compounded into ointments. The odor of tar is often a deterrent to use.

(3) Anthralin is an ancient effective treatment, but it is irritating and stains skin, clothing, and bedding so it is not used very often.

(4) Tazarotene is a retinoid. It treats psoriasis by modulating keratinocyte differentiation and hyperproliferation, as well as by suppressing inflammation. Combining its use with a topical corticosteroid and weekend pulse therapy can decrease irritation.

(5) Topical calcineurin inhibitors such as tacrolimus and pimecrolimus work well on thin lesions in areas prone to atrophy or steroid acne such as the face and body fold areas (axillae, inframammary, abdominal folds, inguinal area, gluteal folds). The burning commonly associated with these agents can be challenging but may be avoided by initial treatment with a corticosteroid and by application to dry skin, not right after bathing. Typically, this burning effect dissipates after several applications.

e. Methotrexate

(1) This folic acid antagonist was approved by the FDA for treatment of psoriasis in 1971.

(2) Commonly used first-line therapy for moderately severe plaque psoriasis, psoriatic arthritis, pustular psoriasis, erythrodermic psoriasis, and palmoplantar psoriasis.

(3) Associated potential side effects limit its use to severe involvement or cases resistant to topical therapies and phototherapy. It is therefore extremely important that methotrexate not be used in patients with contraindications (e.g., pregnancy, breast-feeding, liver disease, alcoholism, immunodeficiency syndromes, leukopenia, anemia, thrombocytopenia) and that screening labs be done prior to the start of the medication, during the initiation of therapy and after dose adjustments.

(4) Usually dosed weekly by mouth or by subcutaneous injections. Liver biopsies are controversial to monitor for liver dysfunction and cirrhosis on methotrexate. Typically, after a cumulative 3 to 4 g of usage, patients are referred to gastroenterology for a discussion about biopsy.

f. Cyclosporine

(1) The therapeutic value of cyclosporine may be related to the downregulation of proinflammatory epidermal cytokines.

(2) It is known to be a highly effective systemic treatment but has a high risk for nephrotoxicity. It is therefore necessary to follow strict monitoring guidelines and to use it ideally under 12 to 18 months. An alternative therapy should be instituted concomitantly, or the psoriasis will recur. When cyclosporine treatment is 6 months or less, it is associated with a low frequency of renal problems, but blood pressure and serum creatinine must be monitored and doses adjusted when indicated.

g. Systemic retinoids (acitretin and etretinate)

(1) Systemic retinoids are an effective treatment for psoriasis, as well as disorders of keratinization and cutaneous lupus.

(2) It decreases inflammation in the epidermis and dermis by interfering with various cytokines.

(3) In contrast to other systemic psoriasis drugs, acitretin is not cytotoxic or immunosuppressive.

(4) The major problem with them is their teratogenicity. Acitretin is converted into etretinate, which has a very long half-life, and a patient cannot become pregnant for 3 years after it is stopped. Therefore, it should not be used in women of childbearing age, unless the woman is absolutely confident that she will not be seeking pregnancy for several years.

(5) Alcohol ingestion can convert acitretin to etretinate and is strongly discouraged.

(6) All of these drugs also have the potential to elevate triglycerides, which may complicate therapy.

(7) Combinations of retinoids with phototherapy can be effective in chronic plaque psoriasis, resulting in lowered cumulative doses of ultraviolet light.

(8) Dose-related side effects include dry lips (or cheilitis), dry skin, pruritus, peeling of the palms and soles, epistaxis, conjunctivitis, and hair loss. All these effects are dose dependent and quickly reversed after drug discontinuation.

(9) The most common systemic effects include headache, arthralgia, myalgia, and fatigue. Skeletal changes after long-term use have been attributed to retinoid, but studies have not supported this theory well.

(10) Elevated liver enzymes are reported in approximately 14% to 35% of patients in US trials. Serum lipid changes (increase in triglycerides, in very low density lipoprotein (VLDL), and in low density lipoprotein (LDL)) are common.

h. Biologics
   (1) Biologics work by impeding certain mechanisms in the autoimmune response characteristic of psoriasis.
   (2) Biologics are distinct from general immunosuppressants because they do not suppress the entire immune system. Instead, they target the specific immune system chemicals involved in producing psoriasis.
   (3) There are multiple biologic agents with unique mechanisms of action used in the treatment of psoriasis. See Chapter 5 to learn more about biologic therapies for psoriasis.

2. Phototherapy
   a. Phototherapy with UVB and photochemotherapy with ultraviolet A (psoralen ingestion with UVA) is a treatment modality for psoriasis that has been available for decades. See Chapter 6 for more information about phototherapy.
   b. Cost-effective but frequently underutilized therapy for psoriasis.
   c. For most people (typically, >75%), sunlight improves psoriasis. Conversely, significant sunburns may cause koebnerization (Figure 8-3) and psoriasis exacerbation.
   d. Studies have shown that suberythrogenic levels can be very effective for clearing psoriasis, but tanning does occur, and the dose must be gradually increased to achieve effective levels.
   e. Maintenance phototherapy after clearing contributes to the length of remission and is necessary for many patients.

G. Patient education and engagement in self-management

1. Nurses play a major role in patient education and engagement in self-management when caring for patients with psoriasis. Patient education is the process by which the nurse produces changes in the patient's knowledge, skills, and attitude necessary for the patient to have the tools they need to address their health condition. Self-management support is defined as the "systematic provision of education and supportive interventions by health care staff to increase patients' skills and confidence in managing their health problems, including regular assessment of progress and problems, goal setting, and problem-solving support." Key issues that nurses should consider addressing with the patient based on individual readiness to learn and engage in self-management are listed in Table 8-2.

H. Follow-up
1. At least once a year—every treatment plan should be reevaluated at least once a year to be sure that it is still working well for the patient and to ensure that there are no concerning side effects.
2. Patients on systemic medications need more frequent follow-up, often every 3 to 6 months with lab checks.
3. The patient should check back sooner if:
   a. There is a lack of response to topical or systemic treatments.
   b. The treatment was working then stopped.
   c. The treatment did not start to work in the time frame that the dermatology provider suggested that it would.
   d. If there is rapid worsening of the condition right away (rapidly spreading rash, pustules, redness covering entire body, fever) since it could indicate pustular or erythrodermic psoriasis. It may also indicate a drug reaction that needs to be addressed right away.

TABLE 8-2 Patient Education and Engagement in Psoriasis Self-care

Key Issues	Teaching Points
Comorbidities	**Psoriatic arthritis** Associated with the cutaneous psoriasis in 7%–26% of cases. Inflammatory arthritis that can be very destructive to joints. Signs and symptoms include pain and swelling, often in the morning ("morning stiffness"). Mild cases treated with NSAIDs. More significant cases treated with disease modifying agents (e.g., methotrexate) or biologics. Report early so appropriate interventions may be started. **Other comorbidities** Metabolic dysfunction, including obesity and metabolic syndrome (diabetes and obesity, ischemic heart disease, hypertension, nonalcoholic fatty liver disease). Subsequent effects on morbidity and mortality. Work with primary care provider (PCP) to optimize cardiovascular and metabolic health through healthy eating, exercise, and possible early intervention in elevated lipids, HTN, elevated blood sugar, etc. Minimize alcohol (alcohol can also trigger psoriasis). **Psychosocial** Depression, anxiety, social isolation, quality-of-life impact. Common in psoriasis. Significant psychosocial burden affecting all aspects of a person's life—relationships, social activities, work, and emotional well-being. The collective effect may be self-perpetuating social withdrawal. Open dialogue about emotional effects. Facilitate healthy emotional and social self-care (e.g., enjoyable activities, support groups, National Psoriasis Foundation, healthy eating and exercise, rest, avoiding excess alcohol and smoking).

TABLE 8-2 (*Continued*)

Key Issues	Teaching Points
Triggers	**Infections** Avoid skin infections, strep throat, and other infections (e.g., good handwashing and other infection prevention techniques when applying topicals, avoiding others that are ill, etc.). Report signs and symptoms of infection so early intervention may help avoid psoriasis exacerbation. **Psychological stress** Emphasize the risk for exacerbations of psoriasis related to worry and stress. See interventions under comorbidities. **Drugs** Patient should be aware that multiple medications may induce psoriasis in some patients—beta-blockers (atenolol), lithium, antimalarials, interferon, NSAIDs, and tetracyclines, so they may need to discuss this with their dermatology provider or PCP. Rapid discontinuation of corticosteroids can lead to exacerbations of plaque and pustular psoriasis. This is why oral prednisone is generally advised to be avoided in patients with psoriasis. Topical steroids should be tapered instead of abruptly stopped. May need to alternate topical steroids with other nonsteroid topicals. **Alcohol and smoking** Help patients understand the impact of alcohol and smoking on psoriasis. Stopping or minimizing alcohol and smoking has the potential to significantly impact the course of the disease. **Trauma—Koebner phenomenon** Condition induced by trauma. Common in psoriasis patients. Can be triggered by various forms of trauma, such as scratching, sunburn, drug eruptions, and tattoos. Patient education is key to preventing this type of trigger.
Treatment Options	80% of psoriasis patients have mild-to-moderate disease, so topical therapies play a central role in the treatment of their psoriasis. Usually start with a single type of therapy. More severe cases (>10% body surface area, severely impaired quality of life, or intractable psoriatic lesions) may require multiple treatment approaches as part of combination, successive, or rotational therapeutic regimens. Main treatment options include topical steroids, topical vitamin D, retinoids, phototherapy, systemic therapies (methotrexate, acitretin, and cyclosporine), and biologic therapies. Other topical therapies include the following steroid-sparing agents: coal tar, calcineurin inhibitors (tacrolimus and pimecrolimus), anthralin, keratolytics such as salicylic acid and tazarotene. In spite of the high efficacy and low side effect profile of topical medications, consistent use is an ongoing challenge. It is essential that patient's questions are answered about use of topical medications. Patients who feel their questions and concerns have been addressed develop a more therapeutic relationship with their health care team. This relationship leads to trust in the treatment plan and ultimately better self-care. Phototherapy is a cost-effective but frequently underutilized therapy for psoriasis. Narrowband UVB is very well tolerated and safe. PUVA has more risks involved but is also very effective for recalcitrant psoriasis. Both can be used as a monotherapy or in combination with topicals or other systemic treatments. All systemic medications have potential risks and therefore require a thorough discussion with the dermatology provider as well as screening tests prior to initiation and in follow-up.
Key Messages to Facilitate Self-care	Emollients play an essential role in controlling psoriasis and preventing exacerbations. Consistency in using medications is key to gaining control of psoriasis. Once controlled, taper topical medications to minimum needed to maintain control. If experiencing a flare, increase topical medications as prescribed to regain control. Topical steroids rarely cause serious side effects if they are used as instructed. A pea-sized amount of topical should cover an area about the size of the palm. Avoid using more than 50 g/wk of very potent topical steroids for more than 2 weeks because of the risk of suppressing the body's ability to make its own steroids. To learn more about different types of topical treatments and their side effects, review the patient handout by the National Psoriasis Foundation titled "Topical Treatments for Psoriasis," which can be accessed at www.psoriasis.org. Phototherapy is an excellent treatment modality but does require time commitment on the part of the patient. It is generally 2–3 times/week for about 8 weeks to achieve 90% or better clearance. Once clear, most patients will taper to maintenance program of every 1–2 weeks for at least 4 weeks. If still doing well, they then work with their dermatology provider to determine how long to continue. Some patients will experience long-term remission following phototherapy. If taking systemic medications (e.g., methotrexate, acitretin, cyclosporine, or a biologic), it is essential for the patient to have regular follow-up visits and tests.

Hypertension (HTN),; Non-steroidal anti-inflammatory drugs (NSAID),; psoralen ultraviolet-A (PUVA),; ultraviolet-B (UVB) RPR – rapid plasma reagin.

II. LICHEN PLANUS

A. Definition

1. LP can be either an acute or a chronic inflammatory disease of the skin, mucous membranes, hair, and nails that may be idiopathic or caused by a drug, contact allergen, or viral infection. Classic cutaneous LP is characterized by flat-topped lesions that are often described using the five Ps—purple, polygonal, pruritic, planar, and papules.

B. Etiology and pathology

1. Thought to be due to an abnormal immune reaction most often provoked by a viral infection (such as hepatitis B or C) or a drug.

2. Research indicates that T cells seem to mistake the skin cells as foreign and attack them, damaging the basal keratinocytes that express altered self-antigens on their surface.

C. Incidence
   1. Occurs worldwide and in all races.
   2. Equally prevalent in males and females.
   3. The exact prevalence is not known. It varies geographically, but the skin disease is reported to affect 0.22% to 1% of adults, and the oral manifestations affect 1% to 4% of the population.
   4. Onset is most often in adulthood.

D. Assessment
   1. Clinical manifestations
      a. Typical LP is characterized by shiny, flat-topped, firm papules varying from a few millimeters to larger plaques (Figure 8-16). They are purple color and frequently have tiny white lines called "Wickham striae."
      b. They may be clustered or widespread, or in lines (linear LP) or circles (annular LP).
      c. Linear LP can be the result of scratching or injuring the skin (Koebner phenomenon).
      d. Most often affects the oral mucosa and the flexor surfaces of the wrists, forearms, and legs.
      e. Genital LP is less common. It can be very painful and have a major impact on QOL (Figures 8-17 and 8-18).
      f. Skin lesions are most often very pruritic.
      g. Oral LP can vary in its presentation but is frequently seen as white, lacy patterns on the buccal mucosa. It may also be seen on the tongue. On the gingiva, it can be atrophic, erosive, or bullous and associated with mild to severe pain (Figure 8-19).
      h. Lichen planopilaris is a variant of LP on the scalp with scaly papules and scarring alopecia.

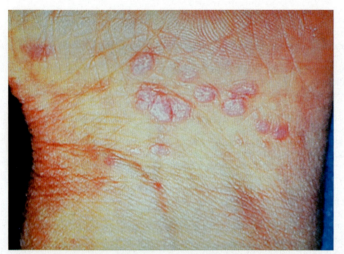

FIGURE 8-16. Lichen planus of the hand and wrist. Note the violaceous color and flat-topped appearance of the lesions. (From McConnell, T. H. (2013). *Nature of disease.* Philadelphia, PA: Wolters Kluwer.)

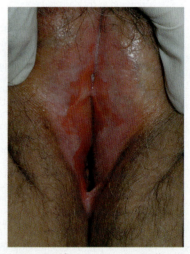

FIGURE 8-17. Nonspecific erosions typically seen in vulvar lichen planus. (From Edwards, L., & Lynch, P. J. (2010). *Genital dermatology atlas.* Philadelphia, PA: Wolters Kluwer.)

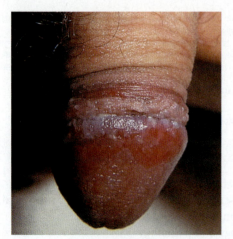

FIGURE 8-18. Uncircumcised penis with erosive lichen planus. (From Edwards, L., & Lynch, P. J. (2010). *Genital dermatology atlas.* Philadelphia, PA: Wolters Kluwer.)

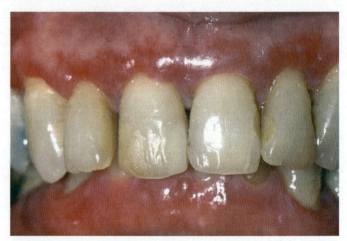

FIGURE 8-19. Oral lichen planus: erythematous, ulcerated, and painful gingival lesions. (Courtesy of Dr. Ralph Arnold, San Antonio, TX.)

i. Nail bed changes include thin nails with longitudinal lines, dystrophy ("pterygium"), splintering, and destruction of the nail fold.

j. Cutaneous LP may resolve spontaneously within 2 years, but oral LP may persist and be more recalcitrant to treatment.

2. Diagnostic tests

a. Most often diagnosed clinically, but 4-mm punch biopsy may be helpful, plus another 4-mm punch biopsy of perilesional skin for direct immunofluorescence when bullous lesions are present.

b. Testing for hepatitis B and C.

c. Patch testing for metal allergies may be helpful for oral LP since it may be a manifestation of an allergy to metallic fillings and other dental restorations.

E. Nursing considerations

1. Medical interventions

a. Corticosteroids

(1) High-potency topical, intralesional, and systemic corticosteroids have all been used effectively for LP.

(2) Mild cases may be treated with topical steroids and sedating antihistamines for itching.

(3) Hypertrophic LP may respond to intralesional corticosteroids or category 1 steroids under occlusion.

(4) In severe cases, systemic corticosteroids are typically used. Moderate doses (30 to 60 mg daily) used for 2 to 6 weeks and then tapered over several weeks to avoid rebound and relapses.

(5) Topical corticosteroids twice daily are first-line therapy for mucosal erosive LP.

b. Topical calcineurin inhibitors, such as tacrolimus and pimecrolimus, are second-line therapies for oral LP.

c. Other nonsteroidal systemic treatments: methotrexate, acitretin, cyclosporine, azathioprine, PUVA, and narrowband UVB have been utilized. Oral metronidazole has been studied as an effective treatment for diffuse LP.

d. Research shows that narrowband UVB may be viewed as an effective treatment for generalized cutaneous LP. It may be especially appropriate when there are contraindications for systemic corticosteroids and other medicines or other immunosuppressive drugs.

2. Patient teaching and engagement: after assessing the patient's readiness to learn and understanding of his/her condition consider offering education on the below topics:

a. Avoid scratching: explain the rational for avoiding scratching due to the pathomechanics of scratching and the risk for koebnerization and lichenification that can worsen pruritus.

b. Utilize cold compresses and cool baths with oatmeal to suppress itch sensation.

c. Discuss purpose of systematic approach to optimal use of topical medications.

d. Review steroid precautions.

e. Advise the patient to complete periodic lab screening as directed by provider if utilizing systemic medications.

f. Discuss rational for consistency in phototherapy.

g. Typically, cutaneous LP resolves within 6 months to a year but is prone to recurrence. Conversely, the hypertrophic type tends to last for years.

3. Follow-up

a. Follow-up with patient in 14 days to assess treatment effectiveness if using topical therapy.

b. Visits every 4 to 8 weeks until condition controlled.

c. When stable, visits every 6 months for reevaluation.

d. More often for exacerbations.

III. PITYRIASIS ROSEA

A. Definition

1. PR is a mild, acute, self-limiting exanthematous eruption characterized by a distinctive morphology of an initial "herald patch" followed by the appearance of oval-shaped salmon-colored papules and macules with a collarette of scaling seen on the trunk and extremities, usually sparing the face, scalp, palms, and soles (Figure 8-20).

B. Etiology and pathology

1. The exact cause is still undetermined, but a viral origin is the most popular hypothesis.

2. Supporters of the viral theory call attention to the prodromal symptoms experienced by some people and the lack of recurrence signifying an immunity being developed.

3. Studies have reported involvement of human herpesvirus 7 (HHV-7) and HHV-6.

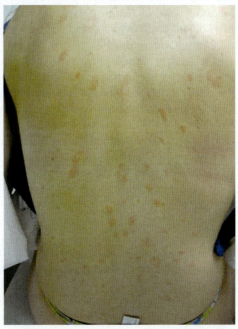

FIGURE 8-20. Pityriasis rosea. (From Goodheart, H. P. (2010). *Goodheart's same-site differential diagnosis: A rapid method of diagnosing and treating common skin disorders.* Philadelphia, PA: Wolters Kluwer.)

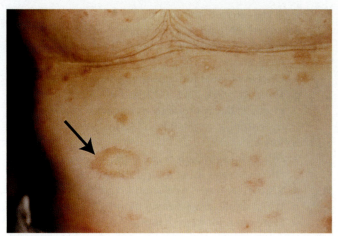

FIGURE 8-21. Pityriasis rosea. Oval herald patch (*arrow*) on the abdomen with a more generalized rash. (From Centers for Disease Control and Prevention Public Health Image Library.)

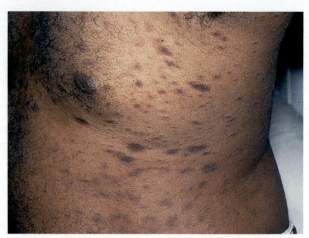

FIGURE 8-22. Pityriasis rosea. Eruption is typically distributed on the chest and/or back in a Christmas tree pattern. (From Goodheart, H. P. (2003). *Goodheart's photoguide of common skin disorders* (2nd ed.). Philadelphia, PA: Lippincott Williams & Wilkins.)

C. Incidence
  1. Multiple studies have tried to establish prevalence. It has been estimated to be 1.31%, but considering the atypical forms that have not been appropriately diagnosed, this is conceivably an underestimation.
  2. Typically occurs in otherwise healthy adolescents and young adults (10- to 35-year-olds).
D. Assessment
  1. Clinical manifestations
    a. Typically begins with a solitary patch on the trunk (more rarely on extremities) called the "herald patch," which is oval, with slightly elevated finely scaling borders (collaret), whereas the center is paler and slightly depressed and it may be the only lesion for about 2 weeks (Figure 8-21).
    b. After herald patch begins to fade, a widespread eruption abruptly develops.
    c. This secondary phase is characterized by patches that are similar to the initial one, but smaller and symmetrically oriented with their long axes along the cleavage lines of the trunk and proximal extremities typically.
    d. Oral lesions are not commonly reported with PR.
    e. Usually, there is an absence of significant systemic symptoms. About 5% of people will experience a mild prodromal phase including a headache, fever, arthralgias, or malaise.
    f. Spontaneous resolution usually in 8 to 12 weeks. Rarely persists over 5 months.
    g. In the typical cases, diagnosis is easy. The differential diagnosis includes guttate psoriasis, secondary syphilis, tinea versicolor, seborrheic dermatitis, nummular eczema, and pityriasis lichenoides chronica.
  2. Diagnostic tests
    a. Testing is usually not necessary after a thorough history and physical are complete, but RPR, KOH, and punch biopsy could be considered.

  3. Nursing considerations
    a. PR is a self-limiting disease, so medical interventions are generally unnecessary.
    b. Best treatment is education and reassurance for the patient.
    c. Pruritus, if present, is usually mild and tolerable.
    d. A Cochrane collaboration article reviewed the literature on various possible treatments used and found the evidence to be inadequate for the efficacy of emollients, topical antihistamines and corticosteroids, sunlight, artificial ultraviolet therapy, systemic antihistamines and corticosteroids, antiviral agents, and intravenous glycyrrhizin.
    e. One study found evidence that oral erythromycin may shorten the course of the rash and alleviate pruritus, but a later study did not confirm the results.
  4. Patient teaching
    a. PR is self-limiting and not dangerous.
    b. Patient may be completely asymptomatic or have some mild itching.
    c. People with darker skin may be at risk of some postinflammatory hyperpigmentation (Figure 8-22).
  5. Follow-up
    a. No follow-up needed unless the condition lasts greater than 5 months or systemic symptoms develop and persist.

IV. KERATOSIS PILARIS

A. Definition
  1. Keratosis pilaris (KP) is a common condition caused by excessive keratinization leading to numerous coarse follicular plugs (Figures 8-23 and 8-24).
B. Etiology and pathology
  1. KP is a genetic condition, but the exact cause has not yet been identified.

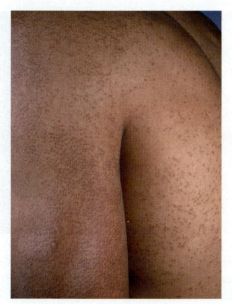

FIGURE 8-23. Shoulders with keratosis pilaris. (From Lugo-Somolinos, A., et al. (2011). *VisualDx: Essential dermatology in pigmented skin*. Philadelphia, PA: Wolters Kluwer.)

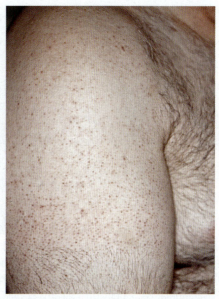

FIGURE 8-24. The discrete lesions of keratosis pilaris are often lifelong and lack the inflammation of folliculitis. (From Craft, N., et al. (2010). *VisualDx: Essential adult dermatology*. Philadelphia, PA: Wolters Kluwer.)

2. The hypothesis is that KP is a disorder of keratinization in which the cells that line the hair follicle form a horny plug instead of exfoliating. This enlarges the pores making them appear more obvious than in the normal skin.
3. Commonly associated with atopic dermatitis.

C. Incidence
1. KP affects nearly 50% to 80% of all adolescents and approximately 40% of adults.
2. Frequently first diagnosed when people are being seen in dermatology for other conditions such as eczema.
3. Frequently primarily a cosmetic concern but medically harmless and often asymptomatic (minor itching is possible).

D. Assessment
1. Clinical manifestations
   a. Primarily found on the lateral upper arms and anterior thighs but may also be seen on the cheeks, upper back, buttocks, and forearms.
   b. May be skin colored, red, or brown.
   c. Keratotic papules on the face may be on a red background that is a variant of KP called keratosis rubra faceii (Figure 8-25).
   d. Worsens in the winter months due to dry air.
   e. Often refractory to treatment.
2. Diagnostic tests
   a. Diagnosis is made by clinical assessment.
   b. Testing is not necessary but punch biopsy could be considered if diagnosis is unclear.

E. Nursing considerations
1. Interventions
   a. Moisturizers alone only somewhat helpful.
   b. Some KP will respond to topical urea or lactic acid creams.
   c. Retinoids may be helpful but easily irritate the skin and should be started at only 1 to 2 times per week.
   d. Inflamed KP, which is often red and itchy, may be treated with a low-dose topical corticosteroid.
2. Patient teaching
   a. KP is genetic and chronic but essentially asymptomatic.
   b. Should not scrub KP or it may become inflamed.
3. Follow-up
   a. No follow-up needed.

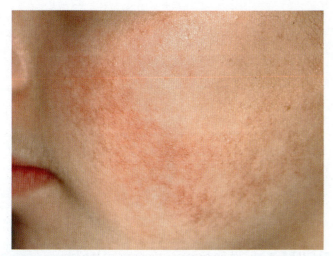

FIGURE 8-25. KP on the face is frequently red, while lesions on the extremities typically are not. (From Craft, N., et al. (2010). *VisualDx: Essential adult dermatology*. Philadelphia, PA: Wolters Kluwer.)

V. LICHEN SIMPLEX CHRONICUS

A. Definition
1. LSC is a common disorder characterized by skin lichenification secondary to excessive scratching and rubbing of the skin (Figure 8-26).

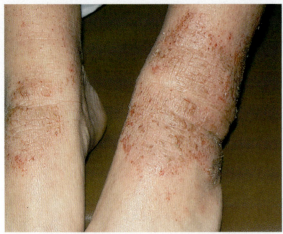

FIGURE 8-26. Lichen simplex chronicus. Lichenified plaques involve the distal pretibial area and ankle. (From Goodheart, H. P. (2003). *Goodheart's photoguide of common skin disorders* (2nd ed.). Philadelphia, PA: Lippincott Williams & Wilkins.)

B. Etiology and pathology
   1. The initial pruritus associated with LSC may be from another skin condition such as atopic dermatitis or psoriasis, a compressed nerve leading to the skin (neuropathic pruritus), or in some cases a psychologically related issue.
   2. Also called neurodermatitis.
   3. Once scratching becomes chronic, the skin thickens as a protective mechanism and develops lichenification (similar to callus that forms on the palms and soles following mechanical trauma) (Figures 8-27 and 8-28).
   4. Lichenification results from thickening of both the epidermis and the stratum corneum.
   5. LSC is frequently very tenacious and tends to recur even if it is responsive to initial treatment.
   6. Longevity seems to be related significantly to the psychological component and how much the person continues to scratch.

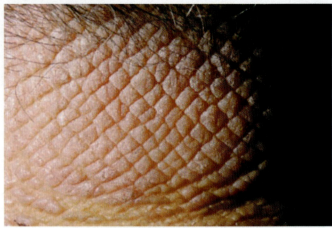

FIGURE 8-28. Lichen simplex chronicus. Chronic "rubbing" of the posterior neck led to lichenification characterized by accentuation and thickening of skin markings. (From Elder, D. E., et al. (2012). *Atlas and synopsis of Lever's histopathology of the skin*. Philadelphia, PA: Wolters Kluwer.)

   7. Itch–scratch cycle plays a dominate role in disease persistence.
   8. The most common sites are the neck, scalp, shoulder, wrist, genital area, and lower leg/ankle.
C. Incidence
   1. It develops predominantly in mid-to-late adult life, but it can also occur in children. When LSC develops in children, it is slightly more likely to occur in boys; when it occurs in adults, it is slightly more prevalent in women.
   2. Recent study finds that having an anxiety disorder is associated with an increased risk of LSC. Researchers recommend combining the management of LSC and psychological disorders to achieve better outcomes.
   3. Anogenital LSC is a common disease. Incidence and prevalence statistics have not been determined (Figures 8-29 and 8-30).

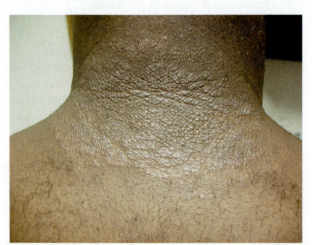

FIGURE 8-27. Lichen simplex chronicus. (From Goodheart, H. P. (2010). *Goodheart's same-site differential diagnosis: A rapid method of diagnosing and treating common skin disorders*. Philadelphia, PA: Wolters Kluwer.)

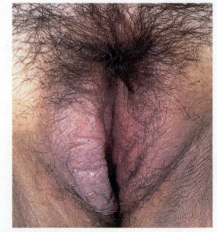

FIGURE 8-29. Lichen simplex chronicus of the labia. Lichenification with excoriations due to scratching. (From Rubin, R., et al. (2011). *Rubin's pathology*. Philadelphia, PA: Wolters Kluwer.)

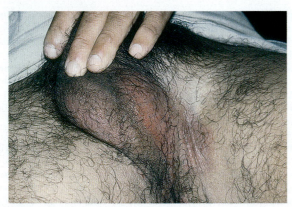

FIGURE 8-30. Lichen simplex chronicus of the testes. (From Goodheart, H. P. (2010). *Goodheart's same-site differential diagnosis: A rapid method of diagnosing and treating common skin disorders.* Philadelphia, PA: Wolters Kluwer.)

D. Assessment
  1. Clinical manifestations
    a. Characterized by the presence of erythematous or hyperpigmented well-defined scaly and thickened papules and plaques with variable degrees of overlying excoriation.
    b. Long-standing LSC may also have hyperpigmentation (Figure 8-31) and hypopigmentation.
    c. Worsens with stress, anxiety, heat, sweating, and irritation from clothing.
  2. Diagnostic tests
    a. Diagnosis is made by clinical assessment.
    b. Testing is not necessary but punch biopsy could be considered if unclear.
E. Nursing considerations
  1. Interventions
    a. Treatment is aimed at reducing pruritus to decrease the urge to scratch since rubbing and scratching cause LSC.

    b. Location, lesion morphology, and extent of the lesions influence treatment.
    c. High-potency topical corticosteroids, intralesional steroids, and topical calcineurin inhibitors (tacrolimus and pimecrolimus) are frequently used. Unlike other conditions where the use of topical steroids is limited to 2 weeks, it is often advised in LSC to use steroids twice a day until the lesions flatten.
    d. Nighttime scratching cannot be controlled with willpower since people are unaware that they are doing it. Using a sedating antihistamine may be very helpful in breaking the itch–scratch cycle (hydroxyzine 10 to 25 mg taken 2 hours before bedtime reduces the risk for morning drowsiness). Increase the dose every 5 to 7 days until nighttime scratching ceases or side effects limit increasing the dose (may require 50 to 75 mg to be effective).
    e. Tricyclic antidepressants (doxepin) may work even better due to its sedating effect and treatment of depression and anxiety.
    f. Selective serotonin reuptake inhibitors (SSRIs) may also be helpful when stress, anxiety, or depression is a significant factor.
    g. Systemic corticosteroids are warranted if not improving after several weeks of topical steroids—40 mg in AM × 7 days, than 20 mg in AM × 7 days.
  2. Patient teaching: after assessing the patient's readiness to learn and understanding of his/her condition, consider offering education on the below topics:
    a. The most important aspect of treatment is to break the itch–scratch cycle or the condition will not improve. Patients must understand the pathomechanisms of the itch–scratch cycle in order to participate in effective self-care.
    b. Untreated LSC will go on indefinitely but may intermittently improve and worsen.
    c. Even with very effective treatment, there is a high likelihood of recurrence if the same triggers are present (underlying disease, warm, sweating, irritation, psychological distress).
    d. Dryness is also a trigger for pruritus so moisturizing several times daily is essential.
    e. Complications include secondary infection, permanent skin color changes, and permanent scarring.
  3. Follow-up
    a. Close follow-up is needed to support consistent follow-through on the treatment plan to break the itch–scratch cycle. People are often much more motivated to optimize treatment when they start to get relief from the condition.
    b. See the person back in clinic in 2 weeks, then again in 1 month. Phone follow-up can also be helpful.
    c. Once the LSC is improved, then other underlying conditions such as atopic dermatitis, psoriasis, and psychosocial issues should be addressed for a long-term plan. Engagement in self-care is essential for long-term success.

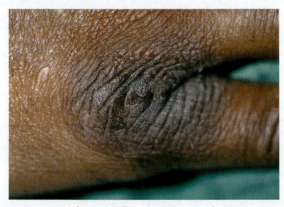

FIGURE 8-31. Lichen simplex chronicus with accentuated skin markings and hyperpigmentation. (From Lugo-Somolinos, A., et al. (2011). *VisualDx: Essential dermatology in pigmented skin.* Philadelphia, PA: Wolters Kluwer.)

BIBLIOGRAPHY

Alai, N. N., & Elston, D. M. (2014). Keratosis pilaris. Retrieved from http://misc.medscape.com/pi/android/medscapeapp/html/A1070651-business.html

Barisic-Drusko, V., Dobric, I., Pasic, A., Palian, D., Jukic, Z., Basta-Juzbasic, A., & Marinovic, B. (1994). Frequency of psoriatic arthritis in general population and among the psoriatics in Department of Dermatology. *Acta Dermato Venereologica. Supplementum, 186*, 107–108.

Barker, S., & Oakley, A. (2014, April). Retrieved from http://dermnetnz.org/acne/eosinophilic-folliculitis.html

Basavaraj, K. H., Ashok, N. M., Rashmi, R., & Praveen, T. K. (2010). The role of drugs in the induction and/or exacerbation of psoriasis, *International Journal of Dermatology, 49*, 1351–1361.

Chuh, A. A., Dofitas, B. L., Comisel, G. G., Reveiz, L., Sharma, V., Garner, S. E., & Chu, F. (2007). Interventions for pityriasis rosea. *Cochrane Database of Systematic Reviews,* (2), CD005068.

Churton, S., Brown, L., Shin, T. M., & Korman, N. J. (2014). Does treatment of psoriasis reduce the risk of cardiovascular disease? *Drugs, 74*, 169–182.

Corrocher, G., Di Lorenzo, G., Martinelli, N., Mansueto, P., Biasi, D., Nocini, P. F., …, Pacor, M. L. (2008). Comparative effect of tacrolimus 0.1% ointment and clobetasol 0.05% ointment in patients with oral lichen planus. *Journal of Clinical Periodontology, 35*(3), 244–249.

Curtis, J. R., Beukelman, T., Onofrei, A., Cassell, S., Greenberg, J. D., Kavanaugh, A., …, Kremer, J. M. (2010). Elevated liver enzyme test among patients with rheumatoid arthritis or psoriatic arthritis with methotrexate and/or leflunomide. *Annals of the Rheumatic Diseases, 69*(1), 43–47.

Drago, F., Broccolo, F., & Alfredo, R. (2008). Pityriasis rosea: An update with a critical appraisal of its possible herpesviral etiology. *Journal of the American Academy of Dermatology, 61*(2), 303–318.

Farber, E. M., Nall, L., & Watson, W. (1974). Natural history of psoriasis in 61 twin pairs. *Archives of Dermatology, 109*(2), 207–211.

Fukamachi, S., Kabashima, K., Sugita, K., Kobayashi, M., & Tokura, Y. (2009). Therapeutic effectiveness of various treatments for eosinophilic pustular folliculitis. *Acta Dermato-Venereologica, 89*, 155–159.

Gladman, D. D., Thavaneswaran, A., Chandran, V., & Cook, R. J. (2011). Do patients with psoriatic arthritis who present early fare better than those presenting later in the disease? *Annals of the Rheumatic Diseases, 70*, 2152–2154.

Gorouhi, F., Davari, P., & Fazel, N. (2014). Cutaneous and mucosal lichen planus: A comprehensive review of clinical subtypes, risk factors, diagnosis, and prognosis. *The Scientific World Journal, 2014*, 1–22.

Gulliver, W. (2008). Long-term prognosis in patients with psoriasis. *The British Journal of Dermatology, 159*(Suppl 2), 2–9.

Henseler, T., & Christophers, E. (1985). Psoriasis of early and late onset: Characterization of two types of psoriasis vulgaris. *Journal of the American Academy of Dermatology, 13*(3), 450–456.

Higgins, E. (2000). Alcohol, smoking and psoriasis. *Clinical and Experimental Dermatology, 25*, 107–110.

Iraji, F., Faqhihi, G., Asilian, A., Siadat, A. H., Larijani, F. T., & Akbari, M. (2011). Comparison of narrow band UVB versus systemic corticosteroids in treatment of lichen planus: A randomized clinical trial. *Journal of Research in Medical Sciences, 16*(12), 1578–1582.

James, W. D., Berger, T. G., & Elston, D. M. (2011). *Andrew's diseases of the skin: Clinical dermatology* (11th ed., pp. 66, 190–198, 248, 410–411). Saunders Elsevier.

Jiaravuthisan, M. M., Sasseville, D., Vender, R. B., Murphy, F., & Muhn, C. Y. (2007). Psoriasis of the nail: Anatomy, pathology, clinical presentation, and a review of the literature on therapy. *Journal of the American Academy of Dermatology, 57*, 1–27.

Kimball, A. B., Gieler, U., Linder, D., Sampogna, F., Warren, R. B., & Augustin, M. (2010). Psoriasis: Is the impairment to a patient's life cumulative? *Journal of European Academy of Dermatology and Venereology, 24*, 989–1004.

Leung, D. Y., Travers, J. B., Giorno, R., Norris, D. A., Skinner, R., Aelion, J., …, Kotb, M., et al. (1995). Evidence for a streptococcal super antigen-driven process in acute guttate psoriasis. *The Journal of Clinical Investigation, 96*, 2106–2112.

Lynch, P. J. (2004). Lichen simplex chronicus (atopic/neurodermatitis) of the anogenital region. *Dermatologic Therapy, 17*, 8–19.

Martin, S. L., McGoey, S. T., Bebo, B. F., & Feldman, S. R. (2013). Patients' educational needs about topical treatments for psoriasis. *Journal of the American Academy of Dermatology, 68*(6), e163–e168.

Mason, A. R., Mason, J., Cork, M., Dooley, G., & Hancock, H. (2003). Topical treatments for chronic plaque psoriasis (Review). The Cochrane Collaboration. Published by John Wiley & Sons, Ltd.

Mumoli, N., Vitale, J., Gambaccini, L., Sabatini, S., Brondi, B., & Cei, M. (2013). Erythrodermic psoriasis. *Quarterly Journal of Medicine, 107*, 4.

Parisi, R., Symmons, D. P., Griffiths, C. E., & Ashcroft, D. M. (2013). Identification and management of psoriasis and associated comorbidity (IMPACT) project team. Global epidemiology of psoriasis: A systematic review of incidence and prevalence. *The Journal of Investigative Dermatology, 133*(2), 377–385.

Pearson, M., Mattke, S., Shaw, R., Ridgely, M., & Wiseman, S. (2007). *Patient self-management support programs: An evaluation.* Retrieved from http://www.ahrq.gov/research/findings/final-reports/ptmgmt/ptmgmt.pdf

PHQ-9 Depression Scale (2015, April 12). AIMS Center: Advancing Integrated Mental Health Solutions. Retrieved from http://aims.uw.edu/resource-library/phq-9-depression-scale

Pongdee, T. (2014). Bleach baths. American Allergy, Asthma & Immunology. Retrieved from http://www.aaaai.org/conditions-and-treatments/library/allergy-library/Bleach-Bath-Recipe-for-Skin-Conditions.asp

Prey, S., Paul, C., Bronsard, V., Puzenat, E., Gourraud, P. A., Aractingi, S., …, Ortonne, J. P. (2010). Assessment of risk of psoriatic arthritis in patients with plaque psoriasis: A systematic review of the literature. *Journal of European Academy of Dermatology and Venereology, 24*(2), 31–35.

Rachakonda, T. D., Schupp, CW, & Armstrong, A. W. (2014). Psoriasis prevalence among adults in the United States. *Journal of the American Academy of Dermatology, 70*, 512–516.

Rapp, S. R., Feldman, S. R., Exum, M. L., Fleischer Jr, A. B., Reboussin, D. M. (1999). Psoriasis causes as much disability as other major medical diseases. *Journal of the American Academy of Dermatology, 41*, 401–407.

Rajendran, P., High, W. A., & Maurer, R. (2014). Eosinophilic folliculitis. Retrieved from http://www.uptodate.com/contents/hiv-associated-eosinophilic-folliculitis?source=machineLearning&search=eosinophilic+folliculitis&selectedTitle=1%7E150&sectionRank=4&anchor=H5#H5

Rasi, A., Tajziehchi, L., & Savabi-Nasab, S. (2008). Oral erythromycin is ineffective in the treatment of pityriasis rosea. *Journal of Drugs in Dermatology, 7*, 35–38.

Sharma, P. K., Yadav, T. P., Gautam, R. K., Taneja, N., & Satyanarayana, L. (2000). Erythromycin in pityriasis rosea: A double-blind, placebo-controlled clinical trial. *Journal of the American Academy of Dermatology, 42*, 241–244.

Shiohara, T., & Kano, Y. (2003). Lichen planus and lichenoid dermatoses. In J. Bolgnia, J. Jorizzo, & R. Rapini (Eds.), *Dermatology* (pp. 175–184). Edinburgh, UK: Mosby.

Szczerkowska-Dobosz, A. (2005). Human leukocyte antigens as psoriasis inheritance and susceptibility markers. *Archivum Immunologiae et Therapia Experimentalis, 53*(5), 428–433.

Tauber, M., Viguier, M., Alimova, E., Petit, A., Lioté, F., Smahi, A., & Bachelez, H. (2014). Partial clinical response to anakinra in severe palmoplantar pustular psoriasis. *The British Journal of Dermatology, 171*(3), 646–649.

Usatine, R. P., & Tinitigan, M. (2011). Diagnosis and treatment of lichen planus. *American Family Physician, 84*(1), 53–60.

Van de Kerkhof, P. C. (2003). Psoriasis. In J. Bolgnia, J. Jorizzo, & R. Rapini (Eds.), *Dermatology* (pp. 125–149). Edinburgh, UK: Mosby.

Vorvick, L. (2012, October). Folliculitis. Retrieved from http://www.ncbi.nlm.nih.gov/pubmedhealth/PMH0001826

Wolff, K., Johnson, R. A., & Saavedra, A. P. (2013). *Fitzpatrick's color atlas* (7th ed., pp. 49–57). United States: The McGraw-Hill Companies.

Woods, G. S., & Reizner, G. (2003). Other papulosquamous disorders. In J. Bolgnia, J. Jorizzo, & R. Rapini (Eds.), *Dermatology* (pp. 158–160). Edinburgh, UK: Mosby.

Zachariae, R., Zachariae, H., Blomqvist, K., Davidsson, S., Molin, L., Mork, C., & Sigurgeirsson, B. (2004). Self-reported stress reactivity and psoriasis-related stress of Nordic psoriasis sufferers. *Journal of the European Academy of Dermatology and Venereology*, *18*(1):27–36.

Zeichner, J. A., Lebwohl, M. G., Menter, A., Bagel, J., Del Rosso, J. Q., Elewski, B. E., …, Tanghetti, E. (2010). Psoriasis Process of Care Consensus Panel. Optimizing topical therapies for treating psoriasis: A consensus conference. *Cutis*, *86*(3), 5–31.

STUDY QUESTIONS

1. A patient with a history of psoriasis on her scalp for years presents with new onset of a rapidly developing rash that is widespread and consists of numerous small papules (about 5 to 10 mm size) with scale. She recently had a sore throat and fever. She most likely has what type of psoriasis?
   a. Plaque
   b. Guttate
   c. Pustular
   d. Inverse

2. Stress, smoking, and alcohol are common triggers for psoriasis.
   a. True
   b. False

3. The Koebner phenomenon is the presence of small bleeding points seen on a psoriatic lesion when the scales are removed.
   a. True
   b. False

4. The lacy white network on the surface of papules, called Wickham striae, is typical and helpful for?
   a. Lichen planus
   b. Lichen simplex chronicus
   c. Atopic dermatitis

5. Where does lichen planus most often present?
   a. Scalp
   b. Nails and joints
   c. Skin and oral mucosa
   d. Genital area

6. What is the primary symptom associated with cutaneous lichen planus?
   a. Scaling
   b. Pain
   c. Crusting
   d. Severe itching

7. Pityriasis rosea generally begins with a solitary scaly patch on the trunk (herald patch), then 2 weeks later, the eruption abruptly worsens with abundant smaller scaly flat lesions that rapidly spread to the trunk and proximal arms and thighs. Patients and parents are often very concerned. The best treatment is usually:
   a. Education and reassurance since pityriasis rosea is self-limiting
   b. Topical steroids
   c. Oral antihistamines
   d. Moisturizer since medications don't really help

8. Your patient has a history of atopic dermatitis since childhood. He is 16 years old now and concerned about small (1 to 2 mm), asymptomatic papules covering both upper arms and thighs. His mom has the same condition. What does he likely have?
   a. Seborrheic keratosis
   b. Acne
   c. Keratosis pilaris
   d. Lichen planus

9. Your patient with lichen simplex chronicus is frustrated by her persistent itching. When you are educating her to maximize her ability to self-manage, you emphasize that the most important aspect of treatment is:
   a. Applying moisturizer
   b. Getting a good night's sleep
   c. Breaking the itch–scratch cycle or the condition will not improve
   d. Taking her antihistamines

10. Lichenification is a condition that develops once scratching or rubbing becomes chronic. The skin thickens as a protective mechanism and develops common characteristics of leather-like hypertrophy with exaggerated skin markings (similar to calluses that form on the palms and soles following mechanical trauma). It is always seen in lichen simplex chronicus but may also be seen with atopic dermatitis and psoriasis.
    a. True
    b. False

Answers to Study Questions: 1.b, 2.a, 3.b, 4.a, 5.c, 6.d, 7.a, 8.c, 9.c, 10.a

Dermatitis/Eczemas

Noreen Heer Nicol

DERMATITIS AND ECZEMA

I. OVERVIEW

A. Dermatitis and eczema are two general terms that are generally interchangeable and describe a particular type of inflammatory response in the skin.

B. Diseases that are considered eczematous disorders are generally characterized by pruritus, lesions with indistinct borders, and epidermal changes.

C. These lesions can appear as erythema, papules, or lichenification of the skin.

D. The disorder presents in an acute, subacute, or chronic phase.

E. The inflammatory process of eczema or dermatitis takes place primarily at the level of the epidermis; however, the dermis can be involved.

F. There are many different types of eczema or dermatitis (Box 9-1, Figure 9-1).

II. COMMON THERAPEUTIC MODALITY

Basic Skin Care for All Patients with Dermatitis or Eczema (Boxes 9-2 and 9-3).

A. Methods of skin hydration and moisturization

B. Proper methods of application of medications

C. Ways to incorporate treatments into daily routines

Tips for All Patients with Dermatitis or Eczema to Reduce Skin Irritation (Box 9-4)

III. RESOURCES FOR ALL TYPES OF DERMATITIS AND ECZEMA (BOX 9-5)

ATOPIC DERMATITIS

I. OVERVIEW

A. Definition

  1. AD is the most common chronic, relapsing inflammatory skin disease of children and is a global health problem.

  2. The disorder leads to pruritus and disruption of the skin surface.

  3. The disease is usually associated with a personal or family history of asthma, allergic rhinitis, or eczema.

B. Etiology

  1. The exact pathogenesis is unknown.

  2. Commonly, there is a family history of AD, asthma, and/or allergic rhinitis and/or food allergy.

  3. Precipitating factors in AD.

    a. Genetic predisposition

    b. Age

Box 9-1. Types of Dermatitis (Eczema)

- **Allergic contact dermatitis (allergic contact eczema).** A red, itchy, weepy reaction where the skin has initially come into contact with a substance that the immune system recognizes as foreign, such as poison ivy or certain preservatives in creams and lotions. This is a delayed hypersensitivity reaction.
- **Atopic dermatitis (atopic eczema).** A chronic skin disease characterized by itchy, inflamed skin associated with a personal or family history of asthma, allergic rhinitis, or eczema.
- **Diaper dermatitis (Diaper rash).** An inflammatory reaction localized to the area of skin usually covered by the diaper. It can have many causes, including infections (yeast, bacterial, or viral), friction irritation, chemical allergies (preservatives, perfumes, soaps, etc.), sweat, decomposed urine, and plugged sweat glands.
- **Dyshidrotic eczema.** Irritation of the skin on the palms of the hands and soles of the feet characterized by clear, deep blisters that itch and burn.
- **Irritant contact dermatitis (irritant contact eczema).** A localized reaction that includes redness, itching, and burning where the skin has come into contact with a substance acting as an irritant such as an acid, a cleaning agent, other chemical, or even water.
- **Neurodermatitis (lichen simplex chronicus).** Scaly patches of the skin on the head, lower legs, wrists, or forearms characterized by skin lichenification secondary to excessive scratching and rubbing of the skin.
- **Nummular eczema (discoid eczema).** Coin-shaped patches of irritated skin—most common on the arms, back, buttocks, and lower legs—that may be crusted, scaling, and extremely itchy.
- **Seborrheic dermatitis (seborrheic eczema).** Yellowish, oily, scaly patches of skin on the scalp, face, and occasionally other parts of the body.
- **Stasis dermatitis.** A skin irritation on the lower legs, generally related to circulatory problems, which often presents with hyperpigmented areas.
- **Xerotic eczema ("xerotic dermatitis," "eczema craquele," "asteatotic eczema," "Winter itch," and "Winter eczema").** Irritated skin that occurs when the skin becomes abnormally dry, itchy, and cracked. It can appear in red bumpy or scaly.

Box 9-2. Patient Education: All Types of Dermatitis and Eczema

- Spend time listening to the patient and/or the parent.
- Individualize treatment.
- Explain the nature of the disease and clarify that the goal is control, not cure.
- Explain the role and the correct use of each therapy, including risks and benefits.
- Demonstrate the technique and how much of various topical agents to apply (e.g., emollients, sealers, medications).
- Reinforce the need to use emollients frequently and liberally.
- Explain the factors that need to be taken into account to decide whether to prescribe topical corticosteroids, topical calcineurin inhibitors, and other systemic therapies:
  ○ Patient's age
  ○ Site to be treated
  ○ Previous response to other therapies
  ○ Extent/severity of disease
- Explain how skin infection (bacterial or viral) can cause deterioration in condition, and teach the signs and symptoms of skin infection.
- Provide written recommendations with step care moving up and down regarding all therapies including bathing and/or showering.
- Include written instructions for prescription as well as over-the-counter products.
- Distribute patient-education brochures.
- Recommend individualized environmental measures to avoid skin irritants and proven allergens.
- Recommend psychosocial support as appropriate.

Adapted from Nicol, N. H. (2005a). Atopic triad: Atopic dermatitis, allergic rhinitis and asthma. *American Journal for Nurse Practitioners*, (Suppl), 36–40; Nicol, N. H. (2005b). Use of moisturizers in dermatologic disease: The role of healthcare providers in optimizing treatment outcomes. *Cutis*, 76(Suppl 6), 26–31; Nicol, N. H., & Ersser, S. J. (2010). The role of the nurse educator in managing atopic dermatitis. In M. Boguniewicz (Ed.), *Immunology and allergy clinics of North America: Atopic dermatitis* (pp. 369–383). Philadelphia, PA: Saunders-Elsevier.

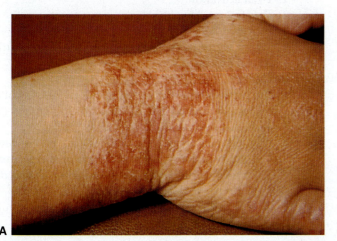
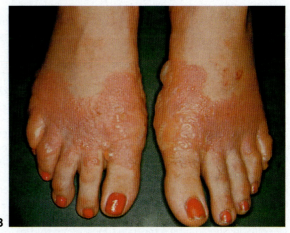

A **B**

FIGURE 9-1. Contact dermatitis. **A.** Allergic contact dermatitis results when a substance comes in direct contact with the skin, leading to a simple inflammatory reaction. **B.** Irritant contact dermatitis results when the substance causes direct skin damage, pain, or ulceration, such as with tight shoes or prolonged use of latex gloves. (From Cohen, B. J., & DePetris, A. (2013). *Medical terminology*. Philadelphia, PA: Wolters Kluwer.)

> **Box 9-3. Basic Principles of Skin Care for Patients with Dermatitis or Eczema**
>
> **Intact and healthy skin is the body's first line of defense. Hydration and moisturization will prevent the breakdown of the skin. "Soak and Seal" is the cornerstone to good daily skin care.**
>
> 1. Soak by taking at least one bath or shower per day; use warm water, for 10 to 15 minutes.
> 2. Use a gentle cleansing bar or wash in the sensitive skin formulation (fragrance-free, dye-free) as needed.
> 3. Seal by patting away excess water and immediately (within 3 minutes) apply moisturizer (fragrance-free moisturizers available in one pound jars or large tubes including Aquaphor ointment, Vaniply ointment, Eucerin Creme (various formulations), Vanicream, CeraVe cream, or Cetaphil cream). Vaseline is a good occlusive preparation to seal in but is most effective after bath or shower. Topical maintenance medications may be used in place of moisturizers or sealer when prescribed.
> 4. Use moisturizers liberally throughout the day. Moisturizers and sealers should not be applied immediately over any topical medication.
> 5. Avoid skin irritants and proven/clinically relevant allergens.
>
> Adapted from Nicol, N. H., & Boguniewicz, M. (2008). Successful strategies in AD management. *Dermatology Nursing*, (Suppl), 3–19.

   c. Emotional stress
   d. Lifestyle
   e. Irritants including course clothing such as wool and some synthetic fabrics, sweating, drying cleansers, cosmetics, or other topical preparations
   f. Climate and extremes in temperature and humidity: hot/humid or cold/dry

> **Box 9-4. Tips for Patients with Dermatitis or Eczema to Reduce Skin Irritation**
>
> • Recognize that skin sensitivity varies among people and according to their health status.
> • Avoid skin irritants and proven/clinically relevant allergens.
> • Learn to read product labels carefully and critically.
> • Use fragrance-free, dye-free products whenever possible. Recognize that even products labeled as for sensitive skin may have a masking or regular fragrance.
> • Add a second rinse cycle to ensure removal of detergent. Changing to a liquid and fragrance-free, dye-free detergent may be helpful.
> • Wear garments that allow air to pass freely to your skin. Open weave, loose-fitting, cotton-blend clothing may be most comfortable.
> • Work and sleep in comfortable surroundings with a fairly constant temperature and humidity level. Humidifiers remain controversial and should be used with great caution and cleaned very routinely when used.
> • Keep fingernails very short and smooth to help prevent damage due to scratching.
> • Carry a small tube of moisturizer/sunscreen at all times. Daycare/school/work should have a separate supply of moisturizer.
> • After swimming in chlorinated pool or using hot tub, shower or bathe using a gentle cleanser to remove chemicals and then apply moisturizer.
>
> Adapted from Nicol, N. H., & Boguniewicz, M. (2008). Successful strategies in AD management. *Dermatology Nursing*, (Suppl), 3–19.

> **Box 9-5. Dermatitis/Eczema Resources and Patient Education**
>
> American Academy of Dermatology
> www.aad.org
> American Academy of Allergy, Asthma, and Immunology
> www.aaaai.org
> American Cancer Society
> www.cancer.org
> American College of Allergy, Asthma, and Immunology
> www.acaai.org
> American Skin Association
> www.americanskin.org
> Centers for Disease Control and Prevention
> www.cdc.gov
> Food Allergy and Anaphylaxis Network
> www.foodallergy.org
> National Eczema Association
> www.nationaleczema.org
> National Eczema Society in the United Kingdom
> www.eczema.org
> National Psoriasis Foundation
> www.psoriasis.org
> National Institute of Arthritis and Musculoskeletal and Skin Diseases (NIAMS)
> www.niams.nih.gov
> The Skin Cancer Foundation
> www.skincancer.org

   g. Proven and clinically relevant environmental allergens (e.g., dust mite, cat, contact allergens including chemicals)
   h. Proven and clinically relevant food allergens (e.g., milk, soy, egg, wheat, fish, and nuts)
C. Pathogenesis
   1. Skin barrier abnormalities.
   2. T-cell activation.
   3. Th1/Th2 cytokine imbalance.
   4. Increased IgE production.
   5. *Staphylococcal aureus* and staphylococcal toxins trigger several processes.
D. Incidence
   1. The prevalence has increased to at least 20% in children and approximately 3% of adults in the United States and other industrialized countries.
   2. Fifty percent of patients with AD go on to develop respiratory manifestations of asthma or allergic rhinitis.
      a. Onset of clinical manifestations before 5 years of age in almost 90% of cases
      b. Almost 75% of all cases clear by adolescence but can reoccur in adults.

II. ASSESSMENT

A. Clinical manifestations
   1. Characterized by basic diagnostic criteria: patient must have three or more basic features (a to d) listed below.
      a. Pruritus

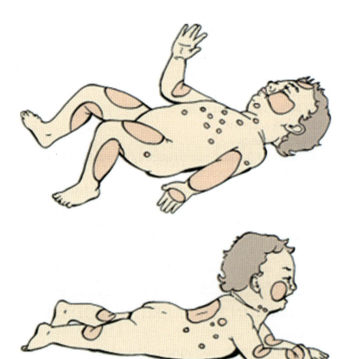

FIGURE 9-2. Distribution of infant atopic dermatitis occurs primarily on the face and scalp and extensor surfaces of the extremities. Diaper areas are usually clear. (From Nettina, S. M. (2009). *Lippincott manual of nursing practice* (9th ed.). Philadelphia, PA: Wolters Kluwer.)

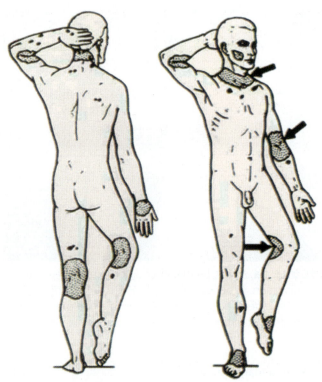

FIGURE 9-4. Distribution of atopic dermatitis in older children and adults typically has involvement of the flexor surfaces (antecubital and popliteal fossa), neck, wrists, and ankles. (Courtesy of Noreen Heer Nicol, PhD, RN.)

b. Typical morphology and distribution:
   (1) Facial and extensor involvement in infants and children. In infants and young children with AD, involvement is commonly present on the scalp, face (cheeks and chin), and extensor surfaces of the extremities (Figures 9-2 and 9-3). Tends to be symmetrical. Is more pronounced in areas not covered by clothing. Diaper area is generally clear in infants.
   (2) Flexural lichenification in adults. Older children and adults typically have involvement of the flexor surfaces (antecubital and popliteal fossa), neck, wrists, and ankles (Figures 9-4 and 9-5). In adults, the hands and feet frequently are involved. The flexor surfaces tend to have greater involvement in older patients.

c. Chronic or chronically relapsing dermatitis
d. Personal or family history of atopy (asthma, allergic rhinitis, AD)
2. Other common skin features associated with AD are listed in Box 9-6.
3. Severity ranges from mild to severe and tends to wax and wane with seasonal variation in select patients, often worsening in the winter due increased dryness.
4. Primary lesions.
   a. Some believe no primary lesion can be identified and that all visible skin lesions in AD are secondary to scratching.
   b. Erythematous papules that may coalesce or dry scaly patches

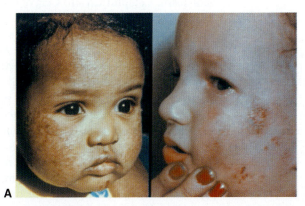
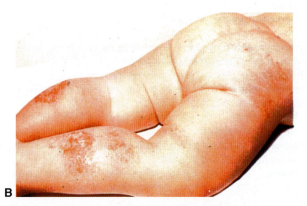

FIGURE 9-3. Infantile atopic dermatitis of the head **(A)** and of the limbs **(B)**. (Courtesy of Schering.)

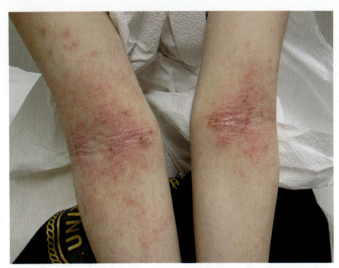

FIGURE 9-5. Atopic dermatitis of antecubital fossae with lichenification. (From Goodheart, H. P. (2010). *Goodheart's same-site differential diagnosis: A rapid method of diagnosing and treating common skin disorders.* Philadelphia, PA: Wolters Kluwer.)

   5. Secondary lesions.
      a. Scale
      b. Excoriations
      c. Lichenification
      d. White dermatographism
   6. Complications.
      a. Secondary bacterial infection usually caused by *S. aureus*
      b. Eczema herpeticum as well as other viral and fungal infections including molluscum and tinea
B. Differential diagnoses
   1. Allergic contact dermatitis
   2. Immunodeficiency
   3. Irritant contact dermatitis
   4. Lichen simplex chronicus
   5. Mollusca contagiosa with dermatitis

Box 9-6.   Skin Features Associated with Atopic Dermatitis

- **Atopic pleat (Dennie–Morgan fold)**—extra fold of skin that develops under the eye
- **Cheilitis**—inflammation of the skin on and around the lips
- **Hyperlinear palms**—increased number of skin creases on the palms
- **Hyperpigmented eyelids**—eyelids that have become darker in color from inflammation or hay fever
- **Ichthyosis**—dry, rectangular scales on the skin
- **Keratosis pilaris**—small, rough bumps, generally on the face, upper arms, and thighs
- **Lichenification**—thick, leathery skin resulting from constant scratching and rubbing
- **Papules**—small raised bumps that may open when scratched and become crusty and infected
- **Urticaria**—hives (red, raised bumps) that may occur after exposure to an allergen, at the beginning of flares, or after exercise or a hot bath

---

   6. Mycosis fungoides (cutaneous T-cell lymphoma)
   7. Nummular dermatitis
   8. Plaque psoriasis
   9. Relative zinc deficiency
   10. Scabies
   11. Seborrheic dermatitis
   12. Tinea corporis
C. Diagnostic tests
   1. Serum IgE tests are frequently elevated but are not helpful diagnostically.
   2. Allergy testing when allergies are suspected. Prick skin testing, patch testing, and in vitro testing can be useful in assessing triggers. Clinical correlation with allergy results and patient's exposure to these triggers are necessary prior to any restrictions.
   3. Skin cultures and sensitivities in cases of suspected secondary infection.

III. COMMON THERAPEUTIC MODALITIES

A. Treatment
   1. Interventions: see Atopic Dermatitis Action Plan (Box 9-7).
      a. Relief of xerosis: soak and seal
         (1) Soak by taking a bath or shower at least once per day. Use warm, not hot, water for 15 to 20 minutes. Avoid scrubbing skin with a washcloth. Bath time should be relaxing and enjoyable for children and adults alike (Figure 9-6).
         (2) Use a gentle cleansing bar or wash such as Dove, Oil of Olay, Eucerin, Basis, Cetaphil, or Aveeno. During a severe flare, limit the use of cleansers to avoid possible irritation. Gentle cleansers are generally perfume-free and dye-free.
         (3) Seal by patting gently away excess water after the bath or shower and immediately applying the moisturizer or the special skin medications prescribed onto damp skin. This will seal in the water and make the skin less dry and itchy. Moisturizers should not be applied over the medications. Vaseline is a good occlusive preparation to seal in the water; however, it contains no water, so it only works effectively after a soaking bath. Recommended moisturizers include Aquaphor Ointment, Eucerin Creme, Vanicream, Cetaphil Cream, CeraVe Cream, or Aveeno Cream (Figure 9-7).
         (4) Wet wrap therapy twice a day when severe or overnight to treat moderate-to-severe AD with multiple excoriations, crusting, and weeping lesions (Box 9-8, Figure 9-8).
            (a) Wet one pair of cotton sleepers, pajamas, or long underwear in warm water, wring out until damp, and put on immediately after applying topical medications.
            (b) Special layering when facial wraps required.
            (c) Place a dry layer on top of the damp ones.
            (d) Not to be used as preventive or maintenance therapy.

Box 9-7. Atopic Dermatitis Action Plan

Basic or Daily Care for Patient with Atopic Dermatitis: "Soak and Seal"

1. Soak by taking at least one bath or shower per day; use warm water, for 10 to 15 minutes.
2. Use a gentle cleansing bar or wash in the sensitive skin formulation (fragrance-free, dye-free) as needed.
3. Seal by patting away excess water and immediately (within 3 minutes) apply moisturizer (fragrance-free moisturizers available in one pound jars or large tubes. Moisturizers include Aquaphor ointment, Vaniply ointment, Eucerin Creme (various formulations), Vanicream, CeraVe cream or Cetaphil cream). A sealer (Vaseline is a good occlusive preparation to seal in and is most effective after bath or shower), or maintenance medication if directed. Use moisturizers liberally throughout the day. Moisturizers and sealers should not be applied immediately over any topical medication.
4. Avoid skin irritants and proven/clinically relevant allergens.

Mild-to-moderate atopic dermatitis

1. Bathe as above for 10 to 15 minutes in comfortably warm water, one to two times a day.
2. Use a gentle cleansing bar or wash in the sensitive skin formulation as needed.
3. Use moisturizers as above to healed and unaffected skin, twice daily especially after baths and at midday total body.
4. Apply to affected areas of the face, groin, and underarms twice daily especially after baths _____ (low-potency topical corticosteroid), or _____ (topical calcineurin inhibitor), or other topical preparation as directed _____.
5. Apply to other affected areas of the body twice daily especially after baths _____ (low- to midpotency topical corticosteroid), or _____ (topical calcineurin inhibitors), or other topical preparation as directed _____.
6. Other medications as directed: _____ (e.g., oral sedating antihistamines, topical or oral antimicrobial therapy)
7. Pay close attention to things that seem to irritate the skin or make condition worse.

Moderate-to-severe atopic dermatitis

1. Bathe as above for 10 to 15 minutes in comfortably warm water, two times a day, in the morning and before bedtime. Your health care provider may recommend dilute bleach baths.
2. Use a gentle cleansing bar or wash in the sensitive skin formulation as needed. May consider an antibacterial cleanser.
3. Use moisturizers as above to healed and unaffected skin, twice daily especially after baths and at midday total body.
4. Apply to affected areas of the face, groin, and underarms twice daily especially after baths _____ (low-potency topical corticosteroid), or _____ (topical calcineurin inhibitors), or other topical preparation as directed _____.
5. Apply to other affected areas of the body twice daily especially after baths _____ (mid- to high-potency topical corticosteroid), or _____ (topical calcineurin inhibitor), or other topical preparation as directed _____.

6. Use wet wraps to involved areas selectively as directed per policy and procedure. Wet wraps are left in place at a minimum of 2 hours. If left in place, need to be rewet every 2 to 3 hours. In general, wet wraps should be removed after 4 hours. If patient falls asleep with wet wraps in place, they may be left on overnight. Stop rewetting during the night. Apply moisturizer to total body after wet wraps are removed.
7. Add other medications as directed: _____ (e.g., oral sedating antihistamines, topical or oral antimicrobial therapy).
8. Pay close attention to things that irritate skin or make condition worse.
9. Step down to moderate plan as above as the skin heals.

Adapted from Nicol, N. H., & Boguniewicz, M. (2008). Successful strategies in AD management. *Dermatology Nursing*, (Suppl), 3–19. This may be modified and used for patient care citing National Jewish Health Atopic Dermatitis Program as source.

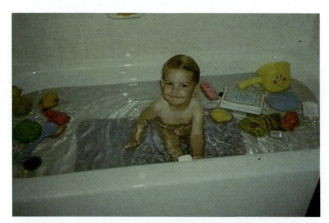

FIGURE 9-6. Soak in warm water for 15 to 20 minutes. (Courtesy of Noreen Heer Nicol, PhD, RN.)

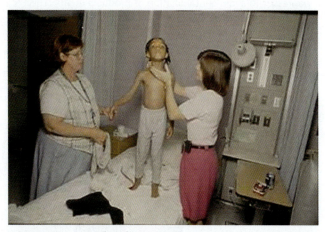

FIGURE 9-7. Seal with appropriate topicals and moisturizers immediately after bathing. (Courtesy of Noreen Heer Nicol, PhD, RN.)

Box 9-8. Wet Wrap Therapy Procedure

- Wet wrap therapy is to be used to relieve inflammation, itching, and burning of atopic dermatitis.
- Wet wraps facilitate the removal of scale and increase penetration of topical medications in the stratum corneum.
- Skin protection provided by the wraps allows healing to take place and cooling of the skin.
- Wet wrap therapy should only be used during flares of atopic dermatitis under the supervision of a health care provider. They should not be used as routine maintenance therapy.

Supplies:

1. Topical medications and moisturizers
2. Tap water at comfortably warm temperature
3. Basin for dampening of dressings
4. Clean dressings of approximate size to cover involved area
   a. ***Face***: 2 to 3 layers of wet Kerlix gauze held in place with SurgiNet.
   b. ***Arms, legs, hands, and feet***: 2 to 3 layers of wet Kerlix gauze held in place with Ace bandages or tube socks, or cotton gloves, or wet tube socks followed by dry tube socks. Tube socks may be used for wraps for hands and feet, and larger ones work as leg/arm covers.
   c. ***Total body***: Combination of above or wet pajamas or long underwear and turtleneck shirts covered by dry pajamas or sweat suit. Pajamas with feet work well for the outer layer.
4. Blankets to prevent chilling
5. Nonsterile gloves if desired

Procedure

1. Be certain that the patient's room is warm and insure privacy. Gather supplies appropriate to the individual.
2. If wraps are to be applied to a large portion of the body, work with two people if possible. It is necessary to work rapidly to prevent chilling.
3. Explain the procedure to the patient and parent.
4. Fill the basin with warm tap water.
5. The patient will have had a 15- to 20-minute soaking bath, in warm water without additional additives, prior to this procedure. Pat skin dry with a towel.
6. Apply the appropriate topical medications to the affected areas and moisturizer to the nonaffected areas immediately after pat drying the skin. Use clean plastic spoons or tongue depressor to avoid contamination of products in jars. This allows large areas to be covered quickly and prevent caregivers from unnecessary exposure to topical medications.

7. Soak the dressings in very warm water, as they cool quickly in this process. Squeeze out excess water. Dressings should be wet, not dripping.
8. Cover an area with wet dressing chosen for the area and the patient. Immediately after wrapping, cover with appropriate dry material such as an Ace bandage, socks, or pajamas. Start at the feet and move upward. Use wet, long underwear or wet pajamas covered by dry pajamas or sweat suit with total body involvement in place of wet gauze.
9. Take steps to avoid chilling. Blanket can be put in a dryer to warm up and cover patient but do not overheat the patient. Wraps can be removed after 2 to 4 hours or can be rewet. A warm blanket and snuggling help pass the time.
10. If the patient is known or suspected to have an infection of the involved areas, place dressings in the appropriate bag and dispose according to the infection control procedure.
11. After all dressings are removed, moisturizers may be applied to the entire body.

Adapted from Nicol, N. H. (1987). Atopic dermatitis: The (wet) wrap-up. *American Journal of Nursing, 87*(12), 1560–1563; Nicol, N. H., & Boguniewicz, M. (2008). Successful strategies in AD management. *Dermatology Nursing,* (Suppl), 3–19; Nicol, N. H., Boguniewicz, M., Strand, M., & Klinnert, M. D. (2014). Wet wrap therapy in children with moderate to severe atopic dermatitis in a multidisciplinary treatment program. *Journal of Allergy and Clinical Immunology: In Practice, 2*(4), 400–406. This may be modified and used for patient care citing National Jewish Health Atopic Dermatitis Program as source.

(e) To be used in conjunction with prescribed topical medications as well as moisturizers.
   b. Decrease inflammation
   (1) Mild-to-moderate strength topical corticosteroids or topical calcineurin inhibitors twice a day as needed. The two topical calcineurin inhibitors drugs, tacrolimus (Protopic) ointment and pimecrolimus (Elidel) cream, are effective in both adults and children without the common side effects of topical steroids such as thinning of the skin and increased skin infections.
   (2) Some patients with AD are sensitive to the ingredients of topical preparations both over the counter or prescription. Cream or ointment vehicles may be used on face and body with a lotion vehicle to scalp.
   (3) Wet wrap therapy may be used with topical corticosteroids in moderate-to-severe AD. They are not to be used as maintenance therapy.

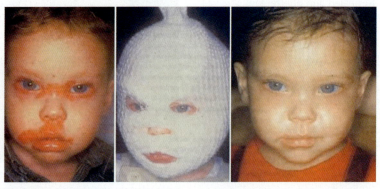

FIGURE 9-8. Wet wrap therapy in atopic dermatitis and play therapy. (Courtesy of Noreen Heer Nicol, PhD, RN, and Barry Silverstein.)

(4) Systemic corticosteroids are likely used too frequently in the treatment of this chronic condition of AD with significant potential of side effects and rebound flaring.

c. Relief of pruritus

(1) Sedating antihistamines such as diphenhydramine (3 to 5 mg/kg/d) or hydroxyzine (1 to 2 mg/kg/d) may help to relieve pruritus.

(2) Use sedating antihistamines at bedtime to decrease itching and to promote more restful sleep.

(3) The relatively low-sedating antihistamine cetirizine may be used to provide relief from pruritus in children as young as 6 months of age during the daytime. The role of nonsedating antihistamines in the treatment of AD remains unclear.

d. Treatment of infections

(1) Topical antibiotic—mupirocin 2% ointment may be applied three times a day to small areas of impetigo. Use three times per day until clearing; never use PRN.

(2) For more widespread infection, use an antistaphylococcal oral antibiotic (e.g., cephalexin 25 to 50 mg/kg/d).

e. Environmental control

(1) Decrease exposure to predisposing factors, which have been evaluated and agreed to by treatment team.

(2) Avoid exposure to anyone with active herpes lesions.

B. Follow-up

1. First follow-up visit in 7 to 14 days to assess treatment effectiveness with patients who have moderate-to-severe disease.

2. Monthly visits until the patient is using primarily moisturizers.

3. When skin condition is stable, visits every 6 months for re-evaluation.

4. As needed for flairs and failure to respond to treatment.

5. AD is usually a long-term condition. Patients may need many repeated treatments before the symptoms go away. And they may return later.

PATIENT EDUCATION
Atopic Dermatitis (SEE BOX 9-2, 9-3, 9-4, 9-5, and 9-7)

• Methods of skin hydration
• Address itch-stratch cycle
• Proper methods of application and amounts of medications
• Signs of skin infection
• Ways to incorporate treatments into daily routines
• Sources of psychosocial support

SEBORRHEIC DERMATITIS

I. OVERVIEW

A. Definition

1. Common chronic dermatitis occurring primarily in areas of increased sebaceous gland concentration resulting in a papulosquamous disorder

2. Occurs in multiple age groups—the infant, the adolescent, and the adult

B. Etiology

1. The exact pathogenesis is unknown.

2. Several factors are associated with the condition including hormonal levels, fungal infections, and nutritional deficits.

3. Occasionally, it may be associated with serious illness and failure to thrive. Rarely, it is an early sign of HIV or other immunodeficiency diseases.

4. Stress can cause flare-ups.

C. Pathogenesis

1. Pathology has been attributed to excessive sebum accumulation on skin surface, but the mechanism for this remains unclear.

2. Occurrence in the neonate is believed to be related to intrauterine exposure to maternal hormones.

3. Occurrence may be linked to a type of yeast, Malassezia furfur. While there are normal levels, there is an abnormal immune response.

4. Immunologic abnormalities linked to T-cell depression and activation of the alternative complement pathway

D. Incidence

1. The incidence in the general population is 2% to 5%.

2. In infants, it tends to regress by 5 to 6 months of age (Figure 9-9).

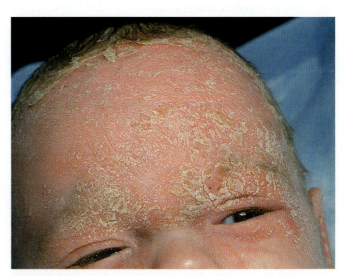

FIGURE 9-9. Severe seborrheic dermatitis with thick, waxy, yellow scale and underlying erythema in an infant. (From Burkhart, C., Morrell, D., Goldsmith, L. A., Papier, A., Green, B., Dasher, D., & Gomathy, S. (2009). *VisualDx: Essential pediatric dermatology.* Philadelphia, PA: Wolters Kluwer.)

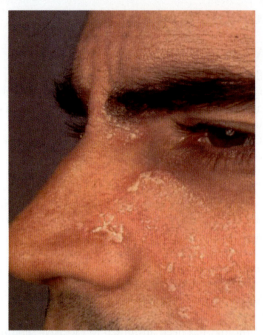

FIGURE 9-10. Seborrheic dermatitis on an adult face. (From Engleberg, N. C., Dermody, T., & DiRita, V. (2012). *Schaechter's mechanisms of microbial disease.* Philadelphia, PA: Wolters Kluwer.)

3. In adolescents and adults, it may improve with age and tends to wax and wane. Most common in adults 30 to 60 years of age (Figure 9-10)

II. ASSESSMENT

A. Clinical manifestations
   1. Minimal to no pruritus in infancy. Adolescents or adults may complain of pruritus.
   2. Lesions are symmetric and typically red with greasy yellow to salmon-colored scale.
   3. Areas of involvement are primarily the scalp, medial eyebrows, central face, retroauricular area, presternal area, or perineum. Seborrheic dermatitis can also affect oily areas of the body, such as the upper chest and back.
   4. Varies from minimal to widespread involvement
   5. Primary lesions—erythematous papules/patches, poorly marginated
   6. Secondary lesions—greasy scale, excoriations if pruritic
B. Differential diagnoses
   1. Allergic contact dermatitis
   2. Atopic dermatitis
   3. Cutaneous candidiasis
   4. Discoid lupus erythematosus, rare in children
   5. Drug eruptions
   6. Irritant contact dermatitis
   7. Nummular dermatitis
   8. Perioral dermatitis
   9. Pityriasis rosea

10. Psoriasis
11. Rosacea, rare under the age of 25
12. Systemic lupus erythematosus, rare in children
13. Tinea infections
C. Diagnostic tests
   1. Usually diagnosed by physical examination, unless another severe systemic disease is suspected
   2. Fungal, viral, and bacterial cultures, as appropriate
   3. Skin biopsy with disease unresponsive to treatment

III. COMMON THERAPEUTIC MODALITIES

A. Treatment
   1. Low-potency topical corticosteroid creams or topical calcineurin inhibitors applied twice daily for several days will usually clear the dermatitis and then used occasionally will control recurrences.
   2. Frequently in infants, tear-free shampoos are adequate to loosen the scales when allowed to remain on the scalp for several minutes and lightly scrubbed with a soft brush to remove the scale. In more difficult cases, scale may be loosened with mineral oil prior to shampooing.
   3. Keratolytic/antiseborrheic or ketoconazole (Nizoral) shampoos may be helpful for adolescents and adults to control scalp scaling.
B. Follow-up
   1. One-week visit to evaluate response, if appropriate
   2. Thereafter, the patient is seen only if the dermatitis does not resolve.
   3. Seborrheic dermatitis is usually a long-term condition. Patients may need many repeated treatments before the symptoms go away. And they may return later.

 PATIENT EDUCATION
Seborrheic Dermatitis

- For infants and children with cradle cap
  ○ Apply baby oil to soften the scale and gently comb out.
  ○ Follow by shampooing with a mild baby shampoo and longer lathering to gently remove the scale.
  ○ Use of an antiseborrheic dermatitis shampoo when milder shampoos are ineffective
  ○ Use prescribed hydrocortisone or an antiyeast cream to areas outside scalp as recommended.
- For adults
  ○ Use of an antiseborrheic dermatitis shampoo containing coal tar, selenium sulfide, or zinc pyrithione on a more frequent basis and longer lathering. Brand names include Selsun Blue, Head & Shoulders, and DHS zinc.
  ○ Use prescribed hydrocortisone or an antiyeast cream to areas outside scalp as recommended.
  ○ Discontinue use of hairsprays and hair pomades with active scalp involvement.

CONTACT DERMATITIS

I. OVERVIEW

A. Definition
   1. Contact dermatitis can be defined and divided on the basis of etiology into two types: irritant contact dermatitis (ICD) and allergic contact dermatitis (ACD).

B. Etiology
   1. Irritant nonallergic contact dermatitis results from direct contact with an irritating substance. Possible irritants are numerous, for example, oil products such as fuels and lubricants, corrosives, detergents, bleaches, ammonia, oven cleaners, ingredients in common skin products, and even water or frequent wetting and drying of skin (Figure 9-11).
   2. ACD affects a limited number of susceptible individuals and is a manifestation of a sensitivity to a substance to which the patient has had previous contact. Possible allergens are many; common examples include fragrances, dyes, nickel, antibiotic ointments or creams, rubber-containing products, formaldehyde, and poison ivy/oak (Figure 9-12).

C. Pathogenesis
   1. ICD from a local irritant is the most common form of contact dermatitis. The intensity of the inflammation is related to the concentration of the irritant and the exposure time.
   2. ACD triggers an immunologic event, which is the result of a type IV delayed hypersensitivity reaction to an allergen.

D. Incidence
   1. Anyone at any time could acquire ICD. Suspect patients working with cleaning agents such as ammonia, bleach, and other wet work and health care workers who work with various lotions, alcohol solutions, and repetitive hand washing and drying. Repeated higher concentrates of

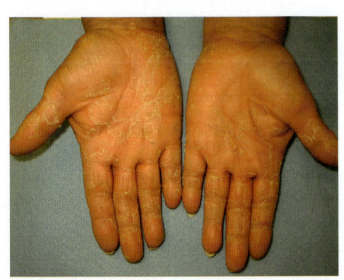

FIGURE 9-11. Irritant contact dermatitis on the hands of a health care worker. (Image provided by Stedman's.)

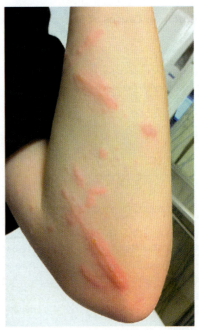

FIGURE 9-12. Allergic contact dermatitis secondary to poison ivy. Erythema and vesicle formation in a linear pattern is characteristic of poison ivy. (Courtesy of Darren Fiore, MD.)

chemicals can cause a contact dermatitis. Approximately 80% of contact dermatitis is irritant in nature.
   2. Individuals must be sensitized to a chemical to acquire contact allergic dermatitis. Patients initially come in contact with a sensitizing agent and have a reaction upon subsequent exposure to the agent. Approximately 20% of contact dermatitis is allergic in nature. Table 9-1 lists some of the most common allergens known to currently cause ACD.

II. ASSESSMENT

A. Clinical manifestations
   1. Irritant contact dermatitis
      a. Can be either acute or chronic. In the acute stage erythema, blister formation, erosion, crusting, shedding, and scaling are seen. The distribution is usually isolated or localized; pruritus is always present.
      b. In chronic contact dermatitis, thickening of skin, scaling, fissures, and crusting are present. Distribution is usually isolated or localized.
   2. Allergic contact dermatitis
      a. Can be either acute or chronic. In acute allergic dermatitis erythema, papules, vesicles, erosion, crusts, and scaling are seen. The dermatosis is usually confined to the area of exposure but can spread to peripheral areas.
      b. In ACD, the patient has been previously exposed to the allergen. This exposure creates a sensitization phase, which results in antigen formation. The resulting sensitized T cells remain in the body. Re-exposure to the antigen in the elicitation phase results in a cutaneous eczematous inflammation. Although

TABLE 9-1 Common Causes of Allergic Contact Dermatitis

Agent	Source
Bacitracin	Topical antibiotic
Balsam of Peru (Myroxylon pereirae)	Fragrance used in perfumes and skin lotions, derived from tree resin
Chromium	Used in tanning of leather Also a component of uncured cement/mortar, facial cosmetics, and some bar soaps
Cobalt chloride	Metal found in medical products; hair dye; antiperspirant; objects plated in metal such as snaps, buttons, or tools; and in cobalt blue pigment
Colophony (rosin)	Fosin, sap, or sawdust typically from spruce or fir trees
Formaldehyde	Preservative with multiple uses, for example, in paper products, paints, medications, household cleaners, cosmetic products, and fabric finishes
Fragrance mix	Group of the eight most common fragrance allergens found in foods, cosmetic products, insecticides, antiseptics, soaps, perfumes, and dental products
Gold (gold sodium thiosulfate)	Precious metal often found in jewelry
Isothiazolinone, methylisothiazolinone, methylchloroisothiazolinone	Preservatives used in many personal care, including wet wipes, household, and commercial products
Neomycin sulfate	Topical antibiotic common in first aid creams and ointments, also found occasionally in cosmetics, deodorant, soap, and pet food
Nickel (nickel sulfate hexahydrate)	Metal frequently encountered in jewelry and clasps or buttons on clothing
Quaternium 15	Preservative found in cosmetic products such as self-tanners, shampoo, nail polish, and sunscreen or in industrial products such as polishes, paints, and waxes
Poison ivy, poison oak, and poison sumac	Plants naturally occurring in many parts of the United States; oily coating from plants of *Toxicodendron* genus
Pramoxine, diphenhydramine	Topical anesthetics, for example, after prolonged use
Thimerosal	Mercury compound used in local antiseptics and formerly in vaccines

these reactions are usually localized, patients who are sensitized to topical medications may develop generalized eczematous reactions.

B. History and physical examination
   1. History of sensitivity to chemicals or substances
   2. Occupation and history of exposure to, for example, neomycin, procaine, benzocaine, sulfonamides, turpentine, balsam of Peru, formalin, chromate, nickel sulfate, cobalt sulfate, *p*-phenylenediamine, and many more.
   3. In an acute exposure, erythema, papules, and edema are present and are usually confined to area of exposure.
   4. In chronic exposure, plaques of lichenification with small, firm, round, or flat-topped papules with mild erythema are present.

C. Differential diagnoses
   1. Asteatotic eczema
   2. Atopic dermatitis
   3. Contact urticaria syndrome
   4. Drug-induced bullous disorders
   5. Drug-induced photosensitivity
   6. Irritant contact dermatitis
   7. Nummular dermatitis
   8. Perioral dermatitis
   9. Phytophotodermatitis
   10. Psoriasis
   11. Scabies
   12. Seborrheic dermatitis
   13. Tinea infections
   14. Transient acantholytic dermatosis

D. Diagnostic tests
   1. Patch testing: to help determine the responsible allergen in ACD and is considered the gold standard for testing. The goal of patch testing is to reproduce the eczema in a controlled process. Small amounts of suspected chemical are applied to the skin, and subsequent examination will reveal reaction. This process must be done in a standardized format to be reliable. The product T.R.U.E. TEST® offers standardized easy-to-use patch testing. Patient counseling of results is key in management. (See Chapter 3.)
   2. Potassium hydroxide preparation and/or fungal culture: To exclude tinea, these tests are often indicated for dermatitis of the hands and feet.
   3. Repeat open application testing (ROAT): To determine whether a reaction is significant in individuals who develop weak or 1+ positive reactions to a chemical
   4. Dimethylglyoxime test: To determine whether a metallic object contains enough nickel to provoke allergic dermatitis. These tests are available to patients as well as health care providers (i.e., Nickel Alert and Nickel Solution). They are very helpful for nickel-allergic patients to participate in determining safe products.
   5. Skin biopsy: May help to exclude other disorders, particularly tinea, psoriasis, and cutaneous T-cell lymphoma

III. COMMON THERAPEUTIC MODALITIES

A. Treatment—See Boxes 9-2, 9-3, 9-4, and 9-5
   1. Eliminate the irritant or allergen when possible.
   2. Topical corticosteroids are used carefully to avoid side effects.
   3. Consider PUVA (psoralen with ultraviolet A) (See Phototherapy Chapter)
   4. In severe cases, a short course of systemic corticosteroids may be required.
B. Follow-up
   1. First follow-up visit in 7 to 14 days to assess treatment effectiveness with patients who have moderate-to-severe disease.
   2. Monthly visits until the patient is using primarily moisturizers.
   3. When skin condition is stable, visits every 6 months for re-evaluation.
   4. As needed for flairs and failure to respond to treatment.
   5. Contact dermatitis, especially ICD, is usually a long-term condition. Patients may need many repeated treatments before the symptoms go away. And they may return later.

PATIENT EDUCATION
Contact Dermatitis

• Avoid any proven and clinically relevant irritants and allergens: do not eliminate things unnecessarily and make daily routines impossible.
• Be sure to have reliable information and sites for proven irritants and allergens.
• Methods of skin hydration and moisturization.
• Proper methods of application and amounts of medications.
• Avoid any activities that dry, heat, or irritate the skin.
• Dress in loose clothing or fabrics that are not irritating to the skin.

DIAPER DERMATITIS OR DIAPER RASH

I. OVERVIEW

A. Definition
   1. An inflammatory cutaneous eruption in the diaper area and one of the leading dermatology disorders that result in childhood dermatology visits. The majority of causes are due to ICD; however, ACD, infection, seborrhea, and psoriasis are other causes.
   2. A number of factors are important in this disease including wetness, friction, inappropriate skin care, microorganisms, antibiotics, and nutritional deficiencies.
B. Etiology and pathogenesis
   1. ICD in the diaper area is caused by an interaction between several factors and is the most frequent cause of diaper dermatitis or rash in the diaper area. Generally, this is seen on buttocks, lower abdomen, genitals, and upper thighs. The skin folds are not usually affected.

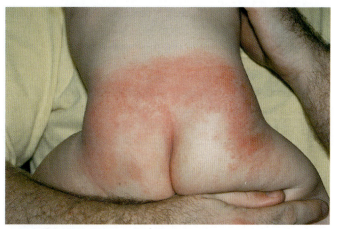

FIGURE 9-13. Irritant contact dermatitis. The patient has diaper rash with an eruption conforming to the shape of a diaper. (From Goodheart, H. P. (2003). *Goodheart's photoguide of common skin disorders* (2nd ed.). Philadelphia, PA: Lippincott Williams & Wilkins.)

Symptoms can vary from mild redness to extremely red, raised, and peeling (Figure 9-13).
   a. Frequent and prolonged skin wetness from occlusion and urine and feces trapped close to the skin
   b. Friction by movement of the skin against skin, the diaper, plastic leg gathers, or fastening tape.
   c. Fecal enzymes causing cutaneous irritation
   d. Oral antibiotic medication administrated for other disorders may predispose a child to diarrhea, which irritated and causes the development of diaper dermatitis.
   2. ACD in the diaper area is far less common than ICD. Itchy, red raised, or scaly areas are present in the areas of the skin that are in contact with the allergen used in the diaper area (Figure 9-14).
   a. Reported allergens include dyes, fragrances, preservatives, neomycin, bacitracin, lanolin, paraben, and other allergens.

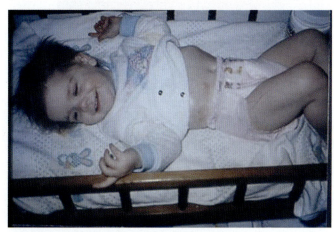

FIGURE 9-14. Allergic contact dermatitis from nickel in pajama snaps in the diaper area. (Courtesy of Noreen Heer Nicol, PhD, RN.)

b. Some baby wipes may contain a preservative, methylisothiazolinone (MI), which may also cause an allergic reaction in certain individuals.

3. Infection

a. If there is frequent and prolonged skin wetness for a prolonged number of days, there is likely to be a secondary *C. albicans* infection (yeast infection). This presents as confluent erythema to dark red with or without satellite papules or lesions. Yeast infections are often found in the skin folds between the thigh and body and in the folds of skin around the genitals (Figure 9-15).

b. Impetigo is a bacterial infection that can develop in the diaper area as well as other areas of the body. It is usually caused by bacteria that normally live on the skin including *Staphylococcus aureus* and group A streptococci; infection can develop when there is a break in the skin. Signs include tiny (1- to 2-mm) raised yellow fluid-filled areas and honey-colored crusted lesions; the lesions may be itchy and/or painful.

c. Other infections include coxsackievirus, human papillomavirus, herpes simplex virus, scabies, and human immunodeficiency virus.

4. Seborrhea or seborrheic dermatitis

a. Seborrhea is a skin condition that causes patches of redness and greasy yellow scaly skin in infants. It is commonly located in the skin folds between the thighs and body and is often found in other areas as well, including the scalp (where it is called "cradle cap"), face, neck, or in other skin folds (e.g., in the armpit, in front of the elbow, behind the knees).

b. Seborrhea is a more common cause of diaper rash/dermatitis.

5. Psoriasis

a. Psoriasis is considered a rare cause of diaper rash/dermatitis.

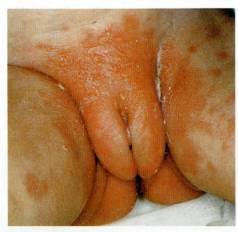

FIGURE 9-15. Diaper dermatitis due to candidal infection. This bright red rash involves the intertriginous folds, with small "satellite lesions" along the edges. (From Fletcher, M. (1998). *Physical diagnosis in neonatology.* Philadelphia, PA: Lippincott-Raven Publishers.)

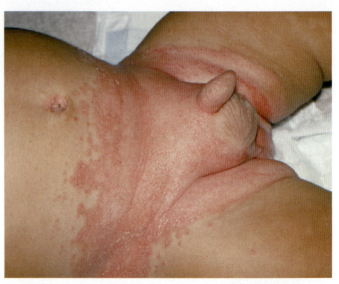

FIGURE 9-16. Psoriasis in the diaper area. These plaques easily could be confused with diaper rash or atopic dermatitis. (From Goodheart, H. P. (2003). *Goodheart's photoguide of common skin disorders* (2nd ed.). Philadelphia, PA: Lippincott Williams & Wilkins.)

b. Psoriasis symptoms often include reddened and silver scaly patches of skin. In the diaper area, the silver scale may be absent (Figure 9-16).

6. Other causes

a. Granuloma gluteale infantum

b. Epidermolysis bullosa

c. Ulcerative hemangioma

d. Infantile granular parakeratosis

e. Langerhans cell histiocytosis

f. Nutritional deficiencies

g. Immune deficiencies

C. Incidence

1. Diaper dermatitis is one of the most frequent skin disorders of infancy, with peak incidence between 9 and 12 months of age. It can start as early as the first week of life.

2. May occur in any child or adult who is incontinent of urine or stool.

II. ASSESSMENT

A. Clinical manifestations (see above with etiology)

1. Erythema with or without papules, erosions, scale, and/or maceration on the lower abdomen, groin, perineum, buttocks, labia majora, scrotum, penis, or upper thigh that initially spares skin creases.

2. Fragile bulla or erosions with a collarette of scale may indicate bullous impetigo.

B. Differential diagnoses

1. Irritant contact dermatitis

2. Atopic dermatitis

3. Cutaneous candidiasis

4. Drug eruptions

5. Allergic contact dermatitis

6. Tinea and bacterial infections

7. Langerhans cell histiocytosis
8. Nummular dermatitis
9. Psoriasis
10. Scabies
11. Seborrheic dermatitis
12. Others, child abuse
13. Human immunodeficiency virus, very rare in infants and children

C. Diagnostic tests
1. Usually diagnosed by physical examination, unless another severe systemic disease is suspected.
2. KOH preparation to skin scrapings to identify *C. albicans* infection.
3. Bacterial, fungal, and viral culture may be needed to rule out secondary infection.
4. Skin biopsy may be required in dermatitis that is unresponsive to therapy to rule out other associated problems particularly in older children or adults.
5. Workup for other systemic diseases as warranted.

III. COMMON THERAPEUTIC MODALITIES

A. Prevention
1. Prevention is the single most important intervention. Most diaper dermatitis is self-limited and may resolve or be prevented quickly with the following steps. Take care with any products that contain preservatives, fragrances, or other additives as they may further irritate the skin. It is important to closely read the ingredient label of all diaper products. The use of superabsorbent disposable diapers has decreased the incidence of the disease.
   a. Airing of the diaper area or frequent diaper changes
   b. Always clean the skin in the diaper area, gently. Use of warm water and a soft cloth is preferable.
   c. Applying barrier creams and ointments (such as petrolatum or zinc oxide) as preventive measures. The ointment or paste should be applied thickly at every diaper change and can be covered with petroleum jelly to prevent sticking to the diaper. The ointment or paste should be long lasting and should stick to irritated or broken areas of skin. It is not necessary to completely clean the ointment or paste off the skin at diaper changes.
2. Always clean the skin in the diaper area, gently. Aggressive cleansing can cause or worsen irritation and delay skin healing. Gentle cleansing with warm water and a soft cloth is usually sufficient. If soap is desired, a mild, fragrance-free product (sample brand names: Dove sensitive or Cetaphil) is recommended. Powders are best avoided.

B. Treatment
1. *C. albicans* diaper dermatitis is treated with a topical antiyeast cream such as nystatin applied TID or with each diaper change. A barrier cream or petrolatum may be placed over the antiyeast cream.
2. In severe dermatitis, hydrocortisone 1% cream twice daily for 1 or 2 days may help to decrease discomfort in between use of other topicals.

C. Follow-up
1. Routine visits for care is sufficient follow-up.
2. In severe diaper dermatitis, a return visit to assess response is recommended.

PATIENT EDUCATION
Diaper Dermatitis or Diaper Rash

• Diaper dermatitis or diaper rash treatment is most effective when a combination of measures is used together. The letters **ABCDE** help to remember all of these measures:
  ○ A = air out the skin by allowing the child to go diaper-free or frequent changes
  ○ B = barrier; use a paste or ointment to protect the skin.
  ○ C = clean; keep the skin clean.
  ○ D = disposable diapers; during an episode of diaper rash, consider using disposable rather than cloth diapers.
  ○ E = educate; educate yourself about how to prevent a recurrence of diaper rash.

NUMMULAR DERMATITIS (NUMMULAR ECZEMA OR DISCOID ECZEMA)

I. OVERVIEW

A. Definition: An inflammatory skin disorder with coin-shaped, usually scaly, lesions generally affecting lower extremities, also referred to as discoid eczema
B. Etiology
1. The exact pathogenesis is unknown.
2. The exudative variant starts acutely and may persist for weeks, months, and rarely years.
3. Secondary infection is common, and sensitivity to contactants is thought to play a role.
C. Pathogenesis
1. The initial plaque may appear at the site of trauma or infection, for example, a thermal burn, scabies infestation, varicose vein surgery, insect bite, or localized ACD site.
2. Severe, extensive nummular dermatitis can be an "id" reaction or an autoeczematization following another type of severe infectious or inflammatory process.
D. Incidence
1. Often appears after a skin injury, such as a abrasion, insect bite, or burn
2. Affects males more than females
3. Men tend to have first outbreaks between 55 and 65 years.
4. Women are likely to have first outbreaks younger between 15 and 25 years.
5. Children are affected less often.
E. Considerations across lifespan
1. The condition is chronic.
2. Plaques may be lichenified.

II. ASSESSMENT

A. Clinical manifestations
1. Characterized by lesions that are 2 to 10 cm or more, distinct, coin shaped or oval, and often distributed symmetrically on the lower legs, arms, backs of hands, and other sites (Figure 9-17)
2. Presents in two forms
   a. Dry, nummular dermatitis, which is usually subacute with erythema and edema
   b. Exudative "wet" nummular dermatitis with vesiculation followed by oozing and scaling
3. Pruritus may be present; color is usually pink to dull red; plaque may be present.
B. History and physical examination
   a. History of psoriasis, AD, and contact dermatitis associated with subsequent nummular eczema.
   b. Lesions may be present for months to weeks.
   c. Change in seasons or excessive cold may initiate nummular eczema.
   d. Coin-shaped, small vesicles and papules with regional clusters of lesions.
C. Differential diagnoses
1. Allergic contact dermatitis
2. Atopic dermatitis
3. Cutaneous T-cell lymphoma
4. Drug eruptions
5. Irritant contact dermatitis
6. Pityriasis rosea
7. Plaque psoriasis
8. Stasis dermatitis
9. Tinea infections, particularly tinea corporis
D. Diagnostic tests
1. Microscopy of skin scrapings to rule out fungal infection.
2. Bacterial, fungal, and viral culture may be needed to rule out secondary infection.

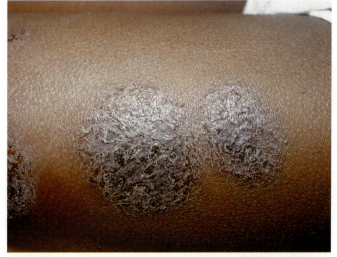

FIGURE 9-17. Nummular eczema with thick, adherent scale crust. (From Lugo-Somolinos, A., Lee, I., McKinley-Grant, L., Goldsmith, L. A., Papier, A., Adigun, C. G., ..., Fredeking, A. (2011). *VisualDx: Essential dermatology in pigmented skin*. Philadelphia, PA: Wolters Kluwer.)

3. Skin biopsy may be required in dermatitis that is unresponsive to therapy to rule out other associated problems particularly in older children or adults.
4. Workup for other systemic diseases as warranted

III. COMMON THERAPEUTIC MODALITIES

A. Treatment—See first section on all eczemas and dermatitis.
1. Therapeutic interventions
   a. Hydration of skin with moisturizing creams and ointments
   b. Use of topical corticosteroids or topical calcineurin inhibitors
   c. Use of topical tar preparations
   d. Use of systemic antibiotics if secondary bacterial infection
   e. PUVA or narrow-band ultraviolet B may be used in very difficult cases.
   f. Resistant lesions may require intralesional corticosteroid injections.
B. Follow-up
1. First follow-up visit in 7 to 14 days to assess treatment effectiveness with patients who have moderate-to-severe disease
2. Monthly visits until the patient is using primarily moisturizers
3. When skin condition is stable, visits every 6 months for re-evaluation
4. As needed for flairs and failure to respond to treatment
5. Nummular dermatitis can be a long-term condition. Patients may need many repeated treatments before the symptoms go away. The symptoms may return later.

PATIENT EDUCATION
Nummular Dermatitis (See Boxes 9-2, 9-3, 9-4, 9-5, and 9-7)

- Methods of skin hydration and moisturization
- Skip any cleansers or topicals that may be drying.
- Proper methods of application and amounts of medications
- Avoid any activities that dry, heat, or irritate the skin.
- Dress in loose clothing or fabrics that are not irritating to the skin.

OTHER COMMONLY SEEN DISORDERS IN PATIENTS WITH ECZEMA COVERED IN THIS TEXTBOOK

i. Lichen simplex chronicus: See Papulosquamous Diseases (Chapter 8).
ii. Keratosis pilaris: See Papulosquamous Diseases (Chapter 8).
iii. Ichthyosis: See Dermatologic Conditions in Children (Chapter 13).

BIBLIOGRAPHY

Akdis, C. A., Akdis, M., Bieber, T., Bindsley-Jensen, C., Boguniewicz, M., Eigenmann, P., ..., Zuberbier, T. (2006). Diagnosis and treatment of AD in children and adults: European Academy of Allergology and Clinical Immunology/American Academy of Allergy, Asthma and Immunology/PRACTALL Consensus Report. *Journal of Allergy and Clinical Immunology, 118,* 152–169.

Berger, T. G., Duvic, M., Van Voorhees, A. S., VanBeek, M. J., Frieden, I. J., & American Academy of Dermatology Association Task Force. (2006). The use of topical calcineurin inhibitors in dermatology: Safety concerns. Report of the American Academy of Dermatology Association Task Force. *Journal of the American Academy of Dermatology, 54*(5), 818–823.

Boguniewicz, M., & Leung, D. Y. M. (2010). Recent insights into AD and implications for management of infectious complications. *Journal of Allergy and Clinical Immunology, 125*(1), 4–13.

Boguniewicz, M., & Leung, D. Y. M. (2011). Atopic dermatitis: A disease of altered skin barrier and immune dysregulation. *Immunological Reviews, 242,* 233–246.

Boguniewicz, M., Moore, N., & Paranto, K. (2008). Allergic diseases, quality of life and the role of the dietician. *Nutrition Today, 43,* 6–10.

Boguniewicz, M., & Nicol, N. (2002). Conventional therapy for atopic dermatitis. *Immunology and Allergy Clinics of North America, 22*(1), 107–124.

Boguniewicz, M., & Nicol, N. H. (2008). General management of patients with atopic dermatitis. In S. Reitamo, T. A. Luger, & M. Steinhoff (Eds.), *Textbook of atopic dermatitis* (pp. 147–164). Andover, UK: Informa UK, Ltd.

Boguniewicz, M., Nicol, N., Kelsay, K., & Leung, D. Y. (2008). A multidisciplinary approach to evaluation and treatment of atopic dermatitis. *Seminars in Cutaneous Medicine and Surgery, 27*(2), 115–127.

Bonamonte, D., Foti, C., Vestita, M., Ranieri, L. D., & Angelini, G. (2012). Nummular eczema and contact allergy: A retrospective study. *Dermatitis, 23*(4), 153–157.

Devillers, A. C. C., & Oranje, A. P. (2012). Wet-wrap treatment in children with atopic dermatitis: A practical guideline. *Pediatric Dermatology, 29*(1), 24–27.

Deleo, V. A., Elsner, P., & Marks, J. G. Jr. (2000). *Contact & occupational dermatology* (3rd ed.). St. Louis, MO: Mosby.

Eichenfield, L. F., Tom, W. L., Chamlin, S. L., Feldman, S. R., Hanifin, J. M., Simpson, E. L., ..., Sidbury, R. (2014). Guidelines of care for the management of atopic dermatitis: Section 1. Diagnosis and assessment of atopic dermatitis. *Journal of the American Academy of Dermatology, 70,* 338–351.

Fonacier, L., Bernstein, D. I., Pacheco, K., Holness, D. L., Blesing-Moore, J., Khan, D., ..., Wallace, D. (2015). Contact dermatitis: A practice parameter-update 2015. *The Journal of Allergy and Clinical Immunology. In Practice, 3*(3 Suppl), S1–S39.

Goldsmith, L. A., Katz, S. I., Gilchrest, B. A., Paller, A. S., Leffell, D. J., & Wolff, K. (2012). *Fitzpatrick's dermatology in general medicine* (8th ed.). New York, NY: McGraw-Hill.

Greaves, M. W., & Leung, D. Y. M. (Eds.) (2000). *Allergic skin disease: A multidisciplinary approach.* New York, NY: Marcel Dekker, Inc.

Gutman, A. B., Kligman, A. M., Sciacca, J., & James, W. D. (2005). Soak and smear: A standard technique revisited. *Archives of Dermatology, 141*(12), 1556–1559.

Iwahira, Y., Nagasao, T., Shimizu, Y., Kuwata, K., & Tanaka, Y. (2015). Nummular eczema of breast: A potential dermatologic complication after mastectomy and subsequent breast reconstruction. *Plastic Surgery International.* Volume 2015, Article ID 209458, 6 pages.

Kapoor, R., Menon, C., Hoffstad, O., Bilker, W., Leclerc, P., & Margolis, D. J. (2008). The prevalence of atopic triad in children with physician-confirmed atopic dermatitis. *Journal of the American Academy of Dermatology, 58,* 68–73.

Klunk, C., Domingues, E., & Wiss, K. (2014). An update on diaper dermatitis. *Clinics in Dermatology, 32,* 477–487.

Leung, D. Y. M. (2013). New insights into atopic dermatitis: Role of skin barrier and immune dysregulation. *Allergology International, 62,* 151–161.

Marks, J. G., & Miller, J. J. (2006). *Lookingbill and Marks' principles of dermatology* (4th ed.). Philadelphia, PA: Saunders-Elsevier.

McCann, S. E., & Huether, S. E. (2014). Structure, function, and disorders of the integument. In S. E. Huether, K. L. McCance, V. L. Brasher, & N. S. Rote (Eds.), *Pathophysiology—The biologic basics for disease in adults and children* (7th ed., pp. 1616–1652). St. Louis, MO: Mosby-Elsevier.

Moore, J. A., Nicol, N. H., & Ruszkowski, A. M. (1995). What patients need to know about patch testing. *Dermatology Nursing, 20*(1), 20–26.

Nicol, N. H. (1987). Atopic dermatitis: The (wet) wrap-up. *American Journal of Nursing, 87*(12), 1560–1563.

Nicol, N. H. (2003). Dermatitis/eczemas. In M. J. Hill (Ed.), *Dermatologic nursing essentials: A core curriculum* (2nd ed., pp. 103–116). Pitman, NJ: Dermatology Nurses' Association.

Nicol, N. H. (2005a). Atopic triad: Atopic dermatitis, allergic rhinitis and asthma. *American Journal for Nurse Practitioners,* (Suppl), 36–40.

Nicol, N. H. (2005b). Use of moisturizers in dermatologic disease: The role of healthcare providers in optimizing treatment outcomes. *Cutis, 76*(Suppl 6), 26–31.

Nicol, N. H. (2009). Assessment of the integumentary system. In J. M. Black, & J. H. Hawks (Eds.), *Medical-surgical nursing: Clinical management for positive outcomes* (8th ed., pp. 1186–1198). Philadelphia, PA: WB Saunders Company.

Nicol, N. H., & Baumeister, L. (1997). Topical corticosteroid therapy: Considerations for prescribing and use. *Lippincott's Primary Care Practice, 1*(1), 62-69.

Nicol, N. H., & Boguniewicz, M. (2008). Successful strategies in AD management. *Dermatology Nursing,* (Suppl), 3–19.

Nicol, N. H., Boguniewicz, M., Strand, M., & Klinnert, M. D. (2014). Wet wrap therapy in children with moderate to severe atopic dermatitis in a multidisciplinary treatment program. *The Journal of Allergy and Clinical Immunology. In Practice, 2*(4), 400–406.

Nicol, N. H., & Ersser, S. J. (2010). The role of the nurse educator in managing atopic dermatitis. In M. Boguniewicz (Ed.), *Immunology and allergy clinics of North America: Atopic dermatitis* (pp. 369–383). Philadelphia, PA: Saunders-Elsevier.

Nicol, N. H., Hanifin, J. M., Tofte, S., & Boguniewicz, M. (2003). Evolution in the treatment of atopic dermatitis: New approaches to managing a chronic skin disease. *Dermatology Nursing, 15*(Suppl 4), 3–19.

Nicol, N. H., & Huether, S. E. (2014). Alterations of the integument in children. In S. E. Huether, K. L. McCance, V. L. Brasher, & N. S. Rote (Eds.), *Pathophysiology-The biologic basics for disease in adults and children* (7th ed., pp. 1653–1667). St. Louis, MO: Mosby-Elsevier.

Nicol, N. H., & Huether, S. E. (2012). Structure, function, and disorders of the integument. In S. E. Huether, K. L. McCance, V. L. Brasher, & N. S. Rote (Eds.), *Understanding pathophysiology* (6th ed., pp. 1038–1069). St. Louis, MO: Mosby-Elsevier.

Nicol, N. H., & Huether, S. E. (2016). Alterations of the integument in children. In S. E. Huether, K. L. McCance, V. L. Brasher, & N. S. Rote (Eds.), *Understanding pathophysiology* (6th ed., pp. 1111–1122). St. Louis, MO: Mosby-Elsevier.

Odhiambo, J. A., Williams, H. C., Clayton, T. O., Robertson, C. F., Asher, M. I., & the ISAAC Phase Three Study Group. (2009). Global variations in prevalence of eczema symptoms in children from ISAAC Phase Three. *Journal of Allergy and Clinical Immunology, 124,* 1251–1258.

Penzer, R., & Ersser, S. J. (2010). *Principles of skin care.* Oxford, UK: Wiley-Blackwell.

Spergel, J. M. (2010). From atopic dermatitis to asthma: The atopic march. *Annals of Allergy, Asthma, and Immunology 105,* 99–109.

Spergel, J. M., & Leung, D. Y. (2006). Safety of topical calcineurin inhibitors in atopic dermatitis: Evaluation of the evidence. *Current Allergy and Asthma Reports, 6,* 270–274.

Tuzun, Y., Wolf, R., Baglam, S., & Engin, B. (2015). Diaper (napkin) dermatitis: A fold (intertriginous) dermatosis. *Clinics in Dermatology, 33,* 477–482.

Weinberg, S., Prose, N. S., & Kristal, L. (2008). *Color atlas of pediatric dermatology* (4th ed.). New York, NY: McGraw-Hill.

Wolff, K., Johnson, R. A., & Saavedra, A. P. (2013). *Fitzpatrick's color atlas and synopsis of clinical dermatology* (7th ed.). New York, NY: McGraw-Hill.

STUDY QUESTIONS

1. The location of the cutaneous manifestations or symptoms of atopic dermatitis varies depending on the age of the patient.
   a. True
   b. False

2. Atopic dermatitis is the most common chronic, relapsing inflammatory skin disease of children. Which of the following diseases is not usually associated with atopic dermatitis?
   a. Asthma
   b. Allergic rhinitis
   c. Food allergies
   d. Discoid lupus

3. The infant with seborrheic dermatitis generally presents with all of the following signs and symptoms *except:*
   a. Erythematous papules
   b. Greasy yellow scale
   c. Intense pruritus
   d. Rash on scalp and forehead

4. A parent can best prevent irritant diaper dermatitis in a healthy 6-month-old infant by:
   a. Changing diapers frequently
   b. Increasing dietary vitamin C intake
   c. Using cloth diapers only
   d. Using commercial diaper wipes regularly

5. Wet wrap therapy:
   a. May promote skin dryness if not used with sufficient emollients
   b. Should not be used over topical corticosteroids
   c. Prevents the healing of excoriated lesions
   d. Is not effective for patients with recalcitrant eczema

6. Which of the following is a frequently described characteristic of nummular eczema?
   a. Coin-shaped lesions
   b. Silver plaque lesions
   c. Fish scale-like lesions
   d. Facial tautness

7. Which of the following is most consistent with proper "soak and seal" method of skin care for atopic dermatitis?
   a. Bath in tepid water for 15 minutes followed by application of moisturizer and then medication applied on top.
   b. Shower in warm water followed by a thorough drying of the skin and then use of moisturizer to the entire body, waiting at least 2 hours to apply topical medications.
   c. Bath in warm water followed by immediate application of anti-inflammatory medications to affected areas and then application of moisturizer to uninvolved areas.
   d. Bath only twice weekly followed by application of topical anti-inflammatory medication to affected areas, then application of moisturizer over the medication.

8. Nummular eczema is an inflammatory skin usually affecting the:
   a. Scalp
   b. Upper extremities
   c. Lower extremities
   d. Torso

9. Patch testing is considered the gold standard to determine if a patient has:
   a. Irritant contact dermatitis
   b. Allergic contact dermatitis
   c. Atopic dermatitis
   d. Nummular eczema

10. Lichenification is:
    a. A prominent clinical feature only during the adult phase of atopic dermatitis
    b. Most evident on the neck and face
    c. An accentuation of skin markings associated with thickening of the skin
    d. Seen only during acute flares of atopic dermatitis

Answers to Study Questions: 1.a, 2.d, 3.c, 4.a, 5.a, 6.a, 7.c, 8.c, 9.b, 10.c

Acne and Other Disorders of the Glands

Sarah W. Matthews • Noreen Heer Nicol

OBJECTIVES

After studying this chapter, the reader will be able to:

- Identify common dermatology disorders of the sebaceous, apocrine, and eccrine glands.
- Recognize the epidemiology, etiology and pathogenesis, diagnostic hallmarks, course and prognosis, clinical presentation, and differential diagnosis for each disease state.
- Describe the common therapeutic modalities for each disease state.
- List the key patient education points and home care considerations for each disease state.

KEY POINTS

- Acne vulgaris is one of the most common skin diseases affecting children and young adults. Good treatment results are usually obtained with proper education and follow-up.
- Distribution of lesions, presence of true comedones, and degree of erythema all aid in differentiation of acne from acne-like disorders.
- Rosacea, unrelated yet often coexisting with acne, does not present with comedones.
- Hidradenitis suppurativa, a chronic, suppurative, scarring disease of apocrine gland-bearing skin, is sometimes associated with severe nodulocystic acne. This disorder is characterized by paired comedones, unlike acne which characteristically has single comedones.
- Primary hyperhidrosis has no known cause but may be brought on by anxiety. Secondary hyperhidrosis has an underlying cause that needs to be found and treated.

I. OVERVIEW

A. The pilosebaceous unit comprises the hair follicle and one or more sebaceous glands attached to it. Sebaceous glands are found in greater numbers on the face, scalp, chest, and anogenital regions. Sebaceous glands are small at birth, enlarge between 8 and 10 years of age with maturation continuing through adolescence, and remain unchanged until later years. They decrease in menopause in females and after the 70th decade in males. As people age, sebum secretion decreases even though the size of sebaceous glands increases. Development of sebaceous glands and sebogenesis are hormone dependent (testosterone, androstenedione, dehydroepiandrosterone).

B. Apocrine gland ducts usually open into the hair follicle above the entrance of the sebaceous glands, but some ducts open directly upon the surface of the skin. Apocrine glands are found in the axillae; around the areolae; the periumbilical, perineal, and circumanal areas; prepuce; scrotum; mons pubis; labia minora; external ear canal; and eyelids. Like sebaceous glands, the activity of the apocrine glands is hormone dependent, but also stimulated by epinephrine and norepinephrine. The apocrine gland secretion is modified by the action of bacteria in the follicular infundibulum causing production of short-chain fatty acids, ammonia, and other odoriferous substances.

C. Eccrine sweat glands are not associated with hair follicles and are found everywhere on the body except for mucocutaneous junctions. They are found in greatest concentration on the palms, soles, axillae, and forehead. Eccrine sweat glands function to help regulate the body's temperature. This is accomplished by the production of eccrine sweat that flows to the skin surface and cools by evaporation. Eccrine sweat is an odorless, colorless, hypotonic solution and is excreted during periods of stress and heat. Axillary eccrine sweat glands contribute to the odor-producing secretion of the apocrine glands by providing a moist environment that is conducive to bacterial proliferation.

SEBACEOUS GLAND DISORDERS: ACNE VULGARIS

I. OVERVIEW

A. Definition: a disease of the pilosebaceous (hair follicle/sebaceous gland) unit where abnormally adherent keratinocytes cause plugging of the follicular duct followed by accumulation of sebum and keratinous debris (Figure 10-1). This results in the formation of microcomedones followed by open and/or closed comedones and/or pustules. In severe acne, cysts or nodules may develop.

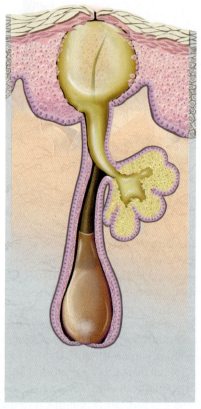

FIGURE 10-1. Acne closed comedone (whitehead). (From Anatomical Chart Company, Wolters Kluwer, 2004.)

BOX 10-1. Approach to the Patient with Acne Vulgaris

- Consider precipitating factors, the type of acne lesions, the severity of acne, the patient's level of emotional distress related to their acne, and the patient's level of engagement in self-care when making treatment decisions.
- Consider the psychosocial implications of moderate-to-severe disease on the patient with acne.
- Manual manipulation of lesions should be avoided. Manipulation increases postinflammatory hyperpigmentation and may lead to scarring.
- Discuss application techniques for various topical medications and products.
- Advise noncomedogenic cosmetic and skin care products. Discuss the use of specific products with each patient. Keep hair oils, spray, and mousse away from face.
- Treatment may take 4 to 6 weeks before effect is seen. Important to stress that acne often flares when treatment started, and disorder may appear to worsen prior to major improvement.
- Review side effects associated with prescribed treatment. Mild reddening or peeling may indicate medication working but needs to be monitored.
- If isotretinoin is being prescribed, strict program requirements are necessary including written and signed consent. Strict pregnancy prevention measures are essential for women. Also, address measures to manage dryness associated with treatment with isotretinoin.

B. Epidemiology
1. Age: affects all ages, with higher incidence (approximately 85%) between ages of 12 and 25.
2. Sex: more severe in males than in females. In males, usually subsides by mid-20s. In females, may occur at any age.
3. Race: lower incidence in Asians and darkly pigmented individuals.
4. Genetic aspects: genetic influence of sebum excretion.
5. Neonatal acne is a response to maternal androgens. Persistence of neonatal acne beyond 12 months of age may be associated with endocrine abnormalities.
6. Other factors (Box 10-1):
   a. Emotional stress exacerbates.
   b. There is good evidence that acne negatively affects quality of life, self-esteem, and mood in adolescents. Acne is also associated with an increased risk of anxiety, depression, and suicidal ideation, highlighting the importance of asking patients with acne directly about psychological issues in order to identify those who might benefit from early psychiatric support.
   c. Occlusion with pressure and friction on skin from headbands, football helmets, hats, tight bras, etc., can exacerbate.
   d. Oil-based cosmetics and hair products can also be responsible for predominantly comedonal acne.
   e. Drugs (such as androgens, ACTH, glucocorticoids, phenytoin, lithium, and isoniazid) and hyperandrogenism may also induce acne.
   f. Science still does not know whether diet and acne are related, and dietary research needs to be read with critical review. Based on the clinical research, it seems prudent to eat a relatively low-glycemic diet rich in colorful fruits and vegetables and omega-3 fats. Some weak evidence has emerged that suggests a possible link between dairy and acne, which warrants further research.
   g. Systemic steroids exacerbate.
C. Etiology and pathogenesis. Basic cause thought to be multifactorial, complex interaction between androgen hormone and bacteria colonization in pilosebaceous units. There are at least four primary contributing factors.
1. Increased sebum production secondary to stimulation by androgenic hormones
2. Abnormal follicular keratinization with the development of a keratin plug at the sebaceous follicle opening
3. Proliferation or bacterial colonization with *Propionibacterium acnes*, an anaerobic bacterium
4. Inflammation
D. Diagnostic hallmarks
1. Distribution: face (which is usually oily), forehead and chin (first areas to be noticed), neck, upper arms, trunk, and buttocks
2. Lesions: comedones (pathognomonic lesions), papules, pustules (Figure 10-2), and inflammatory nodules and cysts
E. Course and prognosis
1. Hormonal factors greatly affect development and course of acne; use of anabolic steroids likely to worsen.

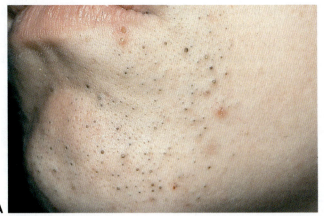 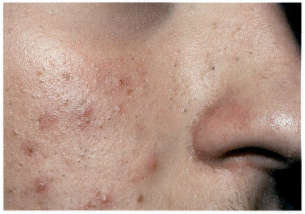

A **B**

FIGURE 10-2. Acne. **A:** Comedones. **B:** Papular and pustular acne. (From Goodheart, H. P. (2008). *Goodheart's photoguide of common skin disorders* (3rd ed.). Philadelphia, PA: Lippincott Williams & Wilkins.)

2. Cystic lesions and severe acne more common in men.
3. In women, activity may peak during a week prior to menses; may clear up or substantially worsen during pregnancy.
4. Presence of cysts and family history of scarring acne are prognostic signs for predicting future severity.
5. Postinflammatory hyperpigmentation or hypopigmentation may persist for months.
6. Cystic acne frequently leads to permanent scarring.

II. ASSESSMENT

A. History
   1. Duration of lesions: weeks to years
   2. Season: may be worse in the fall and winter and better in the summer
   3. Symptoms: lesions may be painful, especially nodulo-cystic type.
B. Clinical presentation
   1. Open comedones (blackheads)—incompletely blocked pores and no scarring
   2. Closed comedones (skin colored)—completely blocked pores and no scarring.
   3. Pustules—plugged duct ruptures with extrusion of keratin plug into surrounding dermis causing inflammatory response and no scarring
   4. Nodules—plugged duct ruptures at the level too deep to result in a visible pustule and no scarring
   5. Cysts—plugged duct ruptures at the level of the sebaceous gland itself and heals with scar formation
C. Clinical manifestations
   1. Neonatal acne
      a. Appears at 2 to 4 weeks of age and lasts until 4 to 6 months.
      b. Lesions are seen primarily on the face, particularly the cheeks, and occasionally on the upper chest and back.
      c. An oily face or scalp may be observed.
      d. Individual lesions are similar to the adolescent acne lesions.

2. Adolescent acne
   a. May first appear at the age of 8 to 10 years, peaks in late adolescence, and may continue until the late 20s or early 30s.
   b. Distribution occurs in areas of high sebaceous activity, such as the face (Figure 10-3), upper chest, and back.
   c. Types of lesions
      (1) Noninflammatory microcomedones
      (2) Noninflammatory comedones
         (a) Closed comedones
         (b) Open comedones
      (3) Inflammatory papules
      (4) Inflammatory pustules
      (5) Inflammatory nodules
   d. Classification of inflammatory acne
      (1) Mild—consists of few to several inflammatory papules or pustules and no nodules
      (2) Moderate—several to many inflammatory papules, pustules, and a few nodules

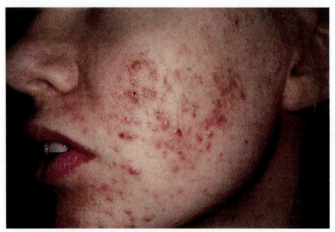

FIGURE 10-3. Papulopustular acne on the face. (From Rosedahl, C. B. (2011). *Textbook of basic nursing.* Philadelphia, PA: Wolters Kluwer.)

(3) Severe—numerous extensive inflammatory papules, pustules, and many nodules
  e. Scarring is common in inflammatory nodulocystic acne and with frequent manipulation of the acne lesions.
D. Atypical findings
  1. Acne conglobata—scarring severe cystic acne with more involvement of the trunk rather than the face (genetically malformed sebaceous follicles present or rarely seen in XYY genotype of tall males who are slightly mentally retarded with aggressive behavior or in polycystic ovary syndrome)
  2. Acne excoriee—individuals neurotically pick at their lesions
  3. Drug-induced acne—acne-like folliculitis without comedones or cysts
E. Differential diagnosis
  1. Folliculitis
  2. Pseudofolliculitis barbae
  3. Acne rosacea
  4. Perioral dermatitis.
F. Laboratory and special tests
  1. No diagnostic testing is generally required, and diagnosis is based on the clinical appearance of the lesions.
  2. Hormonal workup, if needed, for detecting polycystic ovary syndrome.
  3. Hyperandrogenism is evaluated by obtaining blood levels of free testosterone, DHEA, and androstenedione.
  4. Patients being prescribed isotretinoin require the following lab tests before starting treatment and monthly during treatment: complete blood count, platelets, liver function studies, fasting lipid profile, BUN, and creatinine.
  5. Females being prescribed isotretinoin need two negative pregnancy tests prior to initiation of treatment, monthly pregnancy tests during treatment, and a pregnancy test 1 month after the treatment is complete.

III. COMMON THERAPEUTIC MODALITIES

A. Topical therapy which includes products delivered as cleansers and medications
  1. Gentle skin cleansing techniques that use mild soap and water twice a day. Avoid abrasive soaps and cleansers as well as astringents and toners, unless directed. If cleansers with medications are used, caution should be taken to avoid side effects, which include drying and therapy intolerance.
  2. Benzoyl peroxide (2.5% up to 10%): apply once to twice daily for mixed comedones and inflammatory acne as wash, lotion, cream, foam, pads, or gel; side effects include skin irritation, allergic contact dermatitis, and bleaching of clothes. Combining benzoyl peroxide with antibiotics dramatically decreases the incidence of bacterial resistance.
    a. Benzoyl peroxide plus erythromycin—pregnancy (category C)
    b. Benzoyl peroxide plus clindamycin—pregnancy (category C)
  3. Topical antibiotics for inflammatory acne apply once to twice daily as a solution, gel, lotion, or pads; side effects include excessive drying, depending upon vehicle, and emerging bacterial resistance with long-term use.
    a. Erythromycin 2%—pregnancy (category B)
    b. Clindamycin 1%—pregnancy (category B)
  4. Salicylic acid/glycolic acid for mild comedonal acne apply once to twice daily as a cleanser, gel, lotion, or solution to unplug follicles; side effects include mild local irritation.
  5. Azelaic acid 20%—pregnancy (category B). For comedonal and inflammatory acne, apply once to twice daily as an antibacterial of *P. acnes*, to normalize keratinization and for postinflammatory hyperpigmentation; side effects include mild local irritation.
  6. Topical retinoids: apply once daily for comedonal acne to decrease cohesiveness of follicular epithelial cells; side effects include erythema, desquamation, hypo-/hyperpigmentation, and sensitization of skin to sunlight.
    a. Tretinoin (0.025%, 0.05%, 0.1% cream; 0.01%, 0.025% gel; Retin-A Micro 0.04% and 0.1% gel)—pregnancy (category C): not recommended during pregnancy. Unstable in sunlight. Apply at night.
    b. Adapalene (0.1% and 0.3% gel, 0.1% cream, solution, or pledgets)—pregnancy (category C): not recommended during pregnancy. Less irritating than tretinoin or tazarotene and stable in sunlight.
    c. Tazarotene (0.05% and 0.1% gel or cream)—pregnancy (category X). Women of childbearing potential: obtain reliable negative pregnancy test within 2 weeks before starting therapy, use effective contraception during therapy, and begin therapy during normal menses. Stable in sunlight.
  7. Combination therapy
    a. The combination of benzoyl peroxide every morning and a topical retinoid (tretinoin, adapalene, tazarotene) every evening is often effective.
    b. Frequently systemic antibiotics are combined with topical medications.
    c. Combination of topical benzoyl peroxide with both topical and systemic antibiotics is recommended to reduce the development of antibiotic-resistant organisms.
B. Systemic therapy
  1. Antibiotics for inflammatory acne; take one pill or capsule two times per day for a bactericidal effect; side effects include emerging resistance. Pregnancy and nursing mothers: not recommended.
    a. Tetracycline (category D), 250 to 500 mg bid, inexpensive; side effects include photosensitivity, gastrointestinal (GI) upset, candidiasis, tooth discoloration, and enamel hypoplasia (use only in patients >8 years old).
    b. Doxycycline (category D), 50 to 100 mg bid, may be taken with food; side effects similar to tetracycline but with greater photosensitivity.

   c. Minocycline (category D), 50 to 100 mg bid, rare photosensitivity or GI upset; side effects include blue pigmentation, serum sickness-like reactions, and drug-induced lupus.

   d. Erythromycin (category B), 250 to 500 mg bid, may be taken during pregnancy; side effects include GI upset.

2. Isotretinoin (category X) 0.5 to 2.0 mg/kg/d for nodulocystic acne and inflammatory acne recalcitrant to other modes of treatment to normalize keratinization, decrease sebum production, and deplete *P. acnes*; multiple side effects include teratogenicity, cheilitis, conjunctivitis, dry eyes and mouth, pruritus, musculoskeletal pain, and alopecia (Figure 10-4). Strict adherence to pregnancy prevention measures is required as well as monthly pregnancy tests for all women regardless of sexual activity.

3. Oral contraceptives as an adjunct treatment in women for moderate-to-severe inflammatory acne decrease sebum production; side effects include suppressing growth in patients less than 16 years old; contraindicated in males.

4. Spironolactone 50 to 200 mg once daily. Pregnancy (category C). The antiandrogen effects have been shown to cause feminization of the male fetus in animal studies. Used off-label for female acne. Indicated when there are signs of a strong hormonal component such as worsening around menses, acne concentrated in the lower part of the face and upper neck, and/or acne that is recalcitrant to other treatments. Check potassium and creatinine at 1 week after initiation and 1 week after each dose increase. If potassium increases to >5.5 mEq/L or renal function worsens, hold dose until potassium is normal again, then consider restarting at lower dose.

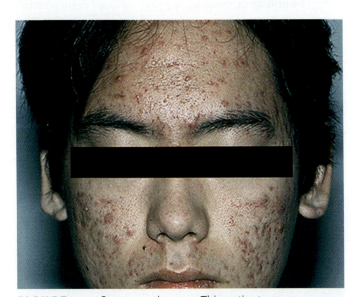

FIGURE 10-4. Severe cystic acne. This patient was subsequently treated with isotretinoin. (From Goodheart, H. P. (2003). *Goodheart's photoguide of common skin disorders.* 2nd ed. Philadelphia, PA: Lippincott Williams & Wilkins.)

C. Follow-up visits
1. Every 4 to 6 weeks until control is obtained.
2. Then every 1 to 3 months particularly if being treated with systemic medication.
3. Patients on isotretinoin are seen monthly during the course of treatment.

PATIENT EDUCATION
Acne Vulgaris

- Do not over wash face; two times per day is recommended.
- Use gentle facial cleanser, not abrasive cleanser.
- Gently clean with hands only; no washcloth.
- Allow 15 to 20 minutes after washing before applying medication to decrease burning/stinging.
- Apply most medications to the entire face; benzoyl peroxide may be used as a spot treatment.
- Recognize that certain soaps, creams, lotions, oil, and cosmetics worsen acne; advise use of noncomedogenic products.

ACNE ROSACEA

I. OVERVIEW

A. Definition: rosacea is a chronic inflammatory disorder involving the flush area of the face associated with diffuse sebaceous gland abnormality and increased reactivity of capillaries that develops over time and is characterized by persistent erythema, papules, tiny pustules, and telangiectasia. There are no blackheads (comedones).

B. Epidemiology
1. Age: most often seen between ages 30 and 50 years but may be seen at any age; peak incidence between 40 and 50.
2. Sex: affects females predominantly; rhinophyma occurs mostly in males.
3. Race: skin phototypes I and II but also in others; rare in Fitzpatrick skin types IV-VI.
4. Genetic aspects: familial predisposition.
5. Other factors: (anything that triggers flushing).
   a. Sun exposure
   b. Stress
   c. Alcohol and hot or spicy foods or drinks
   d. Irritating cosmetics

C. Etiology and pathogenesis
1. Unknown cause, although the hypersensitive skin seen in rosacea in response to environmental triggers seems to be due to dysregulation of the immune systems (innate and adaptive) and the nervous system.
2. Erythema results from dilatation of superficial vasculature of face (atrophy of papillary dermis provides for easier visualization of dermal capillaries).

3. Edema develops as a result of increased blood flow in superficial vasculature (edema may contribute to late-stage fibroplasia and rhinophyma).

D. Diagnostic hallmarks
   1. Distribution: vertical, central third of the face
   2. Lesions: pustules and papules against background of erythema and telangiectasia

E. Course and prognosis
   1. Chronic disease characterized by periodic exacerbations and remissions.
   2. Disease may spontaneously disappear after a few years.

II. ASSESSMENT

A. History
   1. Duration of lesions: days, weeks, and months
   2. Symptoms: episodic facial erythema with increased skin temperature in response to environmental or emotional stimuli
   3. Ocular symptoms

B. Clinical presentation: categorized into four subtypes that are distinguished by the presence of specific primary and secondary characteristics
   1. Erythematotelangiectatic (ETR)
      a. Episodic flushing.
      b. Persistent facial erythema (Figure 10-5). Redness may also involve the peripheral face, ears, neck, and upper chest. Typically, periocular skin is not affected.
      c. Telangiectasias are common but not essential for diagnosis.
   2. Papulopustular (PPR)
      a. Includes all characteristics listed under ETR.

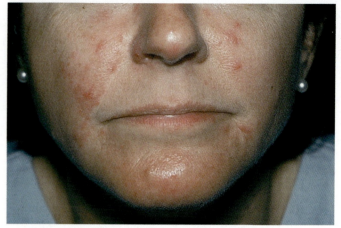

FIGURE 10-6. Rosacea characterized by inflammatory papules and pustules and telangiectasias located on the central third of the face. (From Goodheart, H. P. (2003). *Goodheart's photoguide of common skin disorders*. 2nd ed. Philadelphia, PA: Lippincott Williams & Wilkins.)

      b. Transient papules and/or pustules in the central face.
      c. Severe cases may experience episodes of inflammation that lead to chronic facial edema (Figure 10-6).
   3. Phymatous
      a. Thickened and irregular skin surfaces with nodularities.
      b. Can occur anywhere with a predominance of sebaceous glands but is most common on the nose (Figure 10-7).
      c. Males are most often affected.
      d. Typical age range is from 50 to 70 years.
   4. Ocular
      a. Defined by the National Rosacea Expert Committee as ≥ 1 of the following signs or symptoms: watery or bloodshot appearance, foreign body sensation, burning or stinging, dryness, itching, light sensitivity, blurred vision, telangiectases of the conjunctiva

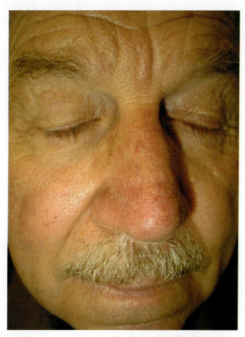

FIGURE 10-5. Erythematotelangiectatic rosacea: background erythema with fine telangiectasias of the central face. Note the lack of inflammatory lesions. (Image provided by Stedman's.)

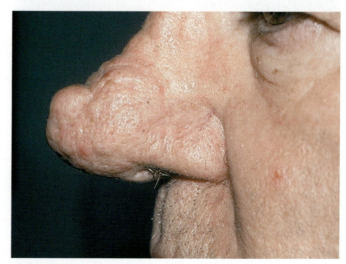

FIGURE 10-7. Acne rosacea with rhinophyma. (From Werner, R. (2012). *Massage therapist's guide to pathology*. Philadelphia, PA: Wolters Kluwer.)

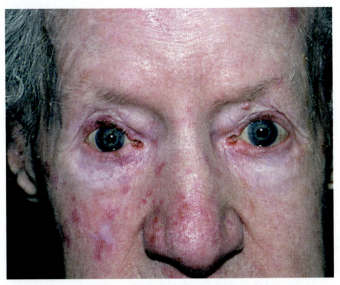

FIGURE 10-8. Ocular rosacea: inflammation of the eyes (conjunctivitis) and lids. This patient also has inflammatory papules and pustules of rosacea on the face. (From Goodheart, H. P. (2003). *Goodheart's photoguide of common skin disorders*. 2nd ed. Philadelphia, PA: Lippincott Williams & Wilkins.)

and lid margin, or lid and periocular erythema (Figure 10-8).

   b. Other signs include blepharitis, irregularity of the eyelid margins, chalazia, and styes.
   c. Ocular involvement is estimated to occur 5% to 50% of patients with cutaneous rosacea and can occur without a diagnosis of skin findings consistent with rosacea.
   d. Rare cases can lead to corneal scaring and decrease visual acuity.
   e. No diagnostic tests; therefore, diagnosis relies on clinical judgment.

C. Atypical findings
   1. Metophyma: enlarged cushion-like swelling of forehead
   2. Blepharophyma: swelling of eyelids related to sebaceous gland hyperplasia
   3. Gnathophyma: swelling of chin

D. Differential diagnosis
   1. Acne vulgaris (comedones and no generalized erythema or telangiectasias).
   2. Seborrheic dermatitis, perioral dermatitis, and systemic lupus (these conditions will not produce characteristic flushing, telangiectasias, papules, and pustules). Be aware that it is not uncommon for seborrheic dermatitis to occur simultaneously with rosacea.
   3. Sarcoidosis (closely mimics with red papules on the face, but manifests in other organs as well).

E. Laboratory and special tests
   1. Bacterial culture if *Staphylococcus aureus* infection is suspected.
   2. Biopsy may be needed if sebaceous hyperplasia is indistinguishable from a basal cell carcinoma due to phymatous changes.

III. COMMON THERAPEUTIC MODALITIES

A. Topical therapy
   1. Metronidazole effective for PPR: twice daily (0.75% cream, lotion, or gel) or 1.0% formulation, once daily; most common side effect is irritation.
   2. Sulfacetamide wash or lotion effective for PPR; side effects: less irritating than metronidazole; contact dermatitis possible. More effective when combined with sulfur.
   3. Azelaic acid 20% cream (category B) applied once daily for PPR. Equivalent to metronidazole in effectiveness.
   4. Ivermectin (1% cream), once daily for PPR (category C). Slightly more effective than metronidazole.
   5. Topical vitamin C antioxidant effect might affect free radical production that might play role in inflammatory reaction of rosacea.
   6. BP–clindamycin cream twice daily—may be effective for both PPR and ETR, but the studies are of poor quality.
   7. Tacrolimus ointment twice daily (category C)—effective for both PPR and ETR.
   8. Pimecrolimus 1% cream twice daily (category C)— effective for both PPR and ETR.
   9. Permethrin 5% cream once daily (category B)—appears to be effective for both PPR and ETR, but the studies are poor.
   10. Brimonidine tartrate 0.5% gel once daily (category B), an alpha adrenergic agonist—for ETR. Effectiveness and safety supported by high-quality evidence.
   11. Oxymetazoline 0.05% solution (prolonged use not advised during pregnancy) twice daily, mix with moisturizer—for ETR.
   12. Cyclosporine 0.05% ophthalmic emulsion shown to be more beneficial than artificial tears for ocular rosacea.
   13. Tretinoin cream or gel (category C) applied once daily for PPR; side effects include delayed onset of effectiveness, dry skin, erythema, and burning/stinging. No good studies showing effectiveness but still commonly used. Clindamycin with tretinoin was not shown to be effective for rosacea when compared to placebo.

B. Systemic therapy is primarily effective for PPR and ocular rosacea: once daily doses dramatically increase the development of bacterial resistance so, when possible, use twice daily regimens or sub–antibactericidal doses.
   1. Tetracycline, 1.0 to 1.5 g per day divided into two to four daily doses until lesions clear; then gradually reduce to 250 mg, twice daily.
   2. Minocycline, 100 mg, twice daily until lesions clear; then gradually reduce to 50 mg, twice daily. Low-dose minocycline is not effective.
   3. Doxycycline, monohydrate formulation, 100 mg, once or twice daily, more consistently effective with fewer gastrointestinal side effects than hyclate form. May also be prescribed at anti-inflammatory dose of 40 mg daily or 50 mg every other day.

4. Clarithromycin, 250 to 500 mg, twice daily.
5. Ivermectin. Limited data on oral treatment.
6. Oral isotretinoin (effective for ETA, PPR, and ocular rosacea), 0.3 mg/kg, in individuals with severe disease not responding to antibiotics. Moderate to high-quality evidence.
C. Cosmetic surgery
1. Residual redness and telangiectasia, after maximum response obtained medically, improves with laser therapy.
2. Irreversible fibrotic changes, such as rhinophyma, do not respond well to medical therapy; refer for surgery or laser therapy.

PATIENT EDUCATION
Rosacea

- Avoid triggers (both exposures and situations that can cause a flare-up of the flushing and skin changes in rosacea):
  - Sun exposure: always apply nonirritating sun block when outdoors; wear hats.
  - Stress: autonomic activation increases flushing.
  - Alcohol consumption: not a cause; aggravates with peripheral vasodilation.
  - Spicy foods: aggravate through autonomic stimulation.
  - Cleansers, lotions, and cosmetics: use nonirritating, hypoallergenic, and noncomedogenic.
- Avoid rubbing, scrubbing, or massaging face; tends to irritate reddened skin.
- Avoid applying corticosteroids to skin without health care provider's specific instructions.
- If exercise results in flushing, exercise in cool environment; don't overheat.
- Keep diary of flushing episodes and factors.
- Access National Rosacea Society, www.rosacea.org, 1-888-NO-BLUSH, 600 S. Northwest Hwy, Suite 200, Barrington, Il 60010.

APOCRINE GLAND DISORDERS: HIDRADENITIS SUPPURATIVA

I. OVERVIEW

A. Definition: hidradenitis suppurativa (HS), also known as acne inversa, is a chronic, scarring disease of apocrine gland-bearing skin caused by intense inflammation following follicular obstruction on "inverse" areas of the body (axillae, beneath breasts, groin, upper and inner thighs, and buttocks).
B. Epidemiology
1. Race: all races, more severe in people of color
2. Age: appears after puberty; most cases in second and third decades of life
3. Sex: anogenital involvement seen more often in males and axillae involvement seen more often in females

4. Genetic aspects
   a. Clustering in families
   b. Mother–daughter transmission observed
   c. Genetic predisposition to acne
5. Other factors
   a. Obesity
   b. Apocrine duct obstruction
   c. Secondary bacterial infection
C. Etiology and pathogenesis
1. Unknown cause but the immune system has been demonstrated to have an important role in this inflammatory disease as demonstrated in both experimental and clinical studies.
2. Keratinous plugging of apocrine duct.
3. Dilatation of apocrine duct and hair follicle.
4. Severe inflammatory changes limited to single apocrine gland.
5. Bacterial growth in dilated duct.
6. Ruptured duct/gland results in extension of inflammation/infection.
7. Extension of suppuration/tissue destruction.
8. Ulceration and fibrosis and sinus tract formation.
D. Diagnostic hallmarks
1. Distribution: axillae, anogenital regions, the scalp, and under female breasts.
2. Lesions: highly characteristic double comedone blackheads with two or more surface openings that communicate under the skin. Abscesses and nodules are moderately to exquisitely painful.
3. Draining sinus tracts.
E. Course and prognosis
1. Progressive and relentless
2. Course varies from recurrent self-healing tender red nodule to diffuse, painful abscess formation.
3. Secondary bacterial infection probably major cause of exacerbations

II. ASSESSMENT

A. History
1. Intermittent pain
2. Marked point tenderness related to abscess formation
3. Contributing factors: smoking, sweating, obesity, and hormonal changes
B. Clinical presentation
1. Initial lesion—inflammatory, tender nodules (Figure 10-9)
2. Eventually—abscesses (red, hot, painful, discharging lumps) and sinus tracts with pus drainage (Figures 10-10 and 10-11)
3. Finally—fibrosis, hypertrophic, and keloidal scars and contractures
C. Associated findings
1. Cystic acne
2. Pilonidal sinus
D. Differential diagnosis
1. Furuncle/carbuncle
2. Lymphadenitis
3. Ruptured cysts

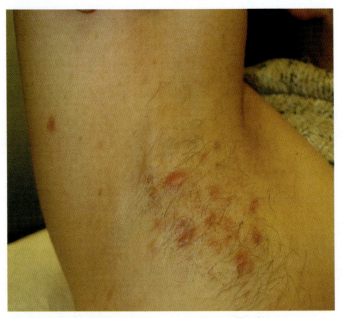

FIGURE 10-9. Hidradenitis suppurativa: axilla. (Image provided by Stedman's.)

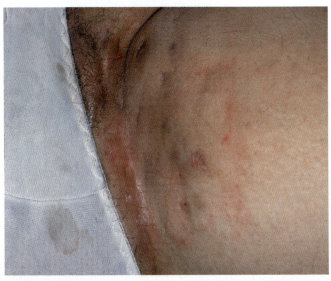

FIGURE 10-11. Inguinal hidradenitis. (From Goodheart, H. P. (2003). *Goodheart's photoguide of common skin disorders.* 2nd ed. Philadelphia, PA: Lippincott Williams & Wilkins.)

4. Cat-scratch disease
5. Sinus tracts and fistulas associated with ulcerative colitis and regional enteritis
E. Laboratory and special tests
  1. Cultures may show a variety of pathogens that secondarily infect lesions.

III. COMMON THERAPEUTIC MODALITIES

A. Topical therapy
  1. Aluminum chloride 20% nightly under occlusion until controlled then one to two times per week for maintenance.

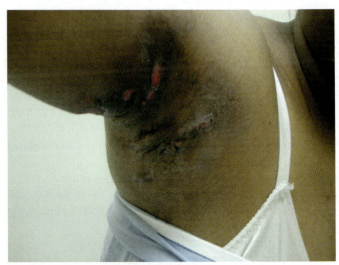

FIGURE 10-10. Axillary hidradenitis suppurativa. (From Goodheart, H. P. (2010). *Goodheart's same-site differential diagnosis: A rapid method of diagnosing and treating common skin disorders.* Philadelphia, PA: Wolters Kluwer.)

2. Tretinoin cream (0.05%) may prevent duct occlusion; side effects include irritation; use only as tolerated.
3. Clindamycin solution applied twice daily—effective for superficial pustules and likely for colonization but not effective for deep nodules and cysts; well tolerated.
B. Intralesional therapy
  1. Acute painful lesions: injections
    a. Nodules—intralesional triamcinolone (3 to 5 mg/mL) diluted with lidocaine
    b. Abscesses—intralesional triamcinolone (3 to 5 mg/mL) diluted with lidocaine followed by incision and drainage of abscess fluid
C. Systemic therapy
  1. Oral antibiotics: helpful for chronic low-grade disease. Use until lesions resolve in conjunction with intralesional injections in early inflammatory lesions to hasten resolution. Benefits of tetracycline antibiotics may be primarily due to anti-inflammatory effects versus antibacterial effects. Combined rifampin and clindamycin are more effective against the common microbes associated with HS.
    a. Clindamycin 300 mg twice daily with rifampin 600 mg daily
    b. Tetracycline—250 to 500 mg, four times per day
    c. Minocycline—100 mg, two times per day
    d. Doxycycline—50 to 100 mg, two times per day
  2. Retinoids
    a. Oral isotretinoin, 1 mg/kg/d for 20 weeks, appears useful in early disease with only inflammatory cystic lesions in which undermining sinus tracts have not developed or when combined with surgical excision of individual lesions. Not useful in more severe disease (only 18% achieve significant improvement).
    b. Acitretin 0.25 to 0.88 mg/kg/d. Significantly more effective than isotretinoin (73% with significant

improvement, 23% with moderate improvement). May only be used in men and sterilized or postmenopausal women.

3. Biologics
   a. Infliximab 5 mg/kg at weeks 0, 2, and 6 and then maintenance therapy every 6 to 8 weeks
   b. Adalimumab 40 to 80 mg, in a frequency ranging from weekly to every other week

D. Surgical management
   1. Incise and drain abscesses.
   2. Excise chronic recurrent, fibrotic nodules, or sinus tracts.
   3. Complete excision of axilla or involved anogenital area may be required for severe, extensive, chronic disease.

PATIENT EDUCATION
Hidradenitis Suppurativa

- Wash with antiseptics, antibacterial soaps, or acne preparations to reduce skin carriage of bacteria.
- Avoid roll-on deodorants.
- Decrease friction and moisture.
- Avoid constrictive clothing.
- Lose weight, if obese.
- Minimize heat buildup and sweat.

ENDOCRINE GLAND DISORDERS: PRIMARY HYPERHIDROSIS

I. OVERVIEW

A. Definition: in some people, the secretion of sweat occurs far higher than needed to keep a constant temperature. This condition is referred to as hyperhidrosis (Figure 10-12).

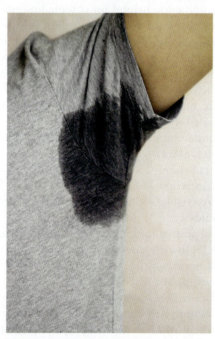

FIGURE 10-12. Axillary hyperhidrosis. (Copyright R. Small, MD.)

B. Epidemiology
   1. Age: 0.5% to 2.8% of the population affected; usually appears during the second or third decade of life.
   2. Sex: not a known factor.
   3. Race: not a known factor.
   4. Genetic aspects: positive family history in 30% to 50% suggests genetic factor.
   5. Other factors: disease is worse in the obese.

C. Etiology and pathogenesis
   1. Cause unknown
      a. May be related to a dysfunction of the sympathetic nervous system and hypothalamus coupled with input from the anterior cingulate cortex of the limbic system leading to neurogenic overactivity of sweat glands in affected area
   2. Eccrine gland has secretory coil and duct.
      a. Secretion of eccrine sweat involves secretion of ultrafiltrate by secretory coil in response to acetylcholine (released from sympathetic nerve endings) and reabsorption of sodium by ductal portion (surface sweat is hypotonic).
      b. Proximal (coiled) duct functionally more active than distal (straight) portion.

D. Diagnostic hallmarks
   1. Distribution: locations
      a. Palmar (hands)
      b. Axillary (armpits)
      c. Plantar (feet)
      d. Facial (face)
      e. Truncal (trunk)
      f. General (over the whole body)
   2. Sweating: can be induced by thermal stimuli and by emotional stress
      a. Emotional sweating stops during sleep.
      b. Thermal sweating occurs even during sleep.

E. Course and prognosis
   1. Persists during lifetime
   2. Exerts negative impact on lives of affected
   3. Triggered by anxiety; rarely associated with psychiatric disorders
   4. Consequences: odor, dehydration, skin maceration, and possible secondary skin infections

II. ASSESSMENT

A. History
   1. Duration: appears suddenly or continuously without any obvious reason
   2. Season: elicited by high outside temperatures
   3. Symptoms: excessive perspiration, nervousness, and anxiety elicit or aggravate sweating; hands feel not only moist but also cold.

B. Clinical presentation
   1. Affected areas often pink or bluish white
   2. Skin, especially on the feet, may be macerated.
   3. Fissured and scaling

C. Typical findings
   1. Facial hyperhidrosis (forehead)

2. Palmar hyperhidrosis (hands)
3. Axillary hyperhidrosis (armpits)
4. Plantar hyperhidrosis (feet)
5. Other locations
   a. Trunk
   b. Thighs
D. Differential diagnosis
   1. Secondary (generalized) disease cause known as part of underlying condition
      a. Hyperthyroidism or similar endocrine diseases
      b. Endocrine treatment for prostatic cancer or other types of malignancies
      c. Severe psychiatric disorders
      d. Obesity
      e. Menopause
E. Laboratory and special tests
   1. None specific except to rule out associated conditions.
   2. Before botulinum toxin type A injection, hyperhidrotic field (particularly in axillary hyperhidrosis) may be visualized using the minor iodine–starch test. In this test, an iodine solution (2 g of iodine in 10 mL of castor oil and alcohol to 100 mL) is painted over the area of the skin to be tested. After it has dried, fine rice or potato starch powder is applied. Sweat causes the mixture to turn dark blue.

III. COMMON THERAPEUTIC MODALITIES

A. Topical therapy
   1. Antiperspirants (first measure due to ease of use, time issues, and cost)
      a. Aluminum chloride (20% to 25%) under occlusion, nightly until controlled then 1 to 3 times/week for maintenance
      b. Sufficient in light-to-moderate cases, repeat regularly
   2. Iontophoresis (often second or third line since it is time consuming, inefficient at times, and expensive)
      a. Low-intensity electric current (15 to 18 mA) supplied by D/C generator, applied to palms or soles immersed in tap water or electrolyte solution. Twenty-minute sessions several times/week to q 1 to 2 weeks
      b. Results vary; difficult to apply in axillary, and impossible to use in diffuse hyperhidrosis of the face or the trunk/thigh region
B. Intradermal therapy
   1. Botulinum toxin type A (BTX-A) (repeat every 6 to 7 months)
      a. For axillae, palms, or forehead, temporarily blocks release of acetylcholine from cholinergic fibers. Inject intradermally at multiple sites of affected area.
         (1) Axillary: inject 10 to 15 sites equally distributed over axilla (Figure 10-13).
         (2) Palmar: injections 2.5 cm apart over palm and along fingers.
C. Surgery

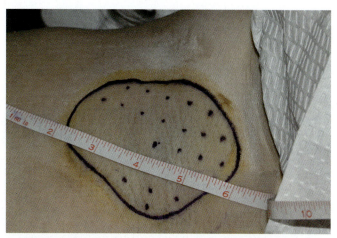

FIGURE 10-13. Injection points marked for botulinum toxin treatment of axillary hyperhidrosis. (Copyright R. Small, MD.)

1. Excision of axillary sweat glands
2. Sympathectomy to interrupt nerve tracks and nodes (ganglia), which transmit signals to sweat glands
   a. Endoscopic thoracic sympathectomy (ETS); less invasive than traditional

 PATIENT EDUCATION
Hyperhidrosis

- Lose weight, if obese.
- Stress management (helps with coping and with disrupting anxiety-sweating circle).

MILIARIA (SEE CHAPTER 13)

BIBLIOGRAPHY

Arndt, K. A., & Hsu, J. T. S. (2007). *Manual of dermatologic therapeutics* (7th ed.). Philadelphia, PA: Lippincott Williams & Wilkins.

Batra, R. S. (2007). Acne. In K. A. Arndt, & J. T. S. Hsu (Eds.), *Manual of dermatologic therapeutics* (7th ed., pp. 3–17). Philadelphia, PA: Lippincott Williams & Wilkins.

Bhate, K., & Williams, H. C. (2013). Epidemiology of acne vulgaris. *British Journal of Dermatology, 168*(3), 474–485.

Bhate, K., & Williams, H. C. (2014). What's new in acne? An analysis of systematic reviews published in 2011–2012. *Clinical and Experimental Dermatology, 39*(3), 273–277.

Blok, J. S., van Hattem, S., Jonkman, M. F., & Horvath, B. (2013). Systemic therapy with immunosuppressive agents and retinoids in hidradentitis suppurativa: A systematic review, *British Journal of Dermatology, 168,* 243–252.

Callen, J. P., Jorizzo, J. L., Zone, J. J., & Piette, W. W. (2009). *Dermatological signs of internal disease* (4th ed.). Philadelphia, PA: Saunders-Elsevier.

Craven, R., Hirnle, C., & Jensen, S. (2013). *Fundamentals of nursing: Human health and function* (7th ed.). Philadelphia, PA: Lippincott Williams & Wilkins.

Eichenfield, L. F., Fowler, J. F., Jr., Fried, R. G., Friedlander, S. F., Levy, M. L., & Webster, G. F. (2010). Perspectives on therapeutic options for acne: An update. *Seminars in Cutaneous Medicine and Surgery, 29*(2 suppl 1), 13–16.

Gill, L., Williams, M., & Hamzavi, I. (2014). Update on hidradenitis suppurativa: Connecting the tracts. *F1000 Prime Reports, 6,* 112.

Goldsmith, L. A., Katz, S. I. Gilchrest, B. A., Paller, A. S., Leffell, D. J., & Wolff, K. (2012). *Fitzpatrick's dermatology in general medicine* (8th ed.). New York, NY: McGraw-Hill.

Grossi E, Cazzaniga, S., Crotti, S., Naldi, L., Di Landro, A., Ingordo, V., ... the GISED Acne Study Group. (2014). The constellation of dietary factors in adolescent acne: A semantic connectivity map approach. *Journal of the European Academy of Dermatology and Venereology.* doi: 10.1111/jdv. 12878. [Epub ahead of print].

Harvey, A., & Huynh, T. T. (2014). Inflammation and acne: Putting the pieces together. *Journal of Drugs in Dermatology, 13*(4), 459–463.

Lwin, S. M., Kimber, I., & McFadden, J. P. (2014). Acne, quorum sensing and danger. *Clinical and Experimental Dermatology, 39*(2), 162–167.

Marks, J. G., & Miller, J. J. (2006). *Lookingbill and Marks' principles of dermatology* (4th ed.). Philadelphia, PA: Saunders-Elsevier.

McCann, S. E., & Huether, S. E. (2014). Structure, function, and disorders of the integument. In S. E. Huether, K. L. McCance, V. L. Brasher, & N. S. Rote (Eds.), *Pathophysiology—The biologic basics for disease in adults and children* (7th ed., pp. 1616–1652). St. Louis, MO: Mosby-Elsevier.

Melnik, B. C., John, S. M., & Plewig, G. (2013). Acne: Risk indicator for increased body mass index and insulin resistance. *Acta Dermato-Venereologica, 93*(6), 644–649.

Nicol, N. H. (2009). Assessment of the integumentary system. In J. M. Black & J. H. Hawks (Eds.), *Medical-surgical nursing: Clinical management for positive outcomes* (8th ed., pp. 1186–1198). Philadelphia, PA: WB Saunders Company.

Nicol, N. H., & Huether, S. E. (2014). Alterations of the integument in children. In S. E. Huether, K. L. McCance, V. L. Brasher, & N. S. Rote (Eds.), *Pathophysiology—The biologic basics for disease in adults and children* (7th ed., pp. 1653–1667). St. Louis, MO: Mosby-Elsevier.

Nicol, N. H., & Huether, S. E. (2012). Structure, function, and disorders of the integument. In S. E. Huether, K. L. McCance, V. L. Brasher, & N. S. Rote (Eds.), *Understanding pathophysiology* (6th ed., pp. 1038–1069). St. Louis, MO: Mosby-Elsevier.

Nicol, N. H., & Huether, S. E. (2012). Alterations of the integument in children. In S. E. Huether, K. L. McCance, V. L. Brasher, & N. S. Rote (Eds.), *Understanding pathophysiology* (6th ed., pp. 1070–1082). St. Louis, MO: Mosby-Elsevier.

Penzer, R., & Ersser, S. J. (2010). *Principles of skin care.* Oxford, UK: Wiley-Blackwell.

Schalock, P. C. (2007). Rosacea and perioral (periorificial) dermatitis. In K. A. Arndt, & J. T. S. Hsu (Eds.), *Manual of dermatologic therapeutics* (7th ed., pp. 174–179). Philadelphia, PA: Lippincott Williams & Wilkins.

Two, A. M., Wu, W., Gallo, R. O., & Hata, T. R. (2015). Rosacea. Part 1. Introduction, categorization, histology, pathogenesis, and risk factors. *Journal of the American Academy of Dermatology, 72*(5), 749–758.

Villasenor, J., & Kroshinsky, D. (2011). Acne and related disorders. In P. C. Schalock, J. T. S. Hsu, & K. A. Arndt (Eds.), *Lippincott's primary care dermatology* (pp. 50–67). Philadelphia, PA: Lippincott Williams & Wilkins.

Weinberg, S., Prose, N. S., & Kristal, L. (2008). *Color atlas of pediatric dermatology* (4th ed.). New York, NY: McGraw-Hill.

Wolff, K., Johnson, R. A., & Saavedra, A. P. (2013). *Fitzpatrick's color atlas and synopsis of clinical dermatology* (7th ed.). New York, NY: McGraw-Hill.

Yazdanyar, S., & Jemec, G. B. (2011). Hidradenitis suppurativa: A review of cause and treatment, *Current Opinion in Infectious Diseases, 24*(2), 118–123.

Yin, N. C., & McMichael, A. J. (2014). Acne in patients with skin of color: Practical management, *American Journal of Clinical Dermatology, 15*(1), 7–16.

STUDY QUESTIONS

1. Acne affects people of all ages, with a higher incidence between the ages of 12 and 25. Which of the following statements about the epidemiology of acne is *true*?
   a. Genetics has no impact on sebum excretion.
   b. Acne is more often severe in males than in females.
   c. Stress is not a factor in the severity of acne.
   d. There is a higher incidence of acne in African Americans.

2. An adolescent women with a 3-year history of acne presents to the clinic. The diagnostic hallmarks that indicate she is likely to have persistent severe acne include:
   a. Distribution primarily on the face and neck
   b. Comedones, papules, and pustules
   c. The presence of cysts and a family history of scarring acne
   d. Acne that peaks during the week before her menses

3. One of the main reasons the FDA strictly controls the use of isotretinoin is the risk for severe birth defects. Pregnancy tests are required every month while taking isotretinoin, except if the patient is 100% abstinent.
   a. True
   b. False

4. Prescribing antibiotics for acne increases the risk that the patient will develop bacterial resistance. Which of the following medications is often added to a patient's acne regimen to decrease the risk of bacterial resistance?
   a. Tretinoin
   b. Salicylic acid
   c. Azelaic acid
   d. Benzoyl peroxide

5. Rosacea is characterized by four subtypes: erythematotelangiectatic, papulopustular, phymatous, and ocular.
   a. True
   b. False

6. Lifestyle can have a significant impact on rosacea. When educating a patient with rosacea, important teaching points include:
   a. Clean the face well with a washcloth and use an astringent to remove all makeup and oils.
   b. Avoid topical corticosteroids, alcohol and spicy foods since they tend to worsen rosacea.
   c. Small amounts of sun may be helpful for clearing rosacea, similar to acne and dermatitis.
   d. Getting overheated while exercising may negatively impact rosacea, but there is no evidence indicating that foods have an impact.

7. Hidradenitis is a chronic, suppurative, recurring inflammatory disease that:
   a. Affects the eccrine gland follicles primarily on the scalp and under breasts
   b. Is most often seen in prepubescent children
   c. Is primarily caused by bacteria
   d. Presents in skin that contains apocrine glands, with the axilla and groin most frequently affected

8. A 23-year-old man has severe hidradenitis that is painful and has caused scaring in the bilateral axillae and groin area. He has not responded well to topical clindamycin, doxycycline, or intralesional steroid injections. Of the four treatments listed below, which would likely be the next choice?
   a. Phototherapy
   b. Methotrexate
   c. Infliximab
   d. Azelaic acid

9. Which of the following statements regarding the epidemiology of primary hyperhidrosis is *true*?
   a. There is a positive family history in 30% to 50% of cases.
   b. Primary hyperhidrosis is more common in whites.
   c. Primary hyperhidrosis is more common in men.
   d. Primary hyperhidrosis is not associated with obesity.

10. Typical first-line therapy for hyperhidrosis is:
    a. Botox
    b. Doxycycline
    c. Topical aluminum chloride 20%
    d. Iontophoresis

Answers to Study Questions: 1.b, 2.c, 3.b, 4.d, 5.a, 6.b, 7.d, 8.c, 9.a, 10.c

Infections

Theresa Coyner • Katrina Nice Masterson

OVERVIEW

Infections in the skin may range from superficial to deep and may be caused by bacteria, fungi, or viruses. These infections may occur in otherwise healthy individuals.

BACTERIAL INFECTIONS

I. IMPETIGO

A. Definition: a common, contagious, superficial skin infection caused by streptococci, staphylococci, or both
  1. Bullous impetigo (Figure 11-1)
    a. Etiology
      (1) Caused by group II *Staphylococcus aureus*.
      (2) Usually not secondarily contaminated by streptococci.
      (3) Colonization of the respiratory tract precedes colonization of the skin by days.
    b. Pathophysiology
      (1) Begins as small vesicles.
      (2) Evolves into sharply demarcated bullae without erythematous halo, which eventually rupture.
      (3) Nikolsky sign not present.

(4) Shallow erosions result within 1 to 2 days.
(5) Typically occurs on the face in infants and children but may infect any surface and any age group.
(6) Heals with hyperpigmentation with dark-skinned individuals.
(7) Characteristic honey-colored crust.
  2. Nonbullous impetigo (Figure 11-2)
    a. Etiology
      (1) Caused by beta-hemolytic streptococci.
      (2) Begins with exposure to *Streptococcus*, which enters the skin via areas of minor trauma.
      (3) Often becomes secondarily contaminated with staphylococcus.
    b. Pathophysiology
      (1) Begins as a small vesicle or pustule.
      (2) After rupture, a moist, erythematous base is exposed.
      (3) Characteristic honey-colored crust.
      (4) Satellite lesions may appear beyond the periphery.
      (5) Generally heals without scarring.
  3. Ecthyma (Figure 11-3)
    a. Etiology
      (1) Caused by *Streptococcus pyogenes* and rapidly contaminated with staphylococcus.
      (2) Considered an ulcerated form of nonbullous impetigo.
    b. Pathophysiology
      (1) Begins like nonbullous impetigo but extends into the dermis.
      (2) Shallow ulcer is formed. Generally, 1 to 10 lesions will be present.
      (3) Lesion crusts over with a purulent, necrotic base.
      (4) Most common on lower extremities in children, elderly, and patients with lymphedema.
B. Assessment
  1. History (Box 11-1)
  2. Current health status
  3. Physical examination
    a. Clinical presentation
    b. Evidence of trauma (bites, abrasions, lacerations)
    c. Gram stain
    d. Culture for causative organism(s)

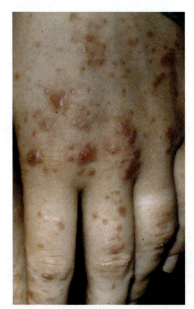

FIGURE 11-1. Bullous impetigo. (Courtesy of Charles E. Lewis, MD.)

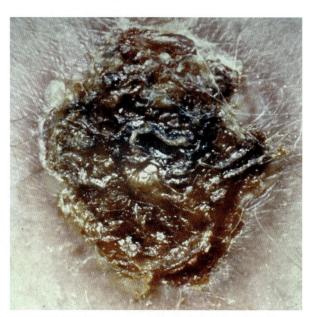

FIGURE 11-3. Ecthyma. (Courtesy of John K. Randall, MD.)

C. Treatment
1. Topical
   a. Mupirocin: apply to lesions tid for 7 to 10 days.
   b. Retapamulin: apply to lesions bid for 5 days.
2. Oral antibiotics for widespread infections
   a. Erythromycin 30 to 50 mg/kg/d every 6 to 8 hours
   b. Cephalexin 25 to 50 mg/kg/d every 6 to 8 hours
   c. Amoxicillin/clavulanate 25 to 45 mg/kg/d every 12 hours
3. Treatment of lesions
   a. Wash with antibacterial soap.
   b. Keep crusts moistened so they can gently be debrided by washing.

PATIENT EDUCATION
Bullous Impetigo

- Infected children should be isolated briefly until treatment is under way.
- Impetigo can spread via fingers, towels, and clothing.
- Sodium hypochlorite (bleach) baths may be helpful.
- ¼ to ½ cup of household bleach added to tub of water.
- Soak for 5 to 15 minutes at a frequency of two times weekly.
- Mupirocin nasal ointment applied to the nares bid × 5 days to reduce colonization.
- Poststreptococcal glomerulonephritis can develop 1 to 3 weeks following impetigo.
- Incidence ranges from 2% to 5% of individuals with impetigo.
- Children and at-risk adults for development of hematuria and edema should be monitored.

BOX 11-1. Taking the History in the Patient with Cutaneous Infection

In addition to a routine history and physical examination, the following issues must be explored:

- Time of onset of lesions (exacerbations, remission, and recurrences)
- Site of onset (pattern of spread or dissemination is important to making correct diagnosis)
- Change (evolution) in lesions (lesions seen on exam may not be the primary lesion)
- Cutaneous symptoms (burning, pruritus, or other discomfort)
- Precipitating factors
- Previous treatment (self-treatment may alter presentation)
- Occupation/hobbies: important to rule out exposure to specific infections
- Family history or close contact exposure to similar symptoms or lesions

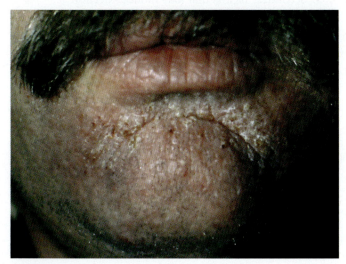

FIGURE 11-2. Nonbullous impetigo. (Courtesy of Charles E. Lewis, MD.)

II. CELLULITIS (FIGURE 11-4)

A. Definition: a diffuse, acute bacterial infection of the skin and subcutaneous tissue
B. Etiology
 1. Group A beta-hemolytic streptococci (erysipelas) or staphylococci most common cause.
 2. Non–group A *streptococcus, Haemophilus influenzae* type B, *Pseudomonas aeruginosa,* and *Campylobacter fetus* may be the etiology in patients with underlying abnormalities of lymphatics or venous drainage.
C. Pathophysiology
 1. Most commonly seen in lower extremities.
 2. Infection spreads locally secondary to the release of enzymes.
 3. Erythema and edema are present.
 4. Skin will be hot and tender to the touch.
 5. Lymphangitic streaks may develop specifically in erysipelas.
 6. Typically occurs near surgical wounds and cutaneous ulcers or may occur in normal skin. It may occur anywhere in immunocompromised patients.
D. Assessment
 1. History (Box 11-1).
 2. Evaluate patient's overall health status.
 3. Physical examination.
  a. Pain
  b. Erythema
  c. Increased warmth to palpation
  d. Edema
  e. Fever
  f. Assess for preexisting lesion
  g. Lymphadenopathy

 4. Diagnostic tests.
  a. CBC with differential
   (1) Mild leukocytosis with increase in neutrophils
   (2) Mildly elevated sedimentation rate
  b. Bacterial culture
E. Treatment
 1. Staphylococcal or streptococcal organisms.
  a. Dicloxacillin 500 to 1,000 mg every 6 hours
  b. Cephalexin 500 mg every 8 hours
 2. Recurrent disease: prophylactic antibiotics.
 3. Surgical debridement may be indicated if pockets of purulent material are present.

PATIENT EDUCATION
Cellulitis

- Burow solution, comprised of an aqueous solution of aluminum acetate (available over the counter), compresses may help alleviate discomfort.
- Leg elevation may hasten recovery.
- Open wounds should be cleansed with a normal saline irrigation using a 30-gauge syringe attached to an 18-gauge angiocatheter.

III. FURUNCLE/CARBUNCLE (FIGURE 11-5)

A. Definition: Furuncle is a boil. Carbuncle is an aggregation of interconnected furuncles that drain through several openings in the skin.
B. Etiology
 1. Staphylococcal infection
 2. May be secondary to ingrown hair or obstruction of sebaceous gland
C. Pathophysiology
 1. Abscess of the skin and subcutaneous tissue
 2. Central necrosis and suppuration seen
 3. Secondary factors that may induce infection
  a. Scratching
  b. Friction
  c. Infestation

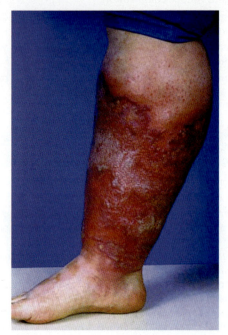

FIGURE 11-4. Cellulitis. (From Elder, D. E., et al. (2012). *Atlas and synopsis of lever's histopathology of the skin.* Philadelphia, PA: Wolters Kluwer.)

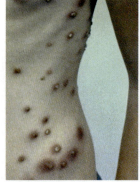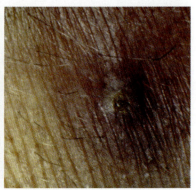

FIGURE 11-5. Furunculosis/furuncle. (Courtesy of John K. Randall, MD.)

d. Pressure from restrictive clothing

e. Chemical irritation

f. Hyperhidrosis

g. Occlusion of the follicle with ointments

4. Lesions

   a. Primary lesion: small, painful, indurated nodules.

   b. Evolves to elevated, tender lesion with shiny erythema and intense pain.

   c. Mature lesion.

     (1) Fluctuant with yellow or creamy white discharge

     (2) Central necrosis

   d. May spontaneously rupture.

   e. Single or multiple lesions may be present.

5. Systemic signs

   a. Fever

   b. Malaise

   c. Regional adenopathy

D. Assessment

1. History (Box 11-1)

2. Physical examination

3. Note location: lesions commonly seen on the back of the neck, face, buttocks, thighs, perineum, breasts, or axillae.

4. Evaluate the appearance of the lesion(s).

5. Distinguish between furuncle and ruptured epidermal cyst (cyst will have keratinous material).

6. Evaluate the presence of predisposing conditions.

   a. Occlusion, especially in hyperhidrosis

   b. Follicular abnormalities

   c. Colonized skin in patient with atopic dermatitis and scabies

7. Diagnostic tests

   a. Gram stain

   b. Bacterial culture

E. Treatment

1. Warm compresses

2. Incision, drainage, and packing to promote continuous drainage

3. Antibiotics appropriate for organism cultured

PATIENT EDUCATION
Furuncle/Carbuncle

- Patients should avoid constrictive clothing.
- Antibacterial soaps in patients with hyperhidrosis may be considered.
- Bleach baths may help to prevent recurrence.

IV. ERYTHRASMA

A. Definition: superficial bacterial infection of skin in intertriginous areas

B. Etiology

1. *Corynebacterium minutissimum* invades the stratum corneum.

2. Growth favored by warm, moist environment.

C. Pathophysiology

1. Lesions most common in the groin but may be seen in any intertriginous area.

2. Irregular erythematous plaque with well-defined borders.

3. Fine scale may cover the lesion.

4. Older lesions will fade to a brown color.

D. Assessment

1. History (Box 11-1)

2. Clinical examination.

   a. Assess for signs of hyperhidrosis.

   b. Assess for signs of poor personal hygiene.

3. Assess for risk factors including diabetes mellitus, obesity, and exposure to humid climate conditions.

4. Diagnostic tests.

   a. Gram stain

   b. Wood's lamp will fluorescence bright coral red.

E. Treatment

1. 11% to 20% topical application of aluminum chloride

2. 2% clindamycin HCl topical solution

3. 2% erythromycin topical gel or solution

PATIENT EDUCATION
Erythrasma

- Erythrasma can be a chronic intermittent condition.
- Weight loss is recommended for obese patients.
- Cotton underwear is recommended, especially boxer shorts for men if erythrasma occurs in the groin area.
- Daily washing includes antibacterial soap, pat dry, and use of a handheld hair dryer on cool setting to dry intertriginous areas thoroughly.

V. PITTED KERATOLYSIS (FIGURE 11-6)

A. Definition: noninflammatory bacterial infection on the soles of the feet and/or palms

B. Etiology

1. Causative agent is either *Micrococcus sedentarius* or *Corynebacterium*.

2. Produce proteolytic enzymes that digest the stratum corneum.

C. Pathophysiology

1. Crater-like pits will occur on weight-bearing areas of the feet.

2. Pits are 1 to 7 mm in diameter.

3. Erosions may rarely occur.

4. No erythema will be present.

D. Assessment

1. History (Box 11-1)

2. Clinical examination

   a. Assess for the characteristic craters.

   b. Assess for the presence of hyperhidrosis and malodor.

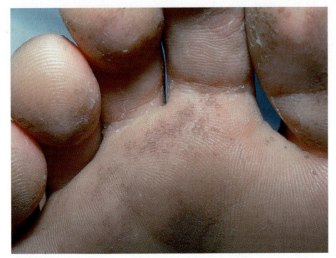

FIGURE 11-6. Pitted keratolysis. (From Burkhart, C., Morell, D., Goldsmith, L. A., et al. (2009). *VisualDx: Essential pediatric dermatology.* Philadelphia, PA: Lippincott Williams & Wilkins.)

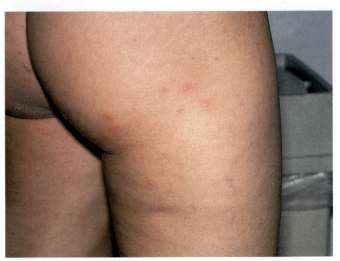

FIGURE 11-7. Folliculitis. (From Goodheart, H. P. (2003). *Goodheart's photoguide of common skin disorders* (2nd ed.). Philadelphia, PA: Lippincott Williams & Wilkins.)

3. Diagnostic tests
   a. Generally, none are performed as this is a clinical diagnosis.
   b. Wood's lamp will not demonstrate fluorescence.
E. Treatment
  1. 10 to 25% aluminum chloride solution applied topically
  2. 2% clindamycin HCl topical solution
  3. 2% erythromycin topical solution

PATIENT EDUCATION
Pitted Keratolysis

- Feet should be kept dry and clean by washing at least daily with antibacterial soap and drying thoroughly.
- Cotton socks should be worn or socks specifically designed to wick moisture away from the skin; change socks daily or more frequently.
- Shoes should be allowed to dry thoroughly prior to the next wear.

VI. FOLLICULITIS (FIGURE 11-7)

A. Definition: inflammation of the hair follicle
B. Etiology
  1. Causative organisms include staphylococcus, dermatophytes, *Klebsiella*, *Proteus*, *Enterobacter*, and *Pseudomonas*.
  2. Drug-induced folliculitis most commonly occurs with use of corticosteroids.
C. Pathophysiology
  1. Organisms gain access to the hair follicle due to chemical irritation, physical injury, or occlusion: specifically with topical steroid.
  2. Inflammation may be superficial to deep.
  3. Pseudofolliculitis barbae caused by shaving.
    a. More common in individuals with tightly curled spiral hair

D. Assessment
  1. History (Box 11-1).
  2. Assess shaving practices.
  3. Lesions (Table 11-1).

TABLE 11-1 Folliculitis Types, Clinical Presentation, and Treatment

Type	Clinical Presentation	Treatment
Dermatophyte folliculitis	Erythematous papules and pustules in the beard area with crusting.	Itraconazole 200 mg bid for 1 wk/mo for 2 mo Terbinafine 250 mg/d for 2–3 wk Griseofulvin microsized 500–1,000 mg/d for 4–6 wk Griseofulvin ultramicrosized 500–700 mg/d for 4–6 wk
Pityrosporum folliculitis	Follicular-based papules and pustules predominantly on the back, chest, and shoulders. Very pruritic.	Topical antifungals Fluconazole 100–200 mg/d for 3 wk Itraconazole 200 mg/d for 1–3 wk
Drug-induced folliculitis	Erythematous follicular papules and pustules located on the trunk, shoulders, and upper arms. Acute onset.	Stop the offending medication Topical benzoyl peroxide or clindamycin
Gram-negative folliculitis	Hot tub folliculitis caused by *Pseudomonas aeruginosa*. Lesions will be pink to erythematous follicular papules and pustules that will appear edematous.	Ciprofloxacin 500 mg bid for 7 d
Bacterial folliculitis	Perifollicular papules and pustules on an erythematous base.	Treatment should be based upon culture results Topical benzoyl peroxide Topical clindamycin Doxycycline 100 mg daily to bid for 2 wk

4. Diagnostic tests
   a. Gram stain
   b. Culture
   c. Histologic analysis
E. Treatment (Table 11-1)

PATIENT EDUCATION
Folliculitis

- Occlusive topical steroids should not be used when folliculitis is present.
- Constrictive clothing is to be avoided.
- Use of a chemical depilatory may be considered.
- All shaving techniques must be done with care; an electric razor should be used if possible. Avoid twin, triple, and quadruple blades as these pull and cut the hair below the skin surface. Wet the area to be shaved with warm water and lather with a thick shaving gel. Shave with the grain of the hair. Replace shaving blades frequently as they dull quickly.
- Cool compresses may be applied after shaving.
- Glycolic acid lotion may be used to reduce hyperkeratosis (elevated bumps).

VII. INFECTIONS WITH POTENTIAL LIFE-THREATENING COMPLICATIONS

A. Meningococcemia (Figure 11-8)
   1. Definition: gram-negative diplococcus skin infection
   2. Etiology
      a. Causative organism is *Neisseria meningitides*.
      b. Transmitted by respiratory secretions.
      c. Present in 10% to 20% of population.
   3. Pathophysiology
      a. Colonization occurs in nasopharyngeal area.
      b. Systemic invasion causes bacteremia.

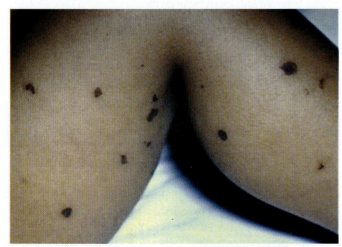

FIGURE 11-8. Meningococcemia. (Courtesy of John K. Randall, MD.)

c. Organism invades endothelial cells of small vessels and releases endotoxin.
   d. Cytokines are released causing hypotension, decreased cardiac output, and increased endothelial permeability.
   e. Thirteen strains of *N. meningitides* and serotypes A, B, C, Y, and W-135 can cause meningococcemia.
   f. Predominantly affects young adults and children.
4. Assessment
   a. History (Box 11-1).
   b. Assess for sudden onset of fever, headache, nausea, vomiting, and stiff neck.
   c. Lesion assessment.
      (1) Rash occurs in 70% of cases.
      (2) Range from pink macules, erythematous papules, to purpuric lesions.
      (3) Petechiae and ecchymosis may occur.
      (4) Purpuric lesions will have central gunmetal gray discoloration.
   d. Diagnostic tests
      (1) Blood culture
      (2) CSF culture
      (3) Gram stain
      (4) Histologic analysis: leukocytoclastic vasculitis and thrombi
5. Treatment
   a. High-dose penicillin, chloramphenicol for penicillin allergic patients, or third-generation cephalosporin

PATIENT EDUCATION
Meningococcemia

- Triage nurses should have high degree of suspicion for patient calls with symptoms of rash, fever, headache, and stiff neck. Urgent visit or refer to emergency department.
- Vaccine is available protecting against serotypes A, C, Y, and W-135.
- Household members, day caregivers, and close personal contacts should be treated prophylactically with rifampin.

B. Staphylococcal Scalded Skin Syndrome (SSSS) (Figure 11-9)
   1. Definition: staphylococcal epidermolytic toxic syndrome also known as Ritter disease
   2. Etiology
      a. Epidermolytic toxin acts as a toxin and elicits an antibody reaction.
      b. Antibody is present in 75% of people over age 10.
      c. Affects young children, immunosuppressed individuals, and patients with chronic renal failure.
   3. Pathophysiology
      a. Begins with a staphylococcal infection of the conjunctivae, throat, nares, or umbilicus.
      b. Toxin is filtered through glomeruli.

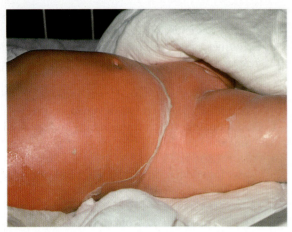

FIGURE 11-9. Staphylococcal scalded skin syndrome (SSSS). (From Burkhart, C., Morell, D., Goldsmith, L. A., et al. (2009). *VisualDx: Essential pediatric dermatology*. Philadelphia, PA: Lippincott Williams & Wilkins.)

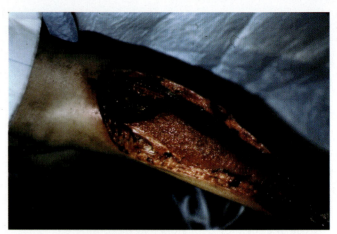

FIGURE 11-10. Necrotizing fasciitis, postoperative. (Courtesy of John K. Randall, MD.)

c. Individuals with poor renal clearance or low glomeruli filtration rate may develop the toxin systemically.

d. Toxin acts in the epidermis affecting cell-to-cell adhesion.

4. Assessment
   a. History (Box 11-1)
   b. Lesions
      (1) Initially tender, erythematous skin with sandpaper-like appearance.
      (2) Skin wrinkles and bullae occur, followed by peeling layers of the skin.
      (3) Nikolsky sign will be present.
      (4) Yellow crusting will occur followed by skin drying and cracking.
      (5) Skin re-epithelializes in 7 to 10 days.
   c. Diagnostic tests
      (1) Culture of the conjunctivae, nose, throat, and bullae. Often negative in children.
      (2) Histologic analysis: dermal–epidermal separation.

5. Treatment.
   a. Hospitalization and IV therapy may be needed.
   b. Nafcillin 100 to 200 mg/kg/d IV.
   c. Less severe cases managed at home with oral antibiotics: dicloxacillin 25 mg/kg/d or cephalosporin for 1 week.

PATIENT EDUCATION
Staphylococcal Scalded Skin Syndrome
- Signs of dehydration must be assessed.
- All medical and skin care needs individual recommendations.

C. Necrotizing Fasciitis (Figure 11-10)
   1. Definition: soft tissue infection causing local tissue necrosis and life-threatening sepsis

2. Etiology
   a. Type 1: polymicrobial infection including aerobic and anaerobic organisms
   b. Type 2: *Streptococcus pyogenes* or staphylococcus
   c. *Vibrio vulnificus* and *Aeromonas hydrophila*, both waterborne organisms, may rarely cause the condition.

3. Pathophysiology
   a. Initially appears as a cellulitis.
   b. Substances produced by the organism resist phagocytosis.
   c. Pyogenic exostosis induces cytokines that mediate fever, shock, and tissue injury.
   d. More common in elderly or individuals with chronic conditions. May occur in healthy individuals.
   e. Extremities are most likely involved.

4. Assessment
   a. History (Box 11-1).
   b. Assess for the presence of chronic conditions, specifically diabetes, arterial disease, alcohol abuse, and malnutrition.
   c. Assess vital signs: fever often absent initially, and tachycardia will be present.
   d. Skin changes.
      (1) Initially tender, erythematous, and swollen.
      (2) Rapidly progresses from reddish purple appearing to gray-blue in poorly defined patches.
      (3) Violaceous bullae may develop.
      (4) Thin, malodorous fluid results from necrosis of fascia and fat.
      (5) Subcutaneous tissue will feel hard and wooden.
   e. Critical diagnostic signs.
      (1) Severe pain out of proportion to the initial clinical signs
      (2) Vital sign abnormalities
      (3) Presence of hemorrhagic bullae indicating occlusion of deep vessels in the fascia
   f. Diagnostic studies
      (1) Coagulopathy, increased WBC with leukocytosis, and elevated creatinine kinase.
      (2) Culture.

(3) MRI or CT scan may indicate depth of tissue involvement.

(4) Histologic analysis: frozen tissue will have massive polymorphonuclear infiltration.

5. Treatment.
   a. Prompt and frequent surgical debridement
   b. Broad-spectrum antibiotics
      (1) Type 1: polymicrobial: combination of ampicillin/sulbactam or piperacillin plus clindamycin plus ciprofloxacin
      (2) Type 2: streptococcal: penicillin plus clindamycin; staphylococcal: cefazolin plus vancomycin plus clindamycin

PATIENT EDUCATION
Necrotizing Fasciitis

- Prompt suspicion of pain that is out of proportion to initial clinical signs.
- Nutritional support is required.
- Scrupulous wound care is required.

VIRAL INFECTIONS

I. WARTS

A. Definition: benign viral epidermal growths
B. Etiology/pathophysiology
   1. Human papillomavirus (HPV).
   2. Infects the keratinocytes of the epidermis. Does not extend into the dermis.
   3. Transmitted by touch.
   4. Variable course. May resolve spontaneously or last a lifetime.
   5. Regression of the virus dependent of the cell-mediated immune response.
   6. Often occur at sites of prior trauma.
   7. Most common in children and young adults but may occur at any age.
   8. More severe in patients with impaired immunity.
C. Common warts: verruca vulgaris (Figure 11-11)
   1. Elevated and well circumscribed.
   2. Irregular shape with hyperkeratotic surface.
   3. Minute papillary projections can be visualized.
   4. Obscure normal skin lines.
   5. Vary in size from 1 mm to over 10 mm.
   6. May proliferate and coalesce (mosaic wart).

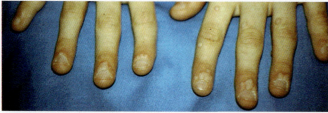

FIGURE 11-11. Common warts: verruca vulgaris. (Courtesy of John K. Randall, MD.)

7. Color ranges from flesh toned, gray, and brown.
8. Black dots seen on the surface are not "seeds" but thrombosed small capillaries.
9. Common sites.
   a. Hands: HPV types 2, 4, and 29
   b. Periungual: often secondary to nail biting
   c. Plantar surface: HPV type 1. Often secondary to communal moist environments
D. Assessment (Box 11-1).
E. Treatment.
   1. Treatment ranges from attempting to activate an immune response to tissue destruction.
   2. All treatments have the potential to cause some level of discomfort and scar.
   3. Salicylic acid 17% to 40%. Creams, liquid, ointments, and plasters available.
   4. Liquid nitrogen applied via spray or cotton applicator. One to three freeze–thaw cycles extending 2 mm beyond the wart diameter.
   5. Laser therapy: various modalities can be used.
   6. Bichloroacetic acid applied to plantar surface only. Protect surrounding skin with a light coat of petrolatum. Lightly curette the surface of wart prior to applying the acid. Cover with dry dressing.
   7. Cantharidin—will create an allergic reaction with significant blistering. Apply to wart surface, allow to dry, and cover with occlusive dressing for 2 to 6 hours.
   8. Imiquimod 5%—apply small amount nightly to wart surface and cover with Band-Aid.
   9. Immunotherapy: squaric acid dibutylester (SADBE) or diphenylcyclopropenone (DCPC). Patient is sensitized with a 1% solution applied to the upper inner arm. When irritation occurs, a 0.1% solution is applied to the wart surface.
   10. *Candida albicans* skin test antigen. 1:1 mixture combined with lidocaine. Injection of 0.1 mL of solution into the wart surface and the intradermal margins of the wart.
   11. Duct tape. Apply to wart for 7 days. Remove the tape, soak, and gently pare the wart.
   12. Electrocautery. Wart and surrounding skin anesthetized. Curette the wart and cauterize. A smoke evacuator should be used to reduce inhalation of viral particles.
   13. Resistant warts.
      a. Blunt dissection
      b. 5-Fluorouracil cream
      c. Intralesional bleomycin: 3 mL of normal saline mixed to 15-unit vial; additional 12 mL of normal saline added. Inject a minute amount (0.1 mL) into the wart surface.

II. VERRUCA PLANA (FLAT WARTS) (FIGURE 11-12)

A. HPV types 3, 10, 28, and 49
B. Slightly raised, irregular, smooth, or slightly hyperkeratotic surface
C. Multiple lesions
D. Flesh colored to slightly pink
E. Prevalent in patients with compromised immunity

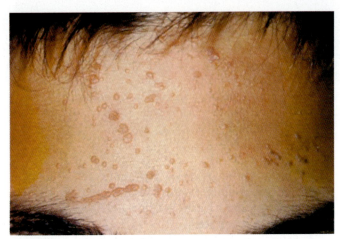

FIGURE 11-12. Flat warts: verruca plana. (From Elder, D. E., et al. (2012). *Atlas and synopsis of lever's histopathology of the skin*. Philadelphia, PA: Wolters Kluwer.)

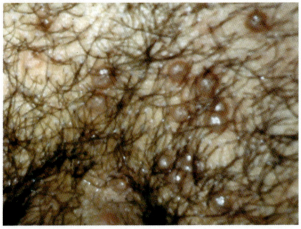

FIGURE 11-13. Molluscum contagiosum: pubic. (Courtesy of Charles E. Lewis, MD.)

F. Common locations
  1. Dorsal hands
  2. Face
  3. Areas routinely shaved
G. Treatment
  1. Topical retinoid cream applied nightly
  2. Liquid nitrogen
  3. Laser
  4. Low levels of electrocautery
  5. 5% fluorouracil cream
  6. 5% imiquimod cream

PATIENT EDUCATION
Verruca

- Treatments for verruca have the potential to scar the skin.
- All treatments will have some level of discomfort.
- Numerous treatments may be needed.
- 5% fluorouracil should be avoided in children.
- Bichloroacetic acid should only be used on the plantar surface.
- Topical retinoids, bleomycin, and 5% fluorouracil should not be used in pregnancy.
- Patients sensitized to SADBE or DCPC may have contact dermatitis to any area the chemical contacts. It should be applied during office visits, not at home.
- Behavior changes to avoid nail biting with periungual lesions.
- Shaving to be avoided in areas where warts are present. If patients refuse to stop shaving, they should use a disposable razor and shave the areas where warts are present last.

III. MOLLUSCUM CONTAGIOSUM (FIGURE 11-13)

A. Definition: benign tumor of the skin
B. Etiology/pathophysiology
  1. Double-stranded DNA cowpox virus.

  2. Spread is by touch and autoinoculation by scratching.
  3. In general, casual contact is a mode of transmission in children and sexual contact in adults.
  4. Lesions are discrete ranging in size from 2 to 5 mm with central umbilication.
  5. Core of the lesion (molluscum body) contains a white substance.
  6. Lesions may be much larger in immunocompromised individuals.
  7. Location: in children, on the face, trunk, extremities, and intertriginous areas. Lesions located in the genital area should arouse suspicion of sexual abuse. In adults, on the face, trunk, extremities, and genitalia.
  8. Atopic individuals are at risk for dissemination of lesions.
  9. Resolves spontaneously in 6 to 9 months, but lesions may remain up to 4 years.
C. Treatment (see treatment options under verruca)
  1. Curettage: scraping individual lesions
  2. Liquid nitrogen
  3. Topical retinoid cream
  4. Salicylic acid
  5. Cantharidin
  6. Laser
  7. 5% imiquimod cream
D. Assessment (Box 11-1)

PATIENT EDUCATION
Molluscum Contagiosum

- Teens and young adults with genitalia lesions should be screened for other sexually transmitted infections.
- School policies may require lesions to be covered.
- Close contacts and family members instructed to monitor for development of lesions.
- All treatments may cause irritation, discomfort, and the potential to scar the skin.

IV. CONDYLOMA ACUMINATUM (FIGURES 11-14 AND 11-15)

A. Definition: sexually transmitted HPV lesions
B. Etiology/pathophysiology
 1. Most common is HPV types 6 and 11. Other subtypes may occur. Types 16 and 18 are associated with neoplasms and dysplasia.
 2. Generally asymptomatic, but pruritus may occur.
 3. Minor trauma during sexual activity allows the virus entry into the skin.
 4. Immunosuppressed and pregnant individuals are most susceptible.
 5. Lesions range from single soft papules to multiple growths. They may coalesce and present as cauliflower-like masses.
 6. Lesions present on the penis, scrotum, anus, and urethra in males.
 7. Lesions present on the vulva, vagina, cervix, and perianal areas in females.
 8. Virus can be transmitted to newborn during vaginal delivery.
 9. Subclinical infections (no visible lesions) may be identified by application of 5% acetic acid. This will cause whitening of the lesions.
 10. Association of HPV with subsequent head, neck, and throat cancers.
C. Assessment
 1. History (Box 11-1)
 2. Diagnostic tests
  a. Serology tests
  b. Cervical Pap smear in women. ViraPap for specific hybridization to determine specific subtypes
  c. Anal smears in both men and women
  d. Lesion biopsy
D. Treatment: often difficult to eradicate
 1. 80% trichloroacetic acid or 90% bichloroacetic acid applied to the lesion. Surrounding skin should be protected by thin coating of petrolatum. After light frosting occurs, a baking soda paste is applied to neutralize.
 2. 5% imiquimod applied to the lesions two times weekly.
 3. Sinecatechin 15% ointment. Apply topically tid for 2 to 4 months.
 4. Podophyllin 10% to 25% compounded in tincture of benzoin, 0.5% solution, 0.15% cream. Podophyllin is a plant compound that halts cell mitosis leading to tissue destruction. Apply to lesion, allow to dry, and wash off in 1 hour.
 5. Podofilox 0.5% gel or solution applied every 12 hours × 3 days then off 4 days.
 6. 5% fluorouracil cream.
 7. Liquid nitrogen.
 8. Light cautery.
 9. Excision.
 10. Ablative laser treatment.

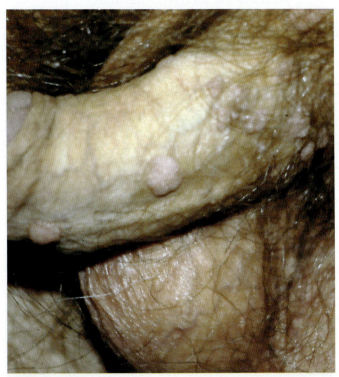

FIGURE 11-14. Condyloma acuminatum: penis. (Courtesy of Charles E. Lewis, MD.)

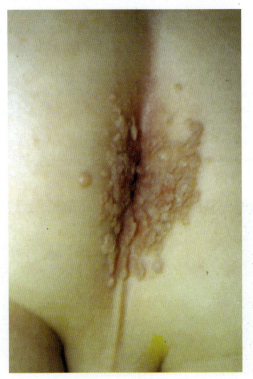

FIGURE 11-15. Condyloma acuminatum: perianal. (Courtesy of Charles E. Lewis, MD.)

PATIENT EDUCATION
Condyloma Acuminatum

• Treatment irritation is expected.

• Imiquimod, sinecatechin, and podophyllin must have irritation to provide any benefit. These medications should not be used in the urethra, vagina, cervix, and anal area.

• Patients should have full sexually transmitted disease screenings including gonorrhea, syphilis, and chlamydia.

• Podophyllin and 5% fluorouracil are contraindicated in pregnancy.

• Condoms do not entirely prevent transmission of the virus.

• HPV vaccination is recommended for all adolescents, male and female. Gardasil is protective against HPV types 6, 11, 16, and 18. Cervarix is protective for females against HPV types 16 and 18.

V. HUMAN HERPESVIRUS (HHV) (FIGURES 11-16 AND 11-17)

A. Definition: viral infection of the skin
1. There are eight herpesviruses. Herpes simplex virus types 1 and 2 (HSV1 and HSV2), varicella-zoster virus (VZV), Epstein-Barr virus (EBV), cytomegalovirus (CMV), and human herpesvirus 6, 7, and 8
B. Etiology/pathophysiology
1. HSV1 spreads by direct contact with contaminated secretions. HSV2 spread by secretions during sexual contact. HSV1 generally oral and HSV2 genital, but with oral/genital contact, HSV2 may be oral and vice versa.
2. Primary, latent, and recurrent infection types.
C. Virus replicated at site of infection (primary) then travels retrograde to dorsal root ganglia (latent). Virus can be reactivated spontaneously or by a stimulus (recurrent).
D. Primary infection
1. May be asymptomatic.
2. Elevated IgG antibody titer.
3. Severity will increase with advanced age and suppressed immune status.
4. Symptoms occur 3 to 7 days after contact.
   a. Tenderness, pain, mild paresthesias, and burning prior to appearance of lesions.

b. Localized pain, tender lymphadenopathy, and flu-like symptoms may occur.
E. Recurrent infection
1. Exacerbating factors.
   a. Sunlight
   b. Trauma
   c. Stress
   d. Menses
   e. Systemic infection
2. Not all individuals will have recurrence.
3. Prodrome
   a. Duration 2 to 24 hours with symptoms similar to that of primary infection.
   b. Recurrent lesions may occur within 12 hours of prodromal symptoms.
   c. Increased frequency of recurrences with HSV2 infections.
F. Assessment
1. History (Box 11-1)
2. Assess overall health of patient.
3. Diagnosis is generally made on clinical presentation.
   a. Grouped vesicles on an erythematous base.
   b. Vesicles quickly open leaving erosions.
   c. Crusting may occur.
   d. Lasts 2 to 6 weeks.
   e. Heals without scarring.
4. Laboratory tests.
   a. Tzanck smear: multinucleated epithelial giant cells
   b. Biopsy of intact lesion
   c. Viral culture
   d. Direct immunofluorescence
   e. Serology: Western blot for HSV antibodies and other tests available for type-specific virus

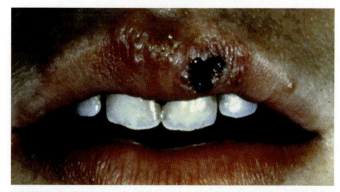

FIGURE 11-16. Human herpesvirus (HHV): lips. (Courtesy of Charles E. Lewis, MD.)

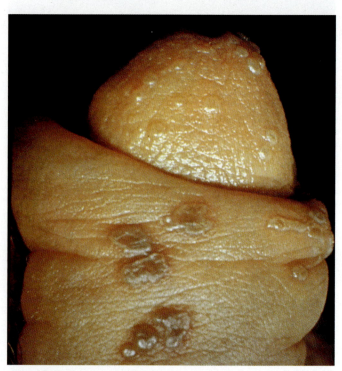

FIGURE 11-17. Human herpesvirus (HHV): penis. (Courtesy of John K. Randall, MD.)

TABLE 11-2 Herpes Simplex Virus Treatment

	Acyclovir	Valacyclovir	Famciclovir
First episode	400 mg tid × 7–10 d 200 mg 5 times daily for 7–10 d	1 g bid × 7–10 d	250 mg tid × 7–10 d
Suppression	400 mg bid	500 mg bid	250 mg bid
Episodic	400 mg tid × 5 d 800 mg bid × 5 d 800 mg tid × 3 d	500 mg bid × 3 d 1 g daily × 5 d	125 mg bid × 5 d 1,000 mg bid × 1 d 500 mg × 1 d then 250 mg bid × 2 d

G. Treatment
   1. Symptom control with cool moist compresses of water or Burow solution.
   2. Topical antivirals less effective than oral medications. Applied every 2 hours.
      a. Acyclovir cream
      b. Penciclovir cream
      c. Docosanol cream (available OTC)
      d. Acyclovir/hydrocortisone: applied five times daily for 5 days
   3. L-Lysine has no research data demonstrating effectiveness.
   4. Systemic antivirals.
      a. Acyclovir.
      b. Valacyclovir.
      c. Famciclovir.
      d. See Table 11-2 for dosing regimens.
H. Other cutaneous types of herpetic infection (Figure 11-18)
   1. Herpes whitlow: infection of the fingertip, often common in health care providers.

   2. Herpes gladiatorum: infection in athletes involved in direct skin-to-skin contact; common in wrestlers.
   3. Eczema herpeticum: widespread HSV infection in atopic patients. Symptoms can range from mild to severe (Figure 11-19).

PATIENT EDUCATION
Herpes Viruses

- Herpes simplex virus is definitely transmitted during active infections and the prodrome period. There may be transmission during times there are no symptoms.
- Condom use during sexual activity is highly recommended.
- Individuals with frequent recurrence should be on suppressive therapy for at least 1 year.

VI. VARICELLA-ZOSTER VIRUS (VZV) (FIGURE 11-20)

A. Definition: an acute vesiculobullous eruption seen in a dermatomal distribution that rarely crosses the midline
B. Etiology
   1. Caused by reactivation of varicella virus acquired during an episode of (or exposure to) chickenpox.
   2. Virus lies dormant in nerve root ganglion until reactivated.
   3. Occurs in 10% to 20% of all persons and can occur in all ages with incidence increasing with age.

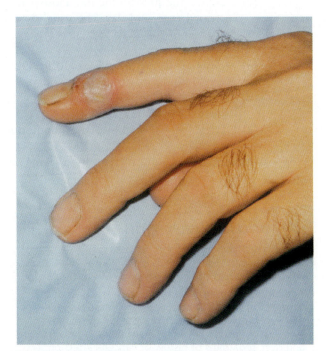

FIGURE 11-18. Herpes whitlow: index finger. (From Berg, D., & Worzala, K. (2006). *Atlas of adult physical diagnosis*. Philadelphia, PA: Lippincott Williams & Wilkins.)

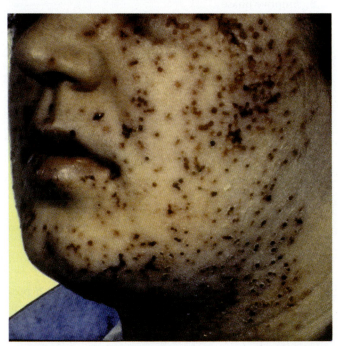

FIGURE 11-19. Eczema herpeticum. (Courtesy of John K. Randall, MD.)

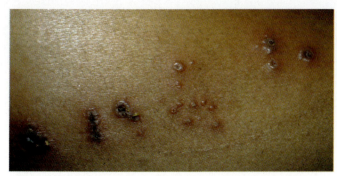

FIGURE 11-20. Varicella-zoster virus (VZV). (Courtesy of Charles E. Lewis, MD.)

C. Pathophysiology
1. Factors that reactivate the virus
   a. Age
   b. Immunosuppressive medications
   c. Lymphoma and other cancers
   d. Fatigue
   e. Emotional upset
   f. Radiation
2. Preeruptive symptoms (localized to dermatome): precede eruption 4 to 5 days
   a. Pain: may be severe simulating pleurisy, myocardial infarction, abdominal disease, or migraine headache.
   b. Pruritus or burning.
   c. Tenderness or hyperesthesia.
   d. Urinary hesitancy or retention involves S2, S3, and S4 nerves.
   e. Flu-like symptoms.
   f. Regional lymphadenopathy may be present.
3. Eruptive phase
   a. Generally limited to a single dermatome
   b. Rare bilateral symmetrical or asymmetrical dermatomes (may signal presence of underlying malignancy)
   c. Viremia (appearance of 20 to 30 scattered vesicles, outside the dermatome); seen in approximately 50% of patients
   d. Eruption
      (1) Begins with erythematous, swollen plaques of various sizes
      (2) Spreads to involve dermatome
      (3) Vesicles with purulent fluid form 3 to 4 days after appearance of erythema
      (4) Vesicular eruption may continue for up to 7 days.
      (5) Rupture of vesicles leads to erosion and crusting.
      (6) Elderly or debilitated patient may have a prolonged and difficult course of infection and may also have prolonged pain (postherpetic neuralgia) for several months.

D. Assessment
1. History (Box 11-1)
2. Current health status of patient
3. Clinical presentation of lesions (particularly if atypical presentation)
4. Diagnostic tests for atypical presentation
   a. Viral culture
   b. Direct fluorescent antigen assay
   c. Quantitative polymerase chain reaction for detection of VZV DNA
E. Treatment
1. Acyclovir 800 mg five times daily for 7 days
2. Valacyclovir 1,000 mg every 8 hours for 7 days
3. Famciclovir 500 mg every 8 hours for 7 days
4. Cool compresses
5. Burow compresses
F. Postherpetic neuralgia treatment
1. Topicals
   a. Lidocaine 2% or 10% gel or 5% patch
   b. Capsaicin 0.05% ointment, 0.075% cream, or 8% patch
   c. Systemic agents
      (1) Gabapentin 300 mg/day increasing 300 mg daily. Usual dose 1,800 to 3,600 mg/day
      (2) Pregabalin 150 mg/day in divided dose increasing up to 30 mg/day within 1 week. Can be increased up to 600 mg/day after 2 to 4 weeks
      (3) Tricyclic antidepressants
         (a) Amitriptyline 10mg initially increased until desired effect up to 100mg nightly.
         (b) Nortriptyline 10 to 25 mg nightly. May be increased up to 25 mg/week. The usual dose is 30 to 75 mg nightly
         (c) Desipramine 10 to 25 mg/day. Dose may be increased every 3rd day. The usual dose is 50 to 150 mg/day.
      (4) Opioid analgesics
         (a) Morphine: 10 mg at night or 10 to 30 mg every 12 hours; maximum dose 200 mg/day
         (b) Tramadol: 100 to 400 mg/day in divided doses at least 4 hours apart
         (c) Oxycodone: 10 mg bid; maximum dose 60 mg/day
         (d) Methadone: 5 mg at night up to 15 mg/day

PATIENT EDUCATION
Varicella-Zoster Virus

- Individuals with zoster are only contagious to individuals who have not had either the varicella virus or the vaccine.
- Advisory Committee on Immunization Practices of the Centers for Disease Control and Prevention recommends VZV vaccine given subcutaneously as a 0.65-mL dose (Zostavax) in all immunocompetent adults aged 60 years and over, regardless of history of varicella infection.

FUNGAL INFECTIONS

I. DERMATOPHYTES

A. Definition: known as tineas; superficial infections of the skin and responsible for the vast majority of skin, hair, and nail infections

B. Etiology

1. Dermatophytes produce enzymes that break down keratin. Organism invades and survives on dead keratin (stratum corneum).

2. Dermatophytes cannot survive on mucosal surfaces, which are devoid of keratin.

3. Occasionally will undergo deep invasion, especially in immunocompromised individuals.

4. Some patients may have genetic predisposition to dermatophyte infections.

C. Pathophysiology

1. Lesions vary in presentation and may resemble other dermatoses, leading to misdiagnosis.

2. Classification

   a. Genera
      (1) *Trichophyton*
      (2) *Microsporum*
      (3) *Epidermophyton*
   b. Transmission modes
      (1) Anthropophilic: human to human
         (a) Mild inflammatory response
      (2) Zoophilic: animal to human
         (a) Intense inflammatory response
      (3) Geophilic: soil to human or animal
         (a) Moderate inflammatory response
   c. Body region
      (1) Tinea corporis: nonhairy parts of the body, face, neck, and extremities
      (2) Tinea cruris: groin and inner thigh
      (3) Tinea capitis: scalp
      (4) Tinea manuum: hands
      (5) Tinea pedis: feet
      (6) Tinea unguium (onychomycosis): nails
      (7) Tinea barbae (tinea sycosis): beard
   d. Hair invasion types
      (1) Endothrix pattern: fungal elements inside the hair follicle
      (2) Ectothrix pattern: fungal elements inside and on the surface of the hair follicle

D. Assessment

1. History (Box 11-1)

2. Inspect skin and mucous membranes

3. Assess for cervical lymphadenopathy with scalp involvement

4. Lesions

   a. Tinea corporis: annular lesion with central clearing and active leading edge of infection with scale. Lesions may also appear arcuate, circinate, and oval (Figure 11-21). Lesions treated with topical corticosteroids may have no scale (tinea incognito).

   b. Tinea cruris: erythematous plaque in the groin with well-demarcated scaly border. Skin within the plaque may have a red-brown appearance. Vesicles may be present at the outer border (Figure 11-22).

   c. Tinea manuum: lesions on the dorsal aspect will appear as tinea corporis. Lesions on the palm will be hyperkeratotic with scale (Figure 11-23).

   d. Tinea pedis: lesions on the dorsal aspect will appear as tinea corporis. Lesions on the sole will be hyperkeratotic with scale in moccasin-type distribution. Web spaces of the toes may have vesicles, fissures, and maceration (Figure 11-24).

   e. Tinea barbae: lesions will be follicular-based pustules often eroded (Figure 11-25).

   f. Tinea unguium: hyperkeratosis of the nail, separation of the distal plate (onycholysis), subungual white debris, and yellowing of the distal plate (Figure 11-26)

   g. Tinea capitis (Figure 11-27)
      (1) Most common organism in North America is *Trichophyton tonsurans*.
      (2) Five patterns of presentation
         (a) Noninflammatory black dot (the color of dot dependent upon hair color). Hair will be broken off at follicle, scalp scale will be present, and large areas of alopecia will be present.
         (b) Kerion: areas of alopecia with boggy and purulent plaque. Abscess may be present (Figure 11-28).
         (c) Seborrheic dermatitis type: fine white scale with tiny perifollicular pustules.
         (d) Pustular: discrete pustules without scaling.
         (e) Favus: thick yellow crusts composed of hyphae and skin debris. Scarring alopecia is common. The causative organism is *T. schoenleinii*.

   h. Variants
      (1) Tinea profunda: granulomatous or verrucal appearance
      (2) "Two feet and one hand syndrome": diffuse hyperkeratosis of one palm and both soles

5. Diagnostic tests

   a. Potassium hydroxide wet mount (KOH); take specimen from active border of lesion.

   b. Wood's lamp
      (1) *T. schoenleinii* will fluoresce pale green.
      (2) *Microsporum audouinii* will fluoresce yellow green.

   c. Fungal culture

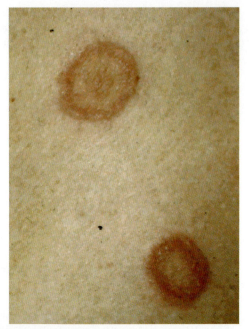

FIGURE 11-21. Tinea corporis. (Courtesy of Charles E. Lewis, MD.)

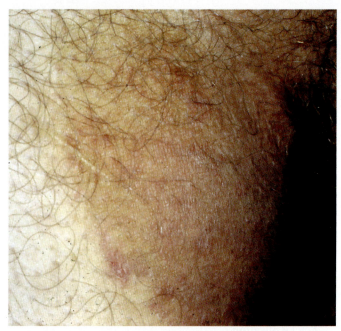

FIGURE 11-22. Tinea cruris. (Courtesy of John K. Randall, MD.)

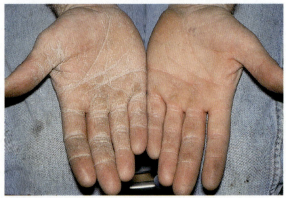

FIGURE 11-23. Tinea manuum. (From Goodheart, H. P. (2003). *Goodheart's photoguide of common skin disorders* (2nd ed.). Philadelphia, PA: Lippincott Williams & Wilkins.)

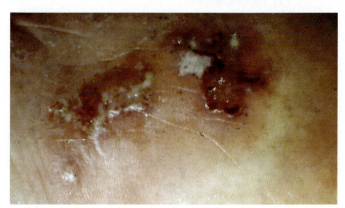

FIGURE 11-24. Tinea pedis. (Courtesy of Charles E. Lewis, MD.)

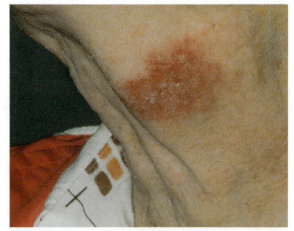

FIGURE 11-25. Tinea barbae. (From Berg, D., & Worzala, K. (2006). *Atlas of adult physical diagnosis*. Philadelphia, PA: Lippincott Williams & Wilkins.)

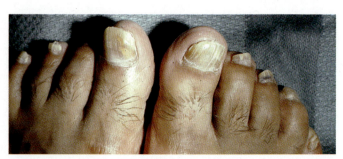

FIGURE 11-26. Tinea unguium. (Courtesy of John K. Randall, MD.)

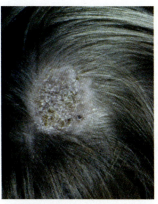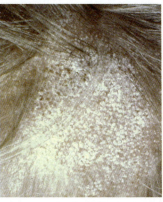

FIGURE 11-27. Tinea capitis. (Courtesy of John K. Randall, MD.)

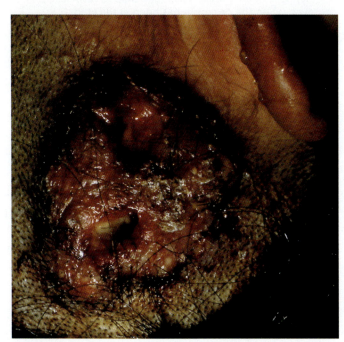

FIGURE 11-28. Kerion. (Courtesy of John K. Randall, MD.)

E. Treatment
  1. Topicals
    a. Allylamines
    b. Azoles
    c. Ciclopirox
    d. Tavaborole 10% nail solution
  2. Shampoos: may help to decrease the fungal load in tinea capitis but ineffective for cure
    a. Ketoconazole 2%
    b. 1% to 2.5% selenium sulfide
    c. 1% to 2% zinc pyrithione
  3. Oral antifungals (Table **11-3**)

> ◯ **PATIENT EDUCATION**
> *Dermatophytes*
>
> - Topicals should be used for at least 2 to 4 weeks for cure.
> - Shampoos need at least 5-minute contact time on the scalp prior to rinsing.
> - Griseofulvin should be taken with a high-fat meal to facilitate absorption.
> - Itraconazole should be taken with a full meal. Grapefruit juice should be avoided.
> - *T. tonsurans* spores remain viable on inanimate objects, such as combs and brushes, and clothing, such as hats. All articles should be cleaned thoroughly and not shared with other family members.
> - Family members of patients with tinea capitis should be assessed for asymptomatic carriers.
> - Tinea pedis may have a high degree of recurrence. Inform patients to wear moisture-wicking socks and change them frequently. Wear well-ventilated shoes. Sandals should be worn in locker rooms and on pool decks.
> - Patients with tinea cruris should wear cotton underwear.

II. TINEA VERSICOLOR (PITYRIASIS VERSICOLOR) (FIGURE 11-29)

A. Definition: superficial, chronic fungal infection seen on upper trunk, arms, or neck
B. Etiology
  1. Caused by *Pityrosporum orbiculare* or *Pityrosporum ovale* (*Malassezia furfur*)
    a. Part of normal skin flora
    b. Concentrated in areas with increased sebaceous activity
  2. Factors contributing to fungal proliferation
    a. Heat/humidity
    b. Cushing disease
    c. Pregnancy
    d. Malnutrition
    e. Burns
    f. Corticosteroid therapy
    g. Immunosuppression
    h. Oral contraception

TABLE 11-3 Oral Antifungals to Treat Tinea Capitis

Medication	Dosage	Duration
Griseofulvin microsize	Adults: 500 mg/d PED: 10–20 mg/kg/d	6–8 wk Or at least 2 wk after resolution of symptoms
Griseofulvin ultramicrosize	Adults: 375 mg/d PED: 5–15 mg/kg/d	6–8 wk Or at least 2 wk after resolution of symptoms
Terbinafine	<20 kg: 62.5 mg/d 20–40 kg: 125 mg/d Over 40 kg: 250 mg/d	2–4 wk Or at least 2 wk after resolution of symptoms
Itraconazole	Oral suspension: 3–5 mg/kg/d Oral capsules: 10–20 kg: 100 mg every other day 21–30 kg: 100 mg daily 31–40 kg: 100 mg and 200 mg on alternate days 41–50 kg: 200 mg daily Over 50 kg: 200–300 mg daily	4–6 wk Or at least 2 wk after resolution of symptoms

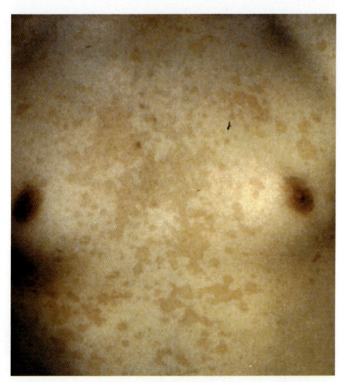

FIGURE 11-29. Tinea versicolor. (Courtesy of John K. Randall, MD.)

C. Pathophysiology
   1. Characteristic lesions and distribution. Generally on the trunk spreading to the neck, upper arms, and abdomen. Occasionally will involve the face, dorsal hands, and legs.
   2. Postpubertal and mature individuals more susceptible.
   3. Pruritus may be present, especially during sweating.
   4. Lesions more prominent in summer due to tanning of noninvolved skin.
D. Assessment
   1. History (Box 11-1).
   2. Current health status.
   3. Evaluate affected skin sites.
   4. Clinical manifestations.
      a. Multiple, small, circular macules of varying color
      b. Lesions enlarge radially
      c. Red to fawn-colored macules, patches, or follicular papules
      d. Slightly scaly
      e. Papular, nummular of confluent
   5. Diagnostic tests
      a. KOH: typical spaghetti-and-meatballs appearance of rod and spores.
      b. Wood lamp: generally will fluoresce a pale, yellow-whitish appearance.
E. Treatment
   1. Ketoconazole 2% shampoo: lather and leave on 5 minutes then rinse × 3 days.
   2. Selenium sulfide shampoo: lather and leave on 5 minutes then rinse × 3 days.

3. Selenium sulfite 2.5% lotion: apply daily for 10 minutes then rinse off × 7 days. Alternative: apply at night and wash off in the AM, weekly × 4 weeks.
4. Terbinafine spray: apply bid × 1 week.
5. Topical antifungal cream: apply bid × 2 to 4 weeks.
6. Itraconazole: 200 mg/day for 7 days.
7. Fluconazole: 300 to 400 mg for 1 day; repeat in 2 weeks.

PATIENT EDUCATION
Tinea Versicolor

• Tinea versicolor has a high degree of recurrence.
• Hypopigmented lesions will take time to resolve, even when the organism has been eradicated.
• Do not consume grapefruit juice with itraconazole.
• Itraconazole should be taken with a full meal.

III. CANDIDIASIS (MONILIASIS, THRUSH) (FIGURES 11-30 AND 11-31)

A. Definition: skin, mucous membrane, and internal infection caused by proliferation of normal flora in the mouth, vaginal tract, and intestinal tract
B. Etiology
   1. *C. albicans*: yeast-like fungus; most common cause of superficial and systemic fungal infections
   2. Factors predisposing to proliferation of organisms
      a. Pregnancy
      b. Oral contraceptives
      c. Antibiotic therapy
      d. Diabetes
      e. Skin maceration
      f. Topical steroids
      g. Some endocrinopathies
      h. Immunocompromised
   3. Infects outer layers of epithelium of mucous membranes and stratum corneum of the skin
C. Pathophysiology
   1. Candidiasis of moist areas
      a. Vulvovaginitis
         (1) Heat/moisture increases the risk of infection.
         (2) Menstruation may worsen symptoms.
         (3) May coexist with *Trichomonas*.
      b. Oral candidiasis
         (1) Seen in infants and adults
         (2) Causative factors: diabetes, depressed cell-mediated immunity, advanced age, cancer, prolonged steroid therapy, chemotherapy, broad-spectrum antibiotics, and AIDS
         (3) Tongue involved in an acute infection: extending into the esophagus and trachea
         (4) Localized, firmly adherent plaques characteristic of chronic infection

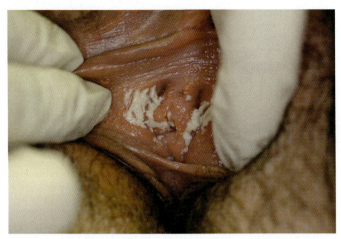

FIGURE 11-30. Vulvovaginitis. (From Kroumpouzos, G. (2013). *Text atlas of obstetric dermatology*. Philadelphia, PA: Wolters Kluwer.)

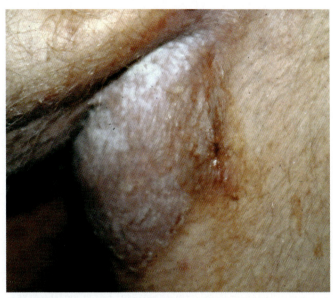

FIGURE 11-32. Intertrigo. (Courtesy of John K. Randall, MD.)

   c. Intertrigo (Figure 11-32)
     (1) Occurs in large skin folds.
     (2) Heat and moisture provide environment for proliferation of organisms.
     (3) Poor hygiene and inflammatory diseases also increase the risk of infection.

D. Assessment
  1. History (Box 11-1).
  2. Current health status.
  3. Evaluate skin and mucous membranes.
  4. Clinical presentation.
    a. Pustules (satellite lesions)
    b. Erythematous, moist, glistening plaques extending beyond the limits of opposing skin folds
    c. Painful fissuring

5. Pruritus and discharge are initial signs of infection.
6. Edema, erythema, and erosion of mucous membranes and external genitalia.
7. Satellite lesions may develop.
8. Diagnostic tests.
    a. KOH
    b. Wood lamp
    c. Fungal culture

E. Treatment
  1. Vulvovaginitis
    a. Azole vaginal creams
    b. Oral azoles: fluconazole 150 mg × 1
    c. Nystatin vaginal tabs
  2. Oral candidiasis
    a. Nystatin oral suspension
    b. Clotrimazole troche
    c. Oral azoles: 200 mg/daily for 2 weeks
  3. Intertrigo
    a. Maintain dryness
    b. Burow compresses
    c. Antifungal creams
    d. Oral azoles

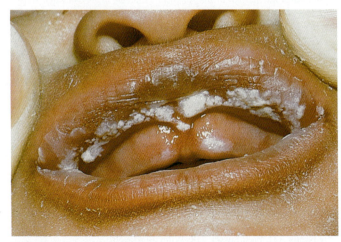

FIGURE 11-31. Oral candidiasis. (From Stedman's medical dictionary (2007). *Stedman's medical dictionary for the health professions and nursing, illustrated*. Philadelphia, PA: Wolters Kluwer.)

 PATIENT EDUCATION
Intertrigo

- Patients should wash the affected area daily with antibacterial soap or benzoyl peroxide wash. Pat dry and use handheld hair dryer on cool setting to thoroughly dry the area.
- Cotton underwear should be worn.

BIBLIOGRAPHY

Amagi, M., & Stanley, J. R. (2012). Desmoglein as a target in skin disease and beyond. *Journal of Investigative Dermatology, 132*(3), 776–784.

Bader, M. (2013). Herpes zoster: Diagnostic, therapeutic, and preventive approaches. *Postgraduate Medicine, 125*(5), 78–91.

Bangert, S., Levy, M., & Hebert, A. A. (2012). Bacterial resistance and impetigo treatment trends: A review. *Pediatric Dermatology, 29*(3), 243–248.

Bhanusali, D., Coley, M., Sliverberg, J. I., Alexis, A., & Sliverberg, N. B. (2012). Treatment outcomes for tinea capitis in a skin of color population. *Journal of Drugs in Dermatology, 11*(7), 852–856.

Braunstein, I., Wanat, K. A., Abuaboura K., McGowan, K. L., Yan, A. C., & Treat, J. R. (2013). Antibiotic sensitivity resistance patterns in pediatric staphylococcal scalded skin syndrome. *Pediatric Dermatology, 31*(3), 305–308.

Centers for Disease Control and Prevention (CDC) Advisory Committee on Immunization Practice. (2013). Recommended adult immunization schedule: United States. *Annals of Internal Medicine, 158*(3), 191–199.

Chen, N., Yang, M., He, L., Zhang, D, Zhou, M., & Zhu, C. (2010). Corticosteroids for preventing post-herpetic neuralgia. *Cochrane Database Systematic Reviews*, (3), CD005582. doi: 10.1002/14651858/CD005582.pub4

de Sá, D. C., Lamas, A. P. B., & Tosti, A. (2014). Oral therapy for onychomycosis: An evidence-based review. *American Journal of Clinical Dermatology, 15*(1), 17–36. doi: 10.1007/s40257-013-0056-2

Derry, S., Sven-Rice, A., Cole, P., Tan, T., & Moore, R. A. (2009). Topical capsaicin for chronic neuropathic pain in adults. *Cochrane Database Systematic Reviews*, (4), CD007393. doi: 10.1002/14651858. CD007393.pub2

Dreyfus, D. H. (2013). Herpesvirus and the microbiome. *Journal of Allergy and Clinical Immunology, 132*(6), 1278–1286.

Elewski, B. E., Hughey, L. C., Sobena, J. O., & Hay, R. (2012). Fungal diseases. In J. L. Bolognia, J. L. Jorizzo, & J. O. Schaffer (Eds.), *Dermatology* (3rd ed., pp. 1251–1284). New York, NY: Saunders/Elsevier.

Elewski, B., Parsier, D., Rich, P., & Scher, R. K. (2013). Current and emerging options in the treatment of onychomycosis. *Seminars in Cutaneous Medicine and Surgery, 32*(2 suppl 1), s9–s12.

Elewski, B., Parsier, D., Rich, P., & Scher, R. K. (2013). Onychomycosis: An overview. *Journal of Drugs in Dermatology, 12*(7), s96–s103.

Gan, E. Y., Tian, E. A. L., & Tey, H. L. (2013). Management of herpes zoster and post-herpetic neuralgia. *American Journal of Clinical Dermatology, 14*(2), 77–85.

Gunderson, C. G., & Martinello, R. A. (2012). A systematic review of bacteremias in cellulitis and erysipelas. *Journal of Infection, 64*(2), 148–155.

Gupta, A. (2013). Systemic antifungal agents. In S. Wolverton (Ed.), *Comprehensive dermatologic drug therapy* (3rd ed., pp. 98–120). New York, NY: Elsevier/Saunders.

Gupta, A. K., Cooper E. A., & Paquet, M. (2013). Recurrence of dermatophyte toenail onychomycosis during long-term follow-up after successful treatments with mono and combined therapy of terbinafine and itraconazole. *Journal of Cutaneous Medicine and Surgery, 17*(3), 201–206.

Gupta, A. K., & Drummond-Main, C. (2013). Meta-analysis of randomized, controlled trials comparing particular doses of griseofulvin and terbinafine for the treatment of tinea capitis. *Pediatric Dermatology, 30*(1), 1–6.

Habif, T. (Ed.). (2010). *Clinical dermatology* (5th ed., pp. 355–381, 419–453, 454–490, 491–543). New York, NY: Mosby/Elsevier.

Hay, R. J., & Adrians, B. M. (2010). Bacterial infections. In T. Burns, S. Breathnach, N. Cox, & C. Griffiths (Eds.), *Rooks textbook of dermatology online* (8th ed., Chapter 30). West Sussex, UK: Wiley-Blackwell.

Idriss, M. H., Khalil, A., & Elston, D. (2013). The diagnostic value of fungal fluorescence in onychomycosis. *Journal of Cutaneous Pathology, 40*(4), 385–390.

Kelly, B. P. (2012). Superficial fungal infections. *Pediatrics in Review, 33*(4), e22–e37.

Kilburn, S. A., Featherstone, P., Higgins, B., & Brindle, R. (2010). Interventions for cellulitis and erysipelas. *Cochrane Database of Systematic Reviews*, (6), CD004299. doi: 10.1002/14651858.CD004299.pub2

Kimbauer, R., & Lenz, P. (2012). Human papillomaviruses. In J. L. Bolognia, J. L. Jorizzo, & J. O. Schaffer (Eds.), *Dermatology* (3rd ed., pp. 1303–1320). New York, NY: Saunders/Elsevier.

Koning, S., van der Sande, R., van Suijlekom-Smit, L. W. A., Morris, A. D., Butler, C. G., Berger, M., & van der Wouden, J. C. (2012). Interventions for impetigo. *Cochrane Database of Systematic Reviews*, (1), CD003261. doi: 10.1002/14651858.CD003261.pub3

Li, M. Y., Jua, Y., Wei, G. H., & Qui, L. (2014). Staphylococcal scalded skin syndrome in neonates: An 8 year retrospective study in a single institution. *Pediatric Dermatology, 31*(1), 127–136.

Li, Q., Chen, N., Yang, J., Zhou, M., Zhou, D., Zhang, Q., & He, L. (2009). Antiviral treatment for preventing postherpetic neuralgia. *Cochrane Database Systematic Reviews*, (2), CD006866. doi: 10.1002/14651858. CD006866.pub2

Magel, G. D., Haitz, K. A., Lapolla, W. J., DiGiorgio, C. M., Mendoza, N., & Tyring, S. K. (2013). Systemic antiviral agents. In S. Wolverton (Ed.), *Comprehensive dermatologic drug therapy* (3rd ed., pp. 121–134). New York, NY: Elsevier/Saunders.

Mendoza, N., Madkan, V., Sra, K., Willison, B., Morrison, L. K., & Tyring, S. K. (2012). Human herpesvirus. In J. L. Bolognia, J. L. Jorizzo, & J. O. Schaffer (Eds.), *Dermatology* (3rd ed., pp. 1321–1344). New York, NY: Saunders/Elsevier.

Millet, C. R., Halpern, A. O., Reboli, A. C., & Heyman, W. R. (2012). Bacterial diseases. In J. L. Bolognia, J. L. Jorizzo, & J. O. Schaffer (Eds.), *Dermatology* (3rd ed., pp. 1187–1220). New York, NY: Saunders/Elsevier.

Mirmirani, P., & Tucker, L. Y. (2013). Epidemiologic trends in pediatric tinea capitis: A population based study from Kaiser Permanente northern California. *Journal of the American Academy of Dermatology, 69*(6), 916–921.

Motaparthi, K., & Hsu, S. (2013). Topical antibacterial agents. In S. Wolverton (Ed.), *Comprehensive dermatologic drug therapy* (3rd ed., pp. 445–459). New York, NY: Elsevier/Saunders.

Phillips, R. M., & Rosen, T. (2013). Topical antifungals. In S. Wolverton (Ed.), *Comprehensive dermatologic drug therapy* (3rd ed., pp. 460–472). New York, NY: Elsevier/Saunders.

Pride, H. B., Tollefson, M., & Silerman, R. (2013). What's new in pediatric dermatology. *Journal of the American Academy of Dermatology, 68*(6), 889 e1–889 e11.

Reglinski, M., & Sriskandan, S. (2014). The contribution of group A streptococcal virulence determinants to the pathogenesis of sepsis. *Virulence, 5*(1), 127–136.

Rich, P., Elewski, B., Scher, R. K., & Parsier, D. (2013). Diagnosis, clinical implications and complications of onychomycosis. *Seminars in Cutaneous Medicine and Surgery, 32*(2 suppl 1), s5–s8.

Scher, R., Rich, P., Parsier, D., & Elewski, B. (2013). The epidemiology, etiology, and pathophysiology of onychomycosis. *Seminars in Cutaneous Medicine and Surgery, 32*(2 suppl 1), s2–s4.

Sheth, P. B., & Landis, M. N. (2013). Topical and intralesional antiviral agents. In S. Wolverton (Ed.), *Comprehensive dermatologic drug therapy* (3rd ed., pp. 473–480). New York, NY: Elsevier/Saunders.

Shimizu, T., & Tokuda, Y. (2010). Necrotizing fasciitis. *Internal Medicine, 49*(12), 1051–1057.

Sterlin, J. C. (2010). Virus infections. In T. Burns, S. Breathnach, N. Cox, & C. Griffiths (Eds.), *Rooks textbook of dermatology online* (8th ed., Chapter 33). West Sussex, UK: Wiley-Blackwell.

Susun, K., Michaels, B. D., Kim, G. K., & Del Rosso, J. Q. (2013). Systemic antibacterial agents. In S. Wolverton (Ed.), *Comprehensive dermatologic drug therapy* (3rd ed., pp. 61–97). New York, NY: Elsevier/Saunders.

Tiwan, A. K., & Lal, R. (2014). Study to evaluate the role of severity stratification of skin and soft tissue infection (SSTIs) in formulating treatment strategies and predicting poor prognostic factors. *International Journal of Surgery*, 12(2), 125–133. doi: 10.1016/j.ijsu. 2013.11.014

Vena, G. A., Chieco, P., Garafalo, A., Bosca, A., & Cassano, N. (2012). Epidemiology of dermatophytoses: Retrospective analysis from 2005 to 2010 and comparison with previous data from 1975. *New Microbiologica*, 35(2), 207–213.

Verrier, J., Krahenbuhl, L, Bontems, O., Fratti, M., Salaman, K., & Monod, M. (2012). Dermatophyte identification in skin and hair samples using a simple and reliable nested polymerase chain reaction assay. *British Journal of Dermatology*, 168(2), 295–301.

Walker, D. H. (2012). Rickettsial diseases. In J. L. Bolognia, J. L. Jorizzzo, & J. O. Schaffer (Eds.), *Dermatology* (3rd ed., pp. 1243–1250). New York, NY: Saunders Elsevier.

STUDY QUESTIONS

1. The infectious organism that causes impetigo is:
   a. *Staphylococcus aureus*
   b. *Streptococcus*
   c. *Enterobacter*
   d. Both a and b
   e. None of the above

2. Impetigo can spread via:
   a. Fingers
   b. Towels
   c. Clothing
   d. All of the above

3. Diagnostic tests for a patient with a suspected cellulitis include a complete blood count demonstrating increased:
   a. Neutrophils
   b. Monocytes
   c. Lymphocytes
   d. Eosinophils

4. A superficial bacterial infection of the skin in an intertriginous area describes:
   a. Ecthyma
   b. Erythrasma
   c. Erysipelas

5. Drug-induced folliculitis most commonly occurs with
   a. Long-term use of oral cephalosporins
   b. Use of phenytoin
   c. Topical use of mupirocin
   d. Topical use of corticosteroids

6. Which one of the following is the causative organism of meningococcemia?
   a. *Neisseria*
   b. *Rickettsia*
   c. Spirochete
   d. *Streptococcus*
   e. None of the above

7. In staphylococcal scalded skin syndrome, Nikolsky sign will be:
   a. Absent
   b. Present

8. The most critical diagnostic sign for necrotizing fasciitis is:
   a. Fever
   b. Bradycardia
   c. Presence of hemorrhagic bullae
   d. Severe pain out of proportion to initial skin findings

9. Warts extend into the dermis.
   a. True
   b. False

10. HPV subtypes associated with neoplasms include:
    a. 3 and 10
    b. 6 and 11
    c. 16 and 18
    d. 28 and 49

11. Appropriate treatment of varicella-zoster virus includes acyclovir:
    a. 200 mg tid for 5 days
    b. 400 mg tid for 5 days
    c. 800 mg five times daily for 3 days
    d. 800 mg five times daily for 7 days

12. Tinea manuum describes a tinea infection of the:
    a. Groin
    b. Feet
    c. Hands
    d. Nails

13. The most common organism causing tinea capitis in North America is:
    a. *Trichophyton tonsurans*
    b. *Trichophyton schoenleinii*
    c. *Microsporum canis*

14. Prodromal symptoms of HSV infection include all of the following *except*:
    a. Flu-like symptoms
    b. Nausea
    c. Paresthesias
    d. Burning sensation

15. Factors that may reactivate herpes zoster include:
   a. Immunosuppressive drugs
   b. Fatigue
   c. Stress
   d. Smoking
   e. a, b, and c
   f. a, c, and d

16. All of the following are characteristics of dermatophyte infections *except*:
   a. Invades the skin and survives on dead keratin
   b. Undergoes deep invasion
   c. Cannot survive on mucosal surfaces

17. Factors contributing to fungal proliferation include all of the following *except*:
   a. Heat and humidity
   b. Pregnancy
   c. Corticosteroid therapy
   d. Age
   e. Malnutrition

18. Factors contributing to the formation of a furuncle include all of the following *except*:
   a. Friction
   b. Hyperhidrosis
   c. Nutritional status
   d. Scratching
   e. Pressure from restrictive clothing

Answers to Study Questions: 1.d, 2.d, 3.a, 4.b, 5.d, 6.a, 7.b, 8.d, 9.b, 10.c, 11.d, 12.c, 13.a, 14.b, 15.e, 16.b, 17.d, 18.c

CHAPTER 12

Bites, Stings, and Infestations

Theresa Coyner • Katrina Nice Masterson

PART I: BITES AND STINGS

OBJECTIVES

After studying Part I of this chapter, the reader will be able to:

- Identify the common manifestations of biting and stinging insects.
- List appropriate avoidance behaviors that may reduce exposure to biting and stinging insects.
- Describe common therapeutic interventions used to return the skin and tissues to preexposure condition.

KEY POINTS

- Incidence of bites and stings can be greatly reduced by avoiding or utilizing protective behaviors when encountering the insects natural habitat.
- Topical application of over-the-counter and household therapies will reduce much of the pain and discomfort of many bites and stings.
- Careful hand washing and reduction of scratching will greatly lessen the chance of secondary infections after insect bites.
- Prompt emergency treatment is indicated for some bites or stings and any anaphylactic reactions.
- Patient and family education must include precautions to be used when sensitivity reactions are identified.

PHYLUM ARTHROPODA

I. OVERVIEW

Humans come in frequent contact with varying numbers of more than one million varieties of insects that inhabit the planet. A limited number of these cause more than a fleeting annoyance or discomfort. Some insects inject venom into humans as a means of self-protection. Others use the human for a blood meal. Although almost everyone has experienced a bite or sting, only about 1% of pediatric and 3% of adult population experiences an allergic reaction. Insects also transmit some diseases (Table **12-1**).

A. Arachnida: a class of eight-legged insects that includes scorpions, spiders, ticks, and mites.

1. Scorpion: *Centruroides sculpturatus* (Figure 12-1)
   a. Found in all continents except Antarctica. In North America, the scorpion is found in Mexico and southwestern states of the United States.
   b. Obtaining a length of 9 mm to 20 cm, it has a forebody, six projecting legs, large anterior claws (pedipolyps), and a hind body with a hooked caudal stinger which it uses to inject venom into its prey.
   c. Major function is control of insect population.
   d. Stings occur most frequently on the legs, thighs, and buttocks of its human victims, often the result of sitting or walking in the scorpion's territory.
   e. Sting produces an immediate sharp burning sensation. Local edema soon surrounds the small puncture wound often followed by skin discoloration. Numbness may extend beyond the puncture site.
   f. The only scorpion in the United States with enough venom to cause serious side effects is the bark scorpion found in the southwest desert. Its bite may produce hypersalivation, tachycardia, decreased blood pressure, peripheral motor symptoms, and severe agitation.
   g. Children due to their size may have a more severe reaction. Debilitated or immunocompromised adults have increased risks of complications of bites. Scorpion bites in the United States rarely are associated with death.
2. Black widow spider: *Latrodectus mactans* (Figure 12-2)
   a. Found in the entire continental United States except Alaska.
   b. The female is 1.5 cm, glossy black with the characteristic red hourglass on the underside of the abdomen. The male of the species is smaller with four pairs of red markings on the abdomen.
   c. Diet consists of insects, centipedes, and other spiders. After mating, the female often ensnares and devours her mate from which she derives the name, black widow.
   d. Often resides in yard debris and wood piles. The spider can also be found inside of homes. It is generally not aggressive. It will bite when threatened or when guarding an egg sac.
   e. The bite feels like a pinprick and leaves a mildly erythematous 3- to 4-mm papule with a central punctum.

TABLE 12-1 Potential Vector Diseases from Blood-Sucking Insects

Insect	Vector Diseases
Flea	Plaque, typhus, tapeworms, filariasis, brucellosis, and melioidosis
Mosquito	Malaria, encephalitis, dengue, and yellow fever
Chigger	Rickettsial typhus, viral encephalitis, and pasteurella plaque
Bedbug	Oriental sore, Chagas disease, Kala-azar, relapsing fever, and perhaps hepatitis B. Note all of which are rare occurrences
Tick—specifically deer tick	Rocky Mountain spotted fever, Lyme disease, and relapsing fever

(1) The injected venom contains α-latrotoxin, which is a neurotoxin that produces massive presynaptic release of acetylcholine.

(2) Diaphoresis and hypertension may occur.

(3) Severe muscle spasms occur within 1 hour of the bite and may mimic myocardial infarction or an acute abdomen.

3. Brown recluse spider: *Loxosceles reclusa* (Figure 12-3)

  a. The highest concentration of spider population is found in Midwest and southern states of the United States.

  b. The spider has a cephalothorax with a characteristic violin-shaped marking, joined to abdomen, and is light to medium brown in color. This violin-shaped marking is not unique to the brown recluse spider. The spider can be identified due to its six eyes as compared to other spiders having eight eyes (two eyes in front and two sets of eyes on the cephalothorax).

  c. Spider prefers an insect diet.

  d. Bites occur most frequently on the extremities of its victim (Figure 12-4).

    (1) Bite may feel like a pinprick or not even noticed by the victim.

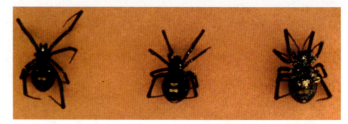

FIGURE 12-2. Black widow spiders: *Latrodectus mactans.* (Courtesy of John K. Randall, MD.)

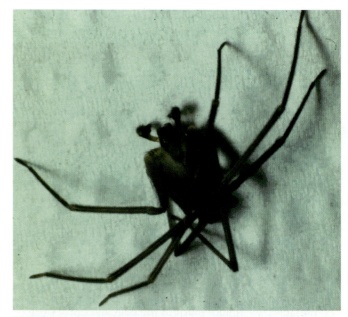

FIGURE 12-3. Brown recluse spider: *Loxosceles reclusa.* (Courtesy of John K. Randall, MD.)

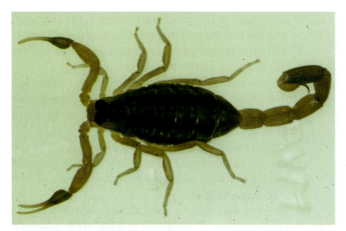

FIGURE 12-1. Scorpion: *Centruroides sculpturatus.* (Courtesy of John K. Randall, MD.)

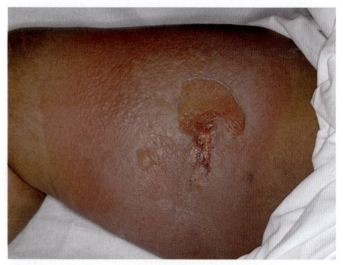

FIGURE 12-4. Brown recluse spider bite on the left lateral thigh. (From Lugo-Somolinos, A., et al. (2011). *VisualDx: Essential dermatology in pigmented skin.* Philadelphia, PA: Wolters Kluwer.)

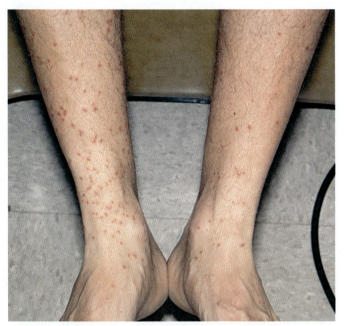

FIGURE 12-5. Chigger bites on the lower legs and ankles. (From Goodheart, H. P. (2003). *Goodheart's photoguide of common skin disorders* (2nd ed.). Philadelphia, PA: Lippincott Williams & Wilkins.)

(2) A coagulotoxin is injected at the time of the bite.
(3) Pain develops 2 to 8 hours after the initial bite.
(4) Presentation is very unpredictable often with the presence of a gray-blue halo surrounding the puncture site within 24 hours.
(5) Early signs of necrosis include hyperesthesia, bullae, cyanosis, red-blue ulcer, and/or painful eschar.
(6) Systemic reactions (loxoscelism) can occur in some victims. This may vary from a mild flu-like presentation to anaphylactic shock. Symptoms caused by coagulotoxin may include deep vein thrombosis, pyoderma gangrenosum, intravascular hemolysis, renal failure, pulmonary edema, and cardiac arrhythmias.

4. Chigger (Figure 12-5)
   a. Present in most grain-growing regions of the United States. They are most prevalent in the south during the summer and fall. They may be known by many other names such as red bugs, jiggers, harvest mites, harvest lice, and harvest bugs.
   b. A barely visible reddish colored mite, the larval stage of the chigger attaches to the skin of the host by means of a hooked mouthpart.
   c. It ingests a blood meal while attached to the human host. The mite does not burrow and releases after engorgement.
   d. Lesions occur most frequently after contact with infested hay or grains. The mite prefers an area where it can feed undisturbed, especially under constrictive clothing.
   e. Pruritic macules or papules up to 5 mm in size are very common after the mite bite. If the individual is sensitized, the eruption may vary from urticarial to a more severe granulomatous reaction. Lesions slowly regress over 1 to 2 months.
5. Tick (Figures 12-6 and 12-7)
   a. Classification: Ixodidae—"hard tick" with hard-like shield with the head visible. Argasidae—"soft tick" with leathery skin and the head hidden by the body of the tick.
   b. This parasite is widespread, preferring thick vegetation or grasses on which to cling when not in contact with an animal or human host.
   c. Most species have three stages in their 2-year life cycle. Larva stage usually hatches in the early spring. The nymph stage in which the tick is about the size of a poppy seed. The adult tick is about the size of an apple seed. Ticks only require one blood meal for each stage of its life cycle. Diseases can be transmitted from tick bites during any of their three life cycle stages.
   d. The tick has four pairs of clawed legs and a specialized mouthpart used for grasping and slicing a hole in its victim to enable the tick to suck blood.

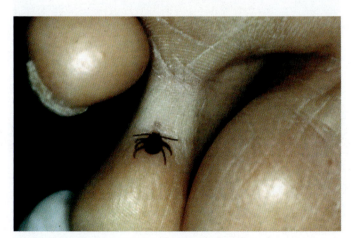

FIGURE 12-6. Tick: Ixodidae on the plantar surface toe. (Courtesy of John K. Randall, MD.)

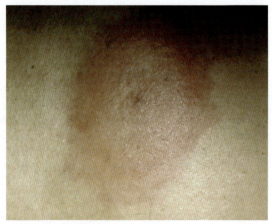

FIGURE 12-7. Tick bite with inflammation. (Courtesy of Charles E. Lewis, MD.)

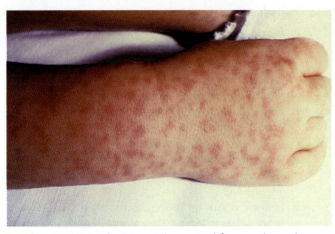

FIGURE 12-8. Rocky Mountain spotted fever rash on the hand and arm. (From Harvey, R. A., & Cornelissen, C. N. (2012). *Microbiology*. Philadelphia, PA: Wolters Kluwer.)

Blood meals are generally provided by small rodents (mice) in the larva stage. Larger mammals (deer and humans) provide the blood meals for the nymph and adult ticks.

 e. Ticks will attach to any exposed skin and often travels under clothing or around body parts until they reach a constricted area. When the tick attaches to the victim, it emits a cement-like substance to help keep the tick adhered to the host.

 f. Rocky Mountain spotted fever (RMSF; Figure 12-8) is a rickettsia disease transmitted to humans after the bite of a deer or dog tick (Box 12-1).

 g. Lyme disease (Figure 12-9) is a spirochete *Borrelia burgdorferi* infection transmitted to humans generally by the bite of a deer tick (Box 12-2).

B. Insecta: class of six-legged insects, many with wings, which includes bees, wasps, and ants. Hymenoptera is a superorder of the class of insects containing wings. Hymenoptera can cause severe hypersensitivity reactions (Box 12-3).

 1. Bumblebee

  a. Largest of the Hymenoptera, the bumblebee is found throughout the United States and is better adapted to cold regions than other bees.

  b. The bumblebee is hairy and usually a black and yellow coloration.

  c. The bee is responsible for pollination of a wide variety of plants.

  d. Generally not aggressive, often stings when its victim disturbs it while walking in patches of clover.

  e. The bee produces one painful, stabbing defensive sting into its victim that may leave behind a barbed stinger. The sting injects formic acid and proteins into its victim. The venom sac is attached to the stinger and will continue to contract and inject additional venom if it is not removed.

  f. The skin lesion is an erythematous papule, which becomes urticarial and edematous. It may remain painful for hours.

BOX 12-1. Rocky Mountain Spotted Fever (RMSF)

RMSF (Figure 12-8) is an infectious disease spread to humans by the bite of a deer or dog tick. Severe headache and fever generally appears after a 2- to 16-day incubation period following transfer of the organism *Rickettsia rickettsii* from the tick. Generally, a tick must be attached to the human host over 24 hours to transmit the infection. However, there are rare cases where the organism can be transmitted in as little as 6 to 8 hours of tick attachment.

The rickettsia are intracellular gram-negative rods that invade endothelial cells. Eighty percentage of victims will have severe headache and fever. A morbilliform rash will start on palms and soles and progresses to a petechial rash on extremities that spreads to the trunk. Myalgias and nausea and vomiting may occur. Children are more commonly affected but fatalities more likely in the elderly.

Diagnosis is made upon clinical presentation, and appropriate antibiotic therapy should be started immediately. Doxycycline is the medication of choice for all nonpregnant individuals despite age. Chloramphenicol is the drug of choice during pregnancy. Use of antibiotic other than doxycycline has an increased risk of death.

Diagnostic tests with highest degree of sensitivity are the indirect immunofluorescence assay (IFA) with rickettsia antigen. An initial serum sample is obtained immediately upon suspicion of RMSF and repeated in 2 to 4 weeks. A fourfold increase is a definitive diagnosis. IgG is negative initially and then will raise in 2 to 4 weeks. IgM starts to elevate in 2 to 4 weeks and may stay elevated for months to years after the tick bite.

RMSF was originally identified in the early 1900s in the Copper Mountain valley in Montana. RMSF cases have occurred throughout the United States with majority of cases occurring in Arkansas, Oklahoma, Tennessee, North Carolina, and South Carolina. Most cases occur during the months of April through September. Prevention is aimed at control of tick populations, avoidance behaviors, and early tick removal.

 2. Honeybee

  a. Found in all of the United States, the honeybee is found in any area with flowers and fruit.

  b. Smaller and somewhat similar in appearance to the bumblebee. It is generally yellow, brown, or gray in color. It measures 1 to 1.5 cm in length.

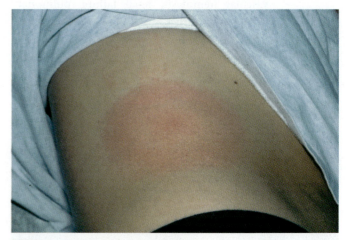

FIGURE 12-9. Lyme disease; erythema migrans. (From Goodheart, H. P. (2003). *Goodheart's photoguide of common skin disorders* (2nd ed.). Philadelphia, PA: Lippincott Williams & Wilkins.)

BOX 12-2. Lyme Disease

Lyme disease (Figure 12-9) is caused by the transfer of the spirochete *Borrelia burgdorferi* to humans by feeding of the deer tick, *Ixodes dammini*, and certain other tick species. The tick is capable of transmitting the disease during any of its stages of development when it varies from poppy seed to sesame seed size. The risk of transmission from an infected attached tick is 0% if less than 24 hours, 12% if 48 hours, 79% in 72 hours, and 94% at 96 hours. The characteristic rash, erythema migrans (EM), occurs in about 60% of patients within 3 days to 4 weeks of the tick bite. The classical presentation is a large circular to oval rash with central clearing (bull's eye). The lesion may enlarge up to 5 cm in size with an irregular margin of erythema surrounding the bite. Satellite lesions may occur with the spread of the lesion. Flu-like symptoms, fever, chills, and myalgias may be present. Administration of doxycycline or amoxicillin at this stage is over 90% effective in curing the condition.

Borrelial lymphocytosis, a bluish-red nodule appearing on either a nipple or an earlobe, is another type of Lyme disease lesion that may rarely occur.

Untreated Lyme disease may eventually develop to chronic or late-stage disease. This condition is characterized by musculoskeletal arthritic changes. Usually, this will be effusion of a large joint. Central nervous symptoms such as lymphocytic meningitis and cranial nerve palsies may also occur. Heart symptoms may include conductive problems such as AV blocks.

Atrophic chronic acrodermatitis (ACA) is a late cutaneous finding in chronic Lyme disease. It is characterized by erythematous to bluish-red discoloration with hyperpigmentation on the lower extremities. Untreated ACA can progress to the atrophic phase where the lower extremity skin is thin with dilated veins.

High-dose penicillin or cephalosporins may be required for treating arthritis or meningitis.

Lyme disease is primarily a clinical diagnosis. If symptoms present less than 30 days, an IgG and Western blot is recommended. If symptoms present greater than 30 days, perform the IgM and the Western blot.

Prevention is aimed at control of tick populations, avoidance behaviors, and early tick removal.

BOX 12-3. Hypersensitivity Reactions to Hymenoptera Venom

Hypersensitivity reactions affect about 5% of the population. Hymenoptera venom from insect stings can cause an immediate type 1 hypersensitivity reaction. This is allergy mediated where a free antigen cross-links to the IgE on mast cells and basophils, which cause release of vasoactive biomolecules. The reaction can be mild causing a localized erythematous wheal at the site of the sting, which may have symptoms of pruritus to pain and localized edema.

IgE will be elevated for several weeks in 20% of adults after following a sting, but generally, this will be asymptomatic.

Type IV hypersensitivity reactions may occur, which is a cell-mediated immune memory response. At least one prior sting is necessary to develop this sensitivity reaction. Sensitivity is more likely to occur with multiple, simultaneous stings. With subsequent stings, mast cell and basophil degranulation occurs resulting in histamine release and inflammatory mediators. Antihistamines may be effective in mild cases. Severe reactions may range from pruritus, flushing, urticaria, and angioedema. Respiratory involvement can include cough and shortness of breath. Cardiovascular involvement may include dizziness, hypotension, decreased consciousness, bradycardia, and arrhythmias. Epinephrine will be needed to treat severe reactions.

The single best predictor of the outcome of a future sting is still the history of reaction to a prior sting. Individuals with an elevated baseline tryptase level above 11.4 ng/mL have a higher incidence of underlying mast cell disorder and may be at higher risk for severe reactions. Individuals with prior severe reactions should be prescribed an epinephrine autoinjector to have available for the possibility of reactions to future stings. They also should be referred to allergy/immunology for evaluation of possible venom immunotherapy (VIT).

c. Very important to pollination, the honeybee is generally not aggressive, unless it perceives a threat.
    (1) Since experiments in Brazil sought to cross the native honeybee with an African cousin, a much more aggressive bee has developed.
    (2) The Africanized honeybee migrated into the United States in the early 1990s.
    (3) This aggressive bee is capable of chasing a fleeing victim for up to one quarter of a mile.
    (4) The sting of this bee is no more venomous than the native honeybee.
  d. If the entire hive is disturbed, a swarm of insects may attack, stinging any body surface. The honeybee may leave a barbed stinger with a venom sac that may continue to inject venom.
  e. The sting produces an edematous erythematous papule.
3. Wasp
  a. The paper wasp lives in communities, while the mud dauber, potter wasp, and digger wasp are solitary.
  b. The wasp has a smooth body that ranges in color from mahogany to black. It ranges from 2 to 5 cm in length. The wasp legs hang down from the body when it flies.
  c. The diet consists of other insects and vegetable matter. Some species are pollinators of crops.
  d. Like other members of Hymenoptera, wasps sting when disturbed or threatened.
  e. Produces a similar lesion to other stings, the venom of all wasps contains histamines and a factor that dissolves red blood cells.
4. Yellow jacket
  a. A member of the wasp family, closely related to the hornet, and widely distributed throughout the United States.
  b. Named for its characteristic yellow markings, it is hairless and has three sets of legs and two sets of wings. It measures 1 to 1.5 cm in length.
  c. The diet consists chiefly of insects and rotting fruit.
  d. Stings may be inflicted on any body part when the nest or individual yellow jacket is disturbed.
  e. Sting is similar to that of the honeybee.
  f. Nests are generally underground or close to the ground and may contain thousands of yellow jackets.
5. Hornet (Figure 12-10)
  a. A member of the wasp family, the hornet, may be found in unique football-shaped nests made of

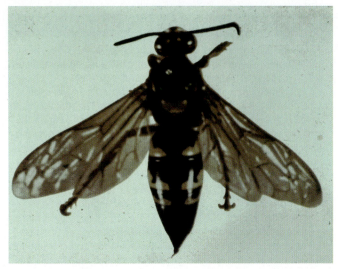

FIGURE 12-10. Hornet. (Courtesy of Charles E. Lewis, MD.)

papery material comprising of masticated plant foliage and wood suspended from a tree limb. The hornet's habitat is more evident in the northern United States.

b. The hornet is about 3 cm in length and is generally white faced with black and white markings on its segments.

c. The diet consists largely of other insects and ripe fruit.

d. The hornet stings to protect its environment and is likely to swarm if the nest is disturbed, whether by accident or intentionally.

e. The sting produces a painful, edematous papule.

6. Ant (Figure 12-11)

a. The wingless member of the order Hymenoptera; the imported fire ant (IFA) is the species most frequently involved in painful stings and allergic reactions. Introduced into the United States from South America; it is prevalent in most of the south.

b. Ants are generally 2 to 5 mm in length, colors varying from tan, red to black. The IFAs live in large colonies, often producing large mounds of dirt or sand especially noticeable after rains.

c. The ant serves a useful purpose as an aerator and mixer of soil. Most species are omnivorous. The IFA can be dangerous to young or injured livestock as well as humans.

d. Walking, gardening, and sitting in the habitat of the ant may result in one or more stings. Multiple stings, with the increased venom load, increase the risk of systemic reaction for small children and debilitated adults.

e. IFA stings create erythematous sterile pustules with high levels of neutrophils. The sterile pustules result from piperidine venom alkaloids.

7. Flea (Figure 12-12)

a. A member of the order of Siphonaptera, fleas can be found all over the world with cat and dog fleas causing the highest proportion of infestation in households. Human fleas are rare in the United States.

b. Wingless, and with three pairs of legs, fleas can jump distances out of proportion to their size.

c. Fleas require a blood meal for survival. However, they can live up to a year without contact with humans or pets.

d. Bites occur most frequently about the ankle of the human but may be scattered in any area as the flea attempts to hide from lights.

e. The bite produces an erythematous papule that may progress to a wheal or blister. Bites may be intensely itchy.

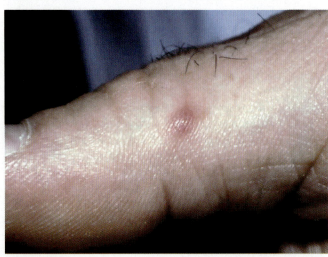

FIGURE 12-11. Fire ant bite on the thumb. (Courtesy of Charles E. Lewis, MD.)

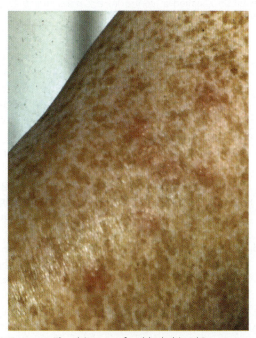

FIGURE 12-12. Flea bites on freckled skin. (Courtesy of Charles E. Lewis, MD.)

8. Sandfly
   a. Sandfly is a colloquial name for the genus of flying biting dipteran. There are many types of dipterans that may be extremely small to as large as a horsefly. The female bites to obtain a blood meal of which the protein is necessary to form her eggs. The sandfly discussed in this section is the type responsible for development of leishmaniasis.
   b. The sandfly consists of four legs and two wings with a proboscis.
   c. The organism that causes leishmaniasis is a protozoa. It exists in two forms: the promastigote and the amastigote. The organism multiplies in the promastigote form in the gut of the sandfly. It then migrates to the proboscis. When the sandfly bites a mammal host, it transforms to the amastigote form.
   d. Types of leishmaniasis include the cutaneous form restricted to the skin, the mucocutaneous form that affects both skin and mucosal surfaces, and visceral leishmaniasis that affects organs of the reticuloendothelial system.
   e. Cutaneous leishmaniasis occurs primarily in the Mediterranean basin, Middle Eastern countries, North Africa, India, and parts of Central and Southern Americas. In the United States, cutaneous forms of leishmaniasis are found in individuals who have traveled to countries where leishmaniasis is endemic or in military personnel who have served terms of duty in the Middle East.
   f. Cutaneous leishmaniasis starts as a small papule that may enlarge into a nodule or plaque. The area further develops into an ulcerated or verrucous lesion with rolled borders. Lesions may be solitary or multiple on exposed skin sites (Figure 12-13).

9. Mosquito
   a. A member of the order Diptera, the mosquito inhabits most of the world where there is sufficient water to permit the hatching phase.
   b. A two-winged, narrow insect with long, slender legs.
   c. The male feeds on nectar, but the female uses her specialized mouthparts to pierce the skin and inject saliva, which inhibits clotting, permitting her to ingest blood. Infectious organisms may be transferred during feeding.
   d. The mosquito will attack any uncovered skin and is able to pierce lightweight clothing.
   e. The bite forms an urticarial papule with intense itching that may begin within 10 minutes and last for days.

10. Bedbug
    a. A member of the order Hemiptera, the bedbug (Figure 12-14) is often far less common than most other insects in the United States. There has been a recent insurgence of bedbugs thought to be due to increase in international travel. *Cimex lectularius* is the bedbug found in tropical climates. *Cimex hemipterus* is the bedbug found in temperate climates.
    b. The bedbug is 2 to 5 mm in length, slightly ovoid and flattened, and brown in color. It resembles an apple seed in appearance.
    c. Blood meals are required every 3 to 5 days as the bug progresses through its multistage development. The adult bedbug can live up to 1 year without a blood meal.
    d. The bedbug pierces the skin with specialized stylets, ingesting blood and dissolved epidermal tissue before releasing. They only feed at night as they hide from bright lights. The victim is rarely aware of the initial bite as the bedbug releases a local anesthetic when biting.

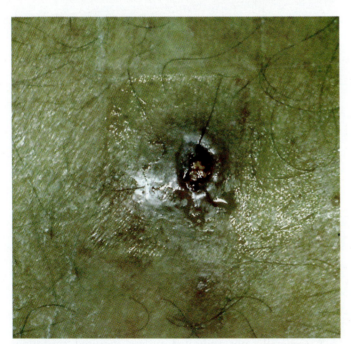

FIGURE 12-13. Cutaneous leishmaniasis. (Courtesy of Charles E. Lewis, MD.)

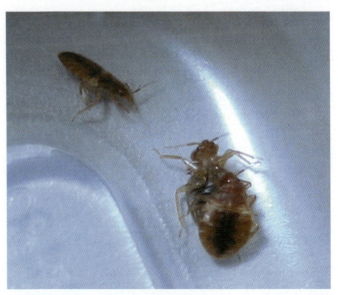

FIGURE 12-14. Bedbugs: *Cimex hemipterus*. (Image provided by Stedman's.)

e. Lesions may occur on any exposed body surface. There is generally a pattern of three linear bites often labeled as "breakfast, lunch, and dinner." The stylets leave behind two red marks that become pruritic papules several minutes after the bite. Depending on the sensitivity of the victim, wheals, vesicles, or hemorrhagic bullae may develop. More severe symptoms including anaphylactic reactions may occur.

PATIENT EDUCATION
Chiggers, Mosquitoes, and Sandflies

- The addition of 1 to 2 teaspoons of chlorine bleach to bathwater before possible exposure may reduce natural body odors that attract the female mosquito.

PATIENT EDUCATION
Ticks

- Meticulous search should be done for ticks on the skin after seeing a tick anywhere.
- Light-colored clothing increases the visibility of ticks upon clothing.
- Clothing sprayed with permethrin may be helpful.
- Tick removal.
- Do not use petroleum jelly, nail polish, and a burnt match as these methods will cause more harm.
- Do not use bare hands to remove ticks.
- Do not compress the body of the tick as it may increase secretion of potentially infectious material.
- Use tweezers to grasp the tick as close to the skin as possible and pull steadily away from the skin. Avoid a twisting motion.
- An alternative technique is to tie a thread tightly around the tick's head as close to the skin as possible and use steady traction to pull away from the skin.
- Another technique is use of a plastic spoon or a plastic card with a "V" cut out of the center. Slide the "V" under the tick and use steady traction to lift the tick away from the skin.

PATIENT EDUCATION
Bees, Wasps, and Hornets

- Perfumes and bright-colored and rough-textured clothing are attractive to bees.
- Beehives and hornets' nests should not be disturbed. Professional exterminators should be contacted for removal.

PATIENT EDUCATION
Ants

- One can observe for characteristic mounds of sand or soil.
- Sandboxes should be checked prior to play sessions for presence of ants.
- Closed-toe footwear will decrease the incidence of ant bites.
- Brushing away ants from the skin with a firm article, such as a credit card, will reduce the likelihood of retaining the ant's head in the skin.

PATIENT EDUCATION
Fleas

- Treatment of pets and other animals will decrease and possibly eliminate fleas and their eggs.

PATIENT EDUCATION
Bedbugs

- When bedbugs are seen, thorough vacuuming behind baseboards, in cracks and crevices, and behind peeling wallpaper may be helpful.
- Bedbugs can be transported in luggage and clothing.
- Professional exterminators will be needed to eradicate bedbugs.
- Infested mattresses should be disposed.

II. ASSESSMENT

A. History and physical examination
1. History of exposure or potential exposure to insect.
2. Presence of one or more lesions with characteristic appearance.
3. Distribution of lesions consistent with biting or stinging habits of insects.
4. Hypertension, tachycardia, and respiratory distress noted with scorpion sting, especially with the presence of hypersalivation.
5. Presence of severe muscle pain or spasms associated with black widow spider bite.
6. Presence of necrosis with brown recluse spider bite.
7. Presence of headache and fever after tick bite.
8. Arthralgia, weakness, and confusion may indicate delayed hypersensitivity reaction.
9. Expressions of feeling of doom may indicate onset of anaphylaxis.

B. Diagnostic tests
1. Generally not indicated unless required to follow course of disease or with specific envenomation.

2. Oxygen saturation may be required with anaphylaxis.

3. Leukocytosis and elevated creatine phosphokinase may be present with the bite of a black widow spider.

4. Hemoglobinemia, thrombocytopenia, and hemoglobinuria may result with envenomation of the brown recluse spider.

5. Positive blood cultures may indicate secondary bacterial infection from any bite, often present with deep tissue necrosis of brown recluse spider bite.

6. About 4 to 6 weeks after the bite of a tick, the ELISA test can be performed. If ELISA is positive or equivocal, the more sensitive Western blot should be performed. IgM will be elevated in 2 to 4 weeks after infectious tick bite. IgG will be elevated in 6 weeks.

III. TREATMENT MODALITIES

A. Local treatment

1. The bites of many insects can be rendered less painful and itching reduced by applying cold compresses.

2. Applying topical antihistamine lotions or systemic antihistamines may reduce the urge to scratch.

3. Topical 1% hydrocortisone may reduce inflammation and pruritus. It is contraindicated with any open areas of skin.

4. Elevation of the affected extremity may reduce edema.

5. Anti-infective topical may reduce incidence of secondary infections when the skin is broken.

6. Keeping the hands and skin clean and trimming nails reduces the risk of secondary infections when the skin integrity is lost.

7. Crotamiton may be helpful in reducing the itch as it has antipruritic properties.

8. Application of a counter irritant such as dilute ammonium solution may decrease itching.

B. Treatments specific to envenomation

1. Scorpion
   a. Treat symptoms of severe agitation, peripheral motor jerking, and hypersalivation as needed.
   b. Be prepared to support respiration.
   c. Anascorp, an antivenom, may be used to reduce symptoms.

2. Black widow spider
   a. Intravenous benzodiazepines to reduce muscle spasms.
   b. Narcotics for pain.
   c. Equine antivenom may be considered up to 48 hours after the bite. Use only if severe pain persists after standard treatment. One ampule diluted in 100 mL of normal saline infused 1 mL/minute over first 15 minutes. Then remainder is infused over 2 to 3 hours. Serum sickness can be a complication.

3. Brown recluse spider
   a. Overaggressive bite management may cause more harm than good.
   b. Tissue necrosis may be treated with dapsone 100 mg/day for 14 days. A G6PD level should be checked prior to administration.
   c. Surgical intervention should be avoided for the first 21 days as toxin remains biologically active in tissues during this time. Generally, surgical intervention should be delayed for 6 to 8 weeks allowing the lesion to stabilize.
   d. After tissue destruction has stopped, skin flaps may be required to repair the defect.

4. Leishmaniasis
   a. Pentavalent antimalarials should be used. Sodium stibogluconate 20 mg/kg/d for 20 days. Meglumine antimoniate 20 mg/kg/d for 20 days.

5. Rocky Mountain spotted fever
   a. Adults and children over 45 kg: doxycycline 100 mg bid for 7 to 14 days or at least 3 days after fever subsides.
   b. Children under 45 kg: doxycycline 2.2 mg/kg/d given bid for 7 to 14 days or at least 3 days after fever subsides.
   c. Doxycycline should be given despite concern about staining of teeth in children. Use of alternate antibiotics may result in an increased risk of death from the condition.
   d. Pregnant women should receive intravenous chloramphenicol sodium succinate 50 to 75 mg/kg/d divided into qid dosing.

6. Lyme disease
   a. Adults: doxycycline 100 mg bid × 21 days, amoxicillin 500 mg tid × 21 days, and cefuroxime 500 mg bid × 21 days.
   b. Children: amoxicillin 50 mg/kg/d × 14 to 21 days and cefuroxime 30 mg/kg/d × 14 to 21 days.

PATIENT EDUCATION
General Information about Bites and Stings

- Bites and stings are avoided by being aware of their natural habitat and use precaution.
- Food and drinks should be covered when eating outdoors.
- Hats and long pants are to be worn and long pants are tucked into socks.
- Application of diethyltoluamide (DEET) to exposed skin may provide protection against mosquitoes, ticks, fleas, chiggers, leeches, and many other biting insects. Concentrations of 10% up to 50% are recommended.
- DEET in concentration of 10% may be applied to children older than 2 months of age, taking caution to avoid the lips and the hands. One must not use DEET in areas that may cause inadvertent introduction into the mouth. DEET is safe to use in pregnancy during the second and third trimesters.
- Concentrations greater than 50% have minimal additional benefit and have a higher probability of increased skin absorption. Regular use should be discussed with the patient's health care providers.

PART II: INFESTATION WITH ECTOPARASITES, SCABIES AND LICE

OBJECTIVES

After studying Part II of this chapter, the reader will be able to:

- Identify the causative ectoparasite in scabies and lice infestations.
- List the most common treatments and cautions for treating infestations.
- List environmental and fomite treatments, which prevent reinfestation.

KEY POINTS

- All cases of very pruritic rashes with intense nighttime itching should raise the suspicion of scabies infestation.
- Calm acceptance of the patient diagnosed with scabies or lice will help the family deal with the social stigma and promote attention to treatment plans.
- Schools and institutions often require complete nit removal before child can reenter the school even when pediculicides are effective.
- Parent education should include methods of eradicating scabies and lice from the home environment to prevent reinfestation.

SCABIES

I. OVERVIEW

The common itch mite, *Sarcoptes scabiei* (Figure 12-15), is responsible for a great deal of misery in every inhabited area of the globe. It is no respecter of social or economic class, sex, gender, age, or standard of personal hygiene.

A. Ectoparasite: *Sarcoptes scabiei*
   1. The mature female mite is about 0.5 mm in diameter.
   2. Only the female mite burrows into the skin.

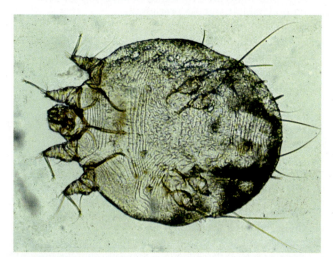

FIGURE 12-15. Scabies mite: *Sarcoptes scabiei*. (Courtesy of John K. Randall, MD.)

BOX 12-4. Immune Response

Immune response is caused by soluble antigen produced when the saliva, body secretions, and feces of the mite come in contact with cellular fluid.

Immune response develops over 4 to 6 weeks with first infestation of the mite.

During the latent period, the mite multiplies.

When the normal allergic response begins, many mites die. Inflammatory response develops.

In the immunocompromised individual, the mite continues to multiply unchecked. This superinfestation is commonly called Norwegian or crusted scabies. Up to a million mites may be present with crusted scabies. Nails may become thickened with white scaly subungual debris.

With the presence of the antigen, future infestations result in pruritus within 24 hours to several days. Past infestation does not confer future immunity.

---

   3. Mites from animals can feed on humans but do not burrow or reproduce in humans.
B. Reproduction
   1. Reproduction takes place on the skin of the host.
   2. The female is impregnated by the male who then dies.
   3. The impregnated female penetrates the skin by producing a secretion that lyses the stratum corneum. This process takes about 45 minutes.
   4. The mature female mite lays up to 4 eggs each day during her 30-day life span. Less than 10% of the eggs develop into mature mites.
   5. The embryo hatches in 3 to 10 days producing a six-legged larva.
   6. The larva goes through two additional shedding stages, finally producing an eight-legged nymph that matures into the adult mite.
   7. Both the larva and the nymph can survive and mature outside of the host.
C. Infestation
   1. Occurs only in close physical contact with a host already infested with the mite or may be transmitted by fomites such as clothing and bed linen.
   2. The mite pushes through the corneocytes into the stratum granulosum.
   3. The motion of the mite is always forward at a rate of 0.5 to 5 mm/day producing an externally visible burrow on the skin of the host.
   4. The burrow may be 5 to 20 mm long, straight, or serpentine in appearance.
D. Immune response (Box 12-4)

II. ASSESSMENT

A. History and physical examination (Figure 12-16)
   1. Very pruritic eruption with increased intensity or symptoms at night.
   2. Family members and household contacts with similar rash and itching.
   3. Presence of papules, pustules, and vesicles.

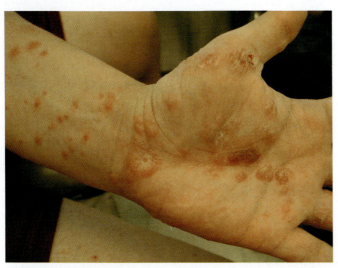

FIGURE 12-16. Scabies rash on the palm. (From Werner, R. (2012). *Massage therapist's guide to pathology*. Philadelphia, PA: Wolters Kluwer.)

4. Presence of a thread-like linear or serpentine-shaped gray-brown or pearly burrow less than 1 mm in width.
5. Lesions tend to be concentrated in the web spaces of the fingers around the wrists, axillae, breasts, areolae, waist, thighs, lower buttocks, and genitalia.
6. In infants and children, the lesion may be nodular and present over the back and on the head.
7. Nodular lesions may be present in the groin or axillae in adults.
8. Lesions in the immunocompromised patient may present with disseminated papular eruption and extensive hyperkeratotic lesions and fissuring, especially on flexor surfaces.

B. Diagnostic tests
1. Mineral oil prep.
   a. Scabies prep using a scalpel blade (premoistened with mineral oil) to scrape a suspected burrow and placing the material on a slide with mineral oil.
   b. Examining the material under the microscope with low magnification.
   c. Presence of the scabies mite, ova, or fecal pellets (scybala) is diagnostic of scabies.
2. Burrow ink test (BIT).
   a. Use of a pen or nonpermanent marker to identify a suspected burrow.
   b. After penetration, the excess ink is removed with an alcohol wipe.
   c. A mineral oil prep is performed as above.
3. Potassium hydroxide (KOH) is generally not used. It will dissolve the keratin but may also dissolve mite pellets.
4. Failure to find mites with scraping can be common and does not rule out a scabies diagnosis.
5. Biopsy.
   a. Seldom used except when lesions are atypical. Scabies mineral oil prep is much more reliable diagnostic test.
   b. Biopsy will demonstrate the presence of eosinophils.

6. Blood tests.
   a. IgE elevated, IgA decreased in crusted scabies.
   b. IgE antibody against recombinant scabies antigen has 100% sensitivity and 93.75% specificity.
   c. Eosinophilia in crusted scabies.
C. Differential diagnosis
1. Unless proven otherwise, all pruritic rashes should raise the suspicion of scabies.
2. Atopic, contact dermatitis, dermatitis herpetiformis, and neurodermatitis may have similar excoriated lesions.

III. TREATMENT MODALITIES

A. Medication
1. Permethrin 5% cream. Acts upon the cell membrane by disabling the sodium transport and decreases polarization of cell membrane. This causes paralysis of the mite.
2. Applied at night massaged into the skin of adults and children from the neck down and washed off in the morning. Generally recommended to repeat in 1 week.
3. Permethrin 5% cream applied from head to toe in infants over 2 months of age and washed off in the morning.
4. 5% to 10% sulfur for pregnant or lactating females and infants under 2 months. Applied nightly for 3 nights and washed off in the morning.
5. Gamma benzene hexachlorine. This is an organochlorine insecticide that inhibits neurotransmission, which induces respiratory and muscular paralysis in mites.
   a. When used properly, it has minimal toxicity but has been associated with seizures and death of an infant.
   b. Distributed throughout the body, slowly metabolized, and stored in fatty tissues and in the brain.
   c. Carries black box warning. It is contraindicated in pregnancy and lactation, and in infants.
   d. 30 mL is the adequate treatment amount for an adult. Apply to the skin at night and wash off in the morning. Second applications should be avoided to reduce chance of neurotoxicity.
6. Crotamiton 10% cream or lotion. This is used to apply to the skin from the neck down at night for 2 to 5 consecutive nights then washed off each AM. Crotamiton is one of the least effective of the current scabies medications. It does though have antipruritic properties and is helpful in some people for this action. Pregnancy category C.
7. Ivermectin. This is available in 3-mg tablets. It acts by binding glutamate-gated chloride ion channels. This creates increased permeability of chloride ions causing hyperpolarization of nerve cells causing death of the mite. It is frequently used to treat scabies, but this use is an off-label indication.
   a. Dose is 200 μg/kg in a single dose repeated in 7 to 10 days.
   b. Pregnancy category C. Manufacturer states that it is not recommended in pregnancy and in children less than 15 kg of weight.

8. Low-dose topical or systemic steroids or oral antihistamines may be needed for treating continued pruritus even after mites have been eradicated.

IV. COMPLICATIONS

A. Intense scratching in response to pruritus may result in secondary bacterial infections.
  1. Antibiotics may be necessary to treat bacterial infections.
B. In the immunocompromised host, the lack of cell-mediated response permits the mite to multiply unchecked.
  1. Hyperkeratotic plaques may form with fissuring.
  2. Normal skin flora then has a portal of entry into the bloodstream.
  3. Once in the bloodstream, normal skin flora may develop into bacteremia, sepsis, and potentially death.
  4. If the normal cell-mediated response does not limit the number of mites, huge numbers may tunnel in and around the fingernails promoting the spread of the mite to other body areas or caretakers.
  5. The hyperkeratosis, fissuring, and numbers of mites make eradication difficult. Appropriate treatment may include alternating permethrin 5% cream and oral ivermectin.

PATIENT EDUCATION
Scabies

• The itching caused by the mite will persist for weeks even after eradication of the mites.
• Fingernails should be kept short to avoid traumatizing the skin when scratching.
• All household contacts and sexual contacts should be treated at the same time.
• Clothing and linen should be changed after overnight or recommended treatment time.
• Clothing is to be washed with hot water wash and dried in hot dryers.
• All nonwashable surfaces are to be vacuumed and then seal and dispose of vacuum bag.
• Fabric articles that cannot be washed or dry cleaned may be encased in plastic for several weeks to avoid reinfestation.
• Medications: topicals should be thoroughly massaged into body crevices (axillae and groin) as well as under fingernails.
• Ivermectin is better absorbed with high-fat meal.

PEDICULOSIS

I. OVERVIEW

Two species of the order Anoplura (Figures 12-17 and 12-18) infest human beings. The louse, which is visible to the naked eye, is endemic to all areas of the globe and is likely responsible or well over 10 million cases of infestation in the United States each year. Although the head louse may be found in all social and economic levels, the body louse and pubic louse

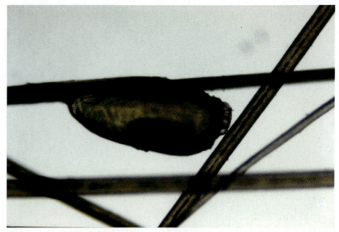
FIGURE 12-17. Pediculosis nit on hair. (Courtesy of Charles E. Lewis, MD.)

are far more prevalent in those with crowded living conditions and uncertain hygiene.

A. Ectoparasite: *Pediculus humanus*
  1. Subspecies *Pediculus humanus corporis* or body louse
  2. Subspecies *Pediculus humanus capitis* or head louse
B. Ectoparasite: *Phthirus pubis*
  1. Commonly called the crab louse
  2. Infests predominately the pubic hairs and other body hair with similar diameter
C. Reproduction
  1. All three types of lice undergo five developmental stages.
    a. The egg or oviposit, which hatches in 5 to 10 days in response to body heat.
    b. Three nymphal stages, which depend on blood meal for survival, develop over the next 8 or 9 days.

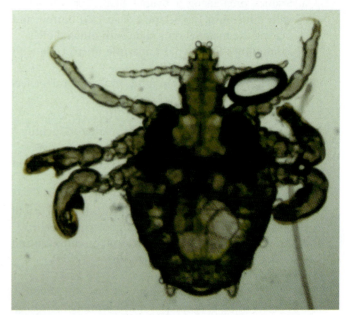
FIGURE 12-18. Pediculosis louse. (Courtesy of John K. Randall, MD.)

c. The adult louse is capable of mating within hours of reaching the adult stage.
2. The adult louse produces 6 to 10 eggs a day and may lay up to 300 eggs during its life span.
3. All require blood meals for survival although they may live off a host for a period of 10 to 30 days if conditions of temperature and humidity are met.
D. Infestation
1. *P. humanus capitis* attaches its oviposit or nit on scalp hair close to the skin.
2. *P. humanus corporis* attaches its oviposit on fabric fibers, particularly the seams of clothing.
3. Phthirus pubis attaches its oviposit on hairs at the skin line of the pubic region, the beard, the eyebrows, the eyelashes, and the axillae.
E. Lesions
1. The head louse produces pruritic red papules above the shoulders, often with dark red spots visible on the neck and shoulders from fecal droppings.
2. The body louse produces an urticarial papule. With extensive infestation, the skin may become dry and scaly with the development of hyperpigmented areas.
3. Pubic lice often produce gray-blue areas called macula cerulea over the trunk and thighs.
F. Immune response (Box 12-4)
1. Develops from saliva injected into the skin when the louse prepares to feed.
2. The saliva prevents blood from clotting while feeding occurs.

II. ASSESSMENT

A. History and physical examination
1. Presence of pruritus, often worse at night
2. Lackluster hair and presence of cervical adenopathy and purulent dermatitis with heavy or prolonged infestation by the head louse
3. Presence of urticarial papules, dry and scaly skin with body louse infestation
4. Presence of macules over the thighs and trunk with infestation by the pubic louse
5. Evidence of louse on the body or in the clothing on close inspection
   a. Presence of fecal droppings in the seams of clothing
6. Presence of the nit on the hair shaft with head and pubic lice
   a. The position of the nit from the skin surface is indicative of the time since attachment, moving with the growing hair.
   b. Nits spread at multiple intervals along the hair shaft indicate prolonged or repeated infestations.
   c. Egg casing distant from the scalp is empty or contains killed ova.
B. Diagnostic tests
1. Visualization of the louse on the skin or clothing, presence of oviposits.
2. Wood light will cause fluorescence of hair infested with head lice.

III. TREATMENT MODALITIES

A. Medication for head lice
1. 1% permethrin lotion and 5% permethrin cream.
   a. Lotion is allowed to remain on the hair for 10 minutes followed by rinse and towel drying with a clean towel.
   b. Cream is allowed to remain on hair overnight followed by rinse and towel drying with a clean towel.
   c. Provides protection from reinfestation for 2 weeks.
2. Malathion 0.5% lotion compounded in isopropyl alcohol 78% and terpineol 12%.
   a. Weak organophosphate that inhibits acetylcholinesterase resulting in neuromuscular paralysis. The alcohol and terpineol have ovicidal and pediculicidal actions to help increase effectiveness.
   b. Similar products were brought to the market prior to 1999 and were removed due to concerns about prolonged application times and flammability issues. They were later reintroduced into the market due to concerns about increases of resistance to other products.
   c. Application to dry hair. Wait 8 to 12 hours and then shampoo. Note—postmarketing studies have demonstrated that 20-minute application time is effective.
   d. Pregnancy category B.
3. Spinosad 0.9% topical.
   a. Action is by excitation of motor neurons resulting in muscle contractions, paralysis, and eventual death of the louse.
   b. Applied to dry hair for 10 minutes. Rinse out and towel dry.
   c. Pregnancy category B.
4. Benzyl benzoate 5% lotion.
   a. Dosage varies according to the length of hair. Ranges from 4 to 6 ounces for hair less than 2 inches in length and up to 32 to 48 ounces for hair longer than 22 inches.
   b. May be used in children over 6 months of age.
   c. Applied to dry hair every 7 days × 2 doses.
   d. Pregnancy category B.
5. Gamma benzene hexachloride 1% shampoo may be used for treatment. 1% lotion may be used for body lice.
   a. Treatment is often less effective than with permethrin.
   b. Apply to wet hair, 15 to 30 mL for short hair, 45 mL for medium length, and up to 60 mL for very long hair.
   c. Allow to remain on the hair for 4 minutes before adding water to work up a lather.
   d. Thoroughly rinse and towel dry.
   e. To reduce chance of excess absorption, wear gloves while applying, avoid getting shampoo on other body parts, and do not apply any occlusive cover.
   f. May require one repeat treatment in 7 to 10 days.
6. Pyrethrin may be used for any type of pediculosis infestation.

a. Available over the counter, this product is less effective than other pediculicides.

b. Apply and wash off after 10 minutes.

c. High potential for misuse due to lack of understanding of the treatment schedule.

d. Chemically related to chrysanthemums and may cause hypersensitivity reactions in some individuals.

e. Pregnancy category C.

7. Ivermectin 0.5% lotion. May be used in adults and children over 6 months of age.

a. Apply to dry hair for 10 minutes, then rinse.

8. Permethrin 5% cream may be used on the body. Apply at night and wash off in the morning. May also be used on the scalp if prior treatment to 1% permethrin has been ineffective.

9. Petrolatum may be applied to eyelashes 2 to 3 times a day to aid in removing lice and nits.

B. Removal of nits

1. Meticulous combing of hair with a special nit comb to remove all nits. Hair should be separated into sections and combed repetitively with nit comb to remove the nits.

2. Shaving the hair will also remove the nits, but this is generally not acceptable to most individuals.

IV. COMPLICATIONS

A. Complications are rare except in debilitated individuals with secondary infections.

B. Potential for some vector diseases.

PATIENT EDUCATION
Pediculosis

- All head coverings such as scarves and caps must be dry cleaned or washed in hot water.

- Combs, brushes, curlers, and hair clips and bows should be washed in hot water.

- Clothing worn by those with heavy body louse infestation may need the additional precaution of ironing seams as this is the attachment area for oviposits.

- All bedding, towels, and worn clothing should be washed in hot water and dried in hot dryer.

- Parents must be instructed about the necessity of thoroughly combing the hair with nit combs. Additionally, it must be reinforced that inspection should be carried out at regular intervals to reduce the possibility of reinfestation.

- Pubic lice in young or adolescent children may indicate sexual activity.

- All infested family members must be treated at the same time.

- Hair conditioners should not be used prior to treatments for lice as the hair conditioner prohibits the treatments from adhering to the hair follicles.

- Resistance to medications is being reported, but many instances of resistance are due to lack of adherence, incorrect treatment, lack of ovicidal or killing properties of the medication, and reinfestation.

BIBLIOGRAPHY

Anderson, R. J., Campoli J., Johar, S. K., Schumacher, K. A., & Allison, E. J. (2011). Suspected brown recluse envenomation: A case report and review of different treatment modalities. *Journal of Emergency Medicine, 41*(2), e31–e37.

Ayoub, N., Maatouk, I., Merhy, M., & Tomb, R. (2012). Treatment of pediculosis capitis with topical albendazole. *Journal of Dermatological Treatment, 23,* 78–80.

Barnes, E. R. & Murray, B. S. (2013). Bedbugs: What nurses need to know. *American Journal of Nursing, 133*(3), 58–62.

Bernardeschi, C., Le Cleach, L., Delaunay, P., & Chosidow, O. (2013). Bedbug infestation. *British Medical Journal, 346(f138),* 1–8, doi: 10.1136/bmj

Biesiada, G. (2010). Lyme disease: Review. *Archives of Medical Science, 8*(6), 978–982.

Bouvresse D. R., Berdjane, Z., Izri, A., Chosidow, O., & Clark, J. M. (2012). Insecticide resistance to head lice: Clinical, parasitological, and genetic aspects. *Clinical Microbiology and Infection, 18,* 338–344.

Burkhart, C. N., Burkhart, C. G. & Morrell S. D. (2012). Infestations. In J. L. Bolognia, J. L. Jorrizzo & J. O. Schaffer (Eds.), *Dermatology* (3rd ed., pp. 1423–1434). New York: Saunders Elsevier.

Burns, D. A. (2010). Diseases caused by arthropods and other noxious animals. In T. Burns, S. Breathnach, N. Cox, & C. Griffiths (Eds.), *Rooks Textbook of Dermatology Online (Chapter 38).* (8th ed.). West Sussex, United Kingdom: Wiley-Blackburn.

Cole, S. W. & Lundquist, L. M. (2011). Spinosad for treatment of head lice infestation. *Annals of Pharmacology, 45,* 954–958.

Dana, A. N. (2009). Diagnosis and treatment of tick infestation and tick-borne diseases with cutaneous manifestations. *Dermatologic Therapy, 22,* 293–326.

Drees, B. M., Calixto, A. P., & Nester, P. R. (2013). Integrated pest management concepts for red imported fire ants Solenopsis invicta (Hymenoptera: Formicidae). *Insect Science, 20,* 429–438.

Elston, D. M. (2010). Tick bites and skin rashes *Current Opinion in Infectious Diseases, 23,* 132–138.

Elston, D. M. (2012). *Bites and stings.* In J. L. Bolognia, J. L. Jorrizzo & J. O. Schaffer (Eds.), *Dermatology* (3rd ed., pp. 1435–1454). New York: Saunders Elsevier.

Elston, D. M. (2013). Systemic antiparisitic agents. In S. Wolverton (Ed.), *Comprehensive Dermatology Drug Therapy* (3rd ed., pp. 135–142). New York: Saunders/Elsevier.

Goddard, J. & Edwards, K. T. (2013). Effects of bed bug saliva on human skin. *Journal of the American Medical Association Dermatology, 149*(3), 372–373.

Golden, D. B. K. (2013). Advances in diagnosis and management of insect sting allergy. *Annals of Allergy, Asthma, and Immunology. 111,* 84–89.

Goldust, M., Rezaee, E., Raghifar, R., & Naghavi-Behzad, M. (2013). Ivermectin vs. lindane in the treatment of scabies. *Annals of Parasitology, 59*(1), 37–41.

Goldust, M., Rezace, E., Raghifa, R., & Hemayat, S. (2013). Treatment of scabies: The topical ivermectin vs. permethrin 2.5% cream. *Annals of Parasitology, 59*(2), 79–84.

Gullan, P. J. & Cranston, P. (Eds). (2010). *External anatomy. An outline of entomology* (4th ed., pp. 23–52). Hoboken, New Jersey: Wiley.

Hahlbolm, D. (2013). Stinging insect allergy. *Advance for NP's and PA's. 4*(3), 19–22.

Hubbard, J. J. & James, L. P. (2011). Complications and outcomes of brown recluse spider bites in children. *Clinical Pediatrics. 50*(3), 252–258.

Juckett, G. (2013). Arthropod bites. *American Family Physician, 88*(12), 841–847.

Krishnan, S. S. & Lockshen, B. N. (2013). Topical antiparasitic agents. In S. Wolverton (Ed.), *Comprehensive Dermatologic Drug Therapy* (3rd ed., pp. 481–486). New York: Elsevier Saunders.

Lane, L., McCoppin, H. H., & Dyer, J. (2011). Acute generalized exanthematous pustulosis and comb-positive hemolytic anemia in a child following loxosceles reclusa envenomation. *Pediatric Dermatology, 28*(6), 685–688.

Losher, D. (2009). A brown recluse spider bite. *Dermatology Nursing, 21*(6), 360–361.

McDade, J., Aygun, B., & Ware, R. E. (2010). Brown recluse spider (loxosceles reclusa) envenomation leading to acute hemolytic anemia in six adolescents. *The Journal of Pediatrics, 156*, 155–157.

Overstreet, M. L. (2013). Tick bites and lyme disease: The need for timely treatment. *Critical Care Nursing Clinics of North America, 25*(2), 165–172.

Roupakias, S. Mitsakous, P., & Al Nimer, A. (2011). Tick removal. *Journal of Prevention Medicine and Hygiene, 52*(1), 40–44.

Rudders, S. A., Clark, S., Wei, W., & Camargo, C. A. (2013). Longitudinal study of 954 patients with stinging insect anaphylaxis. *Annals of Allergy, Asthma, and Immunology, 111*, 199–204.

Shimose, L., & Munoz-Price, L. S. (2013). Diagnosis, prevention, and treatment of scabies. *Current Infectious Disease Reports, 15*, 426–431.

Stanek, G., Wormser, G. P., Gray, J., & Strle, F. (2012). Lyme borreliosis. *The Lancet, 349*, 460–473.

Smith, G. N., Gemmill, I., & Moore, K. M. (2012). Management of tick bites and lyme disease during pregnancy. *Journal of Obstetrics and Gynecology Canada, 34*(11), 1087–1091.

Vinson, S. B. (2013). Impact of the invasion of the imported fire ant. *Insect Science, 20*, 439–455.

Walton, S. F. & Oprescu, F. L. (2013). Immunology of scabies and translational outcomes: Identifying the missing links. *Current Opinion in Infectious Disease, 26*(2), 116–120.

Yavuz, S. T. (2013). Importance of serum basal tryptase levels in children with insect venom allergy. *Allergy, 6*, 386–391.

STUDY QUESTIONS: PART I

1. The clinic triage nurse answers a call from a mother stating that her 4-year-old son has been stung by a bee. She asks what she should do to relieve the pain and itching. Appropriate advice to this parent regarding application of first aid includes which of the following?
   a. DEET to prevent further stings
   b. Cold compresses on the sting area
   c. Bacitracin ointment on the sting area
   d. Mud compresses to "pull out the poison"

2. The vesicles caused by the imported fire ant contain:
   a. Coagulotoxin
   b. Neurotoxin
   c. Purulent material from an infection
   d. Sterile material with many neutrophils

3. Mr. Barnard presents to a dermatology office reporting a new lesion. The lesion is located on his calf and resembles a 5-cm "bull's eye" with central clearing. You suspect this patient might have:
   a. Lyme disease
   b. Rocky Mountain spotted fever
   c. An isolated chigger bite, which has become infected
   d. The bite of a mosquito carrying St. Louis encephalitis

4. One of the most critical questions to ask Mr. Barnard when obtaining his history is with regard to:
   a. Family history of similar lesions
   b. Presence of pain in his extremity
   c. Exposure to a possible tick bite
   d. Recent history of nausea

5. Treatment of Mr. Barnard's condition should include:
   a. Local antibiotics and steroids for the skin lesion
   b. Oral doxycycline for 21 days
   c. Intravenous chloramphenicol
   d. Symptomatic treatment only if fever occurs

6. A patient presents with a grayish-blue halo surrounding a central puncture on her right thigh. The area is slightly edematous and painful. She remembers feeling a mild stinging sensation on her thigh upon awakening the day prior to his visit. You suspect which of the following?
   a. Scorpion sting
   b. Black widow spider bite
   c. Brown recluse spider bite
   d. Sting from a member of the Hymenoptera family

7. A patient presents to the emergency department reporting agonizing muscle spasms after a bite. You suspect which of the following?
   a. Scorpion sting
   b. Black widow spider bite
   c. Brown recluse spider bite
   d. Yellow jacket sting

8. Appropriate treatment for the patient with the muscle spasms includes which of the following?
   a. High-volume infusion of normal saline
   b. Intravenous benzodiazepines
   c. Narcotics
   d. Nitrates

9. Effective methods to remove an attached tick include which of the following?
   a. Burn it with a hot match.
   b. Apply petroleum jelly over the tick.
   c. Grasp the tick with tweezers close to the skin and pull upward.
   d. All of the above.

10. The initial rash associated with Rocky Mountain spotted fever is a morbilliform pattern located on the:
    a. Palms and soles
    b. Trunk
    c. Neck
    d. Face

11. The most reliable predictor of a severe allergic reaction to a future Hymenoptera sting is:
   a. Elevated IgG level
   b. Elevated IgM level
   c. Low serum tryptase level
   d. History of reaction to a previous sting

12. Loxoscelism is a term used to describe the systemic effects caused by which of the following?
   a. Brown recluse spider bite
   b. Rocky Mountain spotted fever
   c. Sting from a Hymenoptera insect
   d. Fire ant stings

Answers to Study Questions Part I: 1.b, 2.d, 3.a, 4.c, 5.b, 6.c, 7.b, 8.b, 9.c, 10.a, 11.d, 12.a

STUDY QUESTIONS: PART II

1. Which one of the following patients would be *most* at risk for developing crusted Norwegian scabies?
   a. A 4-year-old Carrie, who shares a bed with her 6-year-old sister who was just diagnosed with scabies
   b. A 54-year-old Ben, who has poorly controlled type 1 diabetes
   c. A 84-year-old Ed, who takes cyclosporine daily since undergoing renal transplantation
   d. A 65-year-old Bonnie, who was recently diagnosed with a thyroid disorder

2. A mother calls the office stating that the permethrin given 4 days ago for her son is not working, as he is still miserable with itching. An appropriate reply to this parent includes which of the following?
   a. Itching will persist up to 1 month past treating due to the allergic reaction from the scabies saliva.
   b. Her son has probably been reinfected with the scabies mite.
   c. Her son needs a different medication.
   d. She probably did not clean all of the bedding properly.

3. Patient education after a diagnosis of scabies includes which of the following statements?
   a. All household contacts should be treated simultaneously.
   b. All bedding should be washed with hot soapy water and dried in a very hot dryer.
   c. Topical medication should be applied from the neck down in adults, taking care to work the medication under the fingernails and skin crevices.
   d. Keep fingernails cut short to avoid traumatizing the skin if scratching.
   e. All of the above.

4. Sara presents to the dermatology office reporting that her eyes are irritated. Upon close examination, lice are noted on her eyelashes. Appropriate treatment for this condition will be which of the following?
   a. Permethrin 5% lotion applied very carefully to the eyelashes to avoid accidental eye exposure
   b. Petroleum jelly applied to the eyelashes three times daily for 7 to 14 days
   c. Oral ivermectin
   d. Over-the-counter pyrethrin lotion applied one time for 10 minutes and then rinsed

5. The drug that has been documented to cause seizure disorders in some children is:
   a. Pyrethrin.
   b. Permethrin.
   c. Lindane.
   d. Ivermectin.

6. Which of the following statements to explain the rationale for repeated application of a topical antilouse agent is *true*?
   a. Some of the medications are not ovicidal and will need the second treatment for nits that hatch after the first treatment.
   b. Patients may not comb out all of the nits.
   c. There is a high degree of resistance to the available medications.
   d. All of the above.

Answers to Study Questions Part II: 1.c, 2.a, 3.e, 4.b, 5.c, 6.d

CHAPTER 13

Dermatologic Conditions in Children

Emily Croce • Meghan O'Neill

OBJECTIVES

After studying this chapter, the reader will be able to:

- Recognize the skin conditions commonly seen in the pediatric population, including a variety of transient cutaneous conditions in newborns, miliaria, oral candidiasis, ichthyosis, and hemangiomas.
- Describe the factors that may precipitate or contribute to these pediatric skin disorders.
- Discuss the therapeutic interventions frequently used in these pediatric dermatology conditions.
- Identify the important patient teaching issues for these pediatric skin disorders.

KEY POINTS

- Many skin conditions in newborns are transient, self-limiting problems that do not require intervention other than to provide reassurance to parents.
- Genetic skin disorders may present lifelong problems for affected individuals.
- Transient, self-limiting problems that generally do not require intervention other than to provide reassurance to parents include acne neonatorum, acropustulosis of infancy, erythema toxicum neonatorum, harlequin color change, cutis marmorata, sebaceous gland hyperplasia, subcutaneous fat necrosis (if small affected area), sucking blisters, and transient pustular melanosis.
- Miliaria crystallina (self-limited), miliaria rubra (common prickly heat), and miliaria profunda (found in patients who have had several bouts of miliaria rubra) are all sweat-retention diseases related to heat exposure. Miliaria crystallina and rubra are the most common forms seen in the neonatal period.
- Oral candidiasis, also known as oral thrush, is an infection of the oropharyngeal cavity with *Candida albicans*, a yeast commonly seen in the infant period.
- Ichthyosis, which means "fish scale," is a broad category of dermatologic conditions involving varying presentations of excessive scaling of the skin. Major hereditary types, which have been described, include two autosomal recessive congenital ichthyoses (epidermal ichthyosis and lamellar ichthyosis types), ichthyosis vulgaris, and X-linked ichthyosis. Several other, rarer forms exist but are not covered in this chapter.
- Hemangiomas of infancy are common, benign, vascular tumors comprised of endothelial cells. They may be isolated, small, and uncomplicated or may lead to significant cosmetic and/or medical complications and require intervention.

TRANSIENT CUTANEOUS CONDITIONS IN THE NEWBORN

I. OVERVIEW

A. Definition: transient skin conditions that appear and disappear during the first few days to weeks or months of life.

II. EPIDEMIOLOGY

A. Many infants will experience one or more of these conditions.

III. ETIOLOGY AND PATHOGENESIS

A. Infant skin differs from adult skin in that it seems to reflect bodily changes more readily.
B. These conditions are related to one or several of the following influences:
  1. Events occurring during birth
  2. Immaturity of various physiologic systems
  3. Influence of maternal hormones

IV. ASSESSMENT

A. Clinical manifestations
  1. Acne neonatorum (neonatal acne or neonatal cephalic pustulosis) (Figure 13-1)
    a. Presents as multiple, discrete, inflammatory papules and/or pustules on the face, particularly on the cheeks. Occasionally, lesions are also present on the chest, back, and/or groin.
    b. Not considered a true form of acne vulgaris, which also presents with comedones and larger, inflammatory papules
    c. Appears at 2 to 4 weeks of age and may persist for up to 6 months of age. Present in 20% of infants
    d. Thought to be the result of transient, benign increases of circulating androgens in the newborn.

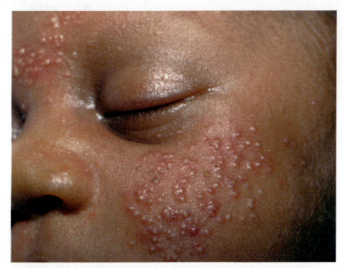

FIGURE 13-1. Neonatal acne (benign cephalic pustulosis) with multiple uniform red papules. (From Lugo-Somolinos, A., et al. (2011). *VisualDx: Essential dermatology in pigmented skin*. Philadelphia, PA: Wolters Kluwer.)

Also potentially related to an inflammatory reaction to *Pityrosporum (Malassezia)* species

   e. A careful history must be obtained to determine whether other virilizing features are present, such as axillary/pubic hair and/or body odor. If present, the child must be referred to a pediatric endocrinologist for further workup.
2. Acropustulosis of infancy (Figure 13-2)
   a. Presents as pustules or vesicles on the palms and soles in recurrent crops and rapidly become pruritic
   b. Pruritus in the neonate may present as an irritable, fretful child.
   c. Lesions may recur every 2 to 4 weeks until 2 to 3 years of age.

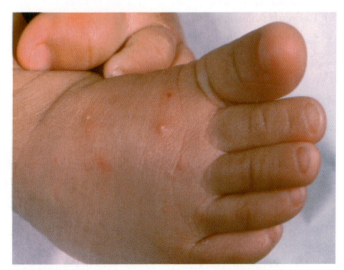

FIGURE 13-2. Scattered papules and pustules on the dorsum of the foot in acropustulosis of infancy. (From Lugo-Somolinos, A., et al. (2011). *VisualDx: Essential dermatology in pigmented skin*. Philadelphia, PA: Wolters Kluwer.)

   d. Sometimes mistaken for scabies infestation
   e. Etiology is unknown.
3. Erythema toxicum neonatorum (Figure 13-3)
   a. A central, 1 to 3 mm, yellowish papule or pustule with a 1 to 3 cm, irregular, macular flare.
   b. Present at 24 to 72 hours of age in approximately half of term infants and typically clear in 4 to 7 days
   c. Lesions are typically seen on the face, may spread to the torso and extremities, and can be seen anywhere except for the palms and soles.
   d. Etiology is unknown.
4. Harlequin color change
   a. Occurs in approximately 10% of healthy infants when placed on one side. Also associated with low birth weight/preterm birth. The gravity-dependent skin develops an erythematous flush, with a simultaneous blanching of the upper side.
   b. A distinct line of demarcation runs along the midline of the body.
   c. Usually subsides within a few seconds of placing the baby in the supine position but may persist up to 30 minutes
   d. Attributed to the immaturity of autonomic vasomotor control. May last up to approximately 3 weeks of age

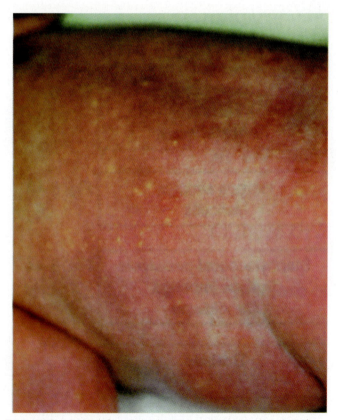

FIGURE 13-3. Erythema toxicum neonatorum showing the usual pattern, with most of the lesions on the trunk and face and fewer on the extremities. (From Fletcher, M. A. (1998). *Physical diagnosis in neonatology*. Philadelphia, PA: Lippincott-Raven Publishers.)

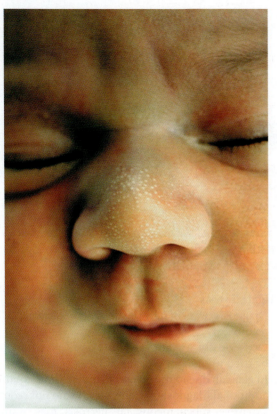

FIGURE 13-4. Milia. (From Jensen, S. (2010). *Nursing health assessment.* Philadelphia, PA: Wolters Kluwer.)

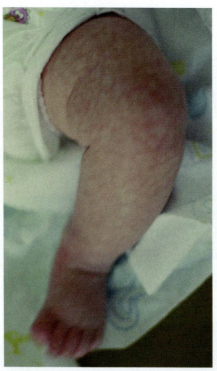

FIGURE 13-5. Cutis marmorata in a 2-month-old baby. (From Salimpour, R. R., Salimpour, P., & Salimpour, P. (2013). *Photographic atlas of pediatric disorders and diagnosis.* Philadelphia, PA: Wolters Kluwer.)

5. Milia (Figure 13-4)
   a. Small retention cysts
   b. One- to two-millimeter pearly white or yellow papules, most commonly on the nose, cheeks, chin, and forehead. Occasionally occur on the torso/extremities
   c. May also occur on the oral mucosa, particularly the palate. These are called Epstein pearls.
   d. Occurs in 40% to 50% of newborns
   e. Usually resolve spontaneously in the first 3 to 4 weeks of life
   f. Milia that are in a widespread or unusual distribution that persist may be associated with other genetic conditions.

6. Cutis marmorata (Figure 13-5)
   a. A physiologic reaction to cold in the newborn with the development of blanching, bluish, reticulated mottling of the skin on the trunk and extremities. Vasoconstriction may also lead to blue hands, feet, and lips, known as acrocyanosis.
   b. Caused by constricted capillaries and venules. Disappears on rewarming
   c. Thought to be caused by immaturity of the autonomic control of skin vascular plexus. More common in preterm infants
   d. Mottling that persists beyond the 6 months of life may be a sign of cutis marmorata telangiectatica congenita, a genetic skin condition that may have additional implications.

7. Sebaceous gland hyperplasia
   a. Follicular, evenly spaced, yellow–white papules where sebaceous gland density is greatest, typically around the nose and upper lip
   b. Differs from milia, which are usually solitary, more discrete, and whiter
   c. Occurs in 21% to 48% of infants.
   d. Resolves by 4 to 6 months.
   e. Hypertrophy of sebaceous glands thought to be the result of maternal and/or fetal stimulation of adrenal glands.

8. Subcutaneous fat necrosis (Figure 13-6)
   a. Sharply circumscribed, indurated, reddish or purple nodules and/or plaques in apparently healthy full-term newborns and young infants. Most commonly on cheeks, back, buttocks, arms, and thighs
   b. Appears within the first 2 weeks of life and resolves over several weeks to months
   c. May heal with atrophy, leaving a skin depression
   d. Extensive subcutaneous fat necrosis can be associated with significant hypercalcemia.
   e. Etiology is unknown. May be related to hypothermia, trauma, asphyxia, or hypercalcemia

9. Sucking blister (Figure 13-7)
   a. Solitary, intact blister or erosion on noninflamed skin of the fingers, dorsum of the dominant hand or wrist, or upper lip
   b. Results from vigorous sucking in the prenatal period
   c. Resolves within a few days

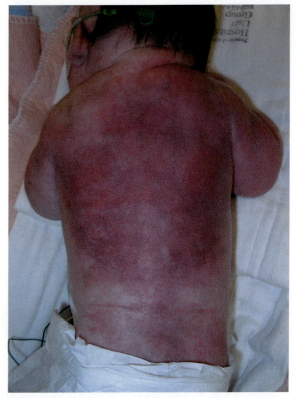

FIGURE 13-6. Subcutaneous fat necrosis of the newborn. (Image provided by Stedman's.)

10. Transient pustular melanosis (Figure 13-8)
    a. Presents at birth as vesicles, pustules, or pigmented macules with a collarette of scale
    b. Seen in less than 1% of newborns. More commonly seen in infants with darker pigment
    c. Pustular lesions typically resolve within 23 to 48 hours, with resultant hyperpigmentation fading over several weeks to months.
    d. Cause is unknown.

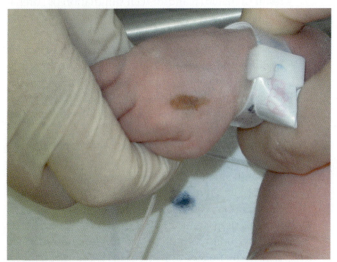

FIGURE 13-7. Sucking blister. The lesion on the left hand of this newborn is the result of sucking that occurred in utero. (Courtesy of Denise A. Salerno, MD, FAAP.)

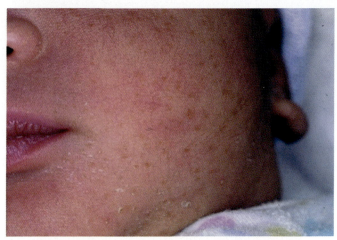

FIGURE 13-8. Transient neonatal pustular melanosis. (Courtesy of Paul S. Matz, MD.)

B. Diagnostic tests
1. Diagnosis is generally made by the lesions' clinical features.
2. Occasionally, a gram stain or Tzanck preparation may be used to rule out infectious causes.
3. In general, due to the benign nature of these conditions, additional diagnostic studies usually are not required.
4. Extensive subcutaneous fat necrosis may warrant a biopsy and serum calcium levels.

V. NURSING CONSIDERATIONS (TABLE 13-1)

A. Interventions
1. Maintain an adequate fluid balance and nutrition in the infant.
2. Instruct and demonstrate appropriate skin care techniques that will keep the skin clean, moisturized, and protected.
3. The majority of these conditions resolve spontaneously and do not require treatment.
    a. In acne neonatorum, most cases require no treatment. For severe and persistent comedonal lesions, azelaic acid 20% cream or the mildest topical retinoid preparations may be considered with close follow-up. Mild inflammatory lesions may be treated with ketoconazole cream. For inflammatory severe and persistent lesions, 2% erythromycin, 1% clindamycin, or 2.5% benzoyl peroxide may be considered with close follow-up. Systemic therapy is avoided when possible, though scarring acne may warrant treatment with oral antibiotics, such as erythromycin.
    b. If acropustulosis of infancy is symptomatic, oral sedating antihistamines (0.6 mg/kg/dose every 4 to 8 hours) may provide relief of itching and may be used in older infants. Potent topical steroids may also be used sparingly for severe cases.

B. Follow-up
1. Follow-up is only necessary if the condition worsens or parents have additional questions.

TABLE 13-1 Nursing Care of Children with Skin Disorders

Nursing Considerations	Goals	Expected Outcomes

Impaired skin integrity related to:
    Environmental agents
    Somatic factors
	Promote healing.
	Eradicate source of skin injury.
		Affected area displays signs of healing.
		Avoids precipitating agents

Potential impaired skin integrity related to:
    Mechanical trauma
    Body secretions
    Infection susceptibility
    Allergenic factors
	Maintain skin integrity.
	Prevent skin breakdown.
	Protect healthy skin.
	Prevent secondary infection.
	Promote general health.
		Skin remains clean, dry, and intact.
		Infection remains confined to primary location.
		Complies with general hygienic measures

Pain related to skin lesions and/or pruritus	Relieve discomfort. Prevent or minimize scratching. Promote rest.	Displays no evidence of discomfort Affected areas remain free of excoriation. Child receives adequate rest.
Potential for infection related to presence of microorganisms	Prevent spread of infection to self and others.	Infection remains confined to primary location.
Body image disturbance related to perception of appearance	Promotion of a positive self-image Provide tactile contact. Support child. Encourage self-care. Educate child on home care.	Verbalizes concerns and feelings Displays signs of comfort Positive response to tactile stimulation Identifies ways to improve appearance Assumes responsibility for care when appropriate Maintains usual activities and relationships

Altered family process related to having a child with a skin condition:
    Child's discomfort
    Time intensive and lengthy therapy
	Support family.
	Educate family on home care.
		Family demonstrates necessary skills.
		Family demonstrates understanding of skin problem and supports child.

PATIENT EDUCATION

Transient Skin Conditions

- Reassure parents regarding the benign nature of these conditions.
- Assure that the child is kept adequately warm, but avoid overdressing or occlusive clothing.

MILIARIA

I. OVERVIEW

Eccrine sweat glands are not associated with hair follicles and are found everywhere on the body except for mucocutaneous junctions. Eccrine sweat glands function to help regulate the body's temperature. This is accomplished by the production of eccrine sweat that flows to the skin surface and cools by evaporation. Eccrine sweat is an odorless, colorless, hypotonic solution and is excreted during periods of stress and heat. Miliaria crystallina (self-limited), miliaria rubra (prickly heat, most common in tropical climates), and miliaria profunda (found in patients who have had several bouts of miliaria rubra) are all sweat-retention diseases related to heat exposure. Miliaria crystallina and rubra are the most common forms seen in the neonatal period. Precipitating factors of these conditions include warming in incubators, fevers, occlusive clothing, dressings, or devices.

A. Definition: Miliaria is an itchy rash caused by inflammation following obstruction and rupture of eccrine sweat glands (Figure 13-9).

II. EPIDEMIOLOGY

A. Age: occurs predominantly in neonates, with a peak in those aged 1 week; but may occur in any age if febrile or recently moved to hot, humid climate
B. Sex: No sex predilection exists.
C. Race: in all races; Asian races produce less sweat and are thus less likely to have miliaria rubra.
D. Other factors
   1. Wearing synthetic clothing, which may irritate the skin
   2. Swaddling too much in clothing or blankets
   3. Lying for prolonged periods in bed or near heat sources (i.e., incubators, heaters, lights, etc.)

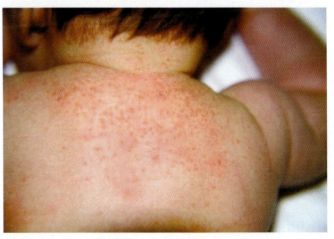

FIGURE 13-9. Miliaria in a 7-day-old infant. (From Salimpour, R. R., Salimpour, P., & Salimpour, P. (2013). *Photographic atlas of pediatric disorders and diagnosis.* Philadelphia, PA: Wolters Kluwer.)

III. ETIOLOGY AND PATHOGENESIS

A. Known causes
   1. Conditions of high heat and humidity that lead to excessive sweating and occlusion of skin. For example, clothing and casts
   2. Normal skin bacteria, such as *S. epidermidis* and *S. aureus,* thought to play role by producing sticky substance, which blocks sweat ducts
   3. Leakage of sweat through walls of duct behind blocked duct responsible for production of miliaria and for further aggravation
   4. Blockage of sweat ducts by dead skin

IV. ASSESSMENT

A. Clinical manifestations
   1. Miliaria crystallina (asymptomatic and self-limited) (Figure 13-10)
      a. Clear, superficial vesicles that are 1 to 2 mm in diameter
      b. Confluent crops without surrounding erythema
      c. On head, neck, and upper part of trunk in infants
      d. On trunk in bedridden, overheated individuals
      e. Lesions rupture easily and resolve with superficial desquamation.
      f. Older lesions will scale.
   2. Miliaria rubra (prickly heat, heat rash) (Figure 13-11)
      a. Uniform, small, erythematous papules and vesiculopapules on a background of erythema
      b. The most common of sweat-retention diseases
      c. Nonfollicular distribution; do not become confluent
      d. Can cause great discomfort; treatment is warranted.
      e. On the neck, groin, and axillae in infants
      f. On covered skin where friction occurs in adults
         (1) Neck
         (2) Scalp

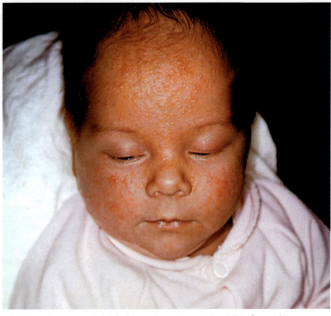

FIGURE 13-11. Prickly heat in a 6-week-old infant. (From Hall, J. C. (2000). *Sauer's manual of skin diseases* (8th ed., p. 407). Philadelphia, PA: Lippincott Williams & Wilkins.)

         (3) Upper part of trunk
         (4) Flexures
         (5) Face and volar areas spared
      g. In late stages, anhidrosis may be observed in affected skin.
   3. Miliaria profunda
      a. Firm, flesh-colored, nonfollicular papules that are 1 to 3 mm in diameter
      b. Erythema is absent.
      c. Primarily on trunk, but can also appear on the extremities
      d. Transient episodes of sweating
      e. Affected skin shows diminished or absent sweating.
      f. May lead to heat exhaustion; treatment is warranted.
      g. Hyperpyrexia and tachycardia are observed when there is heat exhaustion.
B. Diagnostic hallmarks
   1. Distribution: skin folds and on body in areas with friction from clothing.
   2. Lesions: Minute red papules present in very large numbers.
   3. Characteristic intense discomfort; not so much itching as an unbearable prickling sensation
C. History and physical examination
   1. Duration of lesions: 5 to 6 weeks
   2. Season: worse in hot, humid climate
   3. Symptoms: characteristic prickling sensation
D. Atypical findings
   1. Secondary infection appearing as impetigo or as multiple, discrete abscesses
   2. Heat intolerance most likely to develop in miliaria profunda; recognized by anhidrosis or affected skin, weakness, fatigue, dizziness, and even collapse

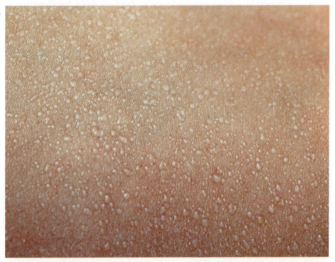

FIGURE 13-10. Miliaria crystallina. Multiple tiny-walled, clear vesicles of varying sizes. (From Burkhart, C., Morrell, D., Goldsmith, L. A., Papier, A., Green, B., Dasher, D., & Gomathy, S. (2009). *VisualDx: Essential pediatric dermatology.* Philadelphia, PA: Wolters Kluwer.)

E. Differential diagnosis
   1. Cutaneous candidiasis
   2. Varicella
   3. Erythema toxicum neonatorum
   4. Folliculitis
   5. Herpes simplex
   6. Pseudomonas folliculitis
   7. Syphilis
   8. Infantile acne
   9. Viral exanthem
F. Diagnostic tests
   1. Clinical diagnosis; laboratory tests not necessary

V. NURSING CONSIDERATIONS (TABLE 13-1)

A. Interventions
   1. Topical therapy
      a. Lotions containing calamine, boric acid, or menthol
      b. Cool wet-to-dry compresses
      c. Frequent showering with bland cleansers (although some discourage excessive use of soap)
      d. Topical corticosteroids
      e. Topical antibiotics if infection is present
      f. Topical application of anhydrous lanolin in patients with miliaria profunda
   2. Systemic therapy
      a. Prophylaxis of miliaria with oral antibiotics is reported.
      b. Oral retinoids, vitamin A, and vitamin C have all been used with variable success.
B. Course and prognosis
   1. May last 5 to 6 weeks despite treatments because plugs formed in sweat duct openings only cast off by outward growth of sweat duct cells, which takes several weeks

---

ORAL CANDIDIASIS

I. OVERVIEW

A. Definition: Oral candidiasis, also known as oral thrush or acute pseudomembranous candidiasis, is an infection of the oropharyngeal cavity with *C. albicans*, a yeast. It is commonly found in infants and also in immunocompromised adults (Figure 13-12).

II. EPIDEMIOLOGY

A. Most common in newborns
B. In adults, most common causes are local or systemic immunosuppression, steroid use, antibiotics, or poorly fitting dentures.

III. ASSESSMENT

A. Physical examination
   1. Infected epithelium appears white, adherent, curd-like papules and plaques and may be able to be scraped off, leaving an inflamed base.
   2. Tongue and buccal mucosa most often affected
B. History
   1. White plaques in the mouth
   2. May have coexisting candidal diaper rash
   3. Mothers of infected newborns may have a history of vaginal candidiasis in late pregnancy.
C. Diagnostic tests
   1. Biopsy
      a. Not recommended
   2. Laboratory tests
      a. Positive KOH or fungal culture

IV. NURSING CONSIDERATIONS (TABLE 13-1)

A. Interventions
   1. Topical therapy—nystatin suspension 1 mL (100,000 units) to each side of the mouth QID or until symptom resolution

---

> **PATIENT EDUCATION**
> *Miliaria*
>
> - Control heat and humidity so that sweating is not stimulated.
> - Treat febrile illness.
> - Remove occlusive clothing.
> - Avoid friction from clothing.
> - Wear clothing and blouses high in cotton and low in synthetics.
> - Limit activity.
> - Stay in air conditioning.
> - Avoid skin irritants.
> - Patients with miliaria profunda are at high risk for heat exhaustion during exertion in hot weather, because ability to dissipate heat by means of evaporation of sweat is impaired.

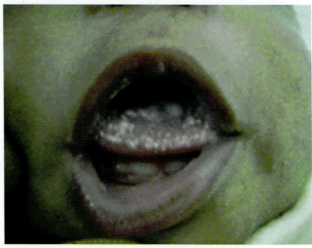

FIGURE 13-12. Thick white patches in the infant with oral candidiasis (thrush). (From Kyle, T., & Carman, S. (2012). *Essentials of pediatric nursing.* Philadelphia, PA: Wolters Kluwer.)

2. Systemic therapy—(full-term neonates) fluconazole 12 mg/kg × 1 day then 6 mg/kg/d for 14 days or until symptom resolution
3. Boil all bottle nipples and pacifiers. Breastfeeding mothers should consider treating their areolae.

B. Course and prognosis
1. In newborns, thrush may clear spontaneously but is more rapidly cleared with treatment.
2. Immunosuppressed patients can experience recurrent and chronic disease.
3. Complications are uncommon.

ICHTHYOSIS

I. OVERVIEW

A. Definition: excessive scaling of the skin. The scale may be "fish scale–like."
1. Several major hereditary types have been described.
   a. Lamellar ichthyosis (LI) and congenital nonbullous ichthyosiform erythroderma (CNIE), both autosomal recessive congenital ichthyoses
   b. Epidermolytic ichthyosis (EI), also known as bullous ichthyosis (BI) or bullous congenital ichthyosiform erythroderma
   c. Ichthyosis vulgaris (IV)
   d. X-linked ichthyosis (XLI)
2. There are several other, rare forms of ichthyosis that have associated abnormalities or are part of specific genetic syndromes such as Netherton syndrome, Sjogren–Larsson syndrome, KID syndrome, Darier disease, and others. They are not described in this chapter due to their rarity and involvement of other body systems beyond skin.

II. EPIDEMIOLOGY

A. IV is common, with 1:250 children having some variant of this disorder from mild to severe.
B. XLI is estimated to occur in 1 in 60,000 males.
C. LI and CNIE appear to occur in approximately 1 per 100,000 live births.
D. The incidence of EI is approximately 1 per 300,000 live births, with 50% of those being new mutations.

III. ETIOLOGY AND PATHOGENESIS

A. IV is inherited as an autosomal dominant disease.
B. XLI is inherited as an X-linked recessive trait that is due to a deficiency of the enzyme steroid sulfatase. Female carriers are asymptomatic.
C. LI and CNIE are inherited in an autosomal recessive trait pattern.
D. Epidermolytic ichthyosis (EI) is inherited as an autosomal dominant disorder.
E. Increased epidermal turnover with excessive production of stratum corneum cells has been demonstrated in LI and EI.
F. In XLI and IV, there appears to be normal epidermal turnover, and the accumulated scale is thought to be due to faulty shedding of the stratum corneum.

IV. ASSESSMENT

A. Clinical manifestations
1. Ichthyosis vulgaris (Figure 13-13)
   a. The skin of the newborn with IV usually remains normal throughout the newborn period.
   b. Manifestations are limited to the skin with fine scales predominately over the legs and buttocks that may be evident by 6 months to 2 years of age.
   c. Dry, follicular, horny plugs (keratosis pilaris) are present on the extensor surface of extremities and may become widespread.
   d. The entire surface of the skin is dry and may be associated with atopic dermatitis.
2. X-linked ichthyosis (Figure 13-14)
   a. Presents in infancy with scales over the posterior neck, upper trunk, and extensor surfaces of the extremities.
   b. Scaling is usually mild during the first 30 days of life, and the skin is a normal color.
   c. As the child ages, the scales become thicker and dirty yellow/brown in color. Antecubital and popliteal areas are often spared as well as the palms and soles.
   d. Corneal opacities are a clinical marker in XLI but are usually not present until adulthood.
   e. Cryptorchidism may occur in as many as 25% of males with XLI, and there is an associated increased risk of testicular cancer.
   f. There may be a history of a prolonged labor before affected individual was born due to the deficiency in steroid sulfatase.
3. LI and CNIE (Figure 13-15)
   a. Large, plate-like, dark scales with or without erythematous skin are present in LI.
   b. In CNIE, generalized fine scales on erythematous skin are present. The erythema may fade as the child ages.

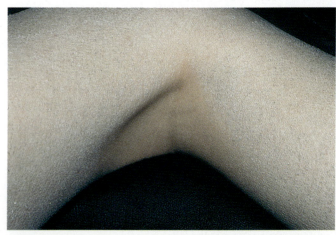

FIGURE 13-13. Ichthyosis vulgaris. This patient has atopic dermatitis and ichthyosis vulgaris lesions that resemble fish scales. Note the characteristic sparing of the popliteal fossa. (From Goodheart, H. P. (2003). *Goodheart's photoguide of common skin disorders* (2nd ed.). Philadelphia, PA: Lippincott Williams & Wilkins.)

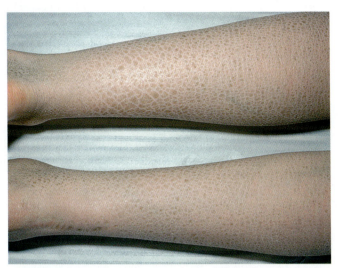

FIGURE 13-14. X-linked ichthyosis typically has large discrete scales compared with ichthyosis vulgaris. (From Burkhart, C., Morrell, D., Goldsmith, L. A., Papier, A., Green, B., Dasher, D., & Gomathy, S. (2009). *VisualDx: Essential pediatric dermatology*. Philadelphia, PA: Wolters Kluwer.)

c. With either condition, the affected infant may be born with a collodion membrane. This is when the infant is born in skin that is a tight, shiny membrane, often likened to plastic wrap or a sausage casing.

d. Facial tautness common may be accompanied by ectropion and eclabium that appear shortly after birth in children with LI.

e. The skin of the palms and soles is generally thickened.

f. Cicatricial alopecia may develop as well as thickening of the nails and inflammation of the nail folds.

g. Heat intolerance is common and due to obstruction of the eccrine glands.

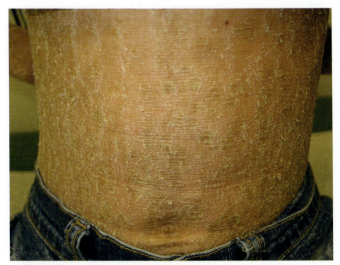

FIGURE 13-15. Lamellar ichthyosis. (Image provided by Stedman's.)

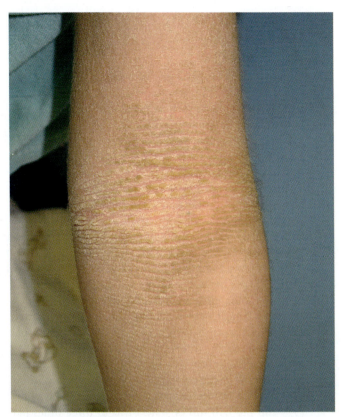

FIGURE 13-16. Epidermolytic ichthyosis with linear scaling reminiscent of "corrugated cardboard." (Image courtesy of CHOP Dermatology.)

4. Epidermolytic ichthyosis (Figure 13-16)

a. Presents at birth with extensive scaling, erythroderma, and recurrent episodes of bullae formation

b. The bullae frequently become infected with *Staphylococcus aureus* causing problems in all ages.

c. With age, the involvement may become more limited in extent, and by school age, thick, warty, malodorous, dirty yellow/brown scales will likely have developed on the palms, soles, elbows, and knees.

d. Flexural areas tend to have greater involvement and frequently become macerated and secondarily colonized with bacteria, producing a foul body odor.

e. Palmoplantar keratoderma affects 60% of patients.

f. After the neonatal period, the mechanobullous component becomes less prominent; however, focal blistering continues.

g. Facial involvement is common, but ectropion does not occur. Nails may become dystrophic due to nail fold inflammation.

B. Diagnostic tests

1. Skin biopsy helps to demonstrate the histologic changes in the epidermis and hyperkeratosis.

2. Measurement of steroid sulfatase activity in red blood cells may be useful in the diagnosis of X-linked ichthyosis.

3. Molecular genetic diagnosis is useful to distinguish the various forms of ichthyosis.

V. NURSING CONSIDERATIONS (TABLE 13-1)

A. Interventions
   1. Skin hydration at least two times daily
   2. Daily use of emollients
      a. Bland emollients such as petrolatum or mineral oil. For example: Aquaphor, Eucerin, Vanicream, CeraVe, Cetaphil, Vaseline, and Aveeno product lines
   3. Keratolytics
      a. Alpha hydroxy acid (lactic acid, urea, glycolic acid) in cream or ointment vehicles. Commercial preparations include Eucerin Plus, Lacticare, Lac-Hydrin, AmLactin, Aqua Glycolic, and Carmol
      b. If available, compounding products of varying concentration is also an option.
   4. Topical retinoids are helpful to some people to remove scaling. These include tretinoin and tazarotene.
   5. Oral retinoids may be used to alleviate the hyperkeratosis. Due to their toxicity, the use is warranted only in patients with severe physical or emotional complications.
   6. Treating active infection with cultures and appropriate antibiotics is of critical importance. Frequency of infection may be minimized by doing dilute bleach baths (1/8 cup per half tub of water) two to three times per week to reduce bacterial colonization of the skin.
   7. Adequate provision of calories in diet, especially protein, and monitoring of child's iron status due to the metabolic drain of erythroderma on a growing child and substantial iron loss in hyperproliferative states
   8. Infants with widespread blistering or collodion membrane are cared for in the NICU with precautions to avoid further trauma to the skin, regulate skin temperature and hydration, as well as prevent infection.
   9. Psychosocial support to deal with issues related to body image, social relationships, and demanding complex therapy
B. Follow-up
   1. One week after discharge from the newborn nursery.
   2. Routine visits for pediatric care and additional visits may be necessary, depending on the severity of the ichthyosis.

PATIENT EDUCATION
Ichthyosis

- Prevent overheating, particularly during strenuous physical activity and/or warm temperatures.
- Bathe with antibacterial soaps or dilute bleach solution to decrease bacterial colonization of skin.
- Consider choice of clothing and shoe wear for children.
- Alert that blistering after infancy often signifies a bacterial infection requiring treatment with an oral antibiotic effective against *S. aureus.*
- Refer to the Ichthyosis Foundation for family support.

HEMANGIOMAS

I. OVERVIEW

A. Definition: benign, vascular tumor comprised of endothelial cells (Figure 13-17)

II. EPIDEMIOLOGY

A. Five to seven percent of newborns have hemangiomas.
B. Approximately 10% of hemangiomas have reached maximal regression with each year of life. For example, 50% of hemangiomas have reached maximal regression by 5 years of age, 90% by 9 years of age, and so on.
C. More common in girls, Caucasians, premature babies, multiple gestations, and in babies whose mothers had maternal hypertension.

III. ETIOLOGY AND PATHOGENESIS

A. The underlying cause of hemangiomas is unknown. Different theories include lack of oxygen to the affected area, trauma to the affected area, and also a small portion of placenta attaching itself to the affected area.

IV. ASSESSMENT

A. Clinical manifestations
   1. Only 20% of hemangiomas are present at birth. The remainder will appear during the first few weeks of life.
   2. Classification of hemangiomas
      a. Superficial hemangiomas—bright red, papular or plaque-like hemangiomas (Figure 13-18)
      b. Deep hemangiomas—blue, nodular hemangiomas (Figure 13-19)
      c. Mixed hemangiomas—contain both a superficial and a deep component (Figure 13-20)
      d. Hemangiomas may be plaque-like/segmental or more discrete.
      e. Rapidly involuting congenital hemangioma (RICH)—fully expressed at birth and quickly involutes

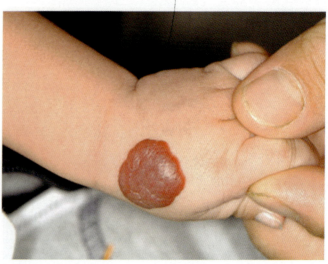

FIGURE 13-17. Cutaneous hemangioma on the hand. (From Nelson, L. B., & Olitsky, S. E. (2013). *Harley's pediatric ophthalmology*. Philadelphia, PA: Wolters Kluwer.)

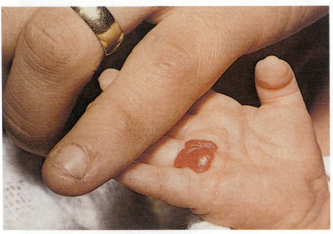

FIGURE 13-18. Superficial hemangioma. (From O'Doherty, N. (1979). *Atlas of the newborn* (pp. 342–345). Philadelphia, PA: JB Lippincott, with permission.)

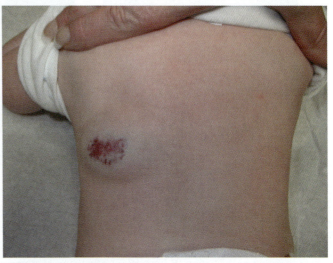

FIGURE 13-20. Mixed hemangioma on the back. These lesions contain both a superficial and a deep component. (Image provided by Stedman's.)

    f. Noninvoluting congenital hemangioma (NICH)—fully expressed at birth but does not resolve over time like typical hemangiomas behave

  3. Characteristics of growth (Figure 13-21)

    a. Rapid growth phase—at 4 to 8 weeks of age, hemangiomas undergo rapid growth that typically continues until the infant is 6 months, with slower growth often continuing until 1 year of age. The rapid growth phase sees the hemangioma growing at a faster rate than the overall growth of the infant. The majority of rapid growth may be complete by 3 months of age.

    b. Stabilization phase—the hemangioma growth slows and approximates the growth rate of the child.

    c. Regression phase—this phase tends to begin sometime in the second year of life with color of the hemangioma fading, followed by flattening of the tumor. This phase slowly continues over a 1- to 10-year period.

  4. Associated complications

    a. Obstruction of a vital function, such as vision, urination, breathing, eating, or defecation (Figure 13-22)

    b. Cardiac, arterial, eye, and reproductive system abnormalities with associated syndromes

    c. High-output cardiac failure and hepatic hemangiomas

    d. Ulceration (Figure 13-23)

    e. Infection

    f. Bleeding

    g. Pain

    h. Undesirable, lasting cosmetic changes such as fibrofatty deposits, stretched skin, and scarring

B. Diagnostic tests

  1. Generally none. Diagnosed by clinical appearance

  2. Occasionally, imaging may be required.

    a. MRI is indicated with midline hemangiomas overlying other defects, such as capillary malformations, sacral dimple, asymmetric gluteal cleft, hair tufts, etc. (Figure 13-24).

    b. Abdominal ultrasound should be performed in patients with 5 or more hemangiomas (hemangiomatosis) to rule out liver hemangiomas (Figure 13-25).

    c. ENT referral with airway evaluation should be obtained for patients with hemangiomas in the "beard distribution" in order to rule out airway obstruction as this may be a medical emergency (Figure 13-26).

    d. Patients with large, plaque-like hemangiomas on the face should be evaluated for PHACE syndrome (Figure 13-27).

    e. Patients with large, plaque-like hemangiomas on the sacral/groin area likely require pelvic/abdominal U/S and/or MRI to rule out associated abnormalities.

  3. Imaging and biopsy may occasionally be required to differentiate hemangiomas from other vascular malformations, lymphatic malformations, or subcutaneous sarcomas.

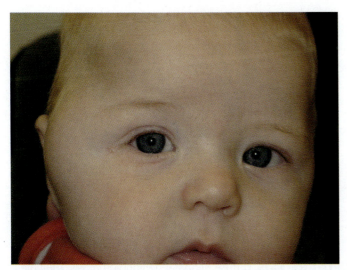

FIGURE 13-19. Deep or subcutaneous hemangioma. Note the normal overlying skin. (Courtesy of Andrea L. Zaenglein, MD.)

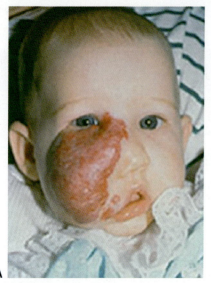 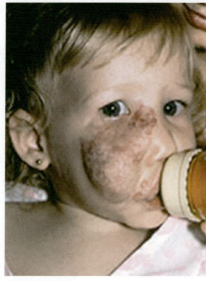 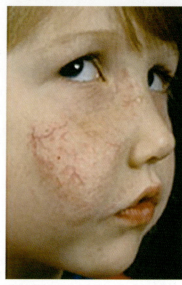

A   B   C

FIGURE 13-21. This girl with a right facial hemangioma demonstrates the three-stage life cycle consisting of rapid growth (**A**, age 3 months), stabilization (**B**, age 18 months), and regression (**C**, age 7 years). (From Thorne, C. H., Gurtner, G. C., Chung, K., Gosain, A., Mehrara, B., Rubin, P., & Spear, S. L. (2013). *Grabb and Smith's plastic surgery*. Philadelphia, PA: Wolters Kluwer.)

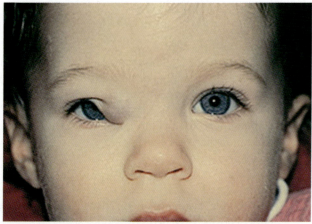

FIGURE 13-22. Hemangioma of the medial upper eyelid. The lesion impairs the visual access and should be treated to prevent long-term vision problems. (From Mulholland, M. W., Lillemoe, K. D., Doherty, G. M., Maier, R. V., & Upchurch, G. R., eds. (2005). *Greenfield's surgery* (4th ed.). Philadelphia, PA: Lippincott Williams & Wilkins, with permission.)

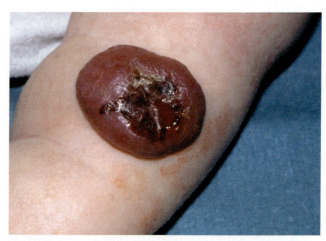

FIGURE 13-23. Ulcerated infantile hemangioma on the arm during the proliferative phase. (From Requena, L., & Kutzner, H. (2014). *Cutaneous soft tissue tumors*. Philadelphia, PA: Wolters Kluwer.)

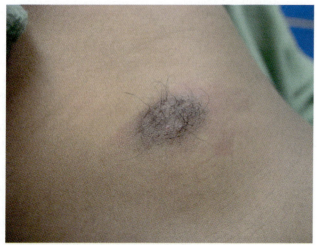

FIGURE 13-24. Lumbar hemangioma. This midline lesion was associated with a dermal sinus and an underlying tethered cord. (Courtesy of Esther K. Chung, MD, MPH.)

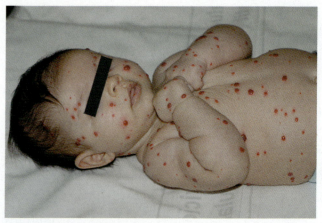

FIGURE 13-25. Diffuse neonatal hemangiomatosis: multiple infantile hemangiomas scattered all over the body surface. (From Requena, L., & Kutzner, H. (2014). *Cutaneous soft tissue tumors*. Philadelphia, PA: Wolters Kluwer.)

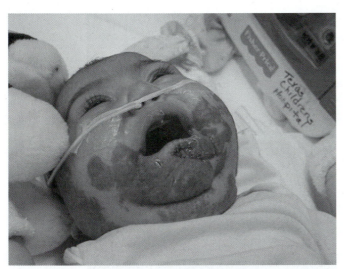

FIGURE 13-26. Segmental mandibular or "beard" hemangioma of infancy in association with hemangioma of infancy of the upper airway. (From McMillan, J. A., DeAngelis, R. D., & Feigin, C. (2006). *Oski's solution.* Philadelphia, PA: Wolters Kluwer.)

V. NURSING CONSIDERATIONS (TABLE 13-1)

A. Interventions

1. In most uncomplicated hemangiomas, the lesions are observed and treated only if complications arise.
2. Measurement of the size of the hemangioma, along with photographs of the lesions at each visit, will document growth and regression.

3. Lesions on the face (particularly forehead, glabella, nose, lips), ears, areolae, and groin are often treated due to potential for disfigurement.
4. Propranolol has become the systemic therapy of choice for most patients requiring medical intervention. After obtaining a thorough cardiac history, auscultating the heart rate and rhythm, and obtaining a blood pressure, the patient is tapered up to a final dose of 2 to 3 mg/kg/d divided BID over a period of several days to a few weeks. The most common side effects are hypotension and decreased heart rate. Hypoglycemia has been reported, so it is recommended to give propranolol after a meal. Propranolol may also "unmask" or aggravate respiratory disease such as asthma and should be used with caution in these patients. It is generally started between 1 and 3 months of age and continued until approximately 1 year of age.
   a. Timolol gel–forming solution, a topical ophthalmic solution for the treatment of glaucoma, may be applied to superficial hemangiomas BID with good results. It does not help with deeper components of hemangiomas but has been shown to reduce the superficial color and some superficial volume.
5. Occasionally, oral or interlesional steroids may be used.
6. Pain management and infection prevention/treatment are often necessary for ulcerated hemangiomas.
7. Vascular-specific pulsed-dye laser is often an effective treatment for ulcerated hemangiomas and for residual erythema after involution of the hemangioma.
8. Hydrocolloid dressings may aid in the resolution of ulcerated hemangiomas.

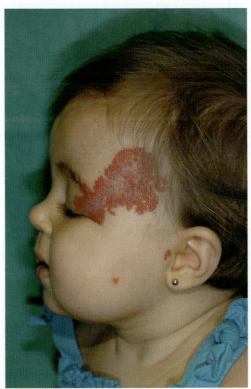
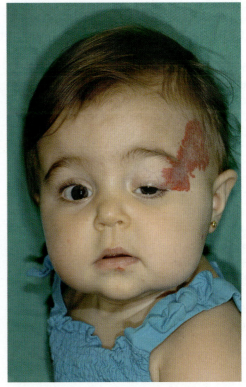

A   **B**

FIGURE 13-27. PHACE syndrome with facial hemangioma. **A, B:** A 6-month-old girl presenting with left facial hemangiomas with secondary ptosis of the left upper eyelid.

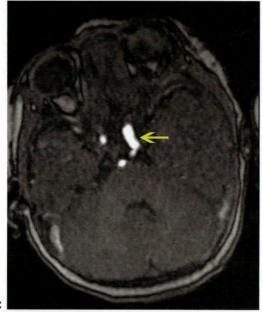
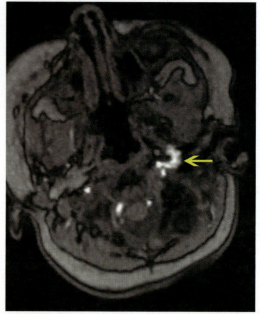

C   D

FIGURE 13-27. (*Continued*) *C, D:* Magnetic resonance images demonstrating an intracranial aneurysm involving the left internal carotid artery extending into the middle cranial fossa (*arrows*). (From Thorne, C. H., Gurtner, G. C., Chung, K., Gosain, A., Mehrara, B., Rubin, P., & Spear, S. L. (2013). *Grabb and Smith's plastic surgery*. Philadelphia, PA: Wolters Kluwer.)

9. Some hemangiomas that ulcerate and do not respond to other therapies may be removed surgically. Additionally, plastic surgery revision may be warranted after maximal involution has occurred if residual cosmetic defects remain.

B. Follow-up

1. Follow closely during rapid growth phase, possibly may need to be seen every month.
2. Once growth is stabilized, time between visits can be lengthened.
3. Children with periorbital hemangiomas should be referred for ophthalmologic evaluation.
4. Children undergoing medical intervention with propranolol will require frequent follow-up visits to assess heart rate, blood pressure, response to therapy, and potential side effects/complications.

Other Common Disorders in Children Covered in This Textbook

- Acne vulgaris—see Chapter 10.
- Atopic dermatitis—see Chapter 9.
- Diaper dermatitis—see Chapter 23.
- Seborrheic dermatitis—see Chapter 9.
- Psoriasis—see Chapter 8.
- Infections—see Chapter 11.
- Bites, stings, and infestations—see Chapter 12.
- Disorders of pigmentation—see Chapter 17.

BIBLIOGRAPHY

Burkes, S. A., Adams, D. M., Hammill, A. M., Chute, C., Eaton, K. P., Welge, J. A., Wickett, R. R., & Visscher, M. O. (2015). Skin imaging modalities quantify progression and stage of infantile haemangiomas. *British Journal of Dermatology, 173*(3), 838–841.

Dixit, S., Jain, A., Datar, S., & Kurhana, V. K. (2012). Congenital miliaria crystallina—A diagnostic dilemma. *Medical Journal Armed Forces India, 68*(4), 386–388.

Dyer, J. A., Spraker, M., & Williams, M. (2013). Care of the newborn with ichthyosis. *Dermatologic Therapy, 26*, 1–15.

Eichenfield, L. F., Frieden, I. J., Mathes, E. F., & Zaenglein, A. L. (2015). *Neonatal and infant dermatology* (3rd ed.). London, UK: Elsevier Saunders.

Enjolras, O. (1997). Management of hemangiomas. *Dermatology Nursing, 9*(1), 11–17.

Filippidi, A., Galanakis, E., Maraki, S., Galani, I., Drogari-Apiranthitou, M., Kalmanti, M., …, Samonis, G. (2013). The effect of maternal flora on *Candida* colonisation in the neonate. *Mycoses, 57*, 43–48.

Fleckman, P., Newell, B. D., van Steensel, M. A., & Yan, A. C. (2013). Topical treatment of ichthyoses. *Dermatologic Therapy, 26*, 16–25.

Ghosh, S. (2015). Neonatal pustular dermatosis: An overview. *Indian Journal of Dermatology, 60*(2), 211.

PATIENT EDUCATION
Hemangiomas

- Review the natural history of hemangiomas.
- State the difficulty in predicting the eventual size, type, final outcome, and need for treatment during the rapid growth phase of the hemangioma.
- Discuss potential complications, as appropriate.
- Review side effects and dosage of any prescribed therapies.
- Teach signs of infection or reaction to additional therapies.

Gomes, M. P. C. L., Porro, A. M., Enokihara, M. M. S. S., & Floriano, M. C. (2013). Subcutaneous fat necrosis of the newborn: Clinical manifestations in two cases. *Anais Brasileiros de Dermatologia, 88*(6, Suppl 1), 154–157.

Masatoshi, J. (2010). Recent progress in studies of infantile hemangioma. *Journal of Dermatology, 37*(4), 283–298.

Neri, I., Balestri, R., & Patrizi, A. (2012). Hemangiomas: New insight and medical treatment. *Dermatologic Therapy, 25*, 322–334.

Paller, A. S., & Manchini, A. J. (2011). *Hurwitz clinical pediatric dermatology* (4th ed.). Edinburgh, UK: Elsevier, Inc.

Paloni, G., Berti, I., & Cutrone, M. (2013). Acropustulosis of infancy. *Archives of Diseases in Childhood. Fetal and Neonatal Edition, 98*, F334–F340.

Rudy, S. J. (1999). Superficial fungal infections in children and adolescents. *Nurse Practitioner Forum, 10*(2), 56–66.

Tawfik, A. A., & Alsharnoubi, J. (2015). Topical timolol solution versus laser in treatment of infantile hemangioma: A comparative study. *Pediatric Dermatology, 32*, 369–376.

Van Praag, M., Van Rooij, R., Folkers, E., Spritzwer, R., Menke, H., & Oranje, A. (1997). Diagnosis and treatment of pustular disorders in the neonate. *Pediatric Dermatology, 14*(2), 131–143.

Weston, W. L., Lane, A. T., & Morelli, J. G. (2002). *Color textbook of pediatric dermatology* (2nd ed.). St. Louis, MO: Mosby Year Book, Inc.

Zuniga, R., & Nguyen, T. (2013). Skin conditions: Common skin rashes in infants. *Family Practice Essentials, 407*, 31–41.

STUDY QUESTIONS

1. Which of the following findings, along with acne neonatorum, would signal the need for a more thorough evaluation and likely referral to an endocrinologist?
   a. Extensive comedonal acne (blackheads)
   b. Early onset of pubic and/or axillary hair
   c. Poor response to initial therapy
   d. Family history of severe acne

2. Cutis marmorata will improve with which of the following interventions?
   a. Rest
   b. Elevation of affected areas
   c. Moving to a warmer environment
   d. Removing excess layers of clothing

3. Which of the following physical findings is associated with harlequin color change?
   a. Bulging veins.
   b. Eyes are two different colors.
   c. Skin is darker on dependent areas.
   d. A white patch on the hair on the scalp.

4. Which of the following subtypes describes miliaria that consists of tiny, clear, vesicular papules that easily, superficially desquamate?
   a. Miliaria crystallina
   b. Miliaria profunda
   c. Miliaria blanca
   d. Miliaria rubra

5. To increase the likelihood of resolution, which of the following interventions should be included in the treatment in infantile oral candidiasis?
   a. Changing diapers frequently
   b. Using BPA-free bottle nipples and pacifiers
   c. Washing hands before feedings
   d. Boiling bottle nipples and pacifiers

6. Which of the following forms of ichthyosis is only found in males?
   a. X-linked
   b. Lamellar
   c. Vulgaris
   d. Bullous

7. Emollients are a hallmark of ichthyosis treatment. Which of the following topical therapies may help to remove some of the excess scale buildup on the skin?
   a. Clindamycin and benzoyl peroxide
   b. Dial soap and bleach baths
   c. Hydrocortisone and tacrolimus
   d. Topical retinoids and keratolytics

8. In addition to asking about side effects and assessing the efficacy of the therapy, which of the following must also be checked prior to initiation and at all follow-up visits for propranolol used in the treatment of hemangiomas of infancy?
   a. Heart rate and blood pressure
   b. Height and blood pressure
   c. Complete blood count
   d. Liver function

9. Which of the following additional tests should a patient with 5 or more hemangiomas undergo?
   a. Eye examination
   b. Abdominal ultrasonography
   c. Sacral magnetic resonance imaging
   d. Electroencephalography

10. Which of the following is a topical therapy option for superficial, uncomplicated hemangioma?
    a. Ammonium lactate
    b. Salicylic acid
    c. Timolol gel
    d. Lidocaine gel

Answers to Study Questions: 1.b, 2.c, 3.c, 4.a, 5.d, 6.a, 7.d, 8.a, 9.b, 10.c

Benign Neoplasms/Hyperplasia

Beth Haney

ACROCHORDONS (SKIN TAGS, PAPILLOMAS, CUTANEOUS TAGS, SOFT FIBROMAS)

I. OVERVIEW

Acrochordons are benign neoplasms. Acrochordons are cosmetic disorders (Figure 14-1).

A. Definition: acrochordons are soft pedunculate, flesh-colored, tan, brown, or pigmented growths, commonly on the neck, shoulders, axillae, groin, inguinal folds, eyelids, upper chest, and trunk. These lesions are asymptomatic but may become irritated or inflamed if exposed to repeated trauma from jewelry, clothing, or opposing skin surfaces.

B. Etiology is not fully understood.

C. Pathophysiology

1. Polyp-type lesion with mildly acanthotic epidermis, a loose, edematous fibrovascular core with mild chronic inflammation and a nerveless dermis

2. Varies in size from 1 to 5 mm although tumors can grow up to 1 cm

3. Single or multiple lesions

D. Incidence

1. Found in approximately 25% of males and females

   a. Increases during middle-aged and older adulthood, pregnancy, acromegaly, menopause, and family history

2. Equal in males and females

3. Associated with obesity

4. Frequently higher in diabetics

5. After the fifth decade, there is no further growth

II. ASSESSMENT

A. History and current health status

B. Diagnosis by clinical presentation: location, color, number, size, irritation, tenderness, and inflammation

C. Biopsy recommended if pigmented or erythematous

III. COMMON THERAPEUTIC MODALITIES

A. Electrodesiccation

B. Scalpel or simple scissor excision at the base of the lesion

C. Cryosurgery

IV. HOME CARE CONSIDERATIONS

A. Wound care (Box 14-1)

B. Control bleeding.

C. Watch for signs of infection.

PATIENT EDUCATION
Acrochordons

- Acrochordons can become easily irritated or infected.
- Patients may avoid complications if they:
  - Cover lesion(s) with bandage when clothing or jewelry irritates the lesion(s).
  - Lose weight if appropriate.
  - Keep skin folds clean and dry.
  - Monitor lesion(s) for changes in size, color, or pain.
  - See a health care provider for lesion removal options.

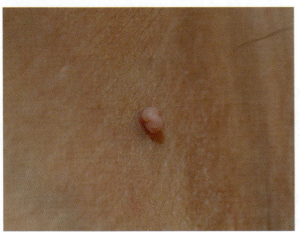
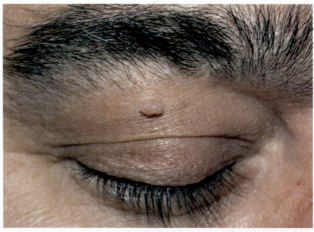

FIGURE 14-1. A: This soft, pedunculated skin tag, or acrochordon, is typical of a fibroepithelial polyp. Skin tags are most common in skinfolds such as the crural crease and axillae. **B:** Eyelid acrochordon. (From Edwards, L., & Lynch, P. J. (2010). *Genital dermatology atlas*. Philadelphia, PA: Wolters Kluwer; Goodheart, H. P. (2003). *Goodheart's photoguide of common skin disorders* (2nd ed.). Philadelphia, PA: Lippincott Williams & Wilkins.)

CALLUSES

I. OVERVIEW

A. Definition: a callus is an elevated superficial, diffusely thickened hyperkeratotic area, usually without a distinct border. Calluses are nontender, but pressure may produce dull pain (Figure 14-2).

B. Etiology
  1. Repeated friction or pressure

C. Pathophysiology
  1. Normal response to friction or pressure; increased activity of keratinocytes in superficial layer of skin leading to hyperkeratosis

D. Incidence
  1. Frequently on palms and weight-bearing surfaces of the foot
  2. Increases with age, women affected more often than men

II. ASSESSMENT

A. Physical examination

B. History of chronic pressure or friction

C. Examination of footwear may assist in assessment.

III. COMMON THERAPEUTIC MODALITIES

A. Topical keratolytics (urea, ammonium lactate), 40% salicylic acid plaster, or ointment.
  1. Use OTC keratolytic preparations as directed. Forms include a patch, lotions, foam, gel, and cream. Apply keratolytic plaster, sticky medicated side to skin, making sure plaster covers the affected area. Cover the plaster with adhesive tape for 1 to 7 days.
  2. Avoid normal skin to prevent irritation and skin damage.
  3. Soak the area in warm water after removing the tape. Rub the soft macerated skin with a rough towel or pumice stone. Reapply the plaster and repeat the process until all hyperkeratotic skin is removed.

BOX 14-1. Wound Care

- Keep dressing dry and in place for 24 to 48 hours as ordered.
- Clean site with soap and water two to three times a day as ordered. Do not apply alcohol or peroxide. Pat site dry.
- Apply antibiotic ointment to keep site moist, two times a day and cover with appropriate dressing.
- If bleeding or oozing occurs at the site, gently apply pressure with a clean gauze for 20 minutes. The bleeding/oozing should stop within 25 minutes; if not, call the office.
- Watch for signs of infection: redness, swelling, pain, heat, pus, and temp greater than 101. Take non-aspirin product for pain and discomfort—Tylenol, if not allergic. Avoid Aleve, Advil, Motrin, ibuprofen, and aspirin products.

Adapted from: Butcher, M. (2013). Assessment, management, and prevention of infected wounds. *Journal of Community Nursing, 27*(4), 25–34.

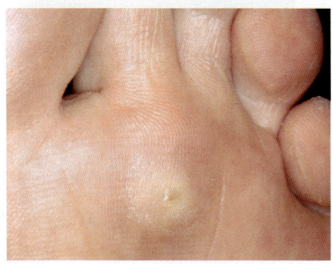

FIGURE 14-2. Corn in a typical location over a metatarsal head. (From Craft, N., et al. (2010). *VisualDx: Essential adult dermatology*. Philadelphia, PA: Wolters Kluwer.)

B. Orthopedic shoes, braces, and support devices to redistribute weight.

C. Epsom salt soaks for 5 to 10 minutes several times a day.

D. Geriatric considerations: salicylic acid treatments can cause breakdown and/or ulceration of thin, atrophic skin, people with diabetes, and those with vascular compromise; use these products with caution. Use of protective padding. Avoid activities that contribute to painful lesion formation.

E. Patient education is similar to recommendations for corns in the next section.

CORNS (CLAVI)

I. OVERVIEW

Corns are found over bony prominences such as the interphalangeal joints of toes (Figure 14-3).

A. Definition: circumscribed, hyperkeratotic, slightly elevated lesion with a central conical core of keratin resulting in a thickening of the stratum corneum. These lesions cause pain and inflammation. "Hard" corns are frequently over the interphalangeal toe joints, especially the fifth toe, and develop under the pressure site from footwear. "Hard" corns are usually painful: dull constant pain or sharp pain when pressure is applied. "Soft" corns appear as whitish thickening, usually in the interdigital spaces between the fourth and fifth toes.

B. Etiology

1. Repeated external pressure creates localized accumulation of keratin.

2. Soft corns result from moisture leading to maceration of the skin and mechanical irritation.

3. Hard corns have a keratin-based core and are usually associated with bony prominences that cause skin to rub on shoe surfaces.

C. Pathophysiology

1. Localized pinpoint accumulation of keratin forms an elongated, hard plug in the horny layer of the epidermis. The plug presses downward on the dermal structure, causing inflammation and irritation of sensory nerves, resulting in marked tenderness.

II. ASSESSMENT

A. Physical examination

B. History related to footwear, working conditions, foot surgery, previous similar lesions

III. COMMON THERAPEUTIC MODALITIES

A. Surgical excision of superficial layer of corn and hard plug in the horny layer

B. Corticosteroids: triamcinolone injection (Kenalog, Aristocort) at base of the corn to relieve pain

C. Topical keratolytics

D. Epsom salt soaks every few hours for 5 to 10 minutes at a time

IV. HOME CARE CONSIDERATIONS

A. Encourage proper-fitting shoes: extra wide for fifth metatarsal corns.

B. Debridement of corn and use of protective padding.

C. Avoidance of activities that cause pain or create lesions.

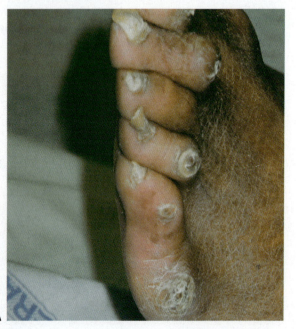
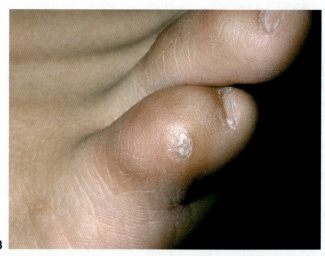

FIGURE 14-3. A: Corns and calluses. **B:** Corn with callus on lateral toe surface. (From Berg, D., & Worzala, K. (2006). *Atlas of adult physical diagnosis*. Philadelphia, PA: Lippincott Williams & Wilkins; and Craft, N., et al. (2010). *VisualDx: Essential adult dermatology*. Philadelphia, PA: Wolters Kluwer.)

CYSTS

I. OVERVIEW

A cyst is a benign, sac-like growth in the skin layers, which originates from the follicle orifice (Figure 14-4). Types of cysts may include epidermal, epidermal inclusion, epidermoid, keratinous, pilar, infundibular, sebaceous, and acne.

A. Definition: a circumscribed lesion with a wall and a lumen that usually contains fluid or solid matter.

B. Etiology: spontaneous, trauma, or congenital.
  1. Cyst wall probably formed from occluded pilosebaceous follicles.
  2. Result of cutaneous surface trauma and a portion of the epithelium is forced into the superficial dermis.

C. Pathophysiology: cyst ruptures and keratin is released, causing an inflammatory foreign body response.

D. Incidence.
  1. Higher incidence in young and middle-aged males; increases with a family history
  2. Multiple lesions (70%)
  3. Solitary (30%)

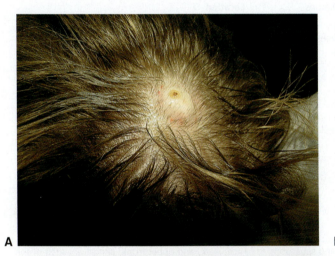

A

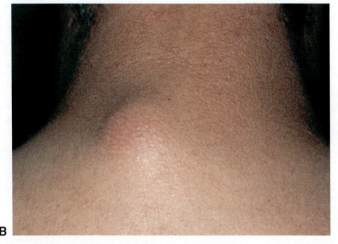

B

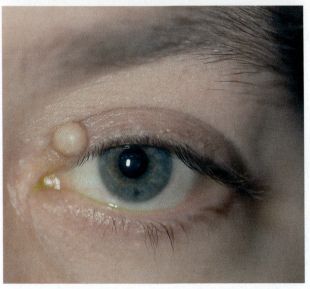

C

FIGURE 14-4. A: Pilar cyst on the scalp. **B:** Epidermoid cyst. These lesions often occur on the back. They appear as smooth, discrete, freely movable, dome-shaped ballotable masses. **C:** Epidermal inclusion cyst showing the typical characteristics of yellow color and telangiectasis. (From Stedman's; Goodheart, H. P. (2003). *Goodheart's photoguide of common skin disorders* (2nd ed.). Philadelphia, PA: Lippincott Williams & Wilkins; and Penne, R. B. (2011). *Wills Eye Institute—Oculoplastics.* Philadelphia, PA: Wolters Kluwer.)

II. ASSESSMENT

Diagnosis by clinical presentation and examination of expressed material confirmation by biopsy (Table 14-1)

A. Location
B. Number
C. Size
D. Firmness
E. Mobility
F. Globular
G. Tenderness
H. Inflammation
I. Infection

III. COMMON THERAPEUTIC MODALITIES

A. Cure by complete excision or punch biopsy for 1- to 2-cm uncomplicated lesions including wall to prevent recurrence
B. Incision and drainage of infected or severely inflamed cysts

C. Intralesional corticosteroid injections (triamcinolone, Aristocort, Kenalog) to decrease lesion size
D. Extraction: comedone extractor for small cysts or milia.

IV. HOME CARE CONSIDERATIONS

A. Wound care (Box 14-1)

PATIENT EDUCATION
Cysts

- Cyst changes, including growth, tenderness, or irritation, need to be monitored.
- Surgical removal may be necessary with close follow-up of healing.
- Health care provider should be consulted with any increased pain that occurs or signs of infection that develop, that is, redness, heat, swelling, and discharge.

TABLE 14-1 Characteristics of Cysts

Type	Common Names	Location
Atheroma Derived from the root sheath of the hair follicle. Globular, elastic, mobile tumor covered with atrophic thin skin, thick wall, filled with keratin, is not connected to the epidermis, and is without external opening. Tender if infected. Baldness over large cyst skin due to follicular pressure damage. No inflammation or proliferation from trauma. No malignant degeneration	Pilar cyst, trichilemmal cyst Archaic names: Wen	>90% Scalp, hair follicle epithelium
Retention cyst Spherical, mobile, firm under tense skin. Ruptures easily by manipulation. Keratinous material can be pressed into the surrounding tissue and then acts as a foreign body and can cause granuloma abscess formation from bacterial infection.	Milia, acne cysts, and traumatic inclusion cysts	Face, trunk, hair follicles areas, scalp, neck, back, and cheeks One millimeter to several centimeters in diameter Cutaneous or subcutaneous—fluctuant, easily movable, tense, swelling Expanded gland duct and foul-smelling rancid lipids and debris will reoccur if wall remains intact.
Sebocystomatosis Central opening exudes a pasty, cheesy odoriferous material composed of keratin and lipid-rich debris	Sebaceous cysts (fat)	Young–middle-aged adults. Scalp, face, neck, upper trunk, scrotum, and vulva
Keratinous cyst Firm, movable, globular, and nontender unless infected. Contents are soft and yellow–white, with a rancid odor	Epidermal and sebaceous	Face, neck, and upper trunk, almost any area of the body
Milium Primary milia arise spontaneously and are keratin filled. Secondary milia arise in pilosebaceous glands or within damaged eccrine sweat gland ducts following subepidermal bulla formation (e.g., epidermolysis bullosa, porphyria cutanea tarda, bullous pemphigoid) or skin radiotherapy. Primary and secondary milia are identical histologically.	Subepidermal cyst	Eyelids, forehead, and cheeks Young to middle-aged men and women and infants Tiny (1–2 mm), superficial, white dome-shaped cysts
Dermoid cyst Present at birth		Deep subcutaneous tissue Walls composed of keratinizing epidermis containing hair follicles, sebaceous glands, and sweat glands
Epidermoid cyst Occurs secondary to traumatic implantation of epidermal cells into the dermis. Contains accumulation of keratin and is encased by a well-formed granular layer of stratified squamous epithelium	Epidermal inclusion cyst	Most common on face, back, chest and base of ears although can occur on almost any skin surface.

Adapted from Goldstein, B. G., & Goldstein, A. O. (2014a). Overview of benign lesions of the skin. Retrieved 27 March, 2014 from http://www.uptodate.com/contents/overview-of-benign-lesions-of-the-skin?source=search_result&search=calluses&selectedTitle=2%7E16#H1101420580; Goldstein, B. G., & Goldstein, A. O. (2014b). Keloids. Retrieved 23 April, 2014 from http://www.uptodate.com/contents/keloids?source=search_result&search=keloid+scar&selectedTitle=1%7E150; Wolff, K., Johnson, R. A., & Saadvedra, A. P. (2013). *Fitzpatrick's color atlas & synopsis of clinical dermatology* (5th ed.). New York, NY: McGraw-Hill; Habif, T. P. (2016). *Clinical dermatology: A color guide to diagnosis and therapy* Philadelphia, PA: Elsevier.

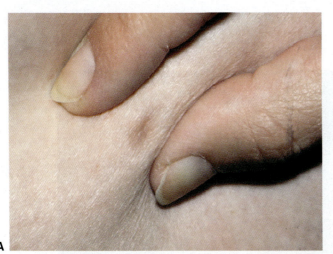 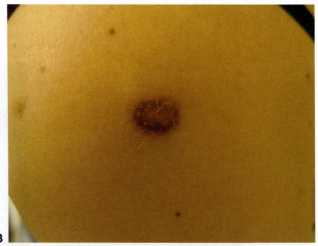

FIGURE 14-5. A: Dermatofibroma: "dimple" or "collar button" sign is elicited on compression of a lesion. **B:** Pigmented dermatofibroma. (From Goodheart, H. P. (2003). *Goodheart's photoguide of common skin disorders* (2nd ed.). Philadelphia, PA: Lippincott Williams & Wilkins; and Stedman's.)

DERMATOFIBROMA (FIBROMA)

I. OVERVIEW

A. Definition: a benign lesion of fibrous connective tissue (Figure 14-5)
B. Etiology
   1. The exact cause is unknown.
   2. Considered to be a late histiocytic reaction to trauma, viral infection, or insect bite.
C. Pathophysiology
   1. Interwoven histiocytes and collagen mesh dermal nodule, with overlying epidermal hyperplasia
D. Incidence
   1. Frequently occurs in middle age; dominant in females
   2. Usually solitary but may be multiple, randomly scattered
   3. Anterior surface of the lower extremities most commonly

II. ASSESSMENT

A. Asymptomatic or may be pruritic, single or multiple, or papule or nodules.
B. Firm, hemispherical disc/dome-shaped borders are ill defined.
C. Color: skin colored, reddish, or tan to brown.
D. Texture of surface may be shiny, dull, scaling, or crusted secondary to trauma from shaving or excoriation.
E. Surrounding ring of pigmentation; 2 to 3 cm and less.
F. Can be found anywhere on trunk or extremities, but commonly on lower legs
G. "Dimples" when gently pinched between the thumb and forefinger (retraction or "dimple" sign)
H. Diagnosis by clinical presentation; confirmation biopsy

III. COMMON THERAPEUTIC MODALITIES

A. Excision for cosmetic reasons only
B. Cryosurgery every 3 to 4 weeks causes gradual involution and elimination of remaining pigment

IV. HOME CARE CONSIDERATIONS

A. The healing area may remain hard if a portion of the fibrous material remains after treatment.
B. Wound care (Box 14-1).

HYPERTROPHIC SCARS

I. OVERVIEW

Hypertrophic scars result from skin trauma in genetically predisposed individuals. Characterized by excess of collagen deposition during wound healing causing an inappropriately large scar usually within 4 weeks of injury. Histologically, hypertrophic scars differ from keloids in that they contain whorls of young, fibrous tissue and fibroblasts in uneven arrangements (Figure 14-6).

II. ASSESSMENT

A. Asymptomatic, pruritic or painful occasionally, and *restricted to the area of injury*
B. Commonly over the sternum, deltoid, mandible, or upper lip but can occur anywhere in predisposed people
C. Less exuberant than keloids
D. Diagnosis by clinical exam, biopsy not warranted unless there is clinical doubt because another procedure to the skin may include further hypertrophic scarring

III. COMMON THERAPEUTIC MODALITIES

A. Involute spontaneously
B. Resolve, mostly or partially, becoming flatter and softer in time without treatment
C. Intralesional glucocorticoid injections
D. Prevention of additional injuries

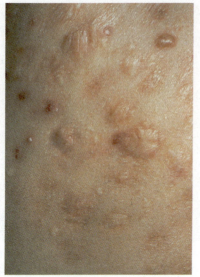 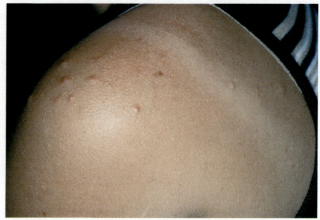

A   B

FIGURE 14-6. A: Hypertrophic scars; characteristic of acne scars that occur on the trunk. **B:** Hypertrophic acne scars are seen on the shoulder of this patient. (From Goodheart, H. P. (2003). *Goodheart's photoguide of common skin disorders* (2nd ed.). Philadelphia, PA: Lippincott Williams & Wilkins.)

KELOIDS

I. OVERVIEW

Keloids are proliferations of connective tissues (collagen) that cause large collagen bundles at the site of a scar or traumatic injuries such as acne, vaccination sites, or thermal or chemical burns. Keloid scars extend in a claw-like fashion beyond the border of original injury and may also develop spontaneously, usually in the presternal area. Keloids may begin years after the original injury and may continue to expand in size for decades (Figure 14-7).

A. Description: nodular, nonencapsulated, highly hyperplastic mass of scar tissue *beyond* injury/trauma border resulting from overproduction of extracellular matrix and dermal fibroblasts.

B. Keloids begin as pink to red, firm, rubbery fibrous plaques with telangiectasias; 3 to 5 weeks to years after trauma. They are smooth, circumscribed, irregularly shaped, and hyperpigmented, sometimes bright red or bluish. May become tender and pruritic, particularly in the early stages of development. Enlargement and extension outside the original area of injury.

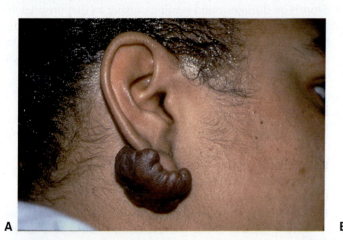 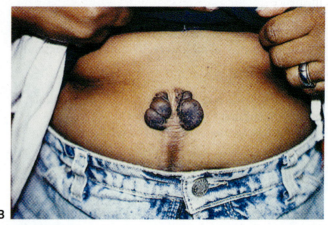

A   B

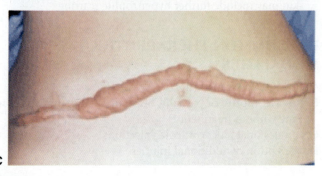

C

FIGURE 14-7. A: Keloid: Developed as a reaction to having her earlobe pierced. **B:** Keloid beyond border of surgical scar. **C:** Keloid scarring, which grows like a tumor and flows over the scar boundary, occurs wherever the skin is breached. Its pathogenesis and treatment are different from those of hypertrophic scars. (From Rubin, E., & Farber, J. L. (1999). *Pathology* (3rd ed.). Philadelphia, PA: Lippincott Williams & Wilkins; and Weber, J., & Kelley, J. (2003). *Health assessment in nursing* (2nd ed.). Philadelphia, PA: Lippincott Williams & Wilkins.)

C. More prevalent among African Americans and people with blood type A.

D. Not present at birth and rare before puberty.

E. Increased prevalence in patients with severe acne and hidradenitis suppurativa.

F. Frequently affected areas are the earlobes (after piercing), face, neck, abdomen, chest, and upper back.

II. ASSESSMENT

A. History of burn, acne, injury, surgery, or other trauma to site

B. Physical exam: location, size, color, tenderness, pain, pruritus, and burning

III. COMMON THERAPEUTIC MODALITIES

A. Prevention by avoiding accidental and intentional skin trauma if prone to keloid

B. Intralesional corticosteroid injections

C. Combination surgical excision and intralesional steroid injections

D. Pulsed dye laser treatment, multiple treatments may be necessary

E. Surgical excision with radiation therapy

F. Radiation therapy to keloids not appropriate for resection

G. Cryosurgery more effective on lesions less than 2 years old

H. Topical silicone gel sheeting may minimize scarring extent and promote gradual resolution

---

PATIENT EDUCATION
Scars and Keloids

- Patients prone to scarring or keloid formation should avoid elective or unnecessary surgery or procedures whenever possible, that is, ear piercing, tattooing, or cosmetic mole removal.
- The injured/scarred area must be protected from further trauma or irritation.
- Wounds should be covered and remain moist to promote healing.
- Avoid sun exposure during healing and posthealing to the area to avoid hyperpigmentation.
- The neck and leg areas should not be shaved while healing as this can irritate pimples or ingrown hairs and cause hypertrophic scar formation.

LIPOMA

I. OVERVIEW

A. Definition: subcutaneous fatty tissue with fine capsule (Figure 14-8). Most common of the benign soft tissue neoplasms

B. Etiology is not well understood.

C. Incidence
   1. Solitary or multiple; asymmetric irregular distribution
   2. Equal sex

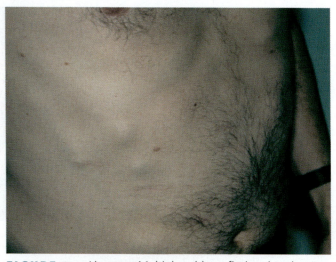

FIGURE 14-8. Lipomas. Multiple rubbery flesh-colored nodules are noted on this patient. (From Goodheart, H. P. (2003). *Goodheart's photoguide of common skin disorders* (2nd ed.). Philadelphia, PA: Lippincott Williams & Wilkins.)

II. ASSESSMENT

A. Soft, rounded, without central pore

B. Freely moveable against overlying skin, slightly compressible

C. Usually small but can enlarge to over 6 cm

D. Frequently occurs on the neck, truck, and extremities most commonly but can occur anywhere

III. COMMON THERAPEUTIC MODALITIES

A. No therapy is necessary when diagnosis is confirmed

B. Surgical excision only if causes pain or is considered disfiguring

SEBACEOUS HYPERPLASIA

I. OVERVIEW

These lesions involve hypertrophy of the sebaceous glands and are generally located on the central face of adults. Etiology unknown. Incidence: seen more often in fair-skinned individuals; these lesions occur after age 30 in 25% of the general population occurs in solid organ transplant recipients (Figure 14-9).

II. ASSESSMENT

A. Solitary lesion, umbilicated and cauliflower-like

B. Multiple soft yellowish and erythematous papules 1 to 3 mm in size, on the forehead and cheeks

C. Surface telangiectasis in the valleys between the small, yellow lobules

D. Asymptomatic; persist unless treated

E. Diagnosis by physical examination

F. Differentiated from basal cell carcinoma (BCC) which usually have recent history of changes and are not yellow in color

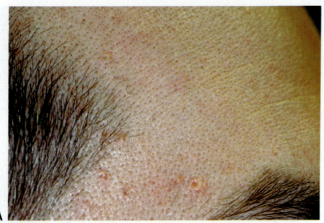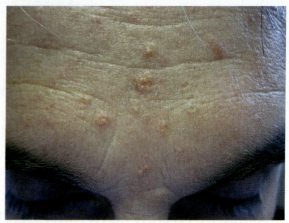

FIGURE 14-9. A: Sebaceous hyperplasia on the temporal area. **B:** Sebaceous hyperplasia on the forehead. Note yellowish papules with dells. (From Goodheart, H. P. (2010). *Goodheart's same-site differential diagnosis: A rapid method of diagnosing and treating common skin disorders.* Philadelphia, PA: Wolters Kluwer.)

III. COMMON THERAPEUTIC MODALITIES

A. No treatment necessary except for patient's request for cosmetic improvement
B. Low-dose isotretinoin (Accutane)
 1. Normal liver function
 2. Not currently pregnant or planning pregnancy for at least 1 month after therapy cessation
 3. Lesions reappear weeks or months after discontinuation of treatment.
C. Light electrocautery
D. Liquid nitrogen cryosurgery
E. Shave excision
F. Carbon dioxide laser
G. Trichloroacetic acid peels

PATIENT EDUCATION
Sebaceous Hyperplasia

- Lesions are benign, but if any changes, visit a health care provider.
- In severe cases, a medication (isotretinoin) may be used to clear up the lesions but will require regular tests and ongoing treatment.
- There are remedies such as peels and laser treatments that may help reduce the lesions.

SEBORRHEIC KERATOSIS

I. OVERVIEW

A. Definition: benign, warty-appearing growths commonly seen on older adults. These lesions are superficial epithelial growths that are raised, well defined, scaly, and hyperpigmented that have a "stuck-on" appearance. Seborrheic keratosis (SK) is the most common benign cutaneous neoplasm (Figure 14-10). Types include seborrheic wart, senile wart, brown wart, and basal cell papilloma.
 1. Slow growing
 2. Round—oval
 3. "Greasy, stuck on the skin"
 4. Hyperkeratotic lesions
 5. Varied size from millimeters to centimeters
 6. Color from flesh colored to brown to black
 7. Common on the face, trunk, shoulders, scalp, and back, although they can appear on any hair-bearing surface
 8. Develop in sun exposed as well as protected areas
 9. Do not contain the human papillomaviruses
B. Tendency to develop SK is an autosomal dominant trait and is extremely common; it has been found in 88% of people older than 65 years and is more prevalent in white-skinned individuals.
C. Pathophysiology: benign proliferations of immature epidermal keratinocytes; keratinization occurs, causing the lesions to become warty, dry, fissured, and at times crumbly appearing. Initially flat, coin-sized lesion with flesh-brown pigmentation that develops into papillomatous hemispherical raised tumors with dark brown to black pigmentation. A keratotic, conical protuberance (cutaneous horn) or open comedones may develop.
D. Incidence: hereditary, common in middle-aged and older adults with onset by age 30; equal sex; more numerous, smaller, and occur earlier in African Americans and Hispanics. A family history predispose to development, although it is not thought to be caused by chronic sun exposure.

II. ASSESSMENT

A. History and current health status
B. Physical exam: location, size, number, appearance, color, borders, pruritus, changes, and irritation—erythema, tenderness, and increased pruritus
C. Diagnosis by clinical presentation and confirmation by biopsy

III. COMMON THERAPEUTIC MODALITIES

A. No treatment is necessary if small and asymptomatic
B. Snip or shave excision
C. Electrodesiccation and curettage
D. Cryosurgery
E. Carbon dioxide laser

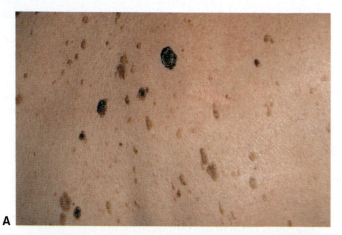

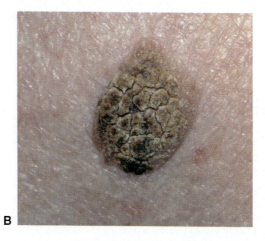

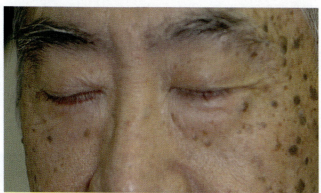

FIGURE 14-10. A: Seborrheic keratoses. These "stuck-on" appearing lesions are most often confused with malignant melanoma by nondermatologists. **B:** Seborrheic keratosis. This lesion has a warty, tortoise shell-like, "stuck-on" appearance. **C:** Seborrheic keratosis. (From Goodheart, H. P. (2003). *Goodheart's photoguide of common skin disorders* (2nd ed.). Philadelphia, PA: Lippincott Williams & Wilkins; and Goodheart, H. P. (2010). *Goodheart's same-site differential diagnosis: A rapid method of diagnosing and treating common skin disorders*. Philadelphia, PA: Wolters Kluwer.)

PATIENT EDUCATION
Seborrheic Keratoses

- Clothing, belts, and razors can easily irritate existing lesions.
- Lesions frequently irritated need to be monitored for bleeding, redness, and changes.
- Lesions can be easily removed with an office procedure when the number is limited.
- Post-treatment area needs to be kept clean, moist, and covered until healed.
- After lesion removal, the sites needs to be monitored for signs of infection.

D. Usually appear around 30 years old
E. Occur most commonly on trunk
F. Virtually all elderly people will have a few lesions.

III. COMMON THERAPEUTIC MODALITIES

A. Electrocautery (cryotherapy is not effective)
B. Laser coagulation
C. Scissor excision

CHERRY ANGIOMA

I. OVERVIEW

A. Definition: the most common vascular malformation is the benign cherry angioma. Histologically, the lesions are made up of numerous moderately dilated capillaries lined with flattened endothelial cells. The stroma is of homogenous collagen and edematous (Figure 14-11).

II. ASSESSMENT

A. Bright red to violaceous or black
B. Dome shaped
C. Tiny to about 3 mm

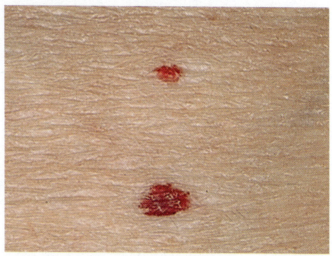

FIGURE 14-11. Cherry angioma. (From Bickley, L. S., & Szilagyi, P. (2013). *Bates' guide to physical examination and history taking* (11th ed.). Philadelphia, PA: Lippincott Williams & Wilkins.)

D. Treatment is only necessary if the condition is bothersome to the patient.

PATIENT EDUCATION

Cherry Angioma

- As these lesions are vascular, the patient needs to avoid picking or irritating the lesions as they will bleed, sometimes profusely.
- Patients should be advised that even after successful treatment, new lesions will likely develop.
- There is no way to prevent lesions.

BIBLIOGRAPHY

Burhan, J. K., & Mak, B. M. (2013). Cyst, sebaceous. In F. J. Domino, R. A. Baldor, J. Golding, J. A. Grimes, & J. A. Taylor (Eds.), *The 5 minute clinical consult* (21st ed., pp. 326–327). Philadelphia, PA: Lippincott Williams & Wilkins.

Butcher, M. (2013). Assessment, management, and prevention of infected wounds. *Journal of Community Nursing, 27*(4), 25–34.

Dunphy, L. M., Winland-Brown, J. E., Porter, B. O., & Thomas, D. J. (2011). *Primary care: The art and science of advanced practice nursing* (3rd ed.). Philadelphia, PA: F.A. Davis and Co.

Feldman, N. J. (2013). Corns and calluses. In F. Domino, R. Baldor, J. Golding, J. A Grimes, & J. S. Taylor (Eds.), *The 5 minute clinical consult 2013* (21st ed., pp. 304–305). Philadelphia, PA: Lippincott Williams & Wilkins.

Goldstein, B. G., & Goldstein, A. O. (2014a). Overview of benign lesions of the skin. Retrieved 27 March, 2014 from http://www.uptodate.com/contents/overview-of-benign-lesions-of-the-skin?source=search_result&search=calluses&selectedTitle=2%7E16#H1101420580

Goldstein, B. G., & Goldstein, A. O. (2014b). Keloids. Retrieved 23 April, 2014 from http://www.uptodate.com/contents/keloids?source=search_result&search=keloid+scar&selectedTitle=1%7E150

Habif, T. P. (2016). *Clinical dermatology: A color guide to diagnosis and therapy* (6th ed.). Philadelphia, PA: Elsevier.

Safoury, O. S., & Ibrahim, M. (2011). A clinical evaluation of skin tags in relation to obesity, type 2 diabetes mellitus, age, and sex. *Indian Journal of Dermatology, 56*(4), 393–397.

Wolff, K., Johnson, R. A., & Saadvedra, A. P. (2013). *Fitzpatrick's color atlas & synopsis of clinical dermatology* (5th ed.). New York, NY: McGraw-Hill.

STUDY QUESTIONS

1. Acrochordons are benign neoplasms and cosmetic disorders with which of the following features?
   a. Soft pedunculate
   b. Flesh colored, tan, or brown
   c. Can evolve into precancerous lesions
   d. A and B
   e. All of the above

2. Calluses are caused by all of the above *except*:
   a. Spontaneous development
   b. External pressure
   c. Repeated friction
   d. All of the above

3. Appropriate treatment for corns includes which of the following?
   a. Surgical excision of superficial layer of corn and hard plug in the horny layer
   b. Corticosteroids: triamcinolone injection (Kenalog, Aristocort) at the base of the corn to relieve pain
   c. Topical keratolytics
   d. Epsom salt soaks every few hours for 5 to 10 minutes at a time
   e. All of the above

4. All of the following are common therapeutic modalities for cysts *except*:
   a. Complete excision and wall removal
   b. Incision and drainage
   c. Intralesional corticosteroid injections
   d. All of the above

5. Dermatofibroma is:
   a. Caused by spontaneous development of localized accumulation of fibroblasts or a reaction to an insect bite
   b. A benign lesion composed of stratum corneum cells
   c. Considered to be an early histiocytic reaction to an insult such as trauma or viral infection
   d. A precancerous lesion that develops from accumulation of keratinocytes

6. Hypertrophic scars can involute spontaneously.
   a. True
   b. False

7. Keloid development can:
   a. Continue in the same area of injury for decades
   b. Never appear on the face
   c. Be found in only the upper third of the chest
   d. All of the above

8. Lipomas are the most common of the benign soft tissue neoplasms.
   a. True
   b. False

9. Characteristics of sebaceous hyperplasia include which of the following?
   a. Small, solitary lesion, umbilicated, cauliflower-like
   b. Multiple soft yellowish and erythematous papules 2 to 3 cm in size, on forehead and cheeks
   c. Surface telangiectasis in the forehead
   d. Painful unless treated
   e. All of the above

10. Seborrheic keratosis is an autosomal dominant trait and is extremely common; it has been found in 88% of people older than 65 years and is more prevalent in white-skinned individuals.
    a. True
    b. False

Answers to Study Questions: 1.d, 2.a, 3.e, 4.d, 5.a, 6.a, 7.a, 8.a, 9.a, 10.a

CHAPTER 15

Photodamage, Photodermatoses, and Aging Skin

Kara Addison • Karrie Fairbrother

OBJECTIVES

After studying this chapter, the reader will be able to:

- Define and list the etiology of photodamage and aging skin.
- Discuss the etiology, pathophysiology, and various treatments of photodermatoses including actinic keratosis, lentigines, polymorphous light eruption, sunburn, porphyria cutanea tarda, and solar urticaria.
- List and promote the widely available methods of protecting the skin from damage by the sun.

KEY POINTS

- Photodamage is a cumulative damage to the skin caused by ultraviolet radiation, which can start as early as childhood and continues through one's entire lifespan.
- Phototoxic and photoallergic reactions occur in the presence of an exogenous agent, which absorbs the ultraviolet radiation. Phototoxicity is more common than photoallergic reaction.
- Sunburn is caused by excessive ultraviolet radiation, which can present with many symptoms including pain, pruritus, edema, vesicles, or bulla.
- Clinical knowledge on the various degrees of risk that accompany many common skin diseases, their behavioral, genetics, environmental causes, and effective treatments needs to be communicated to patients and families.
- Patients require prospective education about skin changes and skin disorders caused by ultraviolet radiation in order to be ready to seek appropriate dermatology care when indicated.
- Nurses are in the best position to educate communities, families, and individuals on the importance of ultraviolet protection.
- The best sunscreens are those that block both ultraviolet A and ultraviolet B rays (broad spectrum). Sunscreen should be used continually throughout a patient's life. No one is too old to slow down skin damage from ultraviolet exposure.

PHOTODAMAGE

I. OVERVIEW

Photodamage is exposure of the skin to ultraviolet (UV) radiation, which causes cumulative damage to all skin types starting in childhood through adult years. Variations in susceptibility, damage classification, presentation, and pathologies can be traced to climate conditions, genetic inheritance, and personal behavior patterns. Systematic treatment options include surgery, a wide variety of chemical applications and injections, cosmetic and laser therapies, and patient education to change the choices that induce preventable damage (Figure 15-1).

A. Definition: a term describing the skin of individuals who have been chronically exposed to UV radiation. The condition is identified by clinical and histologic findings.

B. Etiology (Figure 15-2).
   1. Damage caused by UV exposure starts in early childhood.
   2. The promotion of sun protection is a relatively recent campaign. Many older individuals were unprotected and vulnerable to sunburn in the past.
   3. Both ultraviolet A (UVA) and ultraviolet B (UVB) rays play a significant role in damaging the skin.
   4. Other influences on photodamage include: wind, chemical exposure, and the mechanics of smoking and tobacco smoke.

C. Pathophysiology.
   1. Melanin is the basic physiologic sunscreen in humans. Individuals with less melanin, people with types I, II, and III skin, are more susceptible to burns and damage from the UV radiation. Individuals with more melanin, types IV, V, and VI skin, can also be damaged by UV rays (Table 15-1).
   2. Changes that occur because of sunburn and tanning include:
      a. Impaired immune response secondary to epidermal cell necrosis
      b. Skin pigment darkening; quickly with UVB rays, delayed with UVA rays

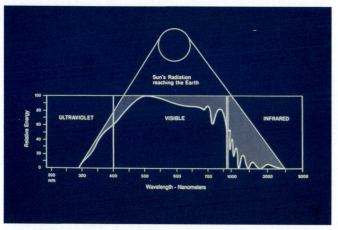

FIGURE 15-1. Solar radiation spectrum. (Copyright 2015 by the American Academy of Dermatology. All rights reserved.)

c. Erythema caused by release of inflammatory mediators, such as cytokines and prostaglandins

d. Genetic changes in the cellular makeup due to UV radiation, increasing the risk of skin cancer

3. Between the ages of 0 and 28 years, the skin absorbs UV radiation while individuals participate in outdoor activities, tan on the beach, or are otherwise exposed. The sunburns and tans are only temporary, but the damage remains.

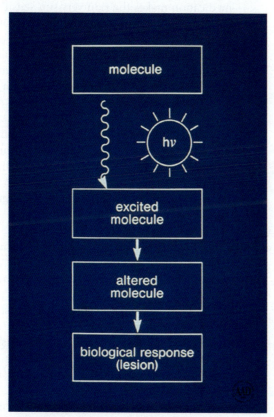

FIGURE 15-2. Induction of a biologic response to solar radiation. (Copyright 2015 by the American Academy of Dermatology. All rights reserved.)

TABLE 15-1 Fitzpatrick Sun-Reactive Skin Types

Skin Type	Skin Color	Tanning Response
Type I	White	Always burn, never tan
Type II	White	Usually burn, tan with difficulty
Type III	White	Sometimes mild burn, tan average
Type IV	Brown	Burns minimally, tan with ease
Type V	Dark brown	Very rarely burn, tans deeply
Type VI	Black	Almost never burns, deeply pigmented

4. As we approach the late 40s to early 50s, unprotected skin becomes leathery, dry, and nodular. Genetic changes caused by the UV radiation exposure begin to evolve.

5. Histologically, the UV-damaged epidermis is generally thicker than unexposed skin and shows some cellular atypia and damage.

6. There is a marked elastosis with a decrease in collagen fibers and bundles in the dermis causing thinned and increasing fragile skin.

7. Telangiectasia and solar lentigines develop with prolonged exposure in sun-damaged skin.

D. Treatment modalities.

1. Surgical treatment.

a. Dermabrasion is a standard method that has been successfully used for many years.

(1) It can be used for the total face or smaller local areas where other methods have not been effective.

(2) Some practitioner believe that elderly skin tends not to heal as well, causing greater incidence of hypertrophic scarring when dermabrasion is utilized.

(3) The older person tends to heal more slowly, leaving the skin open to a greater chance of infection.

b. Aluminum oxide crystal microdermabrasion is a relatively new and popular treatment for facial rejuvenation for damage caused by UV light.

(1) It is a simple, noninvasive procedure that can be repeated as often as every week for 4 to 12 weeks.

(2) The aluminum oxide crystals are used to abrade the skin.

(3) Following the procedure, a mild, transient erythema may occur.

c. Chemical peels.

(1) Phenol or various formulations containing phenol is a method of deeper peel for photodamaged skin.

(a) Side effects: there is a risk of renal toxicity and cardiac arrhythmias from phenol.

(b) Good results have been obtained from monitored use by well-trained practitioner.

(2) TCA is a medium-depth peel. TCA is used in various concentrations, 20% to 50%, to obtain good results in photodamaged skin.

   (a) It is sometimes used with other agents such as Jessner solution.

   (b) Side effects: hypo- or hyperpigmentation, scarring, and infection. Erythema may be persistent.

   (c) Because of potential side effects, physicians may use a decreased concentration or a series of peels.

(3) Alpha hydroxy acids (the most common being glycolic acid) are found in natural sources.

   (a) Lactic acid is found in sour milk, tartaric acid in grapes, and glycolic acid in sugar cane. Cosmetic manufacturers primarily use a synthetic glycolic acid.

   (b) The smaller the molecular structure of the acid, the more it can penetrate the skin. With its two-carbon structure, glycolic acid is the smallest, followed by lactic acid and tartaric acid with three and four carbon atoms, respectively.

   (c) Glycolic acid comes in concentrations of 5% to 99%; 50% to 70% solutions are most commonly used in the physician's office, and 10% to 20% solutions can be found in over-the-counter applications.

   (d) Best results of glycolic peels are seen months after a higher concentration peel.

   (e) Glycolic acid is less sun sensitizing, but a patient should use a good sunscreen when receiving these peels.

d. Collagen injections may be used on the expressive lines and fine-line wrinkles caused by photoaging (Table 15-2).

(1) The patient must have a skin test prior to starting the injections to check for any allergic reactions.

(2) The effects of the collagen injections are not permanent and must be repeated every 6 to 18 months for sustained results.

e. Lipotransfer is the transfer of the patient's own fat from the buttocks or abdomen and injection into the facial expression lines.

   (1) It is a relatively simple procedure done under local anesthesia.

   (2) No skin tests are needed.

   (3) The most commonly injected area is the naso-labial fold.

   (4) Like collagen, it lasts only 6 to 18 months.

   (5) An advantage is that extra fat may be withdrawn and frozen for injection several months later.

2. Topical treatment (retinoids).

a. Tretinoin, a retinoid, applied topically helps to even skin coloring, soften fine wrinkle lines, and increase the formation of blood vessels.

   (1) Tretinoin acts by gently peeling the skin and also by normalizing the epidermal turnover.

   (2) The patient may experience some skin irritation or dryness at first, but this usually subsides.

   (3) When a patient is using a tretinoin, a sunscreen with SPF of 30 or more must be used, as this medication makes the skin very sun sensitive. A cream or lotion is preferred, since gels contain alcohol.

   (4) Before applying tretinoin, the skin should be gently cleansed with warm water and patted dry. Wait 20 to 30 minutes before applying a thin layer to the skin, as skin irritation can occur when applied to damp skin.

   (5) Because of increased sun sensitivity, tretinoin should be applied at night, and a 30 SPF broad-spectrum sunscreen should be applied in the morning.

   (6) Women who are pregnant, or may be pregnant, should not use tretinoin.

3. Cosmetic treatment.

a. Hylan B gels are derived from hyaluronan, a component of all connective tissues.

   (1) Because they are biocompatible, there is no need for skin tests.

   (2) Hylan B gels are water insoluble, they resist degradation, and they are unlikely to migrate.

   (3) There are three hylan B gels with increasingly greater viscosities, so that each is suitable for a different contour, from fine wrinkles to common wrinkles to deep folds.

b. Many over-the-counter products exist that contain alpha hydroxy acids, vitamin C, and niacinamide; however, the skin is unable to absorb these molecules into the collagen layer.

TABLE 15-2 Glogau Photoaging Classification

Type I: No Wrinkles	Type II: Wrinkles in Motion	Type III: Wrinkles at Rest	Type IV: Only Wrinkles
Early photoaging	Early to moderate photoaging	Advanced photoaging	Severe photoaging
Mild pigmentary changes	Early senile lentigines visible	Obvious dyschromia and telangiectasia	Yellow–gray color of skin
No keratoses	Keratoses palpable but not visible	Visible keratoses	Prior skin malignancies
Minimal wrinkles	Parallel smile lines beginning to appear	Wrinkles even when not moving	Wrinkled throughout, no normal skin
Patient age, 20s or 30s	Patient age, late 30s or 40s	Patient age, 50s or older	Patient age, 6th or 7th
Minimal or no makeup	Usually wears some foundation	Always wears heavy foundation	Cannot wear makeup—"cakes and cracks"

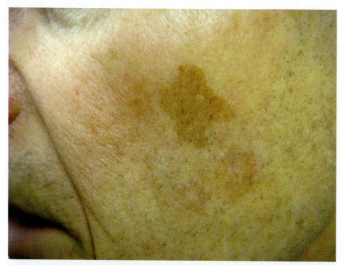

FIGURE 15-3. Solar lentigo. (From Goodheart, H. P. (2010). *Goodheart's same-site differential diagnosis: A rapid method of diagnosing and treating common skin disorders.* Philadelphia, PA: Wolters Kluwer.)

4. Laser therapy can be utilized for a variety of skin-related complications (refer to Chapter 3 for further inquiry).
   a. Telangiectasias on the face, a result of photodamaged skin, may be treated with vascular lesion lasers, such as the pulsed dye, copper bromide, and krypton laser.
   b. Brown macular lesions (solar lentigines; Figure 15-3) may be treated with excellent results with several lasers, one of which is the Q-switched ruby laser.
   c. Rhytides, fine lines around the eyes or upper lip, and scarring may be treated with BBL.

PATIENT EDUCATION
Sunscreens

- **Broad-spectrum designation.** Sunscreens that pass the FDA's broad-spectrum test procedure, which measures a product's ultraviolet A (UVA) protection relative to its ultraviolet B (UVB) protection, may be labeled as "broad-spectrum SPF [*value*]" on the front label. For broad-spectrum sunscreens, SPF values also indicate the amount or magnitude of overall protection. Broad-spectrum SPF products with SPF values higher than 15 provide greater protection and may claim additional uses, as described in the next bullet.
- **Use claims.** Only broad-spectrum sunscreens with an SPF value of 15 or higher can claim to reduce the risk of skin cancer and early skin aging if used as directed with other sun protection measures. Non–broad-spectrum sunscreens and broad-spectrum sunscreens with an SPF value between 2 and 14 can only claim to help prevent sunburn.
- **"Waterproof," "sweatproof," or "sunblock" claims.** Manufacturers cannot label sunscreens as "waterproof" or "sweatproof" or identify their products as "sunblocks," because these claims overstate their effectiveness. Sunscreens also cannot claim to provide sun protection for more than 2 hours without reapplication or to provide protection immediately after application (e.g., "instant protection") without submitting data to support these claims and obtaining FDA approval.
- **Water resistance claims.** Water resistance claims on the front label must indicate whether the sunscreen remains effective for 40 minutes or 80 minutes while swimming or sweating, based on standard testing. Sunscreens that are not water resistant must include a direction instructing consumers to use a water-resistant sunscreen if swimming or sweating.
- **Drug facts.** All sunscreens must include standard "drug facts" information on the back and/or side of the container.
- **Application.** Never spray sunscreen into the face (may be sprayed on the hand and then used on the face), and never spray with someone beneath you "catching" the spray. Adequate spray must be used to make the skin appear uniformly wet.
- *Do not* rub off sunscreen. Inhalation of sunscreen and absorption into the eye membranes is a concern.
- Don't forget to apply an even layer of sunscreen. A patient's handful is usually the correct amount for the body. Put sunscreen on the back of arms and legs, ears, nose, and lips!

PHOTODERMATOSES

I. ACTINIC KERATOSES

A. Definition: Actinic keratoses (AKs) or solar keratosis lesions caused by sun damage are commonly found in elderly patients with skin types I, II, and III. They comprise aggregates of anaplastic keratinocytes confined to the epidermis (Figures 15-4 through 15-7).
B. Etiology.
   1. Sun exposure begins at a very early age, but AKs are not commonly seen in children or teenagers, except in patients with albinism.
   2. AKs are found more in men than women and greatly increase in number with age.
   3. Although they can appear on any sun-exposed area, AKs are most frequently seen in the face, scalp, ears, and arms.
   4. People with blue eyes, fair skin, and albinos are at higher risk to develop AKs. AKs are rarely seen in people with darker skin; types IV, V, and VI.
   5. If left untreated, 10% to 20% of AKs grow through the basement membranes of the epidermal–dermal junction and become squamous cell carcinomas.
   6. Almost 60% of squamous cell carcinomas arise from AKs.
C. Assessment.
   1. Clinically, AKs measure from 2 to 3 mm to 1 to 2 cm. An individual patient may have 1 to more than 100

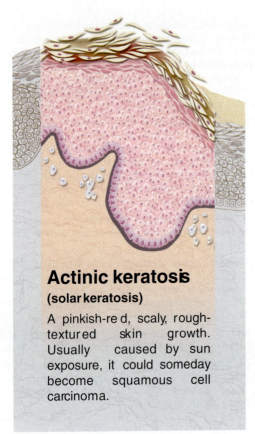

FIGURE 15-4. Diagram illustrating the pathophysiology of actinic keratosis. AKs are aggregates of anaplastic keratinocytes confined to the epidermis. (Provided by Anatomical Chart Co.)

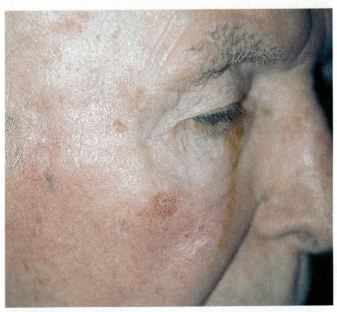

FIGURE 15-5. Multiple actinic keratoses on the cheek and brow with signs of chronic sun damage. (Courtesy of Jurij Bilyk, MD.)

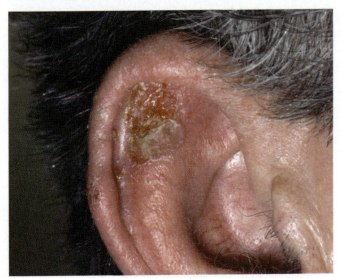

FIGURE 15-6. Bowenoid actinic keratosis. A crusted lesion on the ear helix. (From Elder, D. E. (2014). *Lever's histopathology of the skin*. Philadelphia, PA: Wolters Kluwer.)

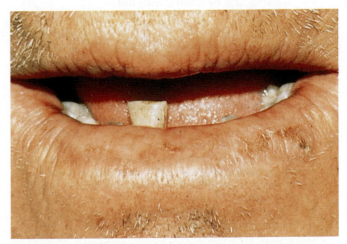

FIGURE 15-7. Actinic cheilitis results from excessive exposure to sunlight and affects primarily the lower lip. Fair-skinned men who work outdoors are most often affected. The lip loses its normal redness and may become scaly, somewhat thickened, and slightly everted. Because solar damage also predisposes to carcinoma of the lip, be alert to this possibility. (From Langlais, R. P., & Miller, C. S. (1992). *Color atlas of common oral diseases*. Philadelphia, PA: Lea & Febiger, used with permission.)

lesions on their body. This generally depends on the type of skin and the amount of sun exposure.

    a. AKs can vary in color from skin colored to a tan or reddish tone.

    b. If they appear the same color as the skin, they must be palpated.

    c. AKs appear are as individual papules that are scaly and rough on the epidermis.

2. A rare variation of the AK is the spreading pigmented AK.

    a. These lesions are usually large in size, over 1 cm.

    b. They may be smooth, slightly scaly, or warty in texture. They are variable in color.

    c. There is a tendency for centrifugal spread.

    d. The spreading pigmented AK is found mostly on the face and can mimic the lentigo maligna in appearance.

3. The lichenoid keratosis resembles a solitary lesion of lichen planus. There is learned discussion whether this is a totally benign lesion or an inflamed AK.

    a. It begins small but can increase in size to 3 to 4 cm and has uneven borders.

    b. The color tends toward red, and it is scaly in texture.

4. Histologically, AKs are well-defined aggregates of abnormal keratinocytes. The epidermis is generally hyperkeratotic.

    a. The nucleus of the keratinocyte is enlarged, hyperchromatic, and irregular in shape. The keratinocyte may be multinucleated.

    b. Cells of the sweat gland ducts and hair follicles tend to be normal.

    c. Changes of solar elastosis often appear in the underlying dermis.

D. Treatment modalities.

1. Several methods for treating AKs are cryosurgery, electrodessication, and chemical peels, using TCA or glycolic acid.

    a. These methods have cure rates of up to 95%.

    b. They are excellent methods for discrete lesions and less diffuse actinically damaged skin.

    c. Cryosurgery and electrodessication are more commonly used for all areas of the body.

    d. Complications of these treatments are hypopigmentation, scarring, infection, and recurrence.

2. Medical treatment.

    a. 5-Fluorouracil (5-FU) 1% to 5% cream or solution and imiquimod 5% are effective for patients with moderate to extensive actinic damage.

        (1) 5-FU is applied one to two times a day for an average of 2 to 4 weeks, followed by 2 weeks of application of a gentle cortisone cream.

    b. Imiquimod 5% is applied three times weekly for 16 weeks. The application of imiquimod results in an 86% reduction of actinic damage.

    c. The skin may become very red and irritated. Therefore, in cases with severe actinic damage, the 5-FU or imiquimod is applied in sections, such as the forehead or left cheek.

    d. Complications of 5-FU and imiquimod treatment include scarring, infection, loss of pigmentation, and recurrence. Also a color difference remains between the normal skin and the actinic-damaged skin after treatment.

    e. Retreatment with 5-FU or imiquimod may be necessary every 3 to 5 years for patients with severe damage, as the AKs will continue to develop.

3. CO_2 dermabrasion is another very effective method of removing multiple AKs.

    a. The patient is generally not incapacitated as long as with the use of 5-FU.

    b. Dermabrasion removes the skin uniformly; therefore, the skin heals uniformly, and the results are cosmetically appealing.

    c. Complications are hypertrophic scarring, hypopigmentation, and infection.

4. Tretinoin has been used in several studies to eradicate AKs from the face and upper extremities.

    a. It has some benefit on early facial AKs, but little effect on extremities.

    b. There is little response by advanced lesions, even after twice a day application of 0.1% tretinoin.

    c. Although there may be some local irritation at the time of treatment, there are no serious or permanent side effects.

5. Photodynamic therapy (PDT) is the newest treatment available.

    a. It is useful for treating multiple lesions.

    b. PDT requires two visits to the dermatologist's office.

        (1) A topical medicine, aminolevulinic acid (ALA), is applied to the AK lesions on the first visit.

        (2) The second visit should be 14 to 18 hours after the application of ALA, when the lesions are exposed to a special blue light for less than 20 minutes.

        (3) The blue light activates the ALA, causing a chemical reaction in the skin that kills the AK cells.

        (4) In between visits, it is important to avoid all sun and UV light exposure.

PATIENT EDUCATION
Photodermatoses

- Any patient who has sun-damaged skin or has a history of AK should see a dermatology provider every 6 to 12 months for a full-body exam or sooner if changes are observed.

- Identification of precancerous lesions (Figure 15-8) is critical to prevent the onset of squamous cell carcinoma.

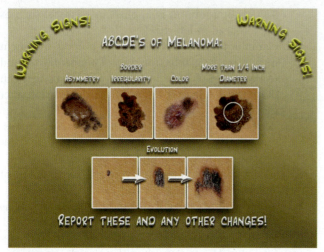

FIGURE 15-8. ABDCE's of melanoma. (Artwork by Elissa Fairbrother, Smack-A-Mole Game.)

II. LENTIGINES

A. Definition: generally pigmented macules that measure 1 to 5 mm. They are rarely seen larger than 1 cm. They are found on normal skin.

B. There are many different varieties of lentigines, but three of the more common ones will be discussed here. These are not sun induced or associated with any systemic disease.

1. Lentigo simplex (juvenile lentigo) appears commonly in children, as the name suggests. However, it can appear on a person at any age.
    a. Clinical features.
        (1) These lesions may occur anywhere on the body and have no particular affinity to the sun-exposed areas of skin.
        (2) They remain small, usually 1 to 5 mm, and few in number.
        (3) The color of the lesions varies from brown to black and is evenly pigmented.
        (4) These lesions are flat and therefore not palpable.
    b. Histologic features.
        (1) The rete ridges are moderately elongated.
        (2) There is increased epidermal hyperplasia and hyperpigmentation.
        (3) The number of melanocytes is increased in the basal cell layer.
        (4) Solar elastosis is absent.
    c. Treatment: juvenile lentigines are benign and may be left untreated.

2. Freckles (ephelides) are found on sun-exposed areas, such as the face, arms, and back of the hands.
    a. Clinical features.
        (1) Freckles are yellow to light brown macules found most frequently in people with light skin and red hair, although any skin type or hair color is susceptible to freckles.
        (2) Although they commonly appear in the summer months, freckles may last all year or throughout the person's life.
        (3) Freckles may measure up to 5 mm and have irregular or well-defined borders.
        (4) Whether their numbers are many or few, they are symmetrical in distribution.
    b. Histologic features.
        (1) The rete ridges are not elongated in freckles.
        (2) Although there is an increase in pigment in the basal cell layer, there does not appear to be an increase in melanocytes.
    c. Treatment: freckles may be left untreated, or they can be removed with the ruby, alexandrite, or Q-switched YAG laser.

3. Lentigines profusa (generalized lentigines) usually appear without any associated abnormality. However, they can rarely occur as a cutaneous sign of a systemic disorder (such as LEOPARD, NAME, or LAMB syndrome) or cardiac, pulmonary, and endocrinologic defects.
    a. Clinical features.
        (1) The lesions usually are present at birth but may not appear until early childhood to early adulthood.
        (2) They appear as 1-mm to 2-cm pigmented lesions that occur anywhere on the body except for the soles of the feet and the buccal mucosa.
        (3) The color varies from dark brown to black.
        (4) The texture of the skin is normal, and the lesions are flat and nonpalpable.
        (5) Lentigines profusa are similar to freckles except for the widespread distribution of the lesion.
    b. Histologic features.
        (1) The rete ridges are slightly elongated.
        (2) There is increased pigment in the melanocytes and an increase in the number of keratinocytes and melanocytes.
        (3) There is no solar elastosis.
    c. Treatment: like all lentigines, these lesions are benign and may be left untreated.

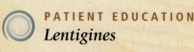

PATIENT EDUCATION
Lentigines

• The sun can darken lentigines and, in the case of freckles, increase their number.

III. POLYMORPHOUS LIGHT ERUPTION (PMLE)

A. Definition: PMLE is a sun-induced allergic reaction to a yet unknown photosensitizer (Figure 15-9).

B. Etiology.

1. Studies are showing some genetic predisposition, but there are no definitive percentages.

2. PMLE can appear anytime, but it is most common before the age of 30 years.

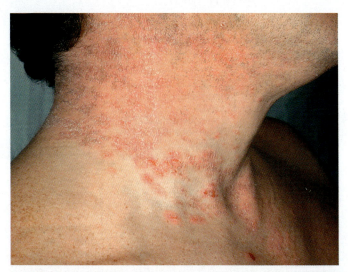

FIGURE 15-9. PMLE on the sun-exposed area of the neck, stopping at the collar line of the shirt. (From Craft, N., Taylor, E., Tumeh, P. C., Fox, L. P., Goldsmith, L. A., Papier, A., …, Rosenblum, M. (2010). *VisualDx: Essential adult dermatology*. Philadelphia, PA: Wolters Kluwer.)

3. In North American and Latin American Indians, PMLE commonly appears in childhood.
4. Although it is present in both sexes, several studies illustrate a greater prevalence in women.
5. PMLE affects all skin types from I through VI.
6. Ten to fifteen percent are found in the Caucasian population.

C. Assessment.
1. Generally, intense pruritus occurs followed by the eruptions of skin lesions.
2. The eruptions may occur several hours or several days after exposure, making diagnosis more difficult.
3. The lesions usually remain 2 to 3 days, with extremes of 24 hours to 10 or more days.
4. The lesions range from small papules and papulovesicles to eczematous reactions, or coalescent papules, which may merge to form plaques.
5. The large papules are pink or red to erythema multiforme-like lesions and usually occur on the face.
6. PMLE lesions are usually confined to sun-exposed areas.
   a. If conditions are such that one involved area is exposed to enough radiation from the sun or artificial sources, another area may flare, even if unexposed. However, the sun-exposed surfaces remain more severe.
7. Occasionally, there is a complete disappearance.

D. Histopathologic characteristics.
1. The small papules and eczematous lesions show epidermal edema, spongiosis of interfollicular epidermis, and occasional vesicle formation. Parakeratosis and acanthosis are frequently present.
2. The large papular lesions show very little epidermal response, but parakeratosis and acanthosis are frequently present.

3. Some edema of the basal cell layer has been noted with both lesions.
4. Both small and large papular lesions show a superficial and deep lymphocytic infiltration in the upper and middle dermis.

E. Treatment modalities.
1. Systemic drugs.
   a. Chloroquine and hydroxychloroquine are most effective.
      (1) Both are quite effective in large papule reactions and in very early small papule-type variants.
      (2) Frequent eye exams are recommended for those taking these drugs more than 2 months beyond the baseline exam.
      (3) Extreme caution must be taken when using these drugs with children, as they are very sensitive.
2. Topical therapy with mild- to high-potency corticosteroids is recommended in short bursts from 3 to 14 days. Be cautious with chronic use due to side effects such as atrophy, telangiectasia, and dependency.
3. Antihistamines should be utilized to help with pruritus and prevention.
4. Studies have been done using PUVA with 8-MOP as a prophylactic to tan and thicken the stratum corneum, with positive results.
5. BB-UVB and NB-UVB have also proved to be effective prophylactic treatments.

 PATIENT EDUCATION
SunAWARE

• The SunAWARE acronym (adapted and expanded here) includes five easy action steps for prevention and early detection of skin cancer:

  ○ **A**void unprotected exposure to sunlight, seek shade, and never indoor tan (Box 15-1). Avoid being outside unprotected when the UV index is above 2 or between the hours of 10 am and 4 pm. Sand, water, and snow increase UV radiation risk due to their reflective properties.

  ○ **W**ear sun-protective clothing, including a long-sleeved shirt (tightly woven), long pants, a wide-brimmed hat (3- to 4-inch brim), and sunglasses year round. Infants should wear bonnets. Clothing with a UPF rating of 50 or higher offers better protection.

  ○ **A**pply recommended amounts of broad-spectrum sunscreen with a sunburn protection factor (SPF) of at least 30 to all exposed skin and reapply every 2 hours, or as needed.

  ○ **R**outinely examine your whole body for changes in your skin and report suspicious changes to a parent or health care provider.

  ○ **E**ducate your family and community about the need to be SunAWARE.

Box 15-1. DNA Position Statement on Indoor Tanning

The Dermatology Nurses' Association (DNA) recognizes the significant public health risks directly related to indoor tanning exposure and recommends the following:

Extensive public health education on the known carcinogenic effects and other associated health risks of artificial UVR and indoor tanning

Partnering with government, industry, agencies such as the CDC and AAD, other medical professionals, and schools to accomplish educational goals

An FDA ban of all nonmedical uses for artificial UVR, including the cosmetic use of indoor tanning beds

Adequate funding to comply with strict enforcement of current indoor tanning guidelines and routine inspection of all indoor tanning equipment

Prohibit use by minors under the age of 18.

Prominent display of warning signs listing the carcinogenic and health risks related to the use of tanning beds

Signed statement by each client that explicitly describes the health risks of indoor tanning

Provision of sanitary eye protection for each client using indoor tanning facilities

Adequate training of all tanning device owners/operators that includes health risks of indoor tanning devices, safe operation and maintenance of equipment, recognition of UVR overexposure and emergency conditions, and first aid/emergency care for burns and UVR-related health injury, that is, disease exacerbations

Establish method to limit exposure time and alert client to end of tanning session.

Prohibit public messages or advertisements promoting the "safety" of indoor tanning.

From Dermatology Nurses Association. (2015). Indoor tanning. Retrieved from: http://www.dnanurse.org/indoor-tanning

IV. PHOTOTOXICITY AND PHOTOALLERGY

A. Definition: photosensitivity reactions are created by combining light, generally UVA, with a photosensitizing chemical (Table 15-3). The two types of photosensitivity reactions are phototoxicity and photoallergy (Table 15-4).

TABLE 15-3 Common Phototoxic Agents, Photoallergens, and Phototoxin

Systemic Agents (Generic Name)	Photoallergens	Phototoxins in the Environment
Amiodarone	Sunscreens:	Coal tar
Benoxaprofen	PABA	Psoralens
Chloroquine	Sulisobenzone (BZP-4)	Tar pitch
Chlorpromazine	Oxygensone (BZP-3)	Perfumes
Chlorpropamide	Cinoxate	Plants (phyto-photodermatitis)
Chlorothiazide	Octyl methoxycinnamate	Angelica
Ciprofloxacin	Homosalate	Celery
Dacarbazine	Octyl salicylate	Cow parsley
Desipramine	Fragrances:	Meadow grass
Diphenhydramine	Musk ambrette	Parsnip
5-Fluorouracil	6-Methylcoumarin	Carrot (wild)
Furosemide	Sandalwood oil	Fig (wild)
Griseofulvin	Antibacterials:	Hogweed
Imipramine	Bithionol	Rue
Itraconazole	Fenticlor	
Ketoprofen	Triclosan	
Nalidixic acid	Dichlorophene	
Naproxen	Tribromo salicylanilide	
Nifedipine	Hexachlorophene	
Piroxicam	Chlorhexidine diacetate	
Promethazine	Others:	
Psoralens	Chlorpromazine	
Quinidine	Hydrochloride	
Quinine	Promethazine	
Retinoids	Thiourea	
Sulfanilamide		
Tetracyclines		
Thiazides		
Tiaprofenic acid		
Tolbutamide		
Vinblastine		

B. Pathophysiology.
1. In order for a reaction to occur, light must be absorbed by the chemical in or on the skin.
2. The chemical may be systemic within the body, or introduced externally to the skin.
3. Although direct sunlight is the major source of light, fluorescent light may also cause response.
4. The clinical pattern of photosensitivity reaction appears on exposed areas of the skin such as the face, particularly the nose and cheeks, the ears, the backs of hands, and the neck area.

TABLE 15-4 Phototoxicity versus Photoallergy

Phototoxicity	Photoallergy
Individual must be exposed to a sufficient amount of photosensitizing chemical at the same time as to the causal wavelength of light.	Individual must be exposed to a sufficient amount of photosensitizing chemical at the same time as to the causal wavelength of light.
Reaction occurs minutes to hours after the first exposure to the sensitizing agent.	Due to a need for prior sensitization, reaction will not occur upon first exposure; a minimum of 24 to 72 hours is required after the combined exposure before the first reaction occurs.
Nonimmunologic reaction	Immunologic reaction
Because of differences in penetration, absorption, and the metabolism of the chemicals in the patient, the reaction can be sporadic.	Photoallergy reactions are less frequent in most patients. The amount of chemical needed to induce a reaction is minimal, and cross-reactivity to other agents is always possible.
Clinically, the patient shows a sunburn, which may even blister. There is peeling and there may be hyperpigmentation. Burning or stinging may be experienced with the reaction.	Clinically, the patient has acute pruritic eruptions or vesicles and papules in areas exposed to light. In patients with chronic reactions, excoriated and lichenified plaques occur.

TABLE 15-4 *(Continued)*

Phototoxicity	Photoallergy
Pathophysiology: a. The phototoxic molecules absorb energy, which is transferred to oxygen molecules; this creates a reactive oxygen species that causes cellular damage. b. A photosensitizer may bind with a biologic substrate, so with the exposure to radiation, the structure of the substrate is altered. Psoralen binding with pyrimidine bases of DNA molecules is an example of this reaction. c. Radiation interacting with phototoxic substances may cause a release of inflammatory mediators. d. A chemical that absorbs radiation may form a photoproduct, which in turn may react with a biologic substrate. Chlorpromazine-induced phototoxicity is an example.	Pathophysiology: a. The systemic or topical chemical absorbs radiation, producing a photoallergen. b. The antigen-presenting cells, such as macrophages and Langerhans, process the photoallergen and introduce it to helper T cells and class II molecules. c. The consequent reaction is the classic type IV delayed hypersensitivity response. d. Photoallergies are most commonly caused by external chemicals and rarely by systemic drugs.
Diagnoses may be facilitated by phototesting. A small area of non–sun-exposed skin is irradiated with gradually increasing amounts of UVB or UVA, until a minimal erythema appears. Usually a lesser dose of UVA irradiation is needed in the phototoxic patient than in the general population where the amount of UVB is the same.	Photopatch testing is a method of confirming photoallergic contact dermatitis. a. Day 1: duplicate sets of photoallergens are applied to the back and covered with an opaque tape. b. Day 2: one set of patches is removed, and sites are exposed to 10 J/cm^2 of UVA or 50% of minimal erythema dose (MED). c. Day 3: both sites uncovered and the reactions are graded. d. Both sites are graded for delayed reaction.

DNA, deoxyribonucleic acid; UVA, ultraviolet A; UVB, ultraviolet B.

5. The most common cause of photoallergic reactions is external exposure to chemicals in the workplace and in rare cases to chemicals in the general environment or in commercially purchased goods.

V. SUNBURN

A. Definition: sunburn is the superficial inflammation of the skin caused by overexposure to UV light from the sun or artificial UV sources.

B. Etiology.
1. Repeated sun exposures and sunburns increase the risk of skin cancer and photoaging.
2. People who are skin types I, II, and III have very little melanin and tend to burn more readily than those with skin types IV, V, and VI.
3. Almost anyone, regardless of skin type or melanin content, can burn if they expose their skin long enough to the UV rays of the sun or to artificial sources.
4. Some drugs, such as tetracycline, sulfonamides, Diabinese, and griseofulvin are photosensitizing. Exposure to UV radiation should be minimized, and sun-protective agents (Box 15-2) should be used.
5. Erythema usually develops 2 to 12 hours after exposure and reaches its greatest severity at 24 hours.

C. Assessment.
1. The skin becomes red, tender to palpation, and warm to touch. In more severe cases, vesiculation appears.
2. There can be extreme burning discomfort accompanying a deeper burn.
3. Overexposure to UV radiation can cause eye damage resulting in painful, gritty eyes, and even temporary blindness.

Box 15-2. Sunscreen Agents

UVA absorbers

Oxybenzone
Sulisobenzone
Dioxybenzone
Methyl anthranilate
Avobenzone
Terephthalylidene dicamphor sulfonic acid
Bis(ethylhexyl)ox phenol methoxyphenyl triazine

UVB absorbers

Para-amino benzoic acid
p-Amyldimethyl-PABA-(padimate A)
Digalloyl trioleate
Triethanolamine salicylate
2-Phenylbenzimidazole-5-sulfonic acid
Ethyl 4-bis(hydroxypropyl)amino benzoate
Octyldimethyl-PABA (padimate O)
Triethanolamine salicylate
2-Ethylhexyl *p*-methoxycinnamate
2-Ethylhexyl salicylate
Glyceryl-PABA
Homomenthyl salicylate
Dihydroxyacetone

Sunscreen stabilizers

Mexoryl SX
Tinosorb
Helioplex

UVA/UVB absorbers

Titanium dioxide
Zinc oxide

From FDA. (2011). Questions and answers: FDA announces new requirements for over-the-counter sunscreen products marketed in the U.S. Retrieved from: http://www.fda.gov/Drugs/ResourcesForYou/Consumers/BuyingUsingMedicineSafely/UnderstandingOver-the-CounterMedicines/ucm258468.htm#Q6_What_are_the_main_points.

4. Other symptoms experienced include headache, chills, malaise, and generalized weakness.

5. After a few days, the vesicles dry, and the skin tightens and peels.

6. The peeling leaves a mottled and sensitive skin underneath.

D. Treatment modalities.

1. The goal of treatment is to reduce discomfort, swelling, and pain.

2. Cool water compresses or cold baths can be helpful in the reduction of heat and pain.

3. The application of steroid lotions, aloe vera, and cooling creams can be helpful.

4. Systematic analgesics such as NSAIDs or acetaminophen will help decrease the pain. In extremely severe cases of sunburn, oral steroids may be necessary.

5. If blisters form, let them break open without manipulation. Clean the area with soap and water. Wet dressings initially may help relieve the pain and risk for infection.

6. If there has been any damage to the cornea of the eye, an ophthalmologist must be consulted.

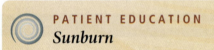

PATIENT EDUCATION
Sunburn

- Sunburned skin will be particularly sensitive to the UV radiation. Further exposure should be absolutely avoided.

VI. PORPHYRIA CUTANEA TARDA

A. Definition: Porphyria cutanea tarda (PCT) is the most common subtype of porphyritic diseases. PCT occurs from a defective enzyme, uroporphyrinogen decarboxylase (UROD), which is produced in the liver. Lack of UROD causes a build of porphyrins in the liver and eventually the skin. The disease is either acquired or autosomal dominant (Figure 15-10).

B. Etiology.

1. The acquired form is usually precipitated by alcohol use. Other triggers include oral contraceptives, smoking, estrogen, environmental exposures, or iron overloading (Habif, 2010).

2. Hepatitis C, HIV, and chronic blood disorders may commonly accompany or precipitate PCT.

3. The disorder frequently occurs sporadically. Onset usually occurs after the age of 40 years in the acquired form. However, PCT usually occurs earlier in life in the inherited form.

4. PCT occurs equally in males and females.

5. Long-wave UV light activates the porphyrins in the skin causing photosensitivity.

C. Assessment.

1. Blistering, skin fragility, and sores frequently occur on sun-exposed areas such as the hands, arms, and face.

2. The bullae heal with erythema, scarring, and milia formation.

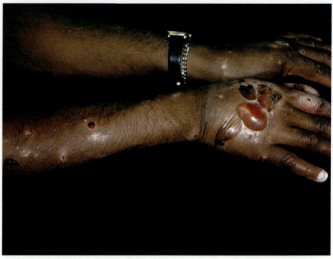

FIGURE 15-10. Blisters and scarring with porphyria cutanea tarda. (From Lugo-Somolinos, A., Lee, I., McKinley-Grant, L., Goldsmith, L. A., Papier, A., Adigun, C. G., …, Fredeking, A. (2011). *VisualDx: Essential dermatology in pigmented skin*. Philadelphia, PA: Wolters Kluwer.)

3. There is hypo- and hyperpigmentation of the sun-exposed areas, particularly the face.

4. Hypertrichoses (hirsutism) is noted in most cases and found generally on the face and the limbs.

5. Scleroderma thickening of the skin may occur in unexposed areas and the face.

D. Pathophysiology.

1. Laboratory findings show:

a. A greatly elevated uroporphyrin excretion (>500 g/24 hours) is found in a 24-hour urine collection. Usually red–brown (tea-colored) urine is observed.

b. Total iron stores are often twice the normal amount in the hepatocytes.

c. Histologic findings reveal subepidermal bullae with little inflammation and thickened capillary walls. Immunofluorescent findings are positive.

2. PCT is one of several porphyrias associated with defective enzymes in the heme biosynthetic pathway.

a. Heme is used in the formation of hemoglobin, cytochromes, and other substances.

b. Porphyrinogens are used in the production of heme.

c. When the metabolic pathway is blocked by a deficiency in the enzyme UROD, the porphyrinogens break up and are therefore oxidized into porphyrins.

d. When there is light absorption, the porphyrin becomes greatly agitated, creating an unstable state.

e. This unstable state causes damage to cells and cell membranes, releasing chemicals that cause inflammation and further tissue damage.

E. Treatment modalities.

1. Abstinence from alcohol is advised.

2. Avoiding Dilantin, diethylstilbestrol, and unnecessary iron intake is recommended, as they can aggravate the disease. And they should never be combined with alcohol.

3. Phlebotomy is the most common treatment for PCT, as it depletes the hepatic iron overload. The recommended procedure is removing 500 mL of blood every 2 weeks, three to four times. Then 500 mL are removed every 3 to 6 weeks, for a total of 10 to 15 pints of blood.

4. Chloroquine in doses of 125 mg twice weekly for 8 to 18 months can help.
   a. Chloroquine is used in low doses (due to hepatotoxicity) and requires baseline and biweekly liver function tests and urinary porphyrin analysis until the uroporphyrin level is less than 100 g/24 hours.
   b. Chloroquine works to release uroporphyrin in the liver tissue, which binds with the hepatic porphyrins, causing them to become more water soluble, and, therefore, increases the urinary output of uroporphyrins.

5. Using the combination of both phlebotomy and chloroquine is more effective than either treatment alone. This combination induces remission in an average of 3.5 months compared to 10.2 months (chloroquine) and 12.5 months (phlebotomy) (Habif, 2010).

PATIENT EDUCATION
Porphyria Cutanea Tarda

- Abstain from alcohol.
- Avoid the use of disease-triggering drugs.

VII. SOLAR URTICARIA

A. Definition: solar urticaria (SU) is an uncommon, IgE-mediated photodermatosis in which UV or visible irradiation causes a wheal and flare response of exposed skin (Figure 15-11).
B. Etiology.
   1. SU occurs in all races and at any age.
   2. Generally, it appears in young adults.
   3. It is slightly more common in females age 10 to 50 years.

4. Susceptibility to this condition may occasionally disappear spontaneously.
C. Assessment.
   1. SU appears within a few minutes of sun exposure.
   2. The symptoms of SU are itching, erythema, burning, and whealing.
   3. After 24 hours, if there is no more exposure to the sun, the lesions and symptoms usually disappear.
   4. The lesions are usually found on the V area of the neck and on the arms.
   5. UVA, UVB, and/or visible light can cause SU.
   6. Phototesting.
      a. Phototesting is used to confirm SU by determining the smallest irradiation dose that causes a wheal or flare response to occur.
      b. This is referred to as the minimal urticarial dose (MUD).
      c. To determine the MUD, readings must be taken immediately after exposure and 6 hours later.
      d. The effectiveness of therapy can be seen in the change of the MUD.
D. Treatment modalities.
   1. The initial method of treating SU is with antihistamines, specifically, H1 receptor antagonists.
      a. Sunlight-induced histamine release is inhibited by antihistamines.
      b. This leads to a decrease in pruritus and prevention of the wheal and flare response.
      c. H1 receptor blockers are prescribed in higher doses than for common allergies.
   2. Less effective therapies, used when the patient is unresponsive to antihistamines, include antimalarials, doxepin, indomethacin, and beta carotene.
   3. PUVA alone, or combined with plasmapheresis, has shown good results.
   4. In recalcitrant cases, cyclosporine and plasmapheresis may be beneficial.
   5. IVIG has been successful in the treatment of severe and resistant forms of SU.

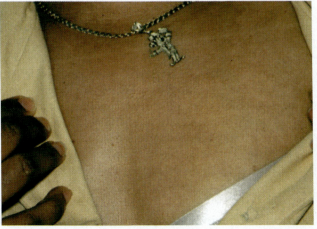
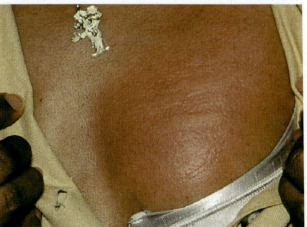

FIGURE 15-11. Solar urticaria induced by UVA light. **A:** Before sun exposure. **B:** After exposure to 15 minutes of sunlight through a glass window. (From Goodheart, H. P. (2003). *Goodheart's photoguide of common skin disorders* (2nd ed.). Philadelphia, PA: Lippincott Williams & Wilkins.)

VIII. CHRONIC ACTINIC DERMATITIS (CAD)

A. Definition: CAD is a syndrome of persistent light reactivity defined by three criteria:
   1. There is commonly an eruption of eczematous character.
   2. Histologically, its appearance is consistent with chronic eczema, with or without lymphoma-like changes.
   3. Photobiologic: there is a reduction in the MED to UVB irradiation.
B. Etiology.
   1. CAD is found more often in males age 63 to 65 years.
   2. It occurs occasionally in young people.
   3. CAD is more prevalent in temperate climates.
C. Assessment.
   1. CAD appears as hyperpigmented patches and scaly, pruritic lichenified plaques.
   2. Generally, they appear on sun-exposed areas, but in acute exacerbation, covered skin may be involved.
   3. In severe cases of CAD, eczematous eruptions may appear.
D. Pathophysiology.
   1. Atypical mononuclear cells may be found in the dermis and epidermis.
   2. There is lymphocytic infiltrate confined to the upper dermis, causing epidermal spongiosis, acanthosis, and sometimes hyperplasia.
E. Treatment modalities.
   1. Broad-spectrum sunscreen and protective clothing are helpful, but not always sufficient.
   2. Avoidance of UV light and sunlight when possible.
   3. Topical steroids and emollients are used to control acute dermatitis.
   4. Occasionally, a short course of oral steroids is given.
   5. In severe cases of CAD, it may be treated with PUVA, or immunosuppressive agents such as cyclosporine, azathioprine, and systemic corticosteroids.

AGING

I. OVERVIEW

A. Intrinsic aging of the skin is genetic in origin, while photoaging is a result of chronic sun exposure and damage.
B. Etiology.
   1. Intrinsic aging.
      a. Skin that has been protected from the sun over the years remains smooth and unblemished.
      b. Due to gravity, hormonal changes, and facial expressions, the facial lines tend to deepen and widen.
      c. There is also atrophy of dermal and subcutaneous tissue.
      d. In comparison, intrinsic aging is exemplified by atrophy, whereas photoaging is hypertrophic.
   2. Photoaging.
      a. Photoaging is due to chronic and continuous overexposure to UVA and UVB rays.

Box 15-3. Ultraviolet-Induced Skin Changes

Texture changes

Solar elastosis
Atrophy
Wrinkles

Vascular changes

Diffuse erythema
Ecchymosis
Stellate pseudoscars
Skin tears
Telangiectasias
Venous lakes

Pigmentation changes

Freckles
Lentigo
Guttate hypomelanosis
Brown and white pigmentation
Poikiloderma of Civatte
Hair follicle prominence

Papular changes

Nevi
Yellow papules and solar elastosis
Favre–Racouchot syndrome (comedones and cysts around the eyes

Adapted from Habif, T. (2010). Light-related disease and disorders of pigmentation. In T. Habif (Ed.), *Clinical dermatology* (5th ed.). Philadelphia, PA: Mosby Elsevier.

---

      b. Elastosis is a result of chronic sun damage characterized by yellowing and coarsening of the skin.
      c. Other sun-induced skin changes include telangiectasias, atrophy of the skin, deep wrinkling, follicular plugging, benign neoplasms, malignant neoplasm, and thickening epidermis (Box 15-3).
C. Treatment modalities.
   1. Collagen injections and lipotransfer can be used on the facial lines.
   2. Different laser procedures may be used to soften the facial lines around the eyes, and upper lip gives very satisfactory results. Lasers can also be used for retexturizing, resurfacing, activating collagen production, and reducing pigmentation issues.
   3. Topical tretinoin and tazarotene creams can be used for wrinkling, tactile roughness, lentigines, freckles, actinic keratosis, telangiectasias, and inflammation.
   4. Utilization of emollients and moisturizing creams can be used to increase skin pliability, decrease inflammation, and improve skin texture.
   5. Plastic surgery procedures such as rhytidectomy (face lifts) and blepharoplasty are available.

II. XEROSIS

A. Definition: xerosis is dry skin that appears when there is dehydration of the stratum corneum (Figures 15-12 and 15-13).
B. Pathophysiology.

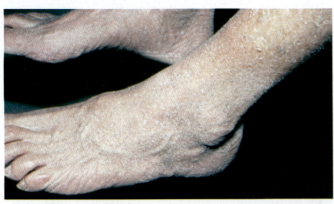

FIGURE 15-12. Xerosis. Dry skin tends to be most apparent on the hands and lower legs. This elderly patient's legs are dry and scaly. (From Goodheart, H. P. (2003). *Goodheart's photoguide of common skin disorders* (2nd ed.). Philadelphia, PA: Lippincott Williams & Wilkins.)

1. Older people have an accelerating decrease in epidermal free fatty acids, compared to younger individuals with similar skin conditions.
2. Xerotic skin has a reduced amino acid content.
3. The lower legs and feet are more commonly affected than the arms among older people.
4. The skin appears dry and scaly.
5. The patient usually complains of dryness and itching.
6. The systemic drying of the skin acids with age is a genetic inheritance.

C. Treatment modalities.
   1. The goal of all treatment is to add water to the skin and its environment.

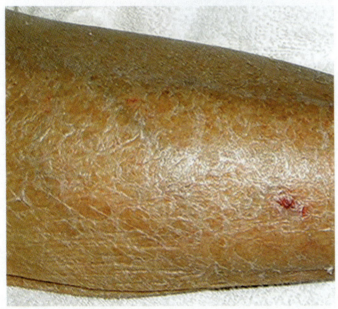

FIGURE 15-13. Moderate xerosis. Dry skin with a scaly, fish-like appearance. Scales are easily rubbed off the skin surface. Treatment is with an exfoliating, emollient, and moisturizing agent. (From Baranoski, S., & Ayello, E. (2015). *Wound care essentials*. Philadelphia, PA: Lippincott Williams & Wilkins.)

2. Room temperatures should be kept cool, and the use of humidifiers encouraged.
3. Warm to cool baths and showers should be taken; hot water should be avoided.
4. Moisturizers should be applied immediately after bathing.
5. Bath oils may be added to the water; however, avoid if high risk for falls.
6. Excessive use of soaps should be avoided, as well as solvents and drying compounds. Gentle nonsoap cleansers such as Cetaphil, Dove, or CeraVe can reduce dryness.
7. Patients should be encouraged to use emollients. Petroleum may be tolerated best by the elderly and should always be applied to moist skin.
8. Where possible, warmer, humid climates are preferable to cold dry regions.
9. For symptomatic xeroses, topical corticosteroid ointments can bring rapid and effective relief.

PATIENT EDUCATION
Xerosis

• Keep the air at home humidified (explain effective ways to the patient to accomplish).
• Take cool baths and apply lubricating agents to the skin.
• Avoid rough or constricting clothing, as it can traumatize dry skin.
• If corticosteroid ointments are being used, luke warm water compresses must be applied 10 to 15 minutes prior to the application of the medication.

III. SEBORRHEIC KERATOSIS

A. Definition: seborrheic keratosis is a benign epithelial lesion (Figure 15-14).
B. Etiology.
   1. Heredity is the most important factor in determining who will develop these keratoses and how many will occur.
   2. Age is the second important factor. Lesions can start to develop as early as the late 20s or early 30s.
   3. Lesions are more commonly seen in people with oily or acne seborrheic skin types.
C. Assessment.
   1. The lesions occur mostly on the scalp, face, neck, and upper trunk and are less common on the appendages.
   2. The color varies from a flesh color to a coal black.
   3. They may be as small as a few millimeters or up to 3 cm in size.
   4. The lesions are usually raised papules or plaques, occasionally appearing as macules.
   5. They can be greasy or warty to the touch.
   6. As they age, they become larger and darker in color.
   7. Occasionally, the keratosis is irritated by clothing or jewelry and becomes inflamed.

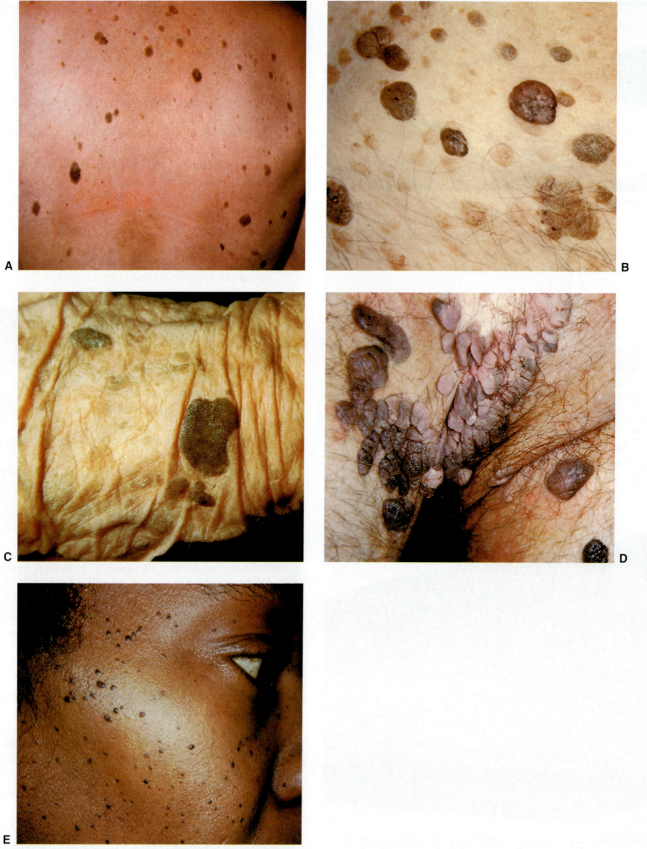

FIGURE 15-14. Seborrheic keratoses **(A)** on the back of an older man; **(B)** close-up of seborrheic keratoses; **(C)** large seborrheic keratosis on older woman's hand; **(D)** multiple seborrheic keratoses on crural area; and **(E)** seborrheic keratoses on the face. (From Hall, B. J., & Hall, J. C. (2010). *Sauer's manual of skin diseases* (10th ed., p. 447). Philadelphia, PA: Lippincott Williams & Wilkins.)

D. Pathophysiology.
1. The melanocytes are small and restricted to the basal cell layer on histologic analysis.
2. There is hyperplasia of the epidermis and adnexal epithelium.
3. There may be an increase of melanin in the keratinocytes, and the granular layer is not prominent.
E. Treatment modalities.
1. The seborrheic keratosis is a benign lesion and may be left untreated.
2. When one becomes inflamed or irritated, it should be removed, usually using cryotherapy, a simple shave or curettage biopsy.
3. Often, patients want them removed for cosmetic reasons, because clothing irritates them, or because they interfere with shaving.
4. Complications of removing these lesions include hypopigmentation, hypertrophic scarring, and infection.

PATIENT EDUCATION
Seborrheic Keratosis

- These lesions are benign and can be left untreated.
- If the lesions become irritated, or if the patient is concerned about melanoma, a dermatologist should be consulted for a thorough examination.

BIBLIOGRAPHY

Adams, L., DiMuzio, A., & Billhimer, W. (2014). Effect of pseudoceramide moisturizer on barrier integrity and treatment of winter xerosis. *American Porphyria Foundation*. doi: 10.1016/j.jaad.2014.01.129

Botto, N. C., & Warshaw, E. (2008). Solar urticarial. *Journal of the American Academy of Dermatology, 59*(6), 909–920. doi: 10.1016/j.jaad.2008.08.020

Ceilley, R. I., & Jorizzo, J. L. (2013). Current issues in the management of actinic keratosis. *Journal of the American Academy of Dermatology, 68*, S28.

Children's Melanoma Foundation. (2014). Sun aware. Retrieved from: http://www.sunaware.org/wp-content/themes/thestation/styles/sunaware/panel1.jpg

Darlenski, R., Surber, C., & Fluhr, J. W. (2010). Topical retinoids in the management of photodamaged skin: From theory to evidence-based practical approach. *British Journal of Dermatology, 163*(6), 1157–1165. doi: 10.111/j.13652133.2010.09936.x

Dermatology Nurses Association. (2015). Indoor tanning. Retrieved from: http://www.dnanurse.org/indoor-tanning

Epstein, E. (2001). *Common skin disorders* (5th ed.). Philadelphia, PA: Saunders.

FDA. (2011). Questions and answers: FDA announces new requirements for over-the-counter sunscreen products marketed in the U.S. Retrieved from: http://www.fda.gov/Drugs/ResourcesForYou/Consumers/BuyingUsingMedicineSafely/UnderstandingOver-the-CounterMedicines/ucm258468.htm#Q6_What_are_the_main_points

Green, A. C., Hughes, M. C., McBride, P., & Fourtanier, A. (2011). Factors associated with premature skin aging (photoaging) before the age of 55: A population-based study. *Dermatology, 222*, 74.

Gruber-Wackernagel, A., Byrne, S. S., & Wolf, P. (2014). Polymorphous light eruption: Clinical aspects and pathogenesis. *Dermatology Clinics, 32*(3), 315–334. doi: 10.1016/j.det.2014.03.012

Habif, T. P. (2010). *Clinical dermatology: A color guide to diagnosis and therapy* (5th ed.). Spain: Mosby Elsevier.

Hadley, J., Tristani-Firouzi, P., Hull, C., Florell, S., Cotter, M., & Hadley, M. (2012). Results of an investigator-initiated single-blind split-face comparison of photodynamic therapy and 5% imiquimod cream for the treatment of actinic keratoses. *Dermatologic Surgery, 38*, 722.

Horner, M., Alikhan, A., Tintle, S., Tortorelli, S., Davis, D., & Hand, J. (2013). Cutaneous porphyrias. Part 1: Epidemiology, pathogenesis, presentation, diagnosis, and histopathology. *International Journal of Dermatology, 52*(12), 1464–1480. doi: 10.1111/ijd.12305

James, W. D., Berger, T., & Elston, D. (2011). *Andrews' diseases of the skin: Clinical dermatology* (11th ed.). Philadelphia, PA: Elsevier Saunders.

Koo, J., Cheung, L., & Lee, S. L. (2007). *Contemporary guide to dermatology*. Newton, PA: Handbooks in Health Care Co.

Lallas, A., Argenziano, G., Moscarella, E., Longo, C., Simonetti, V., & Zalaudek, I. (2014). Diagnosis and management of facial pigmented macules. *Clinics in Dermatology, 32*(1), 94–100. doi: 10.1016/j.clindermatol.2013.05.030

Mayo Clinic. (2015). Diseases and conditions: Sunburn. *Mayo Foundation for Medical Education and Research*. Retrieved from: http://www.mayoclinic.org/diseases-conditions/sunburn/basics/definition/con-20031065

Peris, K., & Fargnoli, M. C. (2015). Conventional treatment of actinic keratosis: An overview. *Current Problems in Dermatology, 46*, 108–114. doi: 10.1159/000366546

Praetorius, C., Strum, R., & Steingrimsson, E. (2014). Sun-induced freckling: Ephelides and solar lentigines. *Pigmented Cell and Melanoma Research, 27*(3). doi: 10.1111/pcmr.12232

Sattler, U., Thellier, V., Sibuad, C., Taieb, S., Mercy, C., Meyer, P. & Meyer, N. (2014). Factors associated with sun protection compliance: Results from a nationwide cross-sectional evaluation of 2215 patients from a dermatological consultation. *British Journal of Dermatology, 170*(6), 1327–1335. doi: 10.1111/bjd.12966

Schulenburg-Brand, D., Katugampola, R., Anstey, A. V., & Badminton, M. N. (2014). The cutaneous porphyrias. *Dermatologic Clinics, 32*(3), 369–384. doi: 10.1016/j.det.2014.03.001

Simpson, S. (2003). Photodermatoses, photodamage, and aging skin. In M. Hill (Ed.), *Dermatology nursing essentials: A core curriculum* (2nd ed., pp. 259–274). New Jersey: DNA.

Uhlenhake, E., Sangueza, O., Lee, A., & Jorizzo, J. (2010). Spreading pigmented actinic keratosis: A review. *Journal of the American Academy of Dermatology, 63*(6), 499–506. doi: 10.1016/j.jaad.2009.07.026

Voelker, R. (2015). Upswing in skin cancer costs. *Journal of the American Medical Association, 313*(4), 348.

Wolff, K., & Johnson, R. (2009). *Fitzpatrick's color atlas and synopsis of clinical dermatology* (6th ed.). New York, NY: McGraw Hill.

Yaar, M., & Glichrest, B. A. (2007). Photoageing: Mechanism, prevention, and therapy. *British Journal of Dermatology, 157*(5), 874–887. doi: 10.1111/j.1365-2133.2007.08108.x

STUDY QUESTIONS

1. When looking for a sunscreen, which of the following must be included on the label for best sun protection?
    a. UVB
    b. Waterproof
    c. Broad-spectrum UVA and UVB
    d. Titanium dioxide

2. Photo damage can result in which of the following?
    a. Skin tags
    b. Telangiectasias
    c. Epidermal thickening
    d. B and C

3. Which of the following is a common treatment for actinic keratosis?
    a. Photodynamic therapy
    b. Cryosurgery
    c. Topical 5-FU
    d. All of the above

4. Which of the following describes polymorphous light eruption?
    a. A sun-induced allergic reaction to a yet unknown photosensitizer
    b. Pigmented macules that occur from photoexposure
    c. Sunburn
    d. UVA exposure with a photosensitizing chemical

5. Preventive photodamage education should include which of the following?
    a. Broad-spectrum sunscreens
    b. Solar-protective clothing
    c. Avoiding the sun between 10 AM and 4 PM
    d. All of the above

6. All of the following are examples of photoaging *except:*
    a. Poikiloderma of Civatte
    b. Telangiectasias
    c. Facial lines tend to deepen and widening due to hormonal changes and gravity
    d. More numerous nevi on sun-exposed surfaces

7. Porphyria cutanea tarda can be diagnosed using which of the following?
    a. Twenty-four-hour collection of urine
    b. Comprehensive metabolic panel
    c. Negative immunofluorescence stain
    d. None of the above

8. When educating a patient on the use of imiquimod or 5-FU, which of the following are important points to discuss?
    a. The skin will become very red, irritated, and painful. Petrolatum jelly, oral pain medications, or topical steroids may be used for pain relief.
    b. In patients with severe actinic damage, treatment may be performed in sections to decrease side effects and pain.
    c. The cream should be applied as many times daily as tolerated for 6 weeks.
    d. A and B

9. Best care for xerosis includes which of the following?
    a. Reduce bathing to one times weekly and apply moisturizer minimally.
    b. Dry skin thoroughly before application of moistures or emollients.
    c. After warm bathing, apply moisturizer within three minutes.
    d. Wear tight warm clothing to decrease moisture loss.

10. Which of the following are the most common complications of treating seborrheic keratosis?
    a. Pigmentation loss and scarring
    b. Increased risk of actinic damage
    c. Infection
    d. B and C

11. Treatment for solar urticaria includes which of the following?
    a. High doses of antihistamines
    b. High doses of antibiotics
    c. Burow solution (1% to 5%) compresses
    d. Application of petroleum jelly

12. Over 45% of actinic keratoses turn into squamous cell carcinoma.
    a. True
    b. False

Answers to Study Questions: 1.c, 2.d, 3.d, 4.a, 5.d, 6.c, 7.a, 8.d, 9.c, 10.a, 11.a, 12.b

CHAPTER 16

Cutaneous Malignancies

Grace Chung

OBJECTIVES

After studying this chapter, the reader will be able to:

- Distinguish between premalignant and malignant skin lesions by different growth patterns and clinical presentations.
- Identify the predisposing factors of cutaneous malignancies.
- Describe the relationship of ultraviolet radiation exposure and genetic mutations in development of cutaneous malignancies.
- Discuss the various treatment options available for patients diagnosed with cutaneous malignant diseases based on clinical and histologic assessment.

KEY POINTS

- Tumors and pigmented lesions of the skin may be benign, premalignant, or malignant.
- Regularly performed visual skin examinations and photoprotective behaviors are the most indispensable and cost-effective preventive measures against development of skin cancers.
- Persistent hyperkeratotic and indurated actinic keratosis lesions should be considered for skin biopsy to rule out skin cancers.
- Squamous cell carcinoma is locally invasive and has potential to metastasize.
- Pearly appearance with telangiectasias is the most common presentation of basal cell carcinoma. A pigmented basal cell carcinoma, however, may resemble other types of growth lesions (e.g., nodular melanoma, pigmented seborrheic keratosis, melanocytic nevus).
- The four types of malignant melanoma include superficial spreading melanoma, nodular melanoma, lentigo maligna melanoma, and acral lentiginous melanoma. The prognosis of a malignant melanoma depends on tumor thickness, depth of invasion, and distant metastasis.
- Cutaneous T-cell lymphoma is a rare type of cancer that originates in white blood cells and typically appears in severely itch skin lesions. Patients with chronic skin rash that delays improvement, progresses through different stages of lesions, and repeated cycles of regression and recurrence should be evaluated for cutaneous T-cell lymphoma.
- Sézary syndrome is an aggressive form of leukemic cutaneous T-cell lymphoma variant.
- Kaposi sarcoma is a multicentric, lymphatic, and vascular epithelial hyperplasia and not a sarcoma of mesenchymal origin.

ACTINIC KERATOSIS

I. OVERVIEW

Actinic keratosis (AK), also called solar keratosis or senile keratosis (nonrecommended synonym), is a premalignant neoplasm of the epidermis. AK presents as a solitary or multiple lesions on sun-exposed areas, and greater than 80% occur on the head, neck, forearms, and dorsal hands. History of AK correlates with increased risk for developing invasive squamous cell carcinomas (SCCs).

A. Definition: AK is a premalignant, atypical proliferation of mutated keratinocytes arising from the basal layer and remaining in the epidermis.

B. Incidence:
1. One of the most commonly seen problems in dermatology visits, affecting more than 58 million people in the United States.
2. The incidence varies by skin type, geographic location, and amount of ultraviolet (UV) radiation exposure.

C. Etiology:
1. Chronic occupational and recreational UV radiation exposure
2. Genetic predisposition: fair skin and family history of skin cancers
3. Genetic disorders: ineffective or interference of DNA repair against skin sun damage (i.e., xeroderma pigmentosum, Bloom syndrome, and Rothmund-Thomson syndrome)
4. Gender (male > female), advancing age, and geographic location
5. History of serious sunburn
6. Immunosuppression in organ transplant recipients and immunomodulatory medication (biologic) users in autoimmune disorders

D. Pathogenesis:
1. Chronic UV radiation exposure, mostly UVB (290 to 320 nm), induces mutation of epidermal keratinocyte DNA.
2. Keratinocyte DNA mutation in the *p53* tumor suppressor gene located on chromosome 17p132 involves in cell cycle regulation, apoptosis (programmed cell death process), and DNA repair.
3. Mutated *p53* gene leads to prolonged cell life span and delayed cell apoptosis, resulting in proliferation and clonal expansion of atypical keratinocytes and formation of AKs.

II. CLINICAL VARIANTS

A. Common AK: few millimeters to 2 cm in diameter, pink or erythematous, keratotic papule or plaque (Figure 16-1)
B. Hypertrophic AK (HAK): tan, white, or gray, thick or exophytic (outward-growing) scaly papule or plaque, with erythematous base (Figure 16-2)
C. Atrophic AK: smooth pink or erythematous macule or patch, with absent keratotic scale
D. Pigmented AK: keratotic scale lying over hyperpigmented macule or patch
E. Cutaneous horn: keratotic projection (exophytic), with the mound of compact keratin resembling the shape of a cone or spicule
F. Actinic cheilitis (solar cheilosis): rough keratotic papule or plaque occurring on the lip; may be cracking (fissuring) or ulcerating

III. LABORATORY AND DIAGNOSTIC TESTS

A. Often clinically diagnosed by visual inspection and palpation.
B. Dermoscopy using handheld device to magnify and illuminate lesions for making clinical diagnosis.
C. Skin biopsy is indicated when diagnosis is uncertain, to get definitive diagnosis and rule out malignancy or differentiate from other nonmalignant growth lesions.

IV. DIFFERENTIAL DIAGNOSIS

Use a fingertip as the diagnostic tool to distinguish AK lesions from common flaky scales on dry skin surface.
A. Inflamed seborrheic keratosis
B. Pityriasis rubra pilaris

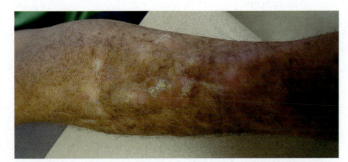

FIGURE 16-1. Actinic keratosis: pink keratotic plaques on this 58-year-old man's forearm. (Courtesy of Grace Chung.)

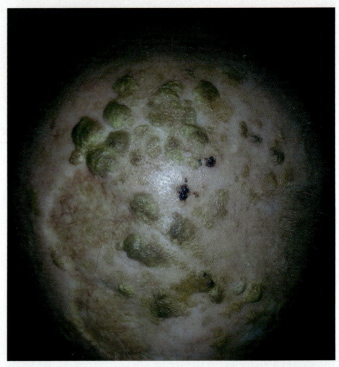

FIGURE 16-2. Hyperkeratotic actinic keratosis. Multiple hyperkeratotic papules and plaques with diffuse actinic damage on this patient's balding scalp. Two scabbed excoriated papules are at the center. (Courtesy of Grace Chung.)

C. Porokeratosis
D. Prurigo nodularis
E. Psoriasis
F. Seborrheic dermatitis
G. Squamous cell carcinoma
H. Superficial basal cell carcinoma (BCC)
I. Viral wart

V. TREATMENT MODALITIES

A. Cryotherapy: most common, first-line treatment option with a cure rate of 98.8%
B. Electrodessication and curettage: ideal treatment for hyperkeratotic AKs and those resembling the presentation of invasive SCC
C. Topical 5-fluorouracil (5-FU): interferes with DNA and RNA synthesis of the mutated keratinocytes by blocking the methylation reaction of deoxyuridylic acid to thymidylic acid
D. Imiquimod (immune response modifier): induces synthesis and release of cytokines such as interferon–tumor necrosis factors (TNF) and interleukins
E. Prevention: sun avoidance, use of sunscreen, photoprotective clothing, and self-screening exam

VI. PROGNOSIS

AKs are premalignant, but they have potential to progress into malignant lesions. Approximately 65% of all SCC and 36% of all BCC are transformed from preexisting AKs.

PATIENT EDUCATION
Actinic Keratosis

- Rough and scaly actinic keratosis (AK) lesions are easier felt than seen.
- AK is a precancerous lesion. Patient should not get confused with the number of AK lesions removed by various types of treatment methods in reporting the history of skin cancer.
- Reasons to remove AK lesions on the skin include cosmetic concerns (unsightliness), frequent irritation, and potential risk of developing into an SCC (rarely BCC).
- Photoprotection is the key in preventing sun damage and future occurrence of AK.

BASAL CELL CARCINOMA

I. OVERVIEW

BCC is the most common nonmelanoma skin cancer (NMSC) in the United States. UV radiation exposure is considered the biggest contributing risk factor for BCC as evidenced by the common sites of occurrence on sun-exposed areas such as the scalp, face, neck, chest, and distal parts of extremities. The malignant nature of BCC is demonstrated by expansive growth, destruction, and invasion of local structures including bone. BCC often remains local with low metastatic potential, and it's highly curable.

A. Definition: BCC is a malignant epithelial neoplasm arising from the basal cells (in the basal layer) of the epidermis and its appendages.

B. Incidence:
1. Over 3.5 million cases of NMSC among more than 2 million people annually.
2. Highest incidence among Caucasians and individuals with fair skin, approximately 75% to 80% of NMSC.
3. Greater than 70% occurrences are on the face, 15% on the trunk, and rare occurrences on non–sun-exposed areas including genital or perianal areas.

C. Etiology:
1. UV radiation exposure
   a. Intermittent episodes of intense UV exposure and recreational sun exposure at any age.
   b. Depletion of earth's protective ozone layer allows dangerous UV rays to penetrate the atmosphere.
2. Ionizing radiation exposure through occupation or therapeutic radiation for disorders such as facial acne, tinea capitis, psoriasis, eczema, or skin cancer.
3. Arsenic and carcinogenic exposures from contaminated drinking water, seafood, agricultural insecticides, or pharmacological mixtures (Fowler solution).
4. Genetic disorders and DNA repair capability:
   a. **Nevoid basal cell carcinoma syndrome (NBCCS)** (also known as Gorlin syndrome)—a rare autosomal dominant genetic disorder, caused by the germline mutations (Figure 16-3)

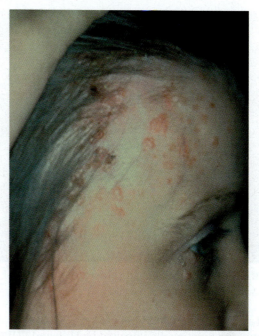

FIGURE 16-3. Nevoid basal cell carcinoma syndrome. (From DeVita, V. T., et al. (2008). *DeVita, Hellman, and Rosenberg's cancer: Principles and practice of oncology*. Philadelphia, PA: Wolters Kluwer.)

   (1) Affected individuals have multiple developmental anomalies in body systems (e.g., skin, bone, endocrine, and nervous system), unusual facial appearance, and predisposition for tumors including multiple BCCs at an early age.
   b. **Xeroderma pigmentosum (XP)**—an autosomal recessive genetic disorder with defective DNA repair mechanism. Inability to repair UV radiation–induced DNA damage and mutations results in development of BCC.
5. BCC may arise in nevus sebaceous, a congenital hamartoma of the skin.

D. Pathogenesis:
1. The mutations in *PTCH1*, *PTCH2*, *SMO* and *SUFU* genes are well known to associate with the development of BCC. Over 70% of BCC development is caused by alteration in *PTCH1* gene on chromosome 9q. *PTCH1* is a tumor suppressor gene, functioning as the controller of proliferation and differentiation.
2. *PTCH1* gene mutation causes loss of normal function and disruption in signaling pathways, resulting in uncontrolled growth in BCC tumorigenesis.
3. The mutations in P53 gene (early during carcinogenesis) and the MC1R gene are uncommonly involved in the development of BCC.
4. UV irradiation–induced skin inflammation: UV exposure results in inflammation of the skin, which leads to increased synthesis of prostaglandin and induction of cyclooxygenase-2 (COX-2). The key role of COX-2 inhibitors induced by the inflammation is to decrease the incidence of carcinogenesis in NMSC.

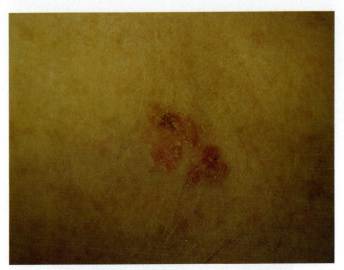

FIGURE 16-4. Superficial basal cell carcinoma. (From Dr. Barankin Dermatology Collection.)

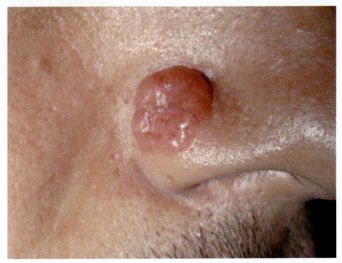

FIGURE 16-5. Nodular basal cell carcinoma. (From Lugo-Somolinos, A., et al. (2011). *VisualDx: Essential dermatology in pigmented skin*. Philadelphia, PA: Wolters Kluwer.)

5. Langerhans cells, found in the basal layer of the epidermis, are functionally impaired by UVB and PUVA treatment leading to morphologic changes within the cell.
   a. PUVA, PUVB, broadband UVB, and narrow band UVB phototherapy are types of UV radiation treatments for many severe skin diseases.
      (1) PUVA is a UV radiation treatment using a photosensitizing agent called Psoralens (P), such as methoxsalen (8-methoxypsoralen), 5-methoxypsoralen, and trisoralen orally or topically. Once the medication is applied (or taken orally 2 hours prior to the treatment), expose the treatment areas of the skin to UVA (long UV wavelength, 320 to 400nm) or UVB (290 to 320nm) in a therapeutic light box, a cabinet containing multiple fluorescent light bulbs to administer controlled amount of UV radiation, 2 to 3 times a week until optimal therapeutic outcomes are achieved.
      (2) Since 2008 however, lack of supplies in Psoralens caused infrequent use of PUVA or PUVB; currently the most common form of phototherapy is Narrowband UVB phototherapy (NB-UVB). NB-UVB (311 to 312mn) is known to have lower risk associated with phototherapy in comparison to formerly used broadband UVB (290 to 320nm).
      (3) Patients must use protective eyewear and cover sensitive skin areas (i.e. face and genitalia) for whole body exposure to limit UV radiation associated irritations, burning, and other damages during the treatment. Currently there are localized treatment instruments available for scalp, extremities, hands and feet.

II. CLINICAL VARIANTS

A. Superficial BCC (Figure 16-4): pearly pink, reddish, or eczematous, with a slightly scaling patch or slightly raised plaque.

B. Papulonodular BCC (Figure 16-5): pearly, shiny, or semi-translucent pink papule or nodule with a crater-like central umbilication and visible surrounding telangiectasia.

C. Sclerotic or morpheaform BCC (Figure 16-6): pale, atrophic, occasionally eroded, or crusting, cicatricial-appearing plaque.

D. Pigmented BCC (Figure 16-7): shiny papule, nodule, or plaque with focally speckled or entirely dark brown, blue-black, or black pigmentation while having pearly, semi-translucent rolled border at the base.

E. Basosquamous cell carcinoma: rarely occurring tumor but aggressive in nature and often classified as an SCC. This type must be confirmed by skin biopsy and histologic study.

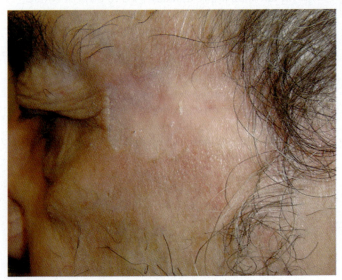

FIGURE 16-6. Morpheaform basal cell carcinoma. (From Khan, F. M., & Gerbi, B. J. (2011). *Treatment planning in radiation oncology*. Philadelphia, PA: Wolters Kluwer.)

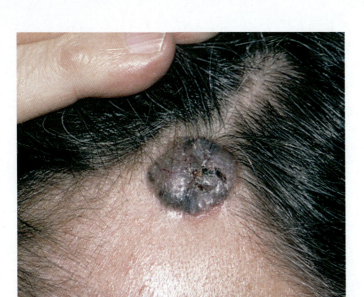

FIGURE 16-7. Pigmented basal cell carcinoma. (From Goodheart, H. P. (2003). *Goodheart's photoguide of common skin disorders* (2nd ed.). Philadelphia, PA: Lippincott Williams & Wilkins.)

III. LABORATORY AND DIAGNOSTIC TESTS

A. Clinical evaluation and skin biopsy for a confirmation of diagnosis.

B. Skin biopsy is highly recommended for patients with atypical features of a lesion for BCC, no prior history of BCC, or other risk factors contributing to possible recurrence of BCC.

IV. DIFFERENTIAL DIAGNOSIS

A. Amelanotic melanoma
B. Dermal nevi
C. Eczema
D. Keratoacanthoma
E. Nodular melanoma
F. Nummular eczema
G. Psoriasis
H. Scar/cicatricial plaque
I. Squamous cell carcinoma

V. TREATMENT MODALITIES

Treatment modalities are decided by the location and size of the tumor.

A. Cryosurgery
  1. A noninvasive procedure using liquid nitrogen.
  2. Useful in small superficial BCC treatment on trunk and extremities.
  3. Liquid nitrogen is administered by cone spray apparatus or by use of cryoprobes that conduct cold evenly.
  4. May result in postinflammatory hypo- or hyperpigmentation (PIH).
  5. No specimen available for evaluation of margins.
B. Electrosurgery (electrodessication and curettage)
  1. Local anesthesia, minimal equipment, and quick office procedure.

2. Useful in treatment of well-differentiated primary BCCs located on trunk and extremities and on patients who are not candidates for invasive surgical procedures.
  3. Disadvantages include lack of specimen for margin evaluation and possible hypertrophic scar development.
  4. Contraindicated in patients with pacemaker or defibrillator implant, BCCs 2 cm or larger, recurrent BCC, or a BCC located in high-risk location for recurrence.
  5. Electrodessication and curettage offers cure rate of 97% to 98%.
C. Carbon dioxide laser (CO_2)
  1. May be used in conjunction with a curette in place of electrocautery.
  2. Advantages include minimal nonspecific thermal injury to adjacent cells with more rapid healing and less pain postoperatively.
D. Surgical excision
  1. Office procedure using local anesthetic
  2. Useful for well-differentiated primary BCC lesions
  3. Provides specimen for random evaluation of surgical margins
  4. Time-consuming procedure requiring surgical skill, assistants, and more equipment
  5. Highly efficacious with cure rate of 96.8% to 99% depends on the types, sizes, depths, and locations of the lesions.
E. Radiation therapy
  1. Superficial x-ray or high-energy electron beam radiation.
  2. Useful for BCCs on the head and neck, with chance of metastasis
  3. May cause radionecrosis over bone
F. Mohs micrographic surgery, named after Frederic Mohs, MD, is defined as excision of skin cancer with histological margin control of deep and peripheral margins.
  1. Office procedure using local anesthesia.
  2. Indications:
    a. Primary BCC on cosmetic sensitive areas (e.g., face and ears).
    b. Morpheaform BCC or tumors with indistinct margins.
    c. Incompletely excised and recurrent BCC.
    d. Certain anatomic areas best treated by the precision of Mohs surgery include central "H" zone of the face comprising the upper lip, nose, medial canthus, and temple.
  3. Tumor is debulked and a layer of tissue is removed to be processed for margin evaluation in an on-site laboratory.
  4. Tissue specimen is marked with color-coding inks to maintain the orientation of the specimen and the defect (surgical site).
  5. The specimen is then frozen, sliced, and fixed on glass slides and treated in series of chemicals for staining.
  6. Surgeon or dermatopathologist reads slides observing the base and epidermal edges of the specimen for the total clearance of the tumor; if BCC persists at one or more color-coded margins, another layer from the corresponding site(s) is harvested from the defect. (Same steps are repeated until the margins are free of tumor.)

7. Precise margin control and conservative removal of the benign skin surrounding the tumor offer advantage in cosmetic sensitive areas and higher cure rate.

8. Disadvantages include possible lengthy procedures with waiting periods; requires special training of surgeon, assistants, and technicians and specialized equipment.

G. Other treatment modalities

1. Topical 5-fluorouracil and imiquimod are effective treatments for superficial BCC and multifocal BCC. May also be used as pretreatment method prior to Mohs or excision surgery for ill-defined BCC lesions on diffuse sun-damaged skin.

2. Photodynamic therapy (PDT) for superficial BCC, which selectively destroys tumor cells by the administration of a photosensitizing topical agent that is activated by light creating oxygen products capable of cell destruction.

a. Beneficial for patients with nevoid BCC syndrome

VI. PROGNOSIS

BCCs' viability is dependent on the integumentary system (e.g., pilosebaceous units and loose connective tissue stroma). Therefore, they have low chance of metastasis and highly curable. Occasionally occurring metastases are associated with long-standing history of neglecting and untreating a large, ulcerating, and aggressively growing, nonhealing lesions.

PATIENT EDUCATION
Basal Cell Carcinoma

- UV radiation exposure, especially a person's life style, habits, and susceptibility to solar radiation, is the biggest contributing factor in developing a BCC.
- Any nonhealing, new-growth lesions on sun-exposed areas should be evaluated for possible nonmelanoma skin cancers such as BCC.
- Cryotherapy and topical agents (e.g., imiquimod, 5-fluorouracil) are effective treatments for superficial BCC without the need to undergo invasive surgical procedures.

SQUAMOUS CELL CARCINOMA

I. OVERVIEW

SCC is the second most common form of skin cancer. SCCs frequently develop on sun-exposed areas due to UV irradiation–induced skin keratinocytes damage and malignant transformation. Unlike BCC, SCC may metastasize via lymphatic or hematogenous spread.

A. Definition: SCC is a malignant epithelial neoplasm arising from the mutated keratinocytes in the epidermal layer of the skin.

B. Incidence:

1. Approximately 20% of NMSC occurrence and over 700,000 case annually

2. Higher incidence among men, advanced age, history of excessive sun exposure, and having multiple AKs

3. Risk factors:
   a. Chronic sun exposure
   b. Immunosuppression
   c. Genetic predispositions
   d. Chemical carcinogen exposures
   e. X-ray irradiation
   f. Geographic factors
   g. Chronic inflammation/nonhealing wounds

C. Etiology:

1. Cumulated dose of UV radiation: excessive UV light absorbed by DNA of keratinocytes results in damage and malignant transformation. Chronic UVB radiation including excessive childhood sun exposure is the most contributory cause of sun damage in cumulative sun exposure.

2. Ionizing radiation.

3. Scar including thermal injury.

4. Chronic inflammation: nonhealing wounds (e.g., chronic ulcer, burns, and infection) and chronic inflammatory dermatoses such as lichen sclerosus et atrophicus. Cutaneous SCC arising from a chronic wound is also known as Marjolin ulcer.

5. Immunosuppression: solid organ transplant recipients, immunosuppressant medication users, HIV infection, and prolonged use of oral prednisone.

6. Genetic disorders: XP, albinism, epidermolysis bullosa (EB) syndrome, epidermodysplasia verruciformis, Fanconi anemia, Fergus-Smith syndrome, dyskeratosis congenital, Rothmund-Thomson syndrome, Bloom syndrome, and Werner syndrome.

7. Human papillomavirus (HPV) infection: HPV-16, HPV-18, HPV-31, HPV-5, and HPV-8. Large group of HPV are DNA tumor viruses that affect the mucosa and skin epithelial layer, resulting in hyperproliferative lesions and development of SCCs.

8. Organic hydrocarbons (coal, tar, pitch, crude, paraffin oil, lubricating oil, fuel oil, anthracene oil, and creosote) and inorganic arsenic. Presence of palmoplantar arsenical keratoses is the clue of arsenic exposure.

9. PUVA: risk increases with number of treatments, previous exposure of ionizing radiation, and history of prior skin cancers.

10. Use of photosensitizing medications: voriconazole, oral contraceptives, and BRAF inhibitors (vemurafenib, dabrafenib)

11. Precursor lesions include solar keratoses, arsenical keratoses, thermal keratoses, chronic radiation keratoses, tar keratoses, chronic cicatrix keratoses, Bowen disease, erythroplasia of Queyrat, and EV (Lewandowsky-Lutz syndrome).

D. Pathogenesis:

1. Chronic UV exposure induces several different cellular responses, including the induction of stress protein, DNA damage repair process, and cytokine production.

2. In dose-dependent DNA damage, affected cells first either undergo apoptosis (cell death as sunburn cells) or cease proliferating (cell cycle arrest) in order to undergo genetic repair process. Then, hyperproliferation and epidermal thickening follow the growth arrest.

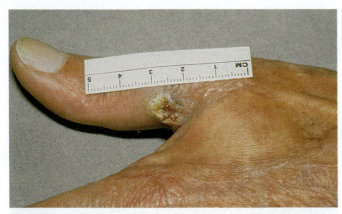

FIGURE 16-8. Invasive squamous cell carcinoma. (From Weisel, S. W. (2013). *Operative techniques in orthopaedic surgery*. Philadelphia, PA: Wolters Kluwer.)

3. In SCC development, accumulated dose of UV radiation exposure induces DNA damage and manifestation of *p53* genetic mutation.
4. Mutated *p53* in basal layer becomes resistant to UV-induced apoptosis and continuously increases the number of mutated *p53* in clonal expansion.
5. Continuous UV irradiation causes second *p53* mutation and gains the growth advantage in squamous cell dysplasia in the epidermal layer.
6. Additional genetic alteration leads to proliferation of neoplastic clone and results in SCC *in situ* at the epidermal surface.
7. Neoplastic tumor progresses to develop invasive property by additional genetic alteration and acquisition of invasive capability to become invasive SCC.
8. Highly differentiated tumors in invasive SCC form epidermal keratinization and invade to the dermis with a broad tumor margin.

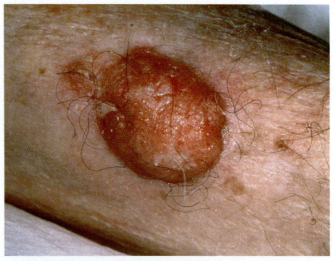

FIGURE 16-9. Nodular squamous cell carcinoma. (From Craft, N., et al. (2010). *VisualDx: Essential adult dermatology*. Philadelphia, PA: Wolters Kluwer.)

9. Continuous progression in tumorigenesis with genetic alteration allows the acquisition of the metastatic capacity in the metastasis of SCC.

II. CLINICAL VARIANTS

A. Invasive SCC (Figure 16-8): dysplastic or malignant keratinocytes involve the full thickness of the epidermis and infiltrate through the basal layer, dermis, or deeper tissues/organs.
  1. Well differentiated: pink, violaceous, or erythematous; firm, indurated papulonodule or plaque, with hyperkeratotic scale
  2. Poorly differentiated: erythematous or pale pink, soft granulomatous papule or plaque may have ulceration, necrosis, or hemorrhaging without hyperkeratosis.
B. Nodular SCC (Figure 16-9): often well-differentiated, pink or erythematous nodule with keratotic scale.
C. SCC *in situ* (Bowen disease) (Figure 16-10): erythematous, crusty, rough, and scaly patch or slightly raised plaque.

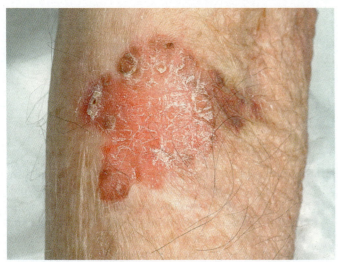

FIGURE 16-10. Squamous cell carcinoma *in situ*. (From Craft, N., et al. (2010). *VisualDx: Essential adult dermatology*. Philadelphia, PA: Wolters Kluwer.)

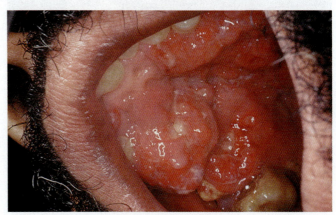

FIGURE 16-11. Oral squamous cell carcinoma. (From DeLong, L., & Burkhart, N. (2007). *General and oral pathology for the dental hygienist*. Philadelphia, PA: Lippincott Williams & Wilkins.)

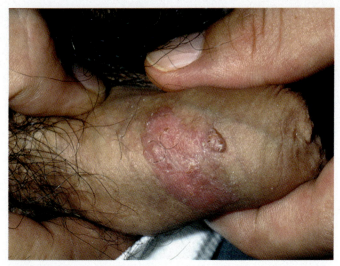

FIGURE 16-12. Penile squamous cell carcinoma *in situ*. (From Craft, N., et al. (2010). *VisualDx: Essential adult dermatology*. Philadelphia, PA: Wolters Kluwer.)

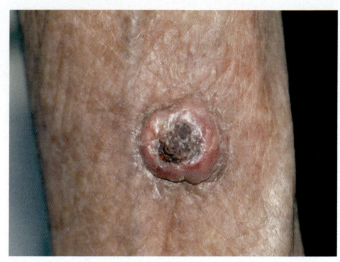

FIGURE 16-13. Keratoacanthoma. (From Goodheart, H. P. (2003). *Goodheart's photoguide of common skin disorders* (2nd ed.). Philadelphia, PA: Lippincott Williams & Wilkins.)

D. Oral SCC (Figure 16-11): pink or pale indurated plaque, ulcer, or nodule developed on the floor of the mouth or on the ventral/lateral side of the tongue. SCC may arise from erythroplakia (premalignant erythematous patches) or leukoplakia (persistent white plaques) of the oral mucosa.

E. Erythroplasia of Queyrat (SCC *in situ* of the glans penis) (Figure 16-12): erythematous, well-demarcated velvety patch or slightly raised plaque.

F. Keratoacanthoma (Figure 16-13): fast-growing (1.5 to 2 cm in 4 to 6 weeks), erythematous, pink, or flesh-colored papule or nodule with central keratotic plug.

G. Verrucous carcinoma (Figure 16-14): indolent form of a well-defined, exophytic, large wart-like papillomatous growth involving oral mucosa (oral florid papillomatosis), anogenital areas (condyloma acuminatum of Buschke-Lowenstein), and plantar foot (epithelioma cuniculatum).

III. LABORATORY AND DIAGNOSTIC TESTS

A. Clinical evaluation and skin biopsy for confirmation of diagnosis

B. Computed tomography (CT) scanning evaluation for possible metastasis to nearby bones and soft tissues for aggressively developing invasive-type SCC lesions

C. Magnetic resonance imaging (MRI) evaluation for possible involvement of perineural, orbital, or intracranial nerves for neurologic symptoms (local paresthesia, numbness, pain, visual changes, etc.)

IV. DIFFERENTIAL DIAGNOSIS

A. Amelanotic melanoma
B. Basal cell carcinoma
C. Hyperkeratotic actinic keratosis
D. Inflamed seborrheic keratosis
E. Merkel cell carcinoma
F. Nummular eczema
G. Paget disease
H. Prurigo nodularis
I. Psoriasis
J. Pyogenic granuloma
K. Traumatic ulcer/chronic inflammation
L. Viral warts (verruca)

V. TREATMENT MODALITIES

A. Mohs micrographic surgery: a treatment of choice for invasive SCC and high-risk SCC. Mohs procedure is particularly preferred for cosmetically sensitive areas on the head and neck.

1. Histopathologic evaluations of entire margins and depth of the specimen are performed during the procedure (repeated process of harvesting specimen from the surgical defect until total clearance).

2. Cure rate for tumors smaller than 2 cm is 98%; decreased cure rate to 75% for tumors larger than 2 cm.

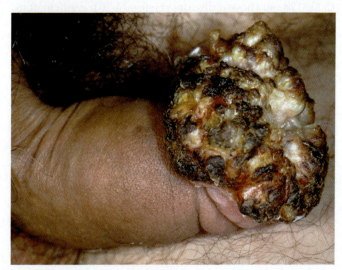

FIGURE 16-14. Verrucous carcinoma. (From Craft, N., et al. (2010). *VisualDx: Essential adult dermatology*. Philadelphia, PA: Wolters Kluwer.)

B. Conventional excision surgery: a typical treatment method for tumors smaller than 2 cm, low-grade, or well-differentiated type on the trunk and extremities.

C. Electrodessication and curettage: treatment for low-grade, small, superficial, and low-risk tumors, preferred on the trunk and extremities.
   1. Less invasive treatment option compared to conventional excision surgery
   2. Useful treatment option for patients in advanced age and poor surgical candidates

D. Cryotherapy: may be effective in treating very small, low-risk, superficial tumors.

E. 5-Fluorouracil (5-FU) and imiquimod topical treatments (biologic modifiers): effective in treating superficial type and early-stage SCC lesions progressing from AK.

F. PDT using photosensitizing agents with blue light (wavelength 400 nm) is effective in destroying skin cancer cells.

G. Radiation therapy is used in combination with other treatment modalities for large tumors; aggressive, recurrent, or inoperative cases; and poor candidates for invasive surgeries.

H. Regional control
   1. Nonpalpable nodes
      a. Close monitoring for lymphadenopathy
      b. Sentinel node biopsy for high-risk SCCs, followed by elective lymph node dissection if node is positive
      c. Radiation to draining (primary echelon) nodes for high-risk lesions
   2. Palpable nodes
      a. Radiation
      b. Surgery
      c. Chemotherapy
      d. Combination of above

VI. PROGNOSIS

The risk of metastasis and prognosis for SCC depend on the size of the tumor, location, depth, perineural involvement, and immunosuppression. SCC lesions developed from ulcerated wounds, chronic inflammation, and recurrent cutaneous lesions are considered high risk for metastasis.

PATIENT EDUCATION
Squamous Cell Carcinoma

- History of chronic UV radiation exposure, including life style, occupational and recreational sun exposure, is the main contributing factor of developing SCC.
- Contact with carcinogenic and arsenic chemicals may contribute to development of SCC *in situ* (Bowen disease).
- SCC occurs most commonly on the head, neck, and arms.
- Chronically inflamed, ulcerated, and nonhealing wounds should be considered for a skin biopsy to exclude SCC (Marjolin ulcer).
- Regular practice of photoprotection (e.g., wearing sun protective clothing, sunglasses, and sunscreen topicals) and seeking treatments for precancerous lesions (AKs) may lead to early detection of SCC and effectively prevent further skin sun damage.

KERATOACANTHOMA

I. OVERVIEW

Keratoacanthoma (KA) is a low-grade, well-differentiated variant of SCC, while the exact classification of the disease is still uncertain and some consider it a benign tumor. KA develops commonly on sun-exposed areas (e.g., head, neck, and extremities). It grows rapidly in 2 to 6 weeks to reach the average size of 0.5 to 2.5 cm in diameter, but it is rarely metastasized. It is manifested as a volcano-like dome-shaped plaque or an exophytic sharply circumscribed, crateriform nodule with central keratotic plug or scale. KA regresses in weeks to months if it is left untreated; however, the regression may result in an irregularly shaped atrophic scar. KA resembles SCC clinically as well as microscopically and is very difficult to distinguish from an invasive SCC.

A. Definition: KA is a rapidly proliferating, highly differentiated tumor of squamous epithelia, with a keratin scale or keratotic plug, arising from the neck of the hair follicle.

B. Etiology: the origin of the KA is still unclear. Below are the proposed etiologies of KA:
   1. Exposure to carcinogenic chemicals such as tar pits.
   2. Smoking
   3. Immunosuppression
   4. HPV infection
   5. Associating with Muir-Torre syndrome (defective DNA mismatch repair gene)

C. Pathogenesis:
   1. Some case studies report KA arises from *p*53 mutation and overexpression of P53 protein in signaling pathway.
   2. Microsatellite instability and mismatch repair deficient in genetic defect may have association with cancer-prone Muir-Torre syndrome.

II. CLINICAL VARIANTS

Clinical presentation of KA resembles SCC, even at the microscopic level; therefore, the differentiation between SCC and KA can be challenging.

A. Clinical stages in KA manifestation:
   1. Proliferative stage: sudden development and growth of firm papule with fine telangiectases for 2 to 4 weeks
   2. Mature stage: formation of a nodular plaque with central keratotic scale or plug
   3. Resolving/involution stage: tumor reabsorption within 4 to 6 months, result in slightly atrophic, depressed, and pale scar

B. Solitary KA (Figures 16-15 and 16-16)
   1. KA centrifugum: solitary lesion that sizes up to 20 cm with simultaneous healing at the center of the lesion. Common sites are on the face, trunk, or extremities.
   2. The giant KA: solitary, rapid-growing large lesion (average 9 cm or more). It's invasive and may involve underlying structures including cartilage.
   3. Subungual KA: rapidly growing, locally aggressive tumor, originating in the nail bed. It's a persistent, tender, swollen, erythematous, and umbilicated lesion, frequently involving the thumb or little finger with potential local bony destruction.

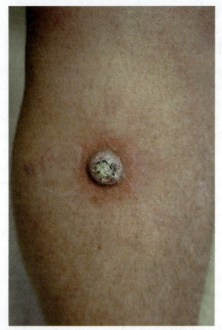

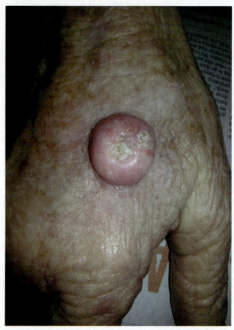

FIGURE 16-15. Keratoacanthoma. An inflamed violaceous nodular plaque with a central keratotic plug. (Courtesy of Grace Chung.)

FIGURE 16-16. Keratoacanthoma. A solitary, pink nodule with central keratin-filled crater. (Courtesy of Grace Chung.)

C. Multiple KAs (Figure 16-17):
  1. Ferguson-Smith (spontaneously regressing multiple KAs): sudden eruption of multiple KAs on sun-exposed areas such as face and extremities. Lesions resolve slowly with potential of recurrence. This condition is hereditary in an autosomal dominant pattern, and the incidence is usually during adulthood (approximately in the third decade of life).
  2. Grzybowski (nonregressing grouped KA): suddenly erupting generalized, disseminated 2- to 3-mm papules resembling milia or early eruptive xanthomas. They involve anywhere on the body including hands and feet, oral mucosa, and larynx. May resolve slowly over many months, and the lesions on the face may result in mask-like facies, ectropion, and atrophic scars.
  3. Muir-Torre syndrome (may have sebaceous differentiation): multiple sebaceous tumors and KA tumors start as erythematous papules and rapidly develop into shiny or flesh-colored nodules with telangiectases and central keratotic plug.

III. LABORATORY AND DIAGNOSTIC TESTS

A. Clinical skin lesion evaluation: rapid growth of exophytic crateriform nodular lesion
B. Confirmation with skin biopsy: complete excisional biopsy, skin full-thickness shave biopsy, or incisional biopsy in order to obtain the full-thickness specimen down to the subcutaneous fat

IV. DIFFERENTIAL DIAGNOSIS

A. Amelanotic melanoma
B. Basal cell carcinoma
C. Merkel cell carcinoma

D. Squamous cell carcinoma
E. Viral wart

V. TREATMENT MODALITIES

Treatment modalities are defined by the location and size of the tumor.
A. Complete excision; close resemblance in clinical and histological appearance of KA and SCC suggests treatment of KA as invasive SCC.
B. Mohs micrographic surgery.
C. Electrodessication and curettage (ED&C).
D. Radiation therapy.
E. Intralesional pharmacologic therapy.

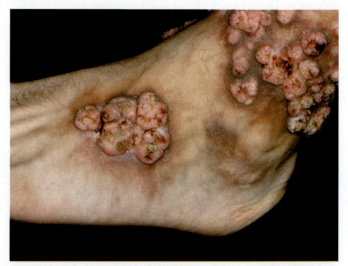

FIGURE 16-17. Multiple keratoacanthoma. (From Craft, N., et al. (2010). *VisualDx: Essential adult dermatology.* Philadelphia, PA: Wolters Kluwer.)

VI. PROGNOSIS

The risk of metastasis is low in KA, but complete excision of the lesion is recommended when there is no clear distinction between KA and SCC. Although some believe that a KA is a benign tumor, it is commonly treated rather than observed for spontaneous resolution. KA has potential for recurrence, but it is highly curable.

PATIENT EDUCATION
Keratoacanthoma

- Keratoacanthoma (KA) is a rapidly growing (in just a few weeks to a few months), nodular skin lesion commonly appearing on sun-exposed areas.
- KA lesions are often described as mild to moderately tender to the touch, little volcano-like nodules with central keratotic scale.
- People with history of excessive sun exposure through geographic location, occupation, recreation, and lifestyle are at risk of developing KA.
- Treatment of KA is preferred over active monitoring to exclude the risk of SCC and minimize the scarring that may result from spontaneous solving.

MALIGNANT MELANOMA

I. OVERVIEW

Cutaneous malignant melanoma (MM) is a potentially life-threatening, dangerous skin cancer. The development of melanoma and its progression can be determined by genetic predisposition and mutation, mutagenic environmental factors, and the host's immune response. Melanoma can be successfully cured when detected and adequately treated early. Melanoma may disseminate to any organ, most commonly in skin and subcutaneous tissue, lymph nodes, lungs, liver, brain, bone, and gastrointestinal tract.

A. Definition: melanoma is a malignant neoplasm of melanocytes (pigment-forming cells) and nevus cells, with a manifestation of irregular size, shape, or atypical pigmentation. It may arise from a preexisting nevus or *de novo* (from a new nevus).

B. Incidence:
1. Melanoma is the most dangerous form of skin cancer.
2. Most common form of malignant disease in young adults between 25 and 29 years old and the second most common form of malignant disease in adolescents.
3. Estimated 9,710 melanoma deaths and 76,100 new cases projected in 2014.
4. Melanoma accounts for approximately 75% of skin cancer–related deaths.
5. The lifetime risk of developing melanoma is 1 in 50 for Whites, 1 in 200 for Hispanics, and 1 in 1,000 for African Americans.
6. Gender difference in melanoma incidence varies by age groups:
   a. Men < women (under 40 years old)
   b. Men > women (over 40; twofold by age 60)

7. The risk of developing melanoma increases with advanced age.
8. The 5-year survival rate is 98% for early detected melanoma before lymph node involvement; the rate decreases to 62% and 16% for regional and distant metastasis, respectively.
9. Risk factors:
   a. History of excessive sun exposure and blistering sunburns
   b. Dysplastic nevi and familial multiple dysplastic nevi syndrome
   c. Multiple moles (>50)
   d. Freckling
   e. Personal and family history of melanoma
   f. Genetic factors: fair skin, red hair, freckles
   g. Socioeconomic status
   h. Immunosuppression
   i. Advanced in age
   j. Gender (male > female)

C. Etiology:
1. Occupational or recreational UV exposure (e.g., outdoor occupations, use of tanning beds, sun bathing)
   a. UVA rays cause skin aging, wrinkling, and DNA damage.
   b. UVB rays cause sunburn and skin DNA damage.
2. Dysplastic nevi (atypical moles) or multiple dysplastic nevi syndrome
   a. Lifetime risk for persons with dysplastic nevi syndrome is greater than 10%.
   b. Persons with congenital melanocytic nevi (moles present at birth) have risk of developing melanoma estimated between 0% and 10% depends on the size and location of the moles.
3. Fair skin, light hair and freckling, and burns easily
   a. Ten times higher risk of developing melanoma for Whites compared to African Americans
   b. More than double the risk of developing melanoma in people who had five or more severe sunburns during childhood and adolescence
4. Personal history of melanoma:
   a. 5% chance of recurrence in persons with history of melanoma
5. Family history of melanoma:
   a. About 10% of people with melanoma have family history of melanoma among their first-degree relatives.
   b. Approximately 10% to 40% of genetic mutation involved in families with high rate of melanoma.
   c. Abnormalities on chromosome 9*p*21 and melanoma-susceptible genes such as *p*16.
6. Genetic disorders such as XP-defective DNA mechanism to repair chronic UV damage led to development of skin cancers including melanoma in sun-exposed areas

D. Pathogenesis:
1. Different sites of the body, different amount of UV radiation, and different genetic makeups and oncogene mutations in each individual result in different types of melanoma.
2. Most common genetic mutations in melanoma involve disorders of the cell cycle pathways and transcriptional control mechanisms.

3. The mutation of *CDKN2A* gene located on chromosome 9*p*21 (codes for *p*16 and *p*14ARF proteins) is highly associated with the predisposition to develop melanoma.

4. The genetic mutation involving *CDKN2A* interferes with *p*53 in cell cycle progression and keeps on producing mutagenic DNA via cell division cycles and allows uncontrolled proliferation of mutated melanocytes.

5. *CDKN2A* involved in germline mutation, which explains the genetic factors in familial melanoma disease.

6. *BRAF* gene mutation is also found in about 40% to 60% of melanomas in intermittently sun-exposed individuals who developed melanoma, more commonly seen in young people.

7. *NRAS*-mutated oncogene is found in 15% to 20% of melanomas, more often in people with later age-at-onset melanomas.

8. *C-KIT*–mutated oncogene is most common in site-specific melanomas such as in mucosal (40%), acral (35%), and sun-damaged skin (25% to 30%) areas.

9. Melanoma is an immunogenic malignant tumor; therefore, complete or partial regression may occur.

II. CLINICAL VARIANTS

A. Superficial spreading melanoma (SSM) (Figure 16-18)
   1. Most common subtype appears on any anatomic surface, but most common on the back for men and the legs for women.
   2. Accounts for 70% of all diagnosed melanoma and is a leading cause of melanoma death for young adults.
   3. It may occur at any age for both men and women, but slightly higher incidence in women.
   4. Commonly appear as well-demarcated, asymmetrical, dark-pigmented macule or a patch or even slightly raised.

5. May arise within preexisting melanocytic nevus or *de novo*, with variegated colors including brown, black, pink, blue, gray, or white areas (possible regression) and with irregular borders.

6. Regression in SSM is a less pigmented area of a dark-pigmented SSM lesion, as a result of host's immune responses trying to destroy it.

B. Nodular melanoma (NM) (Figure 16-19)
   1. The second most common type of melanoma and accounts for 10% to 15% of all melanoma diagnosis.
   2. May develop anywhere on the body and more commonly seen among persons aged 60 years and older.
   3. Sudden appearance of nodular growth, in black, dark brown, or blue colors with well-defined border.
   4. Rapid vertical growth of the tumor warrants deeper invasion and high potential of metastasis with poor prognosis.
   5. Commonly arises *de novo* in uninvolved skin and often delays detection and treatment.
   6. NM is typically a dark-pigmented lesion, but it may appear as a nonpigmented, flesh-colored nodule (amelanotic melanoma; Figure 16-20) or mimicking a scar or a benign cyst (desmoplastic neurotropic melanoma).

C. Acral lentiginous melanoma (ALM) (Figure 16-21)
   1. Typically occurs on the palms, soles, subungual areas, and mucous membranes (mouth, nose, genitalia, anus, and urinary tract) in persons with more pigmented skin, such as Blacks, Asians, and non-White Hispanics. Accounts for 5% of total melanoma occurrence.
      a. 2% to 8% occurrence in Whites
      b. 29% to 72% in dark-skinned persons

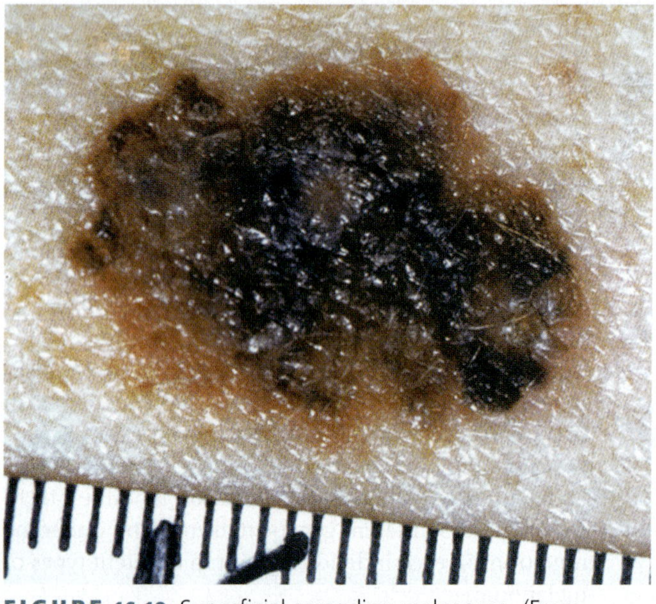

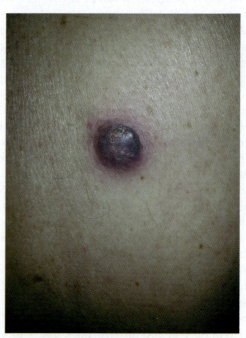

FIGURE 16-19. Nodular melanoma. This melanoma lesion was a 1.2-cm diameter nodule on a man's midback. Its maximum tumor thickness was at least 3.14 mm, with mitotic rate 15/mm², anatomic level IV, and staged as T3aN0M0. (Courtesy of Grace Chung.)

FIGURE 16-18. Superficial spreading melanoma. (From Werner, R. (2012). *Massage therapist's guide to pathology*. Philadelphia, PA: Wolters Kluwer.)

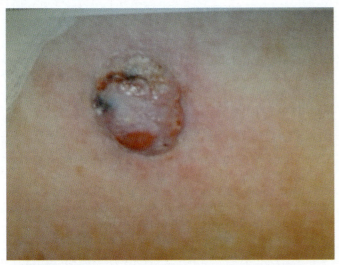

FIGURE 16-20. Amelanotic melanoma. A 2.5-cm diameter, 6.5-mm maximum tumor thickness, hypopigmented nodular amelanotic melanoma on a man's back. This patient's lymph node biopsy showed metastatic melanoma in 2 of 26 nodes. (Courtesy of Grace Chung.)

2. It presents as a flat, tan, brown to darkly pigmented macule or patch.
3. Subungual melanoma is a variant type and appears as dark-pigmented spot or fixed streaks from the proximal nail bed that does not move even with the nail growth.
4. Appearance of pigmented nail fold skin and destruction of the nail plate may indicate advanced ALM.
5. Based on the history of no recent trauma and bleeding under the nail plate (subungual hematoma), nail separating from the nail bed should be evaluated.

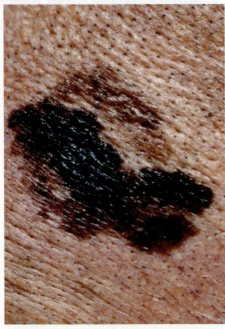

FIGURE 16-22. Lentigo maligna melanoma. (From Penne, R. B. (2011). *Wills Eye Institute—Oculoplastics.* Philadelphia, PA: Wolters Kluwer.)

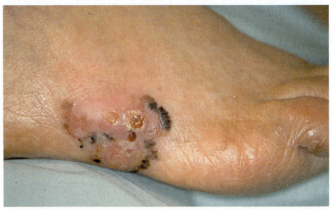

FIGURE 16-21. Acral lentiginous melanoma. (Courtesy of Art Huntley, MD, University of California at Davis.)

6. Mucous membrane involvement is often found in the mouth or inside of the nose, with symptoms including frequent nosebleed, nasal congestion, and pigmented growth or a mass inside the nose and mouth.
D. Lentigo maligna melanoma (LMM) (Figure 16-22)
1. Occurs on exposed surface of the body, often on the face and scalp of elderly persons.
2. Often misdiagnosed as a benign age spot, sun spot, or a lentigo simplex.
3. Typically, gradual growth and evolvement over 10 to 15 years results in irregular pigmentation, shape, and border, but it's not uncommon to see faster-growing LMM in matter of weeks to months.
4. A pigmented LMM patch may evolve into a nodular tumor, but it may also regress and appear as a blue-gray or white lesion.
5. An LMM can give rise to a desmoplastic melanoma, a fibrous tumor that has tendency to grow down and affect nerves of the skin.

III. CLINICAL ASSESSMENT FOR MELANOMA

Early detection and diagnosis are the most critical factors in overall survival rates.
A. Suspected lesions most commonly include asymmetry, border irregularity, color variation, diameter greater than 6 mm, and elevated lesion (ABCDE rule).
B. The most suspicious sign for melanoma is persistently changing (size, color, elevation, itching) pigmented lesion.
C. Other findings that are suspicious include new pigmented lesions after the age of 30 to 40 and multiple halo nevi in mid-to-late adult life.
D. Ulceration correlates with tumor thickness and is a significant feature.
E. Atypical melanoma lesions may appear as nonpigmented, flesh-colored nodules (amelanotic melanoma) or mimicking scars or benign cysts (desmoplastic neurotropic melanoma).
F. Physical examination of the patient with melanoma should include:
1. History of the patient and family, including history of the lesion

2. Computerized digital imaging to allow retrieval and comparison of previously stored images of new and existing lesions (if available)
3. Meticulous skin examination of entire skin surface including the scalp and genitalia
4. Careful palpation of all lymph nodes with special attention to primary draining nodes
5. Body systems evaluation especially of the brain, lungs, bone, gastrointestinal, and constitutional symptoms

IV. LABORATORY AND DIAGNOSTIC TESTS

A. Thorough history taking from patients including onset, duration, changes in color, shape, size, spontaneous bleeding and ulcerating, and evolution of the lesion. Visual inspection and comparison to the criteria of ABCDE rule:
1. Asymmetry (A): mismatching half
2. Border (B): poorly defined, atypical, or irregular border
3. Color (C): variegated shades (e.g., black, blue, reddish brown, tan, white)
4. Diameter (D): frequently greater than 6 mm (may be smaller)
5. Elevation/evolution (E): evolving in color, shape, and size
B. Dermoscopy/epiluminescence microscopy: clinical inspection using handheld magnifying/illuminating device for surface analysis
1. Skin biopsy is strongly recommended for definitive diagnosis and guidance for further follow-up.
2. Determination of the type of skin biopsy is based on the clinical presentation of the suspicious lesion: narrow excision biopsy with safety margin of 2-mm normal skin provides entire lesion or avoid transection of the lesion, adequate specimen for analysis, and staging of the lesion.
3. Incisional biopsy (partial sampling) is acceptable for a lesion with low clinical suspicion and large lesions. Repeat biopsy is suggested if the interpretation (e.g., diagnosis or microstaging) is inconclusive due to the inadequate size of specimen.
4. Chest x-ray and CBC/LDH screening for biopsy are proven invasive melanoma diagnosis.
5. Immunohistochemistry including S100 protein and HMB-45 can be used with panel of antibodies against other tumor markers to help diagnose otherwise nonobvious melanoma (performed by dermatopathologists).
6. Lymphatic mapping with sentinel lymph node biopsy (SLNB) for patients at risk for occult regional lymph node metastases. (Determined and performed by oncologists.)

V. DIFFERENTIAL DIAGNOSES

A. Basal cell carcinoma/pigmented basal cell carcinoma
B. Benign melanocytic nevus
C. Blue nevus
D. Epidermal inclusion cyst
E. Hypertrophic scar
F. Kaposi sarcoma
G. Merkel cell carcinoma
H. Neurofibroma
I. Pigmented seborrheic keratosis
J. Pyogenic granuloma
K. Solar lentigo
L. Spitz nevus
M. Verruca vulgaris

VI. STAGING CLASSIFICATION

A. Summary of 2010 American Joint Commission on Cancer (AJCC) Melanoma Staging System
1. The tumor–node–metastasis (TNM) system by the AJCC is the primary guideline for cancer staging and widely used (Table 16-1 and Box 16-1).
2. 2010 AJCC melanoma staging system update: primary tumor mitotic rate (T1 mitoses/mm^2) replaced Clark level of invasion as the primary criterion for staging and prognosis and predictor for survival. The presence of tumor ulceration remains as the criterion for adverse predictor for survival.
3. Tumor ulceration, a condition that has missing parts of the epidermis of the primary tumor, indicates deeper tissue involvement and greater chance of metastasis compared to nonulcerated tumors. This is determined by pathologists through microscopic examination of the tissue.
4. T is for classifying the tumor based on its three features: thickness (Breslow depth in millimeters [mm]), mitoses, and ulceration.
N is for indicating involvement of the echelon (nearby) lymph nodes.

TABLE 16-1 American Joint Committee on Cancer Melanoma Staging System, 2010[a]

Clinical Stage	Primary Tumor (T)	Regional Lymph Nodes (N)	Distant Metastasis (M)
0	Tis	N0	M0
IA	T1a	N0	M0
IB	T1b T2a	N0	M0
IIA	T2b T3a	N0	M0
IIB	T3b T4a	N0 N0	M0 M0
IIC	T4b	N0	M0
III	Any T	N1, N2, or N3	M0
IV	Any T	Any N	M1

[a]Clinical staging includes microstaging of the primary melanoma and clinical/radiologic evaluation for metastases. By convention, it should be used after complete excision of the primary melanoma with clinical assessment for regional and distant metastases.

Box 16-1. American Joint Committee on Cancer Tumor–Node–Metastasis Definitions

Primary Tumor (T)

TX Primary tumor cannot be assessed (e.g., curettaged or severely regressed melanoma)

T0 No evidence of primary tumor

Tis Melanoma *in situ*

T1 Melanomas 1.0 mm or less in thickness

T2 Melanomas 1.01 to 2.0 mm

T3 Melanomas 2.01 to 4.0 mm

T4 Melanomas more than 4.0 mm

Note: a and b subcategories of T are assigned based on ulceration and number of mitoses per mm^2, as shown below:

Classification	Thickness (mm)	Ulceration Status/Mitoses
T1	≤1.0	a: w/o ulceration and mitosis < 1/mm^2 b: with ulceration or mitoses ≥ 1/mm^2
T2	1.01–2.0	a: w/o ulceration b: with ulceration
T3	2.01–4.0	a: w/o ulceration b: with ulceration
T4	>4.0	a: w/o ulceration b: with ulceration

Regional Lymph Nodes (N)

NX Patients in whom the regional nodes cannot be assessed (e.g., previously removed for another reason)

N0 No regional metastases detected

N1–3 Regional metastases based upon the number of metastatic nodes and presence or absence of intralymphatic metastases (in-transit or satellite metastases)

Note: N1 to N3 and a to c subcategories assigned as shown below:

N Classification	No. of Metastatic Nodes	Nodal Metastatic Mass
N1	1 node	a: micrometastasis[a] b: macrometastasis[b]
N2	2–3 nodes	a: micrometastasis[a] b: macrometastasis[b] c: in-transit met(s)/ satellite(s) without metastatic nodes
N3	4 or more metastatic nodes, or matted nodes, or in-transit met(s)/satellite(s) with metastatic node(s)	

Distant Metastasis (M)

M0 No detectable evidence of distant metastases

M1a Metastases to the skin, subcutaneous, or distant lymph nodes

M1b Metastases to the lung

M1c Metastases to all other visceral sites or distant metastases to any site combined with an elevated serum LDH

Note: Serum LDH is incorporated into the M category as shown below:

M Classification	Site	Serum LDH
M1a	Distant skin, subcutaneous, or nodal metastasis	Normal
M1b	Lung metastases	Normal
M1c	All other visceral metastases Any distant metastasis	Normal Elevated

[a]Micrometastases are diagnosed after sentinel lymph node biopsy and completion of lymphadenectomy (if performed).

[b]Macrometastases are defined as clinically detectable nodal metastases confirmed by therapeutic lymphadenectomy or when nodal metastasis exhibits gross extracapsular extension.

Used with permission of the American Joint Committee on Cancer (AJCC), Chicago, Illinois. The original and primary source for this information is the AJCC Cancer Staging Manual, Seventh Edition (2010), published by Springer Science+Business Media. Any citation or quotation of this material must be credited to the AJCC as its primary source. The inclusion of this information herein does not authorize any reuse or further distribution without the expressed, written permission of Springer, on behalf of the AJCC.

M is for indicating the metastatic status and involvement of distant sites.

5. Mitotic rate indicating the cell division of the tumor and the tumor thickness (Breslow depth) are the primary predictors of the survival.

6. The metastatic lymph nodes are determined by sentinel lymph node dissection (SLND) or elective lymph node dissection (ELND) of the echelon lymph nodes to examine the presence of the melanoma.

   a. Macrometastases can be palpated by physical examination of the lymph nodes.

   b. Micrometastases are detected only by microscopic evaluation after SLN biopsy.

7. Metastasis to distant sites of skin and other vital organs is also screened by the level of serum lactate dehydrogenase (LDH). LDH elevation may indicate the metastatic disease status. Staging 0 to IV on the basis of the new TNM staging system:

   a. Stage 0 (TisN0M0): melanoma *in situ*. Tumor is confined to the epidermis.

   b. Stage I melanoma: determined by the presence or absence of mitoses and ulceration. There are no other indications of regional lymph node involvement or distant metastasis.

      (1) Stage IA, T1aN0M0: tumor 1 mm or smaller without mitosis or ulceration

      (2) Stage IB, T1bN0M0: tumor 1 mm or smaller with mitosis or ulceration

   c. Stage II melanoma: determined by the status of tumor thickness and ulceration. There are no other indications of regional lymph node involvement or distant metastasis.

      (1) Stage IIA: T2bN0M0 or T3aN0M0

      (2) Stage IIB: T3bN0M0 or T4aN0M0

      (3) Stage IIC: T4bN0M0

   d. Stage III melanoma: determined by the level of lymph node metastasis. There are no other indications of distant metastasis.

(1) Stage IIIA: T1-T4aN1aM0 or T1-T4aN2aM0

(2) Stage IIIB: T1-T4bN1aM0, T1-T4bN2aM0, T1-T4aN1bM0, T1-T4aN2bM0, or T1-T4a/bN2cM0

(3) Stage IIIC: T1-4bN1bM0, T1-4bN2bM0, or T1-4a/bN3M0

e. Stage IV melanoma: staging is determined by the location of sites of the metastases (e.g., skin, soft tissue, distant lymph nodes, and vital organs including liver, lungs, bones, and brain) and level of serum LDH.

(1) M1a: tumor metastasis to distant skin, the subcutaneous layers, or lymph nodes; serum LDH is normal.

(2) M1b: tumor metastasis to lungs; serum LDH is normal.

(3) M1c: tumor has metastasis to vital organs other than lungs; serum LDH is normal or elevated.

VII. METASTATIC AND RECURRENT MELANOMA

A. Local recurrence is related to tumor thickness and defined as a recurrence in close proximity to the surgical scar or site of primary cutaneous melanoma (3% rate).

B. In-transit metastases/satellites are small cutaneous tumors present in the dermis and subdermal between the primary melanoma site and the draining nodal basin.

C. Lesions occurring within 2 cm of primary tumor are termed satellites, whereas in-transit metastases are more than 2 cm from site.

D. Regional lymph node metastasis
   1. Highly predictive of visceral metastases
   2. Risk varies based on tumor thickness of primary

E. Distant metastasis is most frequently to nonvisceral sites, skin, subcutaneous tissue, and distant lymph nodes.

F. Late recurrences occur 10 or more years after initial diagnosis and treatment.

VIII. THERAPEUTIC MODALITIES BY STAGE

A. Stage 0 (Melanoma *in situ*) Complete excision with safety margins: wide local excision surgery (WLE) with appropriate benign margins (depends on the size and thickness of the tumor)
   1. Melanoma *in situ*: 0.5-cm normal skin safety margin
   2. Melanoma tumor less than 1 mm: 1-cm horizontal and vertical margin
   3. Melanoma tumor greater than 1 mm: 2- to 3-cm resection margin decided by the anatomical location and conditions

B. Stage I Treatment
   1. SLNB is recommended by AJCC for ulcerated lesion thicker than 1 mm in order to determine the involvement of local lymph nodes and guidance of treatment options.
   2. Free of lymph node involvement leads to WLE surgery with appropriate benign margins (depends on the size and thickness of the tumor).

C. Stage II Treatment
   1. SLNB is recommended before undergoing surgery for determining the involvement of local lymph nodes and guides treatment options.
      a. Sentinel lymph node dissection: use blue dye or radiolabeled colloid injection at the melanoma site and open the close-by lymph node basin to check the presence of melanoma. Free of tumor at the closest lymph node from the primary tumor site suggests negative for metastasis.
   2. WLE surgery with appropriate margins (depends on the size and thickness of the tumor).
   3. Adjuvant therapy is considered for stage IB and stage IIC melanoma (e.g., interferon alfa-2a and interferon alfa-2b), which helps immune system fight the disease and delay or prevent recurrence.
   4. Some clinical trials used vaccine therapy for patients who could not tolerate interferons; no significant increase in survival rate was shown in randomized controlled trials.

D. Stage III Treatment
   1. WLE removal of the primary lesion is recommended for recurrent tumors and in-transit tumors.
   2. Therapeutic lymph node dissection (TLND) of the melanoma affected regional lymph nodes for the patient with palpable lymph nodes for possible macrometastases.
   3. Selected patients will have lymphatic mapping and SLND for determining involvement of sentinel node.
   4. Systemic adjuvant therapy in addition to the surgery with interferons (alfa-2a and alfa-2b), which helps immune system to fight the disease and delay or prevent recurrence.
   5. Radiation adjuvant therapy: may consider use of radiation therapy when the tumor has involved tissues beyond lymph nodes to control further spread of melanoma.
      a. Regional metastasis radiation therapy (in-transit metastasis).
      b. Adjuvant therapy recommended for postsurgical melanoma patients who are free of disease but at high risk for relapse and to complement surgery in the management of melanoma metastatic to lymph nodes.
      c. Stereotactic radiation therapy is considered for brain metastases up to two sites; otherwise, radiation of the entire brain for more than two metastatic tumors.
      d. Palliative radiotherapy for bone metastases.

E. Stage IV Treatment
   1. Surgical removal of metastatic tumors for symptoms treatment
   2. Systemic adjuvant therapy
   3. Chemotherapy
      a. Dacarbazine (DTIC) IV infusion
      b. Temozolomide oral medication for advanced metastatic melanoma

c. IL-2 or IFNa (biochemotherapy) alone or combination treatment with dacarbazine, cisplatin, temozolomide, carmustine, vinblastine, and tamoxifen.

4. Immunotherapies (e.g., IL-2, INF-α2a and ipilimumab): Treatment strategies with vaccines utilizing tumor cells, antibodies, peptides, and dendritic cells.

5. Specific target therapies: Vemurafenib treatment for BRAF mutation genetic signaling pathways in metastatic and unresectable (inoperable) melanoma.

6. Radiation therapy including x-rays and gamma rays targeting cancer cells, and relieve symptoms to control pain in metastatic disease involving the brain

IX. PROGNOSIS

A. Follow-Up Recommendations

1. Follow-up one to four times per year, for 2 years, depending on the thickness of the primary lesion and other risk factors, then one to two times per year thereafter.

2. Post melanoma treatment follow up should be tailored to each patient's history of type and thickness of melanoma, presence of atypical nevi, family history of melanoma, patient anxiety, and patient ability to recognize signs and symptoms of disease.

3. Strong evidence suggests that the majority of metastases and recurrences are discovered by the patient or a family member. Therefore, the patient education program should include how to perform self-conducted skin examination.

PATIENT EDUCATION
Melanoma

- Melanoma is a dangerous type of skin cancer that arises from uncontrolled growth of skin cells that make pigment melanin. It typically appears as a pigmented skin lesion and metastasizes to vital organs, such as liver, lungs and brain, rapidly through the lymphatic system.

- People with multiple moles (more than 50) should be screened for the familial atypical mole and melanoma syndrome.

- Self-screening for melanoma can be guided by the ABCDE rule:
  ○ Asymmetry: irregular shape.
  ○ Irregular, ill-defined border.
  ○ Variegated colors like black, red, brown, blue, and white.
  ○ Diameter noticeably increasing in size.
  ○ Evolution, elevation, enlarging, and changing.

- Avoid excessive sun exposure and use sunscreen (SPF 30 or higher) and reapply every 2 hours while staying in the sun.

- Skin self-examination and clinical skin examination with health care providers are the crucial methods to achieve early detection and treatment of melanoma.

---

4. 5-year and 10-year survival rate: the 5-year survival rate with stages I and II is over 90%, whereas with stage IV, it is approximately 10% to 20%.

CUTANEOUS T-CELL LYMPHOMA

I. OVERVIEW

Cutaneous T-cell lymphoma (CTCL) is a form of non-Hodgkin lymphoma and a type of neoplasm in immune system caused by a mutation of helper (CD4+) T cells. There are various types of CTCLs, but mycosis fungoides (MF) and Sézary syndrome (SS) are the two most common types. CTCL arises primarily in the skin and characterized by remission and exacerbation of skin disease.

A. Definition: CTCL is a malignant disease of T lymphocytes with cutaneous lesions, which arises from proliferation of the cancerous T lymphocytes in the dermis and has tendency to migrate into the epidermis. It progresses gradually through various stages of lesions evolving from a severely pruritic patch to a plaque and to a noduloulcerative lesion and increases the amount of infiltration of malignant T lymphocytes in the skin.

B. Incidence:

1. CTCL represents approximately 4% of all non-Hodgkin lymphoma, with MF comprising the majority of the cases reported.

2. Age-adjusted incidence of 6.4 to 9.6 cases per million people in the United States.

3. Majority of the MF cases are among Whites (approximately 70%), and Blacks, Hispanics, and Asians have about 14%, 9%, and 7%, respectively.

4. Seen in both genders (more frequently in men than in women with 2:1 ratio) with the median age 55 to 60 years old.

C. Etiology: no clear etiopathogenesis has been established, but there are several suggested causative factors of CTCL:

1. Chronic antigen stimulation and accumulation of T-helper memory cells in the skin: Since neoplastic T cells have capability to express antigen-presenting cell (APC) ligands in gene regulation, it may self-stimulate and lead to T-cell expansion in the skin.

2. Infections:
   a. Human T-cell leukemia/lymphoma virus (HTLV1), an exogenous RNA retrovirus.
   b. *Staphylococcus aureus* and other associated enterotoxins may associate with the etiology of MF.
   c. Epstein-Barr virus and cytomegalovirus.

3. Immunosuppression and immunosuppressive therapy in organ transplant patients

4. Genetic factor
   a. Clonal abnormalities in gene expression that separates the entities of MF and SS.
   b. Certain histocompatibility antigens are found with increased frequency in CTCL (e.g., increased expression of cutaneous lymphocyte antigen [CLA] and its ligand E-selectin).

5. Development from other dermatoses as many patients have a preceding eruption of variable duration
   a. Atopic dermatitis is at risk for developing CTCL from chronic stimulation of T cells and possible induction of clonal proliferation.
6. Environmental factors in susceptible host (retrospective studies)
   a. Chemicals (air pollutants, pesticides, solvents and vapors, detergents, disinfectants)
   b. Drugs (tobacco, analgesics, tranquilizers, thiazides)
   c. Occupational exposure (manufacturing especially in petrochemical, textile, metal, and machinery industries)

D. Pathogenesis:
1. Recent studies suggest different origin of the memory T-cell subsets for the MF and SS.
2. MF arises from the background of chronic inflammation. Reactive T cells are found along with dendritic cells and other immune cells such as macrophages, mast cells, and plasma cells.
3. High number of CD8+ cytotoxic T cells (antitumor response) in early skin lesions and advanced tumor lesions in later stage shows significantly decreased cytotoxic T cells.
4. Malignant T cells in the skin involve chemokines, cytokines, and adhesion molecules that facilitate lymphocyte extravasation and migration to the epidermis.
5. As the disease progresses, there is a change in cytokine expression, which correlates with erythroderma, high level of immunoglobulin E, immunosuppression, and susceptibility to bacterial infections in advanced MF and SS.
6. Disease progression in MF and SS has been characterized by altered immune system, such as in T-cell proliferation, accumulation in cytogenetic abnormalities, and apoptosis (programmed cell death); defective/dysfunctional apoptosis expressed by neoplastic T cell has been closely associated with advanced and aggressive disease.
7. Early lesions are often infiltrated with CD8+ cytotoxic T lymphocytes, most likely indicating a mediating antitumor response.
8. Loss of normal immunity with advancing disease compromises antitumor response.

II. CLINICAL VARIANTS AND PRESENTATION

A. Clinical Stages
1. Patch phase (see Figure 4-16)
   a. Lesions typically present in non–sun-exposed areas as dusky red, violaceous, single or multiple scaly macules and patches in various sizes.
   b. Classic distribution is the buttocks, groin, underneath breasts, and axilla, with persistent pruritus.
   c. May be transitory, spontaneously disappearing without scarring.
   d. Phase may last months or years; diagnosis at this stage is often difficult.

B. Plaque phase
1. Plaques may occur from patch-stage lesions or arise from *de novo*.
2. Eruptions are well defined and dusky red and may appear shiny with wart-like infiltrates; a reddish-blue halo may be observed outside the areas of infiltration.
3. As cells proliferate, lesions become firm, and the plaque varies in surface contour.
4. Lesions may spontaneously regress or coalesce into a large plaque and ulcerate or spontaneously disappear.
5. Associating symptoms are scaly scalp with hair loss, thickened and discolored nails, hyperkeratosis, and scaling/fissuring of the palms and soles; risk of misdiagnosing for eczema or psoriasis at this stage.
6. Patient may present with dermatologic emergency as erythroderma, unstable body temperature, weight loss, insomnia, malaise, vasodilation, and exfoliations, which may cause loss of protein, iron, and electrolytes.

C. Tumor phase (T cells lose their affinity for the skin)
1. May occur in CTCL plaques or *de novo*.
2. Lesions appear on the face, back, and body skinfolds as dull reddish brown or purplish red with smooth surface; softly palpable nodular lesions that rapidly grow in size and number.
3. Presentation of the lesions may show secondary infection and excoriation due to severe pruritus. Ulceration and necrosis may occur in later stage.
4. In SS, "red man disease" may occur (Figure 16-23)
   a. Term relates to generalized exfoliating erythrodermic CTCL patients with leukocytes and peripheral blood appearance of "monster" cells.
   b. Intensely pruritic with lymphadenopathy starting either *de novo*, following premalignant eruption, or after established plaque stage of the disease.
5. Different from SS, erythrodermic condition in MF is a progression from the existing lesions, and it has low or no circulating "monster" cell counts.
6. Tumors gradually appear in infiltrative lesions often at the border; may shrink and disappear leaving a pigmented atrophic scar.
7. Widespread CTCL invasion is evidenced by palpable lymph nodes, bone marrow involvement in advanced stages, pulmonary involvement, and osteolytic lesions in the bone with pathologic fractures.
8. Complications of CTCL and cause of death include viral, fungal, and bacterial infections; immunosuppression; and vital organ involvement.

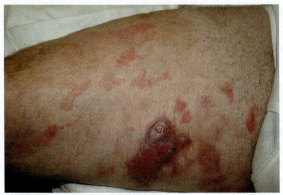
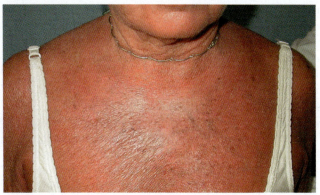

FIGURE 16-23. Sézary syndrome. **A:** Mycosis fungoides patient with cutaneous plaques and a tumor. **B:** Sézary syndrome patient with diffuse erythroderma. (From DeVita, V. T., et al. (2008). *DeVita, Hellman, and Rosenberg's cancer: Principles and practice of oncology*. Philadelphia, PA: Wolters Kluwer.)

III. LABORATORY AND DIAGNOSTIC TESTS

A. Combination of clinical examination and biopsy is necessary for establishing accurate diagnosis.

B. Molecular immunotyping can be helpful in diagnosing CTCL (e.g., CD4+ helper T-cell complex lack in expressing T-cell antigens CD7 and Leu-8).

C. Most sensitive test is Southern Blot test for T-cell antigen receptor rearrangements in peripheral blood (T-cell receptor gene rearrangement test).

D. CBC with determination of absolute lymphocytes count, serum chemistries (including liver and renal function tests), uric acid, LDH and quantitative immunoglobulins, human immunodeficiency virus (HIV), and HTLV-1 testing.

E. Depending on extent of disease, Sézary count, chest radiography, CT scans, PET scans, lymph node or bone marrow biopsy, or as suggested by history or physical examination.

IV. DIFFERENTIAL DIAGNOSIS

A. Allergic contact dermatitis
B. Atopic dermatitis
C. Irritant contact dermatitis
D. Lichen planus
E. Palmoplantar psoriasis
F. Parapsoriasis
G. Pemphigus foliaceus
H. Plaque psoriasis
I. Tinea corporis

V. TREATMENT MODALITIES

A. Skin-directed therapy
1. Topical steroids are the most common treatment, and adjunct treatment with other topicals and systemic therapies at all stages.
2. Phototherapy with UVB.
3. Topical chemotherapy with mechlorethamine (nitrogen mustard HN2).
4. Photochemotherapy.

5. Carbon dioxide laser surgery.
6. Total skin electron beam therapy (limited penetration of electrons spares mucous membranes, bone marrow, gastrointestinal tract, and other vital internal organs). Whole body electron beam irradiation results in 85% complete remission rates with medial survival time of 9 years.
7. Surgical removal of solitary nodule or plaque confined to the skin.
8. Topical or intralesional steroids to control symptoms.

B. Chronic disease (with nodal involvement)
1. Follow protocol for skin-directed therapy.
2. Total skin electron beam therapy followed by topical HN2, phototherapy, or photopheresis to maintain remission. Total skin electron beam therapy is an option for patients with widespread skin lesions or patients who have deficient response to conservative therapies.
3. If necessary, systemic drug such as interferon-α, retinoids, or chemotherapeutic agent such as methotrexate.

C. Postremission maintenance includes topical corticosteroids, nitrogen mustard, interferon (alpha), and phototherapy.

D. Tumors
1. No nodal involvement—as above
2. Histologic nodal involvement
   a. Individualized palliative treatment
   b. Local radiations to local symptomatic disease
   c. Photopheresis
   d. Retinoids/experimental protocols

E. Visceral involvement/Sézary syndrome
1. Individualized palliative treatment
2. Systemic chemotherapy (fludarabine, 2-CDA, chlorambucil, pentostatin)
3. Extracorporeal photopheresis (palliative treatment), whereby leukocytes are selectively removed from peripheral blood by extracorporeal centrifugation technique, exposed to UVA light, and reinfused into the patient.
   a. Causes selective destruction of cancerous cells in the blood
   b. Has been the only single treatment that has been shown to improve survival in patients with Sézary syndrome

4. Immune boosters such as interferon, interleukin-2, and monoclonal antibodies

5. Bone marrow transplant, currently limited by graft versus host disease, offers greatest potential for disease cure.

6. Combinations of skin-directed therapies and biological response modifiers to improve response rates.

7. Recent developments in CTCL therapy include:
   a. Targretin (bexarotene)—a retinoid X receptor–selective retinoid for all stages of CTCL and topical gel formation for the treatment of localized lesions
   b. Ontak (denileukin diftitox): fusion toxin proteins selective for specific T cells; targets malignant T-cell clones
   c. Systemic chemotherapy development including pegylated liposomal doxorubicin, gemcitabine, and pentostatin appears to have greatest potential.

8. Allogenic stem cell transplantation has curative potential for MF and reserved for advanced disease.

VI. PROGNOSIS

The prognosis of CTCL depends on the stage of disease at the time of diagnosis, age, gender, immunocompetence, and the choice and tolerance of the treatments. While there is no cure for MF and SS, the treatment should focus on controlling and limiting the skin lesions, delay the progression, and minimize the recurrence of the disease. The care for the patients should be directed at quality-of-life consideration by optimally treating pruritus and xerosis and prevention of skin infection.

PATIENT EDUCATION
Cutaneous T-Cell Lymphoma

- CTCL is a rare type of cancer that originates in white blood cells and typically appears in severely itch skin lesions.
- Chronic skin rash with delayed improvement, progress through various stages of lesions, and repeated cycles of regression and recurrence should be evaluated.
- Multiple skin biopsies over time may be required to establish the diagnosis.
- Topical corticosteroids are the treatment of choice for early stage of CTCL, and they provide effective adjunct therapy with other topical and systemic treatments in all stages of the disease.
- Avoid hot showers and any skin products that aggravate itching and irritation (e.g., fragranced lotion, alcohol-based skin cleanser).
- Although phototherapy (PUVA, UVB) is known to alleviate some of the itching symptoms associated with CTCL, maintain caution with regard to harmful effects of excessive sun exposure and wear proper sun protective clothing and sunscreen.
- Severely itching, disseminated rash can limit activities of daily living and affect the quality of life. Joining a support group to connect with other people living with CTCL and share experiences may be helpful.

KAPOSI SARCOMA

I. OVERVIEW

Kaposi sarcoma (KS) is an angioproliferative disorder and an opportunistic disease in immunosuppressed hosts. KS is a misnomer as it is not an actual sarcoma (a malignancy of mesenchymal origin). It was first described by Kaposi as idiopathic multiple pigment sarcoma. This multifocal neoplasm is seen primarily as multiple vascular nodules in the skin and other organs. KS is associated with other neoplasms or immune disorders that occur before or after the diagnosis. KS is seen frequently in patients with HIV.

A. Definition: KS is a disease of proliferation in endothelial layer of lymph or blood vessels. Excessive proliferation of spindle cells placed together with other cells such as endothelial cells, inflammatory cells, and fibroblasts in an epithelial layer of the vascular origin results in a formation of a new blood vessel (neoangiogenesis).

B. Incidence:
   1. Incidence of KS varies according to geography.
      a. KS incidence in the United States before the acquired immunodeficiency syndrome (AIDS) epidemic was only 1 for every million people, mostly classic and transplant related.
      b. AIDS epidemic increased KS incidence by 20 times, about 47 cases per million in 1990s, with 1 in 2 chance of developing KS among people infected with HIV. With improving KS treatment options, average KS incidence rate decreased to 6 cases per million each year.
      c. Another higher prevalence is among organ transplant recipients, with the incidence of 1 in 200 people in the United States.
      d. Mostly affects people of either Jewish descent or Mediterranean descent.
      e. In classic KS, two thirds of patients develop lesions only after the age of 50.
      f. Disease is strikingly frequent in a region in Africa that includes Kenya, Tanzania, and Zaire with a frequency of 1.3% to 10% depending on region.
      g. Among people with AIDS, KS predominates in the third and fourth decade with a mean age of 40 years.

C. Etiology (cause may be multifactorial)
   1. Viral
      a. New human herpesvirus (HHV-8/KS) and subsequent identification of humoral immune response to this agent in patients with KS may be causally related to KS.
      b. Causative agents of KS associated with disease among young homosexual men with signs of profound immunosuppression include HIV and other specific serologic association between cytomegalovirus (CMV) and classic endemic KS.
      c. Other causative agents of KS may include various microorganisms such as hepatitis B virus, human papillomavirus (HPV), and *Mycoplasma penetrans* as possible sources of KS.

d. With the replication of retroviral particles in KS lesions, some hypothesize a non-HIV retrovirus etiological linkage to KS.
2. Genetic predisposition
3. Geographic factors
4. Possible hormonal influences
D. Pathogenesis:
1. Classic KS develops slowly and runs a benign course, although, infrequently, rapid courses with involvement of the lung, spleen, heart, and gastrointestinal tract have been reported.
2. In addition to cutaneous lesions, it may develop on mucous membranes of the oral cavity and gastrointestinal tract.

II. CLINICAL VARIANTS

A. Classic (Mediterranean) KS (Figure 16-24)
1. Chronic skin disease affecting predominantly elderly men of Mediterranean, East European, or Jewish heritage with a peak incidence in men after the age of 60. Lesions often appear on the legs.
2. Affected individuals survive an average of 10 to 15 years from diagnosis and most often die from an unrelated cause.
3. Lesions occur most commonly as red or purple nodule or blotch on lower limbs and then upper limbs and may occur on the trunk, head, neck, genitalia, or any skin surface. May appear as blue hues in dark-skinned individuals.
4. Telangiectases may be evident on or near the tumors, ulceration may occur, or the surface may appear verrucous.
5. Lesions may be painful; burning or itching may also be present.
6. Lesions may spontaneously regress as new ones appear; spontaneous remissions have been documented.
7. Occurrence may be in the hundreds in a single patient; nodules may cluster along veins.

B. African or Endemic KS
1. Found in eastern half of African continent near the equator.
2. Described in two distinct age groups
   a. Young adults with a mean age of 35 and a male/female ratio of 13:1
   b. Young children with a mean age of 3 and a male/female ratio of 3:1
3. Most commonly nodular lesions that may regress spontaneously.
4. Florid variety is rapid growing and ulcerated and may bleed with tumors extending deep into the dermis and may involve underlying bone.
5. Infiltrative type is confined to the hand or foot appearing as deeply invasive, fibrotic, indurated tumors with nonpitting edema.
6. Rapidly growing enlarged lymph nodes, often confused clinically with lymphoma, typify lymphadenopathic type of KS occurring in children and young adults.
C. Iatrogenic (Transplant-Related) KS
1. Found in organ transplant patients, particularly renal transplants.
2. Seen in patients receiving chronic immunosuppressive drug therapy. Spontaneous remission after discontinuation of immunosuppressive therapy usually occurs.
D. AIDS-Associated, Epidemic KS (Figure 16-25)
1. KS is often the primary AIDS-defining illness.
2. Sexually transmitted cofactor may play a role in the development of AIDS-KS.
3. Incidence of AIDS-KS continues to rise as more HIV-infected patients progress to AIDS.

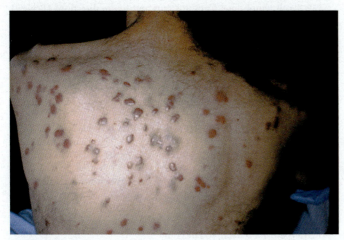

FIGURE 16-24. Kaposi sarcoma. (From Werner, R. (2012). *Massage therapist's guide to pathology*. Philadelphia, PA: Wolters Kluwer.)

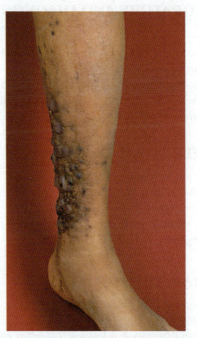

FIGURE 16-25. Kaposi sarcoma. Multiple papules and nodules are present on this patient's leg. (From Goodheart, H. P. (2003). *Goodheart's photoguide of common skin disorders* (2nd ed.). Philadelphia, PA: Lippincott Williams & Wilkins.)

4. Lesions occur in the oral cavity, nose, postauricular, trunk, penis, legs, and feet appearing as small pink macules mimicking insect bites or small brown, tense papules.
5. Examination should include lymph node exam.
6. Macular lesions begin as salmon-colored with a pink halo.
   a. Small, slightly elevated, and round.
   b. Macule becomes purple or brown within a week and halo disappears.
   c. Multiple lesions widely distributed; may demonstrate a mirror-image distribution.
7. Papular and nodular lesions.
   a. May begin as macules.
   b. Facial papules are round and less than 1 cm in size; lesions of the trunk, neck, and extremities are 1 to 2 cm and oblong.
8. Plaques and lymphatic disease.
   a. Large purple plaques containing nodules with hyperkeratosis; resemble psoriasis.
   b. Lymphatic involvement may produce numerous firm, red, round papules with local edema in affected nodal sites.
9. Mucocutaneous and ocular lesions.
   a. Oral involvement most commonly seen as lesions on the palate.
   b. Macular lesions of the conjunctiva are relatively benign.
10. Visceral lesions may affect gastrointestinal tract and lungs as well as the pharynx, heart, bone marrow, urogenital tract, brain, kidney, and adrenal glands.

III. LABORATORY AND DIAGNOSTIC TESTS

A. Combination of clinical assessment and histological conformation by skin biopsy
B. CT scan, bronchoscopy, and endoscopy based on the symptoms and clinical suspicion on other organs' involvement

IV. DIFFERENTIAL DIAGNOSIS

A. Bacillary angiomatosis
B. Blue rubber bleb nevus syndrome
C. Melanocytic nevi
D. Pyogenic granuloma (lobular capillary hemangioma)
E. Tufted angioma

V. THERAPEUTIC MODALITIES

A. There is no curative treatment for KS.
B. Local therapy
   1. Excision of cutaneous lesions (often for cosmesis)
   2. Radiation therapy
   3. Chemotherapy either single or multiagent. Most promising results in use of liposomal encapsulated

doxorubicin and daunorubicin for both AIDs-associated KS and classic KS
4. Systemic treatment of interferon alpha, alone or in combination with cytotoxic therapy or with zidovudine for AIDS-KS
5. Highly active antiretroviral therapy (HAART) for AIDS-related KS

VI. PROGNOSIS

The prognosis is dependent on the size and location of the KS lesions, the function of the immune system, and the comorbidities of the patient. Compromised immune system and underlying comorbidities may cause challenges in making choices for treatment.

PATIENT EDUCATION
Kaposi Sarcoma

- Kaposi sarcoma (KS) typically presents as red or purplish spots and bumps on skin and mucosal layer of the body. It is essential to that a skin biopsy be performed to exclude cutaneous lymphoma.
- KS may also involve internal organs including the intestines, lungs, genitals, and lymphatic system. Associated swelling, bleeding, discomfort, pain, and difficulty breathing depend on the affected organs.

BIBLIOGRAPHY

American Academy of Dermatology (AAD). (2014). Melanoma trends. Retrieved from www.aad.org

American Cancer Society. (2014). Skin cancer prevention and early detection. Retrieved from http://www.cancer.org/cancer/cancer-causes/sunanduvexposure/skincancerpreventionandearlydetection/index

American Joint Committee on Cancer. (2010). *Melanoma of the skin staging* (7th ed.). Chicago, IL: American Cancer Society.

Apisarnthanarax, J., Talpur, R., & Duvic, M. (2002). Treatment of cutaneous T cell lymphoma: Current status and future directions (Review). *American Journal of Clinical Dermatology, 3*(3), 193–215.

Balch, C. M., Ross, M., Buzaid, A. C., Soong, S. J., Atkins, M. B., Cascinelli, N., …, Thompson, J. F. (2001). Final version of the American joint committee on cancer staging system for cutaneous melanoma. *Journal of Clinical Oncology, 19*(16), 3635–3648.

Berg, D., & Otley, C. C. (2002). Skin cancer in organ transplant recipients: Epidemiology, pathogenesis and management. *Journal of the American Academy of Dermatology, 47*(1), 1–17.

Bichakjian, C. K., Halpern, A. C., Johnson, T. M., Hood, A. F., Grichnik, J. M., & Bhushan, R. (2011). Guidelines of care for the management of primary cutaneous melanoma. *Journal of the American Academy of Dermatology, 65*, 1032–1047.

Bouwhuis, S., & Davis, M. D. (2001, June). Sezary syndrome: A summary. *Dermatology Nursing, 13*(3), 205–209.

Chartier, T. K., Aasi, S. Z., Stern, R. S., Robinson, J. K., & Ofori, A. O. (2014). Treatment and prognosis of basal cell carcinoma. *UpToDate.* Retrieved from www.uptodate.com

Chung, G. (2014). A community-based educational intervention to improve melanoma screening among adult Hispanic Americans. Loma Linda University, CA.

Carbe, C., & Bauer, J. (2012). Chapter 113. Melanoma. In J. L. Bolognia, J. L. Jorizzo, & J. V. Schaffer (Eds.), *Dermatology (Bolognia, Dermatology)* (3rd ed.). New York, NY: Elsevier. Ebook ISBN: 9780702051821

Ghadially, R., & Ghadially, F. N. (2002). Keratoacanthoma. In T. B. Fitzpatrick, A. Z. Eisen, K. Wolff, I. M. Freedberg, K. F. Austen, L. A. Goldsmith, & S. L. Katz (Eds.), *Dermatology in general medicine* (5th ed., pp. 865–871). New York, NY: McGraw-Hill.

Grekin, R. C., Samlaska, C. P., & Van-Christian, K. (2000). Epidermal nevi, neoplasms and cysts. In R. B. Odom, W. D. James, & T. G. Berger (Eds.), *Andrew's diseases of the skin clinical dermatology* (9th ed., pp. 820–825, 1082–1087). Philadelphia, PA: WB Saunders Co.

Guill, C. K., & Orengo, I. (2001, June). Cutaneous malignant melanoma. *Dermatology Nursing, 13*(3), 210–213.

Heald, P. W. (2002). Identifying and treating T-cell lymphoma. *Skin Cancer Foundation Journal, XIX*, 39–40.

Heald, P. W., & Edelson, R. L. (1999). Cutaneous T cell lymphomas. In T. B. Fitzpatrick, A. Z. Eisen, K. Wolff, I. M. Freedberg, K. F. Austen, L. A. Goldsmith, & S. L. Katz (Eds.), *Dermatology in general medicine* (5th ed., pp. 1227–1250). New York, NY: McGraw-Hill.

Hoppe, R. T., Kim, Y. H., Kuzel, T. M., Zic, J. A., & Connor, R. F. (2014). Staging and prognosis of mycosis fungoides and Sezary syndrome. *UpToDate*. Retrieved from www.uptodate.com

Jawed, S. I., Myskowski, P. L., Horwitz, S. H., Moskowiz, A., & Querfeld, C. (2014a). Primary cutaneous T-cell lymphoma (mycosis fungoides and Sezary syndrome). Part I. Diagnosis: clinical and histopathologic features and new molecular and biologic markers. *Journal of the American Academy of Dermatology, 70*(2), 205–220.

Jawed, S. I., Myskowski, P. L., Horwitz, S. H., Moskowiz, A., & Querfeld, C. (2014b). Primary cutaneous T-cell lymphoma (mycosis fungoides and Sezary syndrome). Part II. Prognosis, management, and future directions. *Journal of the American Academy of Dermatology, 70*(2), 223–241.

Lange, J. R. (2000). The current status of sentinel node biopsy in the management of melanoma. *Dermatologic Surgery, 26*(8), 809–810.

Langley, R. C., et al. (1999). Neoplasms: Cutaneous melanoma. In T. B. Fitzpatrick, A. Z. Eisen, K. Wolff, I. M. Freedberg, K. F. Austen, L. A. Goldsmith, & S. L. Katz (Eds.), *Dermatology in general medicine* (5th ed., pp. 1080–1116) New York, NY: McGraw-Hill.

Lim, J. L., Asgari, M., Stern, R. S., Robinson, J. K., & Corona, R. (2014). Epidemiology and risk factors for cutaneous squamous cell carcinoma. *UpToDate*. Retrieved from www.uptodate.com

Liskay, A., & Nicol, N. H. (1998). Anatomy and physiology of the skin. In M. J. Hill (Ed.), *Dermatology nursing essentials: A core curriculum* (pp. 3–13), Pitman, NJ: Dermatology Nurses' Association.

Malignant Melanoma-Information for Medical Professionals. (2014). Retrieved from http://skincancer.dermis.net/content/e04typesof/e154/e156/index_eng.html

Melanoma Center. (n.d.). Your Source for melanoma information. Retrieved from http://www.melanomacenter.org/staging/stage4.html

Musse, L. (2002, February). Cutaneous T-cell lymphoma. *Dermatology Nursing, 14*(1), 55.

Padilla, R. S., Robinson, J. K., & Corona, R. (2014). Epidemiology, natural history, and diagnosis of actinic keratosis. *UpToDate*. Retrieved from www.uptodate.com

Petter, G., & Haustein, U. F. (2000). Histologic subtyping and malignancy assessment of cutaneous squamous cell carcinoma. *Dermatologic Surgery, 26*(6), 521–529.

Piepkorn, M. (2001). *A new look at genetics breakthrough in melanoma. Skin Cancer Foundation Journal, XIX*, 46–47.

Rappersberger, K., Stingl, G., & Wolff, K. (1999). Kaposi's sarcoma. In T. B. Fitzpatrick, A. Z. Eisen, K. Wolff, I. M. Freedberg, K. F. Austen, L. A. Goldsmith, & S. L. Katz (Eds.), *Dermatology in general medicine* (5th ed., pp. 1195–1203). New York, NY: McGraw-Hill.

Rigel, D. S. (2001). Melanoma update—2001. *Skin Cancer Foundation Journal, XIX*, 13–14.

Rivas, M. P., & Nouri, K. (2005). Benign and malignant neoplasms. In B. E. Strober (Ed.), *Dermatology 2005 study guide and online practice exam*. Stiefel Laboratories.

Schmid-Wnedtner, M. H., Volkenandt, M., Plewig, G., Berking, C., Baumert, J., Schmidt, M., & Sander, C. A. (2002). Cutaneous melanoma in childhood and adolescence: An analysis of 36 patients. *Journal of the American Academy of Dermatology, 46*(6), 874–879.

Schwartz, R. A., & Stoll, H. L. (1999). Squamous cell carcinoma. In T. B. Fitzpatrick, A. Z. Eisen, K. Wolff, I. M. Freedberg, K. F. Austen, L. A. Goldsmith, & S. L. Katz (Eds.), *Dermatology in general medicine* (5th ed., pp. 840–850). New York, NY: McGraw-Hill.

Sober, A. J., Chuang, T. Y., Duvic, M., Farmer, E. R., Grichnik, J. M., Halpern, A. C., …, Lowery, B. J. (2001). Guidelines of care for primary cutaneous melanoma. *Journal of the American Academy of Dermatology, 45*(4), 579–586.

Sosman, J. A., Atkins, M. B., & Ross, M. E. (2014). Overview of the management of advanced cutaneous melanoma. *UpToDate*. Retrieved from www.uptodate.com

Soyer, H. P., Rigel, D. S., & Wurm, E. M. T. (2012). Chapter 108. Actinic keratosis, basal cell carcinoma and squamous cell carcinoma. In J. L. Bolognia, J. L. Jorizzo, & J. V. Schaffer (Eds.), *Dermatology (Bolognia, Dermatology)* (3rd ed.). New York, NY: Elsevier. Ebook ISBN: 9780702051821

Surveillance Epidemiology and End Results (SEER) Program. (2014). Retrieved from http://seer.cancer.gov/statfactshtml/melan.html

Swanson, N. A., & Johnson, T. M. (1998). Management of basal and squamous cell carcinoma. In C. W. Cummings, J. M. Fredrickson, C. J. Krause, L. A. Harker, & D. E. Schuller (Eds.), *Otolaryngology head and neck surgery* (3rd ed.). St. Louis, MO: Mosby.

Vargo, N. L. (2003). Basal cell and squamous cell carcinoma. *Seminars in Oncology Nursing, 19*(1), 12–21.

Vargo, N. L. (2003). Cutaneous malignancies. In M. J. Hill (Ed.), *Dermatology nursing essentials: A core curriculum* (pp. 119–135). Pitman, NJ: Dermatology Nurses' Association.

Wu, P. A., Stern, R. S., Robinson, J. K., & Corona, R. (2014). Epidemiology and clinical features of basal cell carcinoma. *UpToDate*. Retrieved from www.uptodate.com

STUDY QUESTIONS

1. Which of the following conditions is the most common reason for dermatology visits in the United States?
   a. Malignant melanoma
   b. Basal cell carcinoma
   c. Actinic keratosis
   d. Squamous cell carcinoma

2. Many studies have shown that excessive sun exposure is the most common cause of skin damage and development of skin cancers. Which of the following describes the pathogenesis of basal cell carcinoma?
   a. Accumulative dose of chronic UV radiation exposure induces DNA damage and *p*53 genetic mutation.
   b. Episodes of excessive UV radiation exposure, including childhood history of severe sunburn, induce genetic alteration of *PTCH1* gene on chromosome 9q.
   c. Excessive UV radiation exposure and genetic makeup involving the mutation of CDKN2A gene located on chromosome 9*p*21.
   d. Excessive UV radiation exposure and genetic mutation involving CDKN2A interferes with *p*53 in cell cycle.

3. Assessment of an infiltrative squamous cell carcinoma includes which of the following?
   a. Dome-shaped lesion with central ulceration
   b. Pearly lesion with raised borders with telangiectasias on the surface
   c. Scaly, irregular, raised red patches occurring in actinically damaged skin
   d. Vague, yellowish, scar-like plaque with indistinct margins

4. Which of the following types of cutaneous malignancies grows rapidly from a small papule to a large volcano-like nodule, with a central keratotic plug, in just 2 to 6 weeks?
   a. Keratoacanthoma
   b. Basal cell carcinoma
   c. Mycosis fungoides
   d. Actinic keratosis

5. Which two types of cutaneous malignancies highly resemble each other clinically, as well as histologically?
   a. Actinic keratosis and squamous cell carcinoma
   b. Basal cell carcinoma and malignant melanoma
   c. Mycosis fungoides and Sézary syndrome
   d. Keratoacanthoma and squamous cell carcinoma

6. The American Academy of Dermatology and the American Cancer Society recommend the use of the A (asymmetry), B (border), C (color), D (diameter), and E (evolution) pneumonic to screen for which of the following types of cutaneous malignancy?
   a. Kaposi sarcoma
   b. Malignant melanoma
   c. Cutaneous T-cell lymphoma
   d. Keratoacanthoma

7. Which of the following describes a change in the 2010 American Joint Commission on Cancer Melanoma Staging System, 7th edition?
   a. Tumor thickness is recategorized as 1, 2, and 4 mm.
   b. Tumor characteristic of ulceration became an unremarkable factor.
   c. In-transit metastasis is separated from satellite lesions in staging.
   d. Mitotic rate (T1 mitoses/mm^2) replaced Clark level of invasion as the primary criterion for staging and prognosis.

8. Mr. Jones is a 65-year-old farmer. He is at a dermatology clinic with his wife who is concerned about a changing mole on his back. He describes it as a mole that he has had all of his life, but he has been experiencing increased itchiness, frequent burning-like sensation, and occasional spontaneous bleeding at the mole for the past 6 months. His wife believes the mole has been changing from a smooth-bordered light brown mole to an ill-defined bordered, reddish brown, partially white and black mole. Which of the following is your presumptive diagnosis of this lesion?
   a. Malignant melanoma
   b. Squamous cell carcinoma
   c. Basal cell carcinoma
   d. Kaposi sarcoma

9. Mr. Duke is a 49-year-old AIDS patient with multiple comorbidities, and his medications have been causing frequent adverse reactions. For the past 3 months, his new symptoms include firm, purplish, nontender bumps and reddish patches around his ears, jawline, and chest areas. He is at a dermatology clinic, discussing possible skin biopsy for a diagnosis. Which of the following is your presumptive diagnosis of these lesions?
   a. Malignant melanoma
   b. Squamous cell carcinoma
   c. Basal cell carcinoma
   d. Kaposi sarcoma

10. Mrs. Smith is a 57-year-old renal transplant recipient on immunosuppressant medications. She is at a dermatology clinic reporting a new lesion on her left temple, which was first noted about 4 months ago. She describes it as a shiny, dark brown growth approximately 5 mm in diameter, and it has a semitranslucent border at the base. Which of the following is your presumptive diagnosis of this lesion?

a. Nodular melanoma
b. Nodular squamous cell carcinoma
c. Pigmented basal cell carcinoma
d. Kaposi sarcoma

11. Which of the following genetic diseases is most susceptible to developing both basal cell carcinoma and squamous cell carcinoma?

a. Nevoid basal cell carcinoma syndrome
b. Muir-Torre syndrome
c. Epidermolysis bullosa syndrome
d. Xeroderma pigmentosum

12. Which of the following is optimal patient education for preventing melanoma and nonmelanoma skin cancers?

a. Daily use of multivitamins containing vitamin A and drinking adequate amount of water.
b. Daily physical activities during morning and evening hours only to avoid midday sun exposure.
c. Daily journal writing to count total number of moles, and seeking medical attention when a new mole lesion is noted.
d. Daily use of sunscreen, photoprotective clothing, and performing regular skin self-examination.

Answers to Study Questions: 1.c, 2.b, 3.a, 4.a, 5.d, 6.b, 7.d, 8.a, 9.d, 10.c, 11.d, 12.d

CHAPTER 17

Disorders of Pigmentation and Dermatologic Considerations in Ethnic Skin

Heather Onoday

THE MELANOCYTE

I. OVERVIEW

The melanocyte comprises approximately 5%-10% of the cellular component of the interfollicular epidermis and an equal component of the hair bulb. They are cells of neural crest origin. (Refer to the discussion of melanocyte in the Cells in the Epidermis section in Chapter 1.) Melanocytes reside in the basal layer of epidermis, where they form the epidermal melanin units as a result of the relationship between one melanocyte and 30-40 associated keratinocytes. The ratio of melanocytes to keratinocytes is 1:10 in the epidermal basal layer.

A. Characteristics of the melanocyte
1. Limited in number.
2. Major synthetic product is melanin.
   a. Melanin is the primary determinant of skin color and hair color.
   b. Melanin accounts for racial and ethnic skin pigmentation differences.
   c. Melanin functions to:
      (1) Absorb ultraviolet light
      (2) Protect genome of dividing basal keratinocytes and melanocytes
      (3) Scavenge free oxygen radicals
3. Melanocytes can up- or downregulate pigmentation in response to:
   a. Physiologic stimuli (e.g., production of melanocyte stimulating hormone, MSH)
   b. Environmental stimuli (e.g., ultraviolet radiation).
   c. Pathologic stimuli (e.g., trauma)
B. Hypothesized to contribute to epidermal homeostasis during inflammation

II. DISORDERS OF PIGMENTATION

A. Disorders of pigmentation may present as either hypo- or hyperpigmentation (too much or too little melanin).
1. Can be localized or diffuse
2. Can be acquired or congenital

B. Acquired hypopigmentation
   1. Vitiligo
   2. Postinflammatory (e.g., after laser treatment)
   3. Inflammatory disorders (e.g., psoriasis, atopic dermatitis)
   4. Neoplasms (e.g., cutaneous T-cell lymphoma)
   5. Postinfection
      a. Bacteria: *Treponema pertenue*, *Treponema carateum*, and *Mycobacterium leprae*
      b. Yeast: *Pityrosporum orbiculare*
      c. Protozoan: *Leishmania donovani*
      d. Helminth: *Onchocerca volvulus*
      e. Fungus: tinea versicolor
C. Congenital hypopigmentation
   1. Albinism
   2. Piebaldism
   3. Tuberous sclerosis
   4. Hypomelanosis of Ito (pigmentary mosaicism)
D. Acquired hyperpigmentation
   1. Melasma
   2. Chemically induced
   3. Melanocytic nevi
   4. Ephelides (freckles): small orange-brown or light-brown macules promoted by sun exposure, fading in winter months; usually on face, arms, and back; benign
   5. Fixed drug eruptions or phototoxic eruptions
   6. Café au lait spots: uniformly pale-brown macules seen on any cutaneous surface; present at birth; six or more macules of greater than 1.5 cm would warrant a workup for neurofibromatosis (von Recklinghausen disease)
   7. Postinflammatory (e.g., thermal burns)
E. Diffuse brown hyperpigmentation: Addison disease

DISORDERS OF HYPOPIGMENTATION

VITILIGO

I. OVERVIEW

A distinctive disorder of pigmentation in which the affected epidermis is devoid of one of its three main cell types (melanocytes) leading to a lack of melanin-based pigmentation in those affected areas.

A. Definition: acquired loss of pigmentation characterized histologically by complete absence of melanocytes in association with a total loss of epidermal pigmentation
B. Etiology
   1. Exact pathogenesis is unclear.
   2. Generalized symmetric form. Thought to be an autoimmune disease associated with antibodies (vitiligo antibodies) and cell-mediated cytotoxicity directed against melanocytes.
   3. May be genetic (a predisposing factor); over 30% of affected individuals have reported vitiligo in a parent, sibling, or child; polygenic (i.e., not caused by a single gene defect)
   4. Other theories include cytotoxic mechanisms, an intrinsic defect of melanocytes, oxidant–antioxidant mechanisms, and neural mechanisms.

5. No definitive precipitating factor has been established; anecdotal correlation with the following environmental factors:
   a. Psychological stress
   b. Physical trauma
   c. Pregnancy
   d. Oral contraceptives
   e. Sunlight and artificial ultraviolet light
   f. Illness
      Note: These associations are frequently observed in a high percentage of normal individuals and have not been epidemiologically shown to occur more frequently in patients with vitiligo.
C. Pathophysiology
   1. Caused by a loss of melanin from the epidermis.
   2. A decrease in the number of melanocytes in affected areas.
   3. Pigment loss may be localized, generalized, or universal.
D. Incidence
   1. Worldwide prevalence of vitiligo is between 0.5% and 2%.
   2. Up to 2.16% of children and adolescents are affected with vitiligo.

II. ASSESSMENT

A. History
   1. Ask about initial presentation.
   2. Ask about any somatic complaints or vision problems that may be associated with vitiligo.
      a. Migraines
      b. Decrease in hearing or pain with hearing (melanin may play important role in the structure and function of the auditory system)
   3. Assess other diseases associated with vitiligo
      a. Thyroid disease (hypo- and hyperthyroidism, Grave disease)
      b. Diabetes mellitus
      c. Pernicious anemia
      d. Addison disease
      e. Multiglandular insufficiency syndrome
      f. Alopecia areata
      g. Melanoma
      h. Lupus erythematosus
      i. Rheumatoid arthritis
   4. Diseases that have been reported in patients with vitiligo
      a. Immune deficiency diseases
      b. Multiple myeloma
      c. Dysgammaglobulinemia
      d. Cutaneous T-cell lymphoma
      e. Thymoma
B. Clinical manifestations
   1. Initial presentation and progression: variable; but genital, anal, axillary, and periorbital are often first areas affected.
   2. Usually a depigmented macule or patch (1 to 3 cm)
   3. Distinct margins
   4. Variations in color and margins can occur (margin may be hyperpigmented, hypopigmented, or exhibit erythema, which is suggestive of an inflammatory process).
   5. Face, joints, hands, and legs are the most commonly affected areas (Figure 17-1).

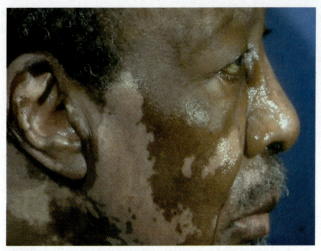

FIGURE 17-1. Vitiligo. (Copyright 2015 by the American Academy of Dermatology. All rights reserved.)

6. Mucous membranes may be affected.
7. Often symmetrical in presentation (Figure 17-2).
8. Classification of patterns of distribution
   a. Localized
      (1) Focal: one or more macules in one area
      (2) Segmental: dermatomal pattern
      (3) Mucosal: localized on mucous membranes
      (4) "Lip-tip" pattern: involves skin around the mouth as well as on the distal fingers and toes; lips, nipples, and genitalia (tip of penis)
   b. Generalized often remarkably symmetrical
      (1) Acrofacial: distal extremities and face
      (2) Vulgaris: diffuse presentation
      (3) Mixed: combination of acrofacial and vulgaris

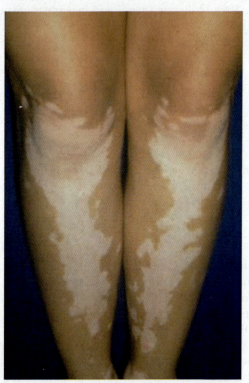

FIGURE 17-2. Vitiligo symmetry. (Copyright 2015 by the American Academy of Dermatology. All rights reserved.)

   c. Universal-depigmented areas cover almost the entire body
9. Associated cutaneous findings
   a. White and prematurely gray hair
   b. Alopecia areata
   c. Halo nevi
C. Differential diagnosis
   1. Piebaldism
   2. Lupus erythematosus
   3. Tinea versicolor (pityriasis versicolor)
   4. Pityriasis alba
   5. Lichen sclerosus et atrophicus
   6. Cutaneous T-cell lymphoma
   7. Sarcoidosis
   8. Scleroderma
   9. Postinflammatory pigmentary alteration (PIPA)
   10. Tuberous sclerosis
   11. Hypomelanosis of Ito
   12. Incontinentia pigmenti

III. COMMON THERAPEUTIC MODALITIES

A. Goals of treatment
   1. Restore normal function to epidermis
   2. Cosmesis
B. Medical therapy: aimed at stimulating proliferation and migration of melanocytes
   1. Topical steroids
      a. Topical class 3 can be employed.
      b. Applied daily for several months or longer.
      c. If pigmentation not seen within 3 months, steroid should be stopped for approximately 6 months and then may be reinstituted or another treatment modality used.
   2. Topical immunomodulators
      a. Seem to be equally effective as topical steroids, especially when used in the face and neck region
      b. Off-label indication for vitiligo
      c. Black box warning for possible risk of cancer
   3. Phototherapy (see Chapter 6, Phototherapy, for comprehensive discussion)
      a. Psoralen plus Ultra Violet A light (PUVA) either topical or systemic.
      b. Topical or systemic PUVA is used two to three times weekly for several months; if no response, stop treatment for at least 6 months before trying again.
      c. UVB narrowband (310- to 315-nm wavelength), two to three times weekly.
      d. UVB narrowband therapy with excimer laser produces monochromatic rays at 308 nm to treat limited, stable patches of vitiligo, treated two to three times weekly, averaging 24 to 48 sessions.
   4. Depigmentation
      a. Used when there is involvement of more than 50% of the skin surface.
      b. Monobenzone (monobenzyl ether of hydroquinone [MBEH]) is applied to skin twice daily until satisfactory depigmentation is achieved.

(1) Frequently requires strength of 20% to 40% to induce necrotic death of melanocytes

   c. Informed consent from the patient as depigmentation is permanent and increases photosensitivity and pruritus.

C. Surgical therapy

   1. Punch grafts: technique similar to hair transplantation
      a. Donor sites are pigmented areas of the skin.
      b. Transplanted into depigmented areas of the skin.
      c. Held in place with pressure dressings.
      d. Repigmentation seen in 4 to 6 weeks after transplantation.
      e. Residual pebbled skin may result, which can be cosmetically unacceptable.

   2. Minigrafts: variant of the punch graft using smaller donor grafts to minimize pebbling

   3. Suction blisters
      a. Epidermal grafts are obtained by vacuum suction.
      b. Blister roof is removed intact and grafted to depigmented site.
      c. Good for large areas of depigmentation.
      d. May be combined with phototherapy.
      e. Repigmentation using this method may cause a mottled appearance.

   4. Autologous cultures
      a. Use autologous cultured melanocytes and keratinocytes from unaffected donor skin.
      b. Applied to recipient sites that have had epidermis removed by suction, cryotherapy, or dermabrasion.
      c. Color may be mottled or incompletely re-pigmented.

   5. Autologous melanocyte grafts
      a. Variant of autologous cultures.
      b. Injected into the depigmented site or used on superficially dermabraded skin.
      c. Culturing melanocytes requires expertise and several months.
      d. Spread of pigmentation is minimal.

   6. Problems with surgical therapies
      a. Graft failure.
      b. Donor sites may become depigmented (isomorphic response).
      c. Risk of infection.
      d. Risk of scarring in donor sites.
      e. May be cost prohibitive.
      Note: Five general options for management are sunscreens, cover-up, repigmentation, minigrafting, and depigmentation.

ALBINISM

I. OVERVIEW

A group of inherited disorders that are characterized by little or no production of melanin

A. Definition: genetically defined defect in the melanocyte system of the eye, skin, or both

B. Etiology

   1. One of four genetic mutations

C. Pathophysiology

   1. Mutations in the gene disrupt the ability of cells to synthesize melanin.

   2. Two classifications
      a. Oculocutaneous albinism (OCA)
      b. Ocular albinism (OA)

D. Incidence

   1. OCA: 1:17,000

   2. OA: not established

II. ASSESSMENT

A. History

B. Clinical manifestations

   1. OCA: diluted skin/hair pigmentation
      a. Skin
         (1) In light-skinned individuals, skin is very light.
         (2) In darkly pigmented individuals, large, pigmented freckles in light-exposed areas may be seen.
      b. Hair
         (1) In darkly pigmented individuals, hair is yellow to yellowish-brown.
         (2) In lighter-skinned individuals, hair may range from white to cream, yellow to yellow-red, to vibrant red.
      c. Eye
         (1) Iris: blue/gray and translucent.
         (2) Retina and choroid: paucity of pigment.
         (3) In darkly pigmented individuals, the iris will be pale blue to cinnamon brown.
         (4) Photophobia and nystagmus seen in all races.
         (5) Visual acuity is decreased.

   2. OA
      a. Decrease or absence of melanin in the iris and retinal pigment epithelium.
      b. Nystagmus present.
      c. Iris translucency may occur.
      d. Decrease in visual acuity.
      e. Hair and skin color are normal.

III. COMMON THERAPEUTIC MODALITIES

A. Treatment goals are surveillance and preventing complications.

B. Sunscreen use.

C. Regular skin inspection for early detection of skin cancers.

D. Appropriate eye protection.

PIEBALDISM

I. OVERVIEW

Congenital absence of melanocytes in affected areas of the skin and hair (depigmentation) that may have spontaneous expansion and contraction

A. Definition: disorder of hypopigmentation, which involves skin and hair only

B. Etiology

   1. Autosomal dominant mutation of the c-kit or SNA12 gene, rare

C. Pathophysiology
  1. Hypomelanosis
  2. Histologically, absence or markedly decreased melanocytes in affected areas
D. Incidence: 1:20,000 births

II. ASSESSMENT

A. History
  1. Screen for deafness.
  2. Screen for congenital megacolon particularly in infants.
B. Clinical manifestations
  1. Characteristic pattern
    a. White forelock
    b. Occasionally white macules/patches on forehead, chin
    c. Lack of pigmentation
      (1) Trunk
      (2) Anterior thorax
      (3) Abdomen
      (4) Midarm to wrist
      (5) Midthigh to midcalf (anterior and posterior)
      (6) Normal pigmentation of hands, upper part of arm, shoulders, upper thighs, and feet to midcalf
  2. Two features to distinguish piebaldism from vitiligo
    a. Presence of islands of normal pigmentation (Figure 17-3) in areas of hypomelanosis
    b. Characteristic distribution
    c. Congenital
    d. Frequently hereditary autosomal dominant pattern can be observed in family members.

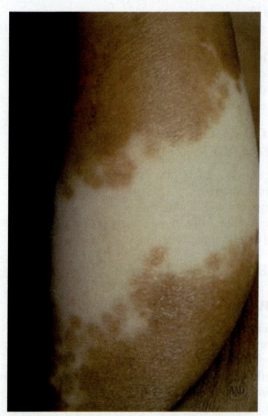

FIGURE 17-3. Piebaldism. (Copyright 2015 by the American Academy of Dermatology. All rights reserved.)

III. COMMON THERAPEUTIC MODALITIES

A. Minigrafts: most successful
B. Culture grafts: not always cosmetically acceptable
C. PUVA: not always cosmetically acceptable

TUBEROUS SCLEROSIS

I. OVERVIEW

Also called tuberous sclerosis complex. Hypopigmentation is one of the earliest clinical signs of tuberous sclerosis.
A. Definition: rare, multisystem, genetic disease that causes benign tumors to grow in the brain and on other vital organs such as the kidneys, heart, eyes, lungs, and skin. Also affects the central nervous system, resulting in symptoms including seizure, developmental delay, and behavioral abnormalities.
B. Etiology
  1. Genetic
C. Pathophysiology
  1. Melanocytes present
  2. Melanosomes in melanocytes decreased and poorly melanized
D. Incidence
  1. 1:6,000 births

II. ASSESSMENT

A. History
B. Clinical manifestations
  1. Common locations
    a. Trunk
    b. Lower extremities
  2. Configurations
    a. Ash leaf spot: lance-ovate (round at one end and pointed at the other); considered as a tertiary feature of tuberous sclerosis (Figure 17-4)
    b. Oval
    c. Polygonal
    d. Shagreen patch area of thickened, elevated pebbly skin, usually found on lower back (Figure 17-5)

FIGURE 17-4. Ash leaf macule, seen in tuberous sclerosis. (Copyright 2015 by the American Academy of Dermatology. All rights reserved.)

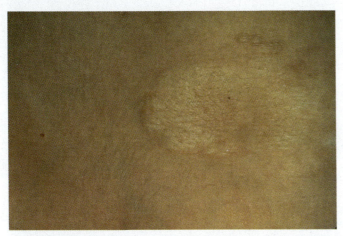

FIGURE 17-5. Shagreen patch, seen in tuberous sclerosis.

3. May see multiple 1- to 3-mm macules ("confetti-like") with poliosis (loss of melanin) of scalp, hair, eyebrows, and eyelashes
4. Hypopigmented spots of the iris and fundus
5. Wood lamp enhances lesions in light-skinned patients.

III. COMMON THERAPEUTIC MODALITIES

None for skin lesions

DISORDERS OF HYPERPIGMENTATION

MELASMA

I. OVERVIEW

Disorders of hyperpigmentation can be caused by any of the following factors: hereditary/developmental, metabolic, endocrine, inflammatory, chemically induced, nutritional, or neoplastic. Melasma is one of the most commonly seen disorders of hyperpigmentation.

A. Definition: acquired, brown hypermelanosis of the face. Also called chloasma faciei
B. Etiology
   1. Secondary to an increase in the number and activity of melanocytes
   2. No known cause. Melasma has been linked to:
      a. Oral contraceptives
      b. Pregnancy
      c. Cosmeceutical or medication (usually a phototoxic or allergic reaction)
      d. Genetic predisposition
      e. Endocrine (progesterone and estrogen both have an effect on melanogenesis)
      f. *Race*
      g. Nutrition
      h. Metabolism
      i. Sunlight
C. Pathophysiology
   1. Epidermal type: melanin is deposited in the basal and suprabasal layers of the epidermis.

2. Dermal type: melanophages in the superficial and deep dermis in addition to epidermal hyperpigmentation.
D. Incidence
   1. Unknown true incidence.
   2. Almost 90% affected are women.
   3. More common in persons of Latino origin living in tropical areas.
   4. Commonly seen in women who are pregnant or using oral contraceptives or hormonal replacement.
   5. Is seen in men, but usually without hormonal factors.

II. ASSESSMENT

A. History: always take a complete history.
B. Clinical manifestations
   1. Symmetrical
   2. Irregular light to dark-brown hyperpigmentation
   3. Seen on the face
      a. Centrofacial
         (1) Most common presentation
         (2) Involves cheeks, forehead, upper lip, nose, and chin
      b. Malar
         (1) Localized to cheeks and nose
         (2) Second most common presentation
      c. Mandibular
         (1) Involves the ramus of the mandible
         (2) Least common presentation
   4. Four types (distinguished with the use of Wood light according to the depth of pigment deposition)
      a. Epidermal: shows enhancement of pigmentation (most common type intense under Wood lamp).
      b. Dermal: no enhancement of color (many melanophages) in the dermis.
      c. Mixed: shows no or slight enhancement of color.
      d. Indeterminate or unapparent—lesions are not discernible under Wood light in skin types V to VI.
   5. Differential diagnosis (partial list)
      a. Drug-induced hyperpigmentation
      b. Pigmented contact dermatitis
      c. Postinflammatory hyperpigmentation
      d. Exogenous ochronosis (blue-black or slate gray hyperpigmented changes secondary to prolonged topical application of hydroquinone, phenol, or resorcinol)

III. COMMON THERAPEUTIC MODALITIES

A. Identify and eliminate causative factors.
B. Medications
   1. Hydroquinone alone (2% to 4% concentrations most commonly used)
   2. Hydroquinone with retinoic acid (retinoic acid enhances epidermal penetration of hydroquinone and reduces the activity of the melanocytes)
   3. Broad-spectrum sunscreen
   4. Topical steroids (alone or in conjunction with hydroquinone, or hydroquinone plus retinoids)
   5. 5-Fluorouracil (effective particularly if patients have actinically damaged skin)

6. Azelaic acid (causes reversible inhibition of tyrosinase; may be used in conjunction with hydroquinone)
C. Possible side effects of topical medications
  1. Hydroquinone therapy
    a. Irritant contact dermatitis
    b. Exogenous ochronosis
    c. Brown discoloration of nails secondary to deposition of hydroquinone oxidated products
    d. Vitiligo in predisposed individual
  2. Topical steroids: hypopigmentation, atrophy
D. Chemical peel (trichloroacetic acid or phenol solution). Phenol peels can cause cardiac, renal, and pulmonary toxicities.
E. Lasers (Q-switched, fractionated nonablative)

CHEMICALLY INDUCED HYPERPIGMENTATION

I. OVERVIEW

Hyperpigmentation has long been associated with exposure to a variety of chemicals.
A. Definition: unusual darkening of the skin as a direct result of exposure to chemicals
B. Etiology
  1. Direct deposition of the chemical into the skin.
  2. Stimulation of melanin formation.
  3. Binding of chemical to melanin.
  4. Production of metabolites or nonmelanin pigment.
  5. Hyperpigmentation may be enhanced by exposure to ultraviolet light.
  6. Offending agents
    a. Antimalarials
    b. Antibiotics
    c. Heavy metals, such as silver
    d. Chemotherapeutic agents
    e. Topical preparations (e.g., tar-containing compounds)
    f. Antiarrhythmic, amiodarone
C. Pathophysiology
  1. Dependent on etiologic agent.
  2. Antimalarials: hyperpigmentation appears in the dermis; may be a combination of melanin and hemosiderin.
  3. Antibiotics: pigmentation depends on presentation; minocycline is used as an example here.
    a. In areas of scarring, such as acne scars, hemosiderin and ferritin are present in macrophages and appear blue-black.
    b. Blue-black, brown, or slate gray patches on extremities have pigmented macrophages that stain for both melanin and iron.
    c. Generalized muddy-brown pigmentation sometimes exacerbated on sunlight-exposed regions.

II. ASSESSMENT

A. History with emphasis on chemical exposure
B. Physical examination
C. Clinical manifestations
  1. May vary, as described.
  2. Skin biopsy may be indicated to confirm diagnosis.

III. COMMON THERAPEUTIC MODALITIES

A. Often persistent.
B. Stop offending agent or exposure if known (particularly drug).
C. Prevent recurrent exposure.
D. Use sunscreens.

NEVI

MELANOCYTIC NEVI

I. OVERVIEW

Nevi, or moles, are benign tumors composed of nevus cells that are derived from melanocytes and can occur anywhere on the cutaneous surface, and except for certain types (large congenital and dysplastic), most nevi have low-malignancy potential.
A. Definition
  1. Nevus cell: larger than melanocyte, may lack dendrites; has more abundant cytoplasm and coarse granules; aggregates in groups or proliferates in basal region at dermoepidermal junction
  2. Types of nevi (Table 17-1)
    a. Common nevi: classified based on location within the skin
      (1) Junction
      (2) Compound
      (3) Intradermal
    b. Special forms
      (1) Congenital (Figure 17-6)
      (2) Halo nevus (Figure 17-7)
      (3) Nevus spilus (speckled lentiginous nevus)
      (4) Becker nevus
      (5) Benign juvenile melanoma (Spitz nevus)
      (6) Blue nevus (Figure 17-8)
      (7) Labial melanotic nevus
B. Etiology
  1. Dependent on type
C. Pathophysiology
  1. Junctional: nevus cells at dermoepidermal junction
  2. Compound: nevus cells at dermoepidermal junction and upper dermis
  3. Dermal: nevus cells in dermis, rarely extends into superficial fat, usually along follicular structures
D. Incidence
  1. Very common
  2. Present in 1% of newborns with incidence increasing throughout infancy and childhood, peaking at puberty

II. ASSESSMENT

A. History.
B. Clinical manifestations (Table 17-1)
C. Dermoscopy
  1. Noninvasive method that allows the *in vivo* evaluation of color and microstructures of the skin.

TABLE 17-1 Types of Nevi

Type	Morphology	Comments
Junctional	Initially 1–2 mm, expanding to 4–6 mm; flat, slightly elevated, smooth surface; sharply circumscribed; uniformly brown, tan, or black	Progression is slow, over decades; may change into compound nevus; rare at birth, develop after 2 years of age
Compound	Slightly elevated, dome-shaped, papule; skin-colored, brown, "halo nevus"; cells at dermoepidermal junction and upper dermis; hair may be present	Generally benign, may be a cosmetic concern
Dermal	Brown or black, but may lighten with age; vary in size, maybe a few millimeters up to a centimeter; dome-shaped nevi are most common; symmetric with smooth surface; white or translucent; surface telangiectasia may make lesion difficult to distinguish from a basal cell carcinoma; may be polypoin or verrucous in appearance; found on trunk, neck, axilla, groin	Elevated lesions often removed due to being prone to trauma; skin-colored border may be present making nevus look similar to a halo nevus; rarely degenerate into a melanoma but should be monitored, nonetheless
Congenital	Present at birth, vary in size from a few millimeters to several centimeters; may cover wide areas of the trunk (bathing suit distribution) extremity, or face; giant hair nevus is the largest form; may see coarse hair in the body of the nevus; uniformly brown or black but may be red or pink; surface flat at birth and becomes verrucous or nodular over time; high risk of degeneration into melanoma in very large lesions	Large, thick lesions—consider removal early due to tendency to become malignant; removal should be done with consideration of cosmesis; all congenital nevi should be checked regularly by a dermatology provider
Nevus spilus	Oval or irregular; hairless lesion that is brown with dots of darker pigmentation present; flat surface with the darker dots with some elevation; range in size from 1 to 20 cm; appear at any age	Degeneration into melanoma not documented; excision for cosmetic reason can be performed
Halo nevus	Can be a compound or dermal nevus that exhibits a skin-colored border(halo); sharply demarcated borders that are round or oval; generally located on the trunk, may occur on the palms or soles; develop spontaneously and frequently in adolescence; may be singular or multiple; incidence of vitiligo may be increased in individuals with halo nevi	Removal indicated if atypical features develop
Becker nevus	Lacks nevus cells; developmental anomaly; presents as a brown macules with a patch of hair or both; usually seen in adolescent males; seen on the shoulder, inframammary area, upper and lower back; vary in size; irregular border that is sharply demarcated	Malignant degeneration has not been reported; lesions are generally too large for excision; hair is sometimes removed for cosmetic reasons
Benign juvenile melanoma (Spitz nevus)	Common in children but can be seen in adults; hairless, red or reddish-brown; dome shaped; surface may be smooth or verrucous; range in size from 0.3 to 1.5 cm; vascular and may bleed with trauma; usually solitary but may be multiple; appear suddenly	Should be biopsied for histologic examination due to risk of malignant transformation
Blue nevus	Common on extremities and dorsum of hands; small, round lesions, slightly elevated; blue in color; appear in childhood	Large lesion may degenerate into a malignant lesion
Labial melanotic macule	Located on the lower lip, exhibit as brown macules; commonly seen in young adult women; do not darken with exposure to sunlight	Do not require removal. May be treated due to cosmetic considerations

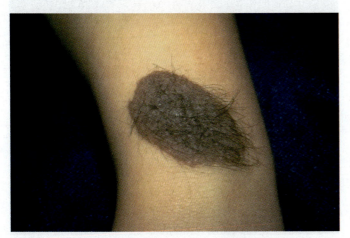

FIGURE 17-6. Congenital nevus. (Copyright 2015 by the American Academy of Dermatology. All rights reserved.)

2. Introduction of this method of observing colors and structure within a nevus, not otherwise visible to the unaided eye, helps to predict the histopathology diagnosis.
D. Longitudinal photography

III. COMMON THERAPEUTIC MODALITIES

A. Common nevi
  1. Suspicious lesions
     a. Should be biopsied; then, any appropriate intervention taken after histology established
     b. Removal for cosmetic purposes
  2. Special forms
     a. Large congenital nevi—2.8% at risk for development of melanoma; surgical removal indicated

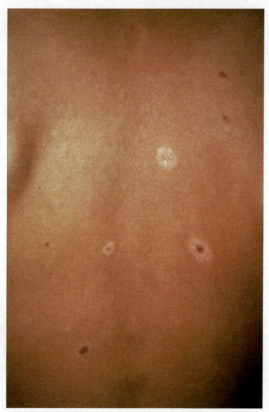

FIGURE 17-7. Halo nevi. (Copyright 2015 by the American Academy of Dermatology. All rights reserved.)

b. Nevus spilus: cosmetic surgical excision, longitudinal evaluation to identify early transformation.

c. Halo nevi: biopsy is unnecessary unless the nevus is otherwise suspicious or has an atypical presentation, atypical history of lesion, or in patients with history of or at high risk for melanoma.

d. Becker nevus (pigmented hairy epidermal nevus)—risk of malignant transformation appears to be very low.

e. Benign juvenile melanoma (Spitz nevus)—requires removal to determine risk.

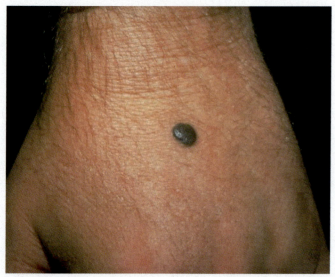

FIGURE 17-8. Blue nevus. (Copyright 2015 by the American Academy of Dermatology. All rights reserved.)

TABLE 17-2 Dysplastic Nevus Syndrome (Familial Dysplastic Nevus Syndrome)[a]

Characteristics	Management
Autosomal dominant Develop melanoma at an early age Predisposition to multiple primary melanomas Tendency to develop superficial spreading melanomas Distinctive large melanocytic nevi present (larger than common moles) (see Figure 17-9) Mixture of colors including tan, brown, pink, and black Irregular and indistinct border, may fade into surrounding skin Surface may be both macular and papular Characteristic presentation: pigmented papule surrounded by a macular collar of pigmentation ("fried egg lesion") Nevi not present at birth; present in midchildhood as common moles, which change appearance at puberty Lesions may continue to appear after age of 40 Lesions occur in sun-exposed areas as well as scalp, buttocks, and breasts	History: document sun exposure, evolution of nevi, family history of melanoma or presence of large number of moles (particularly large moles) Physical examination: entire integument should be examined, including scalp and eyes Examinations should be done at minimum, every 1 yr, or as directed by provider Excisional biopsy should be performed (≥1 DN); total excisional biopsy to avoid recurrence. Consider excision of all new nevi, particularly those in the scalp Photograph total body surface as a baseline for comparison on follow-up Patient education is paramount to compliance with surveillance, treatment, and follow-up; self-examination should be emphasized All family members should be examined on a regular basis for early detection

[a]The identification of the dysplastic nevus (DN) in melanoma-prone families led to the determination that DN are cutaneous. Markers, which identify individuals who are at increased risk for melanoma. DN may be the single most important precursor lesion of melanoma occurring in persons with melanoma-prone families and in persons who lack both a family history of melanoma and a personal history of melanoma.

f. Blue nevus—most commonly benign, biopsy not typically needed unless new or changing. Rare cases of malignant melanoma have been reported arising in association with cellular blue nevi.

g. Labial melanotic macule: removal not necessary unless it has suspicious features.

B. Dysplastic nevus syndrome (Table 17-2)
  1. Excisional biopsy
  2. Photograph for comparison and follow-up (Figure 17-9)

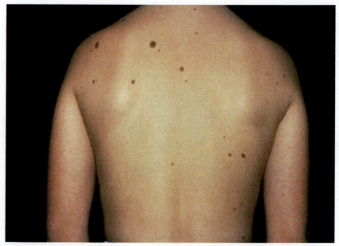

FIGURE 17-9. Dysplastic nevi. (Copyright 2015 by the American Academy of Dermatology. All rights reserved.)

VARIANTS OF ETHNIC SKIN TYPES

I. OVERVIEW

Most skin diseases occur in all types of skin. Fitzpatrick separated skin types by photoresponsiveness; skin types III, IV, V, and VI compose the ethnic population that is being addressed. It is important to recognize normal pigmentation variants in ethnic people in order to distinguish these variations from pathologic conditions.

A. Differences in skin type
   1. Clinical differences that may be appreciated in ethnic skin types include pigment, follicular response, fibroblast hyperresponsivity, curly hair, and ashiness.
      a. Skin pigment or skin color is determined by melanosome/melanin production. Melanosomes in keratinocytes in lighter-skinned individuals are smaller and distributed as membrane-bound complexes. In darker-skinned individuals, such as African Americans, melanosomes tend to be larger and distributed more individually. (Refer to melanin production discussion in Chapter 1.)
      b. Follicular reactivity is common to many dermatologic diseases in darker skin types: follicular accentuation is clearly visible in darker-skinned individuals, as can be seen in pityriasis rosea, atopic dermatitis, nummular eczema, and sarcoidosis.
      c. Fibroblast hyperresponsivity, which is thought to be induced by mast cell/fibroblast interaction and prolonged by a decrease in collagenase activity, leads to another characteristic of darker skin types (typically types IV to VI), in the case of keloid formation.
      d. Curly hair: in people of African descent, hair tends to curl and spontaneously knot and break. Hair can be straightened with chemicals and heat and hot oils and tend to cause hair shaft fracture and scalp scarring, which can result in temporary or permanent alopecia.
      e. Ashiness: those with dark skin may appear "ashy white" when the skin is dry and scaly; although this scaling occurs in lighter skin, it is not as clinically evident.

NORMAL SKIN CHANGES IN DARKER-SKINNED PATIENTS

I. OVERVIEW

A. Definition: pigmentary demarcation lines (PDLs) also described as Voigt and Futcher lines consist of a demarcation between darkly pigmented and lightly pigmented portions of the upper arms in African Americans. For our purpose, we will deal with types A and B PDLs, which are those with sharp transitions.
B. Etiology
   1. Unknown.
   2. One theory suggests that the purpose of PDLs is protective in nature. The dorsal skin is more heavily pigmented to provide protection from UV radiation.

C. Incidence
   1. African descent: 20% to 60%.
   2. Asian descent: less frequent.
   3. Japanese: 4% (more often in women than in men).
   4. Light-skinned individuals: rarely seen.
   5. Evident at birth or is noted in childhood.

II. ASSESSMENT

A. Physical examination
   1. PDL (Futcher, Voigt) lines are distinct lines of demarcation between darkly pigmented skin laterally and lighter skin anteromedially along the length of the arm.
   2. Lines may follow the distribution of spinal nerves.
   3. Lines are clearly seen on the skin.
   4. PDL (Futcher, Voigt) lines can be present on the posteromedial aspect of the lower leg in women of African descent and may be more pronounced during pregnancy.

III. TREATMENT MODALITIES

A. PDLs have no clinical significance other than cosmetic considerations.
B. No treatment needed; no cosmetic treatment options available.

NAIL PIGMENTATION (LONGITUDINAL MELANONYCHIA)

I. OVERVIEW

A. Definition: longitudinal, linear, dark bands, brown to black, found in the nail plates
B. Etiology
   1. Pigmentation is due to increased melanin deposits in the nail plates.
   2. May be associated with melanocytes within the nail matrix.
C. Incidence
   1. African descent: 50%.
   2. May exceed 90% in very dark-skinned individuals.
   3. Ten to twenty percent in Asians.
   4. One percent in light-skinned populations.
   5. Increases with age.
   6. Rate of subungual melanoma is 0.1/100,000 per year.

II. ASSESSMENT

A. Physical examination
   1. Longitudinal, pigmented nail stripes in the nail plates, width varying from one to several millimeters; may be single or multiple in number.
   2. Distribution of nail pigment may be diffuse rather than linear.
   3. Most common in the thumb, index, or middle fingernails.
   4. Use of dermoscopy is encouraged (assessing for asymmetry in structure or color).
B. Diagnosis
   1. Related to distribution and clinical findings.
   2. Melanoma should be considered.

III. TREATMENT MODALITIES

A. No treatment is necessary for benign pigment changes.

B. Biopsy is warranted if suspicion of malignancy is present.

PALMAR AND PLANTAR PIGMENTATION

I. OVERVIEW

In dark skin, the palms and soles are usually lighter in color than the rest of the body. Palmar or plantar pigmentation frequently presents in varying degrees.

II. ASSESSMENT

A. Physical examination

   1. Palmar pigmentation normally occurs in flexural and digital creases.

   2. Small hyperkeratotic papules that evolve into discrete, conical depressions (pits) are also common; limited to palmar and digital creases.

   3. Pigmented macules are commonly seen on the palms and soles of darker-skinned individuals; these lesions are usually multiple, nonerythematous, irregularly shaped with indistinct borders, varying in color from tan to dark brown.

   4. Plantar pigmentation is normally present in those with dark skin; however, it may be present in light skin as well.

B. Diagnosis

   1. Physical examination.

   2. Plantar lesions also may occur in secondary syphilis.

   3. Possibility of melanoma should be considered.

III. TREATMENT MODALITIES

A. None indicated

COMMON DISEASES IN THE DARKER-SKINNED ADULT

I. OVERVIEW

Dermatologic diagnosis is often more difficult to reach in the darker-skinned patient because subtle changes in skin color may be hidden. Pink and light red hues may be totally missed. Dark reds and browns may appear as purple, gray, or black. Patient history, distribution of lesions, and skin surface changes become the most important diagnostic tools.

A. Disorders that may appear differently in persons with darker skin types include atopic dermatitis, pityriasis rosea, psoriasis, and lupus erythematosus.

B. Any inflammatory disease will appear different in more darkly pigmented skin than in lighter skin.

II. ASSESSMENT

A. Follicular prominence in this disease may be more pronounced.

B. Fine scale in darker skin types seen in pityriasis rosea may be better appreciated.

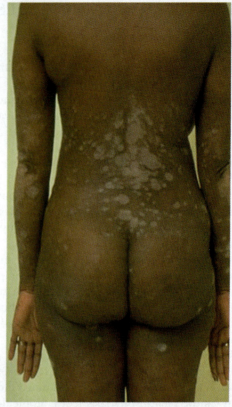

FIGURE 17-10. Psoriasis in darker-skinned individual. (Copyright 2015 by the American Academy of Dermatology. All rights reserved.)

C. Erythema may be less evident.

D. Papular and papulovesicular variants of pityriasis rosea may be more common in darker skin types.

E. Psoriasis plaques may appear more bluish black due to pigment incontinence.

F. All disorders are more likely to elicit postinflammatory hyperpigmentation or hypopigmentation in darker skin types (Figure 17-10).

FOLLICULAR OCCLUSION TRIAD

I. OVERVIEW

The follicular occlusion triad is made up of three diseases that often occur together: hidradenitis suppurativa, acne conglobata, and dissecting cellulitis of the scalp.

A. Definition: hidradenitis suppurativa is a disease involving the apocrine gland–bearing skin of the axilla, groin, inframammary area, and the anogenital region. Symptoms range from mild discomfort to debilitation with extensive scarring, painful draining inflammatory nodules, and the development of sinus tracts. The patient with acne conglobata is affected with multiple open comedones, inflammatory nodules with pus, extensive scarring, and sinus tracts of the back, buttocks, face, and chest. These large comedones tend to have multiple openings. The patient with dissecting cellulitis of the scalp (also known as perifolliculitis capitis abscedens et suffodiens) is plagued by inflammatory nodules, sinus tracts, chronic drainage, crusting alopecia, and scarring. All can be very difficult to treat.

B. Etiology
  1. Predisposing factors
    a. Obesity.
    b. Predisposition to acne.
    c. Obstruction of apocrine duct.
    d. Bacterial infection.
    e. Smoking tobacco may increase severity.
C. Pathophysiology
  1. Apocrine duct plugged with keratinous material
  2. Dilatation of apocrine duct and hair follicle
  3. Severe inflammation of apocrine gland
  4. Bacterial growth in dilated ducts
  5. Extension of inflammation/infection secondary to ruptured duct/gland
  6. Extension of suppuration/tissue destruction
  7. Ulceration and fibrosis/scar
  8. Sinus tract formation
D. Incidence
  1. Onset puberty
  2. May undergo a spontaneous remission with age (over 35)
  3. Men tend to be affected in anogenital area and women in axillae.

II. ASSESSMENT

A. History and physical examination
  1. Intermittent pain, mild to extreme pain.
  2. Multiple inflamed erythematous nodular lesions. Abscesses are frequently recurrent and drain purulent/seropurulent material.
  3. Sinus tracts form and drain pus; fibrosis, hypertrophic, and keloidal scars form; contractures.
  4. Open comedones form. Double comedones may develop even when active nodules are absent.
  5. Lesions may also be found in inguinal folds, gluteal cleft, perineum, or inframammary and may extend over the back and buttocks.
  6. Obesity commonly seen.
  7. Severe cystic acne.
B. Diagnosis
  1. Clinical exam and history
  2. Bacterial cultures from drainage to rule out infected of lesions
    a. *Staphylococcus aureus*
    b. *Staphylococcus milleri*
    c. Anaerobic streptococcus
    d. *Bacteroides* species
    e. *Pseudomonas aeruginosa*

III. THERAPEUTIC MODALITIES

A. Medical
  1. Antibiotics
    a. Early
      (1) Erythromycin
      (2) Tetracycline

      (3) Minocycline
      (4) Intralesional triamcinolone injections
    b. Late
      (1) Maintenance with antibiotics.
      (2) Prednisone.
      (3) Oral retinoids may have limited therapeutic benefit.
      (4) Biologics (e.g., Anakinra) have been used to treat severe forms, however are not FDA approved for this use, though they have demonstrated some limited efficacy in randomized controlled trials.
B. Surgical
  1. Axillary hidradenitis suppurativa may respond well to surgical excision of skin to include the removal or scarring of apocrine sweat glands.
  2. Inguinal: surgical control is more difficult and less successful.
  3. Oral retinoids may have more positive effective in early disease, when combined with surgical excision of individual lesions.

KELOIDS

I. OVERVIEW

Keloids represent exaggeration of the normal fibroblastic process involved in wound healing. Keloids are difficult to treat and commonly recur.
A. Definition: shiny, hyperpigmented, thick, elevated, firm, papules, plaques, and tumors characterized by deposition of excessive amounts of collagen (Figures 17-11 and 17-12)
B. Etiology
  1. Unknown.
  2. Usually occur following injury to skin but may appear spontaneously without apparent skin trauma.
  3. Keloids tend to form in dark-skinned individuals more frequently than in those with light skin.

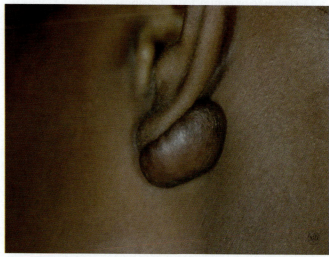

FIGURE 17-11. Keloid. (Copyright 2015 by the American Academy of Dermatology. All rights reserved.)

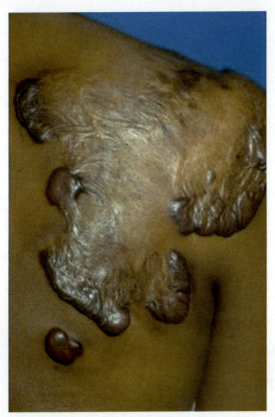

FIGURE 17-12. Keloid. (Copyright 2015 by the American Academy of Dermatology. All rights reserved.)

4. Possible sources of keloid formation: any minor or major surgical procedure, many inflammatory or bullous skin disorders, burns, accidental traumatic events, vaccinations, acne, and secondary infections.

C. Pathophysiology
   1. Exuberant fibrous repair tissue following a cutaneous injury.
   2. Benign growths.
   3. Papules grow into large nodules or plaques, often with claw-like or contracted extensions.
   4. Growth may be slow or become large in a short time.

D. Incidence
   1. Equal incidence in males and females.
   2. More common in Fitzpatrick types IV to VI.
   3. Occur more often on young adults.
   4. Research indicates that keloids are also common in other groups.
      a. Chinese population in Malaysia
      b. Light-skinned people of Finland

II. ASSESSMENT

A. History and physical examination
   1. Usually asymptomatic.
   2. Commonly pruritic; maybe painful, especially with contractures.
   3. Firm, smooth, hairless, shiny, and raised above the surrounding skin surface.

4. May be erythematous; progress to brownish-red hue; become hyperpigmented or hypopigmented over time.
5. Erythema may not be noticed in dark skin.
6. May be linear following traumatic or surgical injury. Sometimes confused with hypertrophic scars.
   a. Keloids differ from hypertrophic scars in that keloidal tissue growth, in a traumatized site, extends beyond the boundary of the injury.
   b. Tissue growth from hypertrophic scar remains confined to the site of original injury.
   c. Hypertrophic scars tend to regress, flatten, and soften spontaneous over time.
   d. Keloids may continue to expand in size for years.
   e. Hypertrophic scars are likely to form soon after injury, whereas keloids may not begin growing until months later.
7. Spontaneous regression is rare in keloids.
8. Common sites: ear lobes, shoulders, upper back, neck, chest, skin overlying the jaw, lateral chest (in women), and regions of higher tension on the skin.

B. Diagnosis
   1. Clinical examination.
   2. Biopsy not warranted; it may induce new or larger scar.

III. THERAPEUTIC MODALITIES

A. Medical
   1. Intralesional corticosteroid injection: triamcinolone, typically once a month to reduce pruritus and sensitivity of lesion, reduce its volume, and flatten it.
   2. Intralesional triamcinolone plus cryotherapy may be slightly more effective. The corticosteroid must be injected directly into the bulk of the keloid.
   3. Corticosteroid injections may cause temporary hypopigmentation at or around the injection site. Usually resolves within a few months.
   4. Atrophy may occur in the surrounding skin if corticosteroid inadvertently infiltrates the surrounding normal tissue.
   5. Interferon injections 0.01 to 0.1 mg three times per week for 3 consecutive weeks.
   6. Silicone gel sheeting for 12 to 24 hours daily for 8 to 12 weeks or longer may flatten keloid.

B. Surgical
   1. Simple surgical excisions. Lesions may grow back larger than the original lesion.
   2. Simple surgical excisions and steroid injections followed by pressure dressing. Pressure dressing is most effective if it is maintained for at least 4 to 6 months after surgery.
   3. Other techniques employed: laser, interferon, tamoxifen, chemotherapeutic agents, imiquimod, calcineurin inhibitors, narrowband UVB, compression therapy, skin grafts, random pattern flaps, and radiation alone or with excision and electrosurgery.

HAIR LOSS

TRACTION ALOPECIA/CENTRAL CENTRIFUGAL CICATRICIAL ALOPECIA

I. OVERVIEW

Hair and scalp disorders that may be related to grooming practices occur more frequently in those with darker skin and curly hair. Hot combing, chemical straightening, braids, and weaves are common methods of hairstyling. However, the repeated process that straightens and makes curly hair more manageable, may also damage the scalp and hair. Traction alopecia and central centrifugal cicatricial alopecia (CCCA), a scarring alopecia, are potential results of using these grooming techniques extensively. Evidence has not clearly demonstrated hot combing as the cause of CCCA, but discussing grooming practices should be part of the history in any instance of alopecia.

A. Definition: traction alopecia is a gradually developing patchy hair loss resulting from the cumulative effects of prolonged traction on the scalp and hair. Traumatic hair loss caused by straightening and styling the hair with a hot comb and the application of oils or pomades has been implicated in CCCA.

B. Etiology
   1. Traction alopecia
      a. Braiding: corn rowing the hair frequently and tightly; sometimes adding jewelry, beads, and synthetic hair.
      b. Weaving: corn rowing the hair, then attaching natural human or synthetic hair to the hair or gluing it to the scalp. May glue human hair strand by strand to natural hair.
   2. CCCA
      a. Heat from the hot comb causes the hair to break. Hot oil flows down the hair shaft damaging the fair follicles. This may contribute to alopecia.

C. Pathophysiology
   1. Damage may occur in the hair follicles with traction alopecia or CCCA.
      a. The individual's hair is braided with or without the addition of human or synthetic hair (Figure 17-13).
      b. Extensive tension is placed on the hair follicle causing follicular erythema and follicular pustules.
      c. Conditions may be exacerbated by oils and pomades.
      d. Follicular atrophy may result in a noninflammatory permanent alopecia.
      e. Commonly affects the frontal and temporal hairline in traction alopecia.
      f. Pulling a heated metal comb from roots to end.
      g. Curling the hair with electric or curling iron heated from 300°F to 500°F
      h. Breakage and rearrangement of hydrogen bonds by the high temperature straightens the hair.
      i. Reverse the process by adding moisture to the hair.

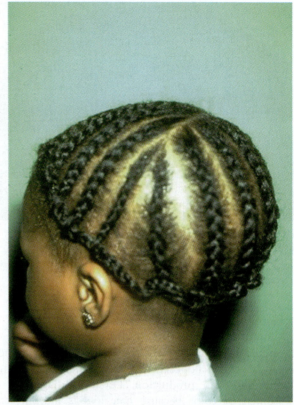

FIGURE 17-13. Braids causing traction. (Copyright 2015 by the American Academy of Dermatology. All rights reserved.)

      j. Burning of skin surface when hot oil flows down the hair shaft causing inflammation, which can lead to postinflammatory pigment changes.
      k. Scarring causes a decrease in the number of hair follicles.
      l. Vertex of scalp (central, frontal, and parietal areas) is most commonly seen in CCCA.

D. Incidence
   1. More common among African American. Can occur in all races.
   2. Prepuberty to older adults.
   3. CCCA pattern of hair loss may also occur in men who do not hot comb their hair but do use oil and pomades. May be clinical alopecia imitators of CCCA.

II. ASSESSMENT

A. History and physical examination
   1. Traction alopecia/CCCA
      a. Hair loss in frontal and temporal hairline in traction alopecia and vertex in CCCA (Figure 17-14).
      b. Lymphocytic perifollicular inflammation may be seen.
      c. Hair breakage at anchoring sites in weaves.
      d. Permanent hair loss/scarring.
      e. Headache due to scalp tension.
      f. Remaining hair may be broken, coarse, or thickened.

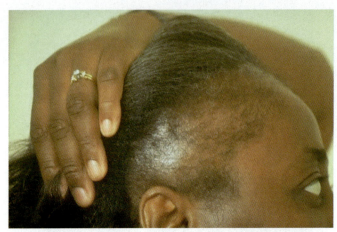

FIGURE 17-14. Central centrifugal cicatricial alopecia. (Copyright 2015 by the American Academy of Dermatology. All rights reserved.)

B. Diagnosis
  1. Clinical examination and history.
  2. Should be distinguished from male pattern baldness (androgenetic alopecia) caused by genetic factors, age, and androgen production. Often misdiagnosed in women of color because hair loss is attributed to grooming causes.
  3. Biopsy can help determine causes of alopecia

III. THERAPEUTIC MODALITIES

A. Punch/follicular grafting and flap rotation techniques of hair transplantation to correct permanent hair loss/scarring

ACNE VENENATA (POMADE ACNE)

I. OVERVIEW

The practice of grooming the hair and scalp with oils and pomades is attributed partly to traditional and cultural beliefs for many African American individuals. Unfortunately, some of these products contribute to acneiform lesions or other sequelae.

A. Definition: follicular-based eruption of closed comedones with occasional papules and pustules
B. Etiology
  1. Prolonged application of oils or oil-based creams to the hair and scalp.
  2. Inflammation occurs around the hair follicle.
C. Pathophysiology
  1. Pomades, which are liquid or solid preparation of mineral, petrolatum, and paraffin (hydrocarbons), straighten hair by plastering it into position.
  2. The heavier solid pomades tend to occlude hair follicles.
  3. Pustules form around the hair follicles producing an inflammatory reaction called folliculitis. The condition worsens as bacterial growth in the follicle increases.

  4. Acne develops on the forehead and temples, clinically similar to acne vulgaris but more monomorphous.
D. Incidence
  1. Adults and children
  2. Infantile acne secondary to pomade application to hair and scalp

II. ASSESSMENT

A. History and physical examination
  1. Uniform open and closed comedones.
  2. Papules, pustules, and cystic nodules may be present.
  3. Hair may be oily.
  4. On examination, may detect exogenous topical material.
  5. Postinflammatory hyperpigmentation may follow acne lesions.
  6. Common sites: scalp, forehead, and temples.
B. Diagnosis
  1. Clinical examination; biopsy is not indicated.

III. THERAPEUTIC MODALITIES

A. Discontinue use of oil-based products; typically resolves within a few months
B. Antibiotics to treat infection, as needed
C. Keratolytics (benzoyl peroxide) or topical retinoids

DISORDERS UNIQUE TO AFRICAN AMERICANS

PSEUDOFOLLICULITIS BARBAE

I. OVERVIEW

Pseudofolliculitis barbae is one of the most troublesome conditions that can affect African American men. A standard treatment is to stop shaving the affected area.

A. Definition: an inflammatory disorder seen in many men of African descent who shave; also known as ingrown hairs
B. Etiology
  1. Hair follicles ingrow curved or tightly coiled.
  2. When the hairs emerge on the skin surface, they have a sharp point caused by shaving, turning the hair back into the skin.
C. Pathophysiology
  1. Tightly coiled hair.
  2. After shaving, the free end may re-enter the skin and incite an inflammatory foreign body reaction.
  3. Also, the top of the coiled penetrating shaft may be shaved off, leaving small pieces of hair in the skin.
  4. An inflammatory reaction occurs due to repeated hair penetrations and hair shaft remnants.
  5. Common sites: chin, upper anterior neck, and mandible. May also develop on legs and axilla from shaving.
D. Incidence
  1. Occurs more frequently in African American men than in White men

II. ASSESSMENT

A. History and physical examination
1. Irritated papular and pustular eruption on the neck, chin, and mandible (Figure 17-15).
2. Keloids can form.
3. Over time, postinflammatory hyperpigmentation occurs throughout the bearded area.
4. Severity: mildly bothersome to severe, scarring eruptions.
B. Diagnosis
1. Clinical examination
2. Bacterial culture yielding *Staphylococcus albus*. The disorder, however, is not primarily infectious.

III. THERAPEUTIC MODALITIES

A. Discontinue shaving the affected area.
B. If unable to stop shaving, use a new razor each time; avoid electric razors.
C. Apply warm, wet towel to beard before shaving.
D. When possible, carefully free ingrown hairs.
E. Use razor that can leave longer extension of hair.
F. Brush beard gently before shaving to dislodge hairs that are attempting to re-enter the skin.
G. May use depilatory creams.
H. Limited success with topical corticosteroids, tretinoin creams, benzoyl peroxide cream or gel, and glycolic cream.
I. Topical or systemic antibiotics can be recommended.
J. Permanent hair reduction with electrolysis or hair laser, though risk of postinflammatory pigment alteration with any treatment that uses thermal energy.

DERMATOSIS PAPULOSA NIGRA

I. OVERVIEW

Dermatosis papulosa nigra is a common, benign condition experienced by many individual with darker skin types, in particular African American adults. It is characterized by growth on the face and neck of multiple pigmented papules. Adults who experience facial lesions also exhibit lesions on the body. Prepubescent children are rarely affected.

A. Definition: stuck-on appearing papules that may be hyperpigmented or the color of the surrounding skin. Lesions are typically 1 to 5 mm in size.
B. Etiology
1. Unclear
2. Possible nevoid condition, hereditary disease, eruptive tumor, or simply a variant of seborrheic keratosis
C. Pathophysiology
1. Histologically, epidermal tumors look similar to seborrheic keratoses with underlying acanthotic epidermis.
2. The keratinocytes are basaloid.
3. Horn cysts may be present.
4. Some lesions are deeply melanin pigmented.
5. They do not spontaneously regress.
D. Incidence
1. Most unique to those of African descent; occurring in up to 35%.
2. Puberty onset.
3. Women are more often affected than men.
4. Prevalence increases with age.
5. Occurrence in other groups: Asian, Hispanic, and those with skin types IV to VI.

II. ASSESSMENT

A. History and physical examination
1. Multiple asymptomatic, brown, tan, or skin-colored papules.
2. Benign lesions can be smooth, rough, or verrucous.
3. Cosmetically unacceptable to the patient.
4. Common sites: face, scalp, neck, back, or chest.
B. Diagnosis
1. The clinical appearance of multiple lesions on the face suggests a diagnosis of dermatosis papulosa nigra. It is rarely biopsied (Figure 17-16).
2. Other tumors may be hidden among the many lesions.
3. Careful physical exam to ensure no other skin tumors go undetected.

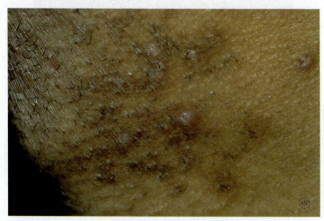

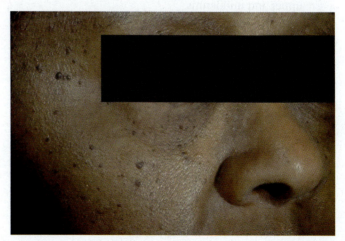

III. THERAPEUTIC MODALITIES

A. The right surgical approach is difficult to decide.
B. Low-energy electrodessication is effective; risk of hyperpigmentation/hypopigmentation.
C. Cryotherapy is not a treatment of choice because of the pigmentation alteration that may be produced.
D. Scissor excision or curettage to excise lesions; causes little bleeding and no postoperative complications.
E. Chemical peels with alpha hydroxy acids will soften and flatten these lesions and seem to prevent new lesions. Risk of pigment alteration.

MELANOCYTIC LESIONS/CONDITIONS COMMON IN THE ASIAN PATIENT

NEVUS OF OTA

I. OVERVIEW

A macular lesion on the side of the face involving the conjunctiva and lids, as well as the adjacent facial skin, sclera, ocular muscles, and periosteum

A. Definition: the nevus of Ota is a facial, dermal melanocytic lesion common in the Asian patient. Nearly all lesions appear before age 30. The incidence in Japanese patients is from 0.1% to 0.2%. Females predominate.
B. Assessment
1. History and physical examination.
   a. Unilateral blue-black or brown pigment.
   b. Usually corresponds to the forehead, temple, eyelid, nose, ear, and/or scalp.
   c. Pigmentation may also be found in the sclera and oral mucosa.
   d. Cosmetically often unacceptable to the patient.
   e. Bilateral occurrence is by age 30 if it happens.
   f. Pigmentation is not necessarily symmetrical.
C. Diagnosis
1. Histologically, melanocytes are found scattered in the upper and middermis.
2. Bilateral nevus of Ota can be confused with nevus of Ota–like macules.
   a. Pigmentation is more intense with bilateral nevus of Ota and more subtle with bilateral nevus of Ota–like macules.
   b. The patient is almost always seen in Asian or darkly pigmented women.
   c. Bilateral nevus of Ota–like macules never appear on the mucosa and are never congenital, whereas both congenital presentations and mucosal pigmentation often occur with bilateral nevus of Ota.

II. THERAPEUTIC MODALITIES

A. Camouflage is the usual approach to treatment of the condition.
B. Laser surgery has been shown to decrease appearance of the pigment of nevus of Ota.

NEVUS OF ITO

I. OVERVIEW

Nevus of Ito is similar in appearance to nevus of Ota, but the characteristic location of nevus of Ota is periocular (Figure 17-17). Nevus of Ito has the distribution of the shoulder and neck.

A. Definition: nevus of Ito is a bluish discoloration of skin, which is innervated by the posterior supraclavicular and lateral brachial cutaneous nerves. Most common in Asians, rare in light-skinned populations.
B. Assessment
1. History and physical examination
   a. Differentiation of epidermal nevus syndrome from hypomelanosis of Ito may be particularly difficult in children in whom there is wide variation in background pigmentation.
   b. The classic lesion has its onset at birth or childhood and shows increased pigmentation in the skin.
   c. Usual distribution on shoulders and neck.
   d. Cosmetically unacceptable to most patients.
   e. Pigmentation is not symmetrical.
   f. Does not regress over time.
C. Diagnosis
1. Histologically, melanocytes are found scattered in the upper and middermis.
2. Lesions typically present as blue macules/patches.

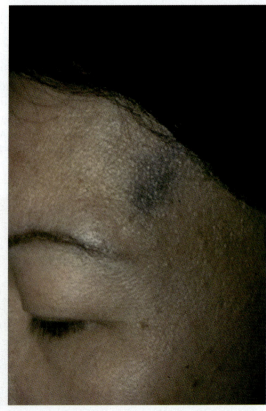

FIGURE 17-17. Nevus of Ota. (Copyright 2015 by the American Academy of Dermatology. All rights reserved.)

II. THERAPEUTIC MODALITIES

A. Camouflage is the usual approach to treatment of the condition.

CONGENITAL DERMAL MELANOCYTOSIS

I. OVERVIEW

The congenital dermal melanocytosis (slate gray nevus, Mongolian spot) presents as a blue-to-gray patch on the sacrum or buttocks of a neonate.

A. Definition: congenital dermal melanocytosis (CDM) is a poorly defined blue-to-gray area of skin discoloration present at birth, usually in the area of the buttocks and lower spine. It may also involve other areas such as the upper back, shoulders, and arms or legs; palms and soles are spared. CDMs are flat birthmarks with wavy borders and irregular shapes, common among people of Asian, East Indian, African, and Latino descent.

B. Assessment
  1. History and physical examination.
    a. The pigmented area has large concentrations of skin cells called melanocytes, with normal skin texture. They commonly appear at birth or shortly after birth and may look like bruises (Figure 17-18).
    b. CDM may cover a large area of the back.
    c. Often appear on the base of the spine, on the buttocks, and sometimes on the ankles or wrists.

C. Diagnosis
  1. Histologic examination of a CDM shows elongated, dendritic, melanin-containing cells scattered lightly throughout the dermis.
  2. The diagnosis of CDM is usually obvious, and a biopsy is not needed. The incidence varies according to the overall depth of this birthmark.
    a. African descent: 90%
    b. Asian: 80%

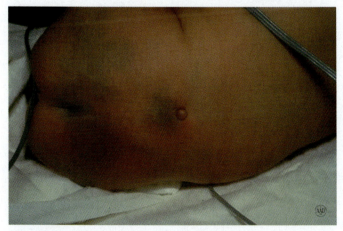

FIGURE 17-18. Congenital dermal melanocytosis. (Copyright 2015 by the American Academy of Dermatology. All rights reserved.)

    c. Latina: 65%
    d. European: 9.5%
  3. The vague resemblance to a bruise has led to concerns of child abuse.

II. THERAPEUTIC MODALITIES

A. No specific treatment is required.
B. The color reaches a peak at 1 to 2 years of age and then begins to fade.
C. The majority of lesions are absent by adolescence.
D. Occasionally, lesions persist to adulthood and are usually localized to the buttocks.

BIBLIOGRAPHY

Allemann, I. B., & Goldberg, D. J. (Eds.) (2011). *Basics in dermatological laser applications* (p. 133). Basel, Switzerland: Karger Medical and Scientific Publishers.

Ardic, F. N., Aktan, S., Kara, C. O., & Sanli, B. (1998). High frequency hearing and reflex latency in patients with pigment disorder. *American Journal of Otolaryngology, 19*(6), 365–369.

Arndt, K. A., Laboit, P. C., Robinson, J. K., & Wintroub, B. U. (1996). *Cutaneous medicine and surgery: An integrated program in dermatology.* Philadelphia, PA: W.B. Saunders Company.

Bigby, M. E., David, A. K., & Brown, A. E. (1994). *Recognition and management of skin diseases in people of color.* Boston, MA: Glaxo Wellcome, Inc.

Blattner, C., Polley, D. C., Ferritto, F., & Elston, D. M. (2013). Central centrifugal cicatricial alopecia. *Indian Dermatology Online Journal, 4*(1), 50.

Boer, J. (2006). Oral retinoids for hidradenitis suppurativa. In G. B. E. Jemec, J. Revuz, & J. J. Leyden (Eds.) *Hidradenitis suppurativa* (pp. 128–135). Berlin/Heidelberg: Springer.

Boissy, R. E., & Nordlund, J. J. (1996). Vitiligo. In K. A. Arndt, P. E. LeBoit, J. K. Robinson, & B.U. Wintroub (Eds.), *Cutaneous medicine and surgery: An integrated program in dermatology* (pp. 1210–1218). Philadelphia, PA: W.B. Saunders Company.

Bolognia, J. L., & Shapiro, P. E. (1996). Albinism and other disorders of pigmentation. In K. A. Arndt, P. E. LeBoit, J. K. Robinson, & B. U. Wintroub (Eds.), *Cutaneous medicine and surgery: An integrated program in dermatology* (pp. 1219–1232). Philadelphia, PA: W.B. Saunders Company.

Bordere, A. C., Lambert, J., & Van Geel, N. (2009). Current and emerging therapy for the management of vitiligo. *Clinical, Cosmetic and Investigational Dermatology, 2,* 15.

Chan, H. H., Alam, M., Kono, T., & Dover, J. S. (2002). Clinical application of lasers in Asians. *Dermatologic Surgery, 28*(7), 556–563.

Cichorek, M., Wachulska, M., Stasiewicz, A., & Tymińska, A. (2013). Skin melanocytes: biology and development. *Advances in Dermatology and Allergology/Postępy Dermatologii I Alergologii. 30*(1):30–41. doi:10.5114/pdia.2013.33376.

Farber, M. J., Heilman, E. R., & Friedman, R. J. (2012). Dysplastic nevi. *Dermatologic Clinics, 30*(3), 389–404.

Fitzpatrick, T. B., & Mihm, M. C. (1971). Abnormalities of the melanin pigmentary system. In T. B. Fitzpatrick, K. A. Arndt, W. H. Clark, A. Z. Eisen, E. J. Van Scott, & J. H. Vaughan (Eds.), *Dermatology in general medicine* (pp. 1591–1637). New York, NY: McGraw-Hill Book Company.

Fitzpatrick, T. B., Johnson, R. A., Polano, M. K., Suurmond, D., & Wolff, K. (1994). *Color atlas and synopsis of clinical dermatology common and serious diseases.* New York, NY: McGraw-Hill, Inc.

Goldstein, A. M., & Tucker, M. A. (2013). Dysplastic nevi and melanoma. *Cancer Epidemiology, Biomarkers and Prevention, 22*(4), 528–532.

Granter, S. R., McKee, P. H., Calonje, E., Mihm Jr, M. C., & Busam, K. (2001). Melanoma associated with blue nevus and melanoma mimicking cellular blue nevus: A clinicopathologic study of 10 cases on the spectrum of so-called 'malignant blue nevus'. *American Journal of Surgical Pathology, 25*(3), 316–323.

Grimes, P. E., & Davis, L. T. (1991). Cosmetics in blacks. *Dermatologic Clinics, 9*(1), 53–68.

Grønskov, K., Ek, J., & Brondum-Nielsen, K. (2007). Oculocutaneous albinism. *Orphanet Journal of Rare Diseases, 2*, 43.

Gul, U., Kilic, A., Tulunay, O., & Kaygusuz, G. (2007). Vitiligo associated with malignant melanoma and lupus erythematosus. *Journal of Dermatology, 34*(2),142–145.

Habif, T. P. (1990). *Clinical dermatology: A color guide to diagnosis and therapy* (2nd ed.). St. Louis, MO: The CV Mosby Company.

Habif, T. P. (2001). *Skin disease: Diagnosis and treatment.* St. Louis, MO: The CV Mosby Company.

Halder, R. M. (1991). Topical PUVA therapy for vitiligo. *Dermatology Nursing, 3*(3), 178–182.

Jefferson, J., & Rich, P. (2012). Melanonychia. *Dermatology Research and Practice, 2012*, 952186.

Johnson Jr, B. L., Moy, R. L., & White, G. M. (1998). *Ethnic skin: Medical and surgical.* St. Louis, MO: Mosby, Inc.

Kruger, C., & Schallreuter, K. U. (2012). A review of worldwide prevalence of vitiligo in children/adolescent and adults. *International Journal of Dermatology, 51*(10), 1206–1212.

Lebwohl, M. G., Heymann, W. R., Berth-Jones, J., & Coulson, I. (2013). *Treatment of skin disease: Comprehensive therapeutic strategies* (4th ed., p. 79, E-book). Netherlands: Elsevier Health Sciences.

McKee, P. H., Calonje, E., & Granter, S. R. (2005a). Cutaneous adverse reactions to drugs and effects of physical agents. In P. H. McKee, E. Calonje, & S. R. Granter (Eds.) *Pathology of the skin with clinical correlations* (3rd ed., pp. 638–642). London, UK: Elsevier.

McKee, P. H., Calonje, E., & Granter, S. R. (2005b). Disorders of pigmentation. In P. H. McKee, E. Calonje, & S. R. Granter (Eds.) *Pathology of the skin with clinical correlations* (3rd ed., pp. 993–997). London, UK: Elsevier.

Montagna, W., Prota, G., & Kenney Jr, J. A. (1993). *Black skin structure and function.* San Diego, CA: Academic Press, Inc.

Njoo, M. D., Westerhof, W., Bos, J. D., & Bossuyt, P. M. M. (1999). The development of guidelines for the treatment of vitiligo. *Archives of Dermatology, 135*(12), 1514–1521.

Onwudiwe, O., & Callender, V. D. (2014). Pomade acne. In *Acneiform eruptions in dermatology* (pp. 155–159). New York, NY: Springer.

Ortonne, J. P., Bahadoran, P., Fitzpatrick, T. B., et al. (2003). Hypomelanosis and hypermelanosis. In I. M. Freedburg, A. Z. Eisen, K. Wolff, et al. (Eds.), *Fitzpatrick's dermatology in general medicine* (6th ed., pp. 836–881). New York, NY: McGraw-Hill.

Rordam, O. M., Lenouvel, E. W., & Maalo, M. (2012). Successful treatment of extensive vitiligo with monobenzone. *Journal of Clinical and Aesthetic Dermatology, 5*(12), 36–39

Rosen, T., & Martin, S. (1981). *Atlas of black dermatology.* Boston, MA: Little, Brown and Company.

Sawada, M., Yokota, K., Matsumoto, T., Shibata, S., Yasue, S., Sakakibara, A., & Akiyama, M. (2014). Proposed classification of longitudinal melanonychia based on clinical and dermoscopic criteria. *International Journal of Dermatology, 53*(5), 581–585.

Thompson, F. V. (1993). Management of a vitiligo patient: A case study. *Dermatology Nursing, 5*(2), 139–144.

Thong, H. Y., Jee, S. H., Sun, C. C., & Boissy, R. E. (2003). The patterns of melanosome distribution in keratinocytes of human skin as one determining factor of skin colour. *British Journal of Dermatology, 149*(3), 498–505.

Torok, H. M., Jones, T., Rich, P., Smith, S., & Tschen, E. (2005). Hydroquinone 4%, tretinoin 0.05%, fluocinolone acetonide 0.01%: A safe and efficacious 12-month treatment for melasma. *Cutis, 75*(1), 57–62.

Torres, J. E., & Sanchez, J. L. (1996). Melasma and other disorders of hyperpigmentation. In K. A. Arndt, P. E. LeBoit, J. K. Robinson, & B. U. Wintroub (Eds.), *Cutaneous medicine and surgery: An integrated program in dermatology* (pp. 1233–1241). Philadelphia, PA: W.B. Saunders Company.

Tsatmali, M., Ancans, J., & Thody, A. J. (2002). Melanocyte function and its control by melanocortin peptides. *Journal of Histochemistry and Cytochemistry, 50*(2), 125–133.

Watt, A. J., Kotsis, S. V., & Chung, K. C. (2004). Risk of melanoma arising in large congenital melanocytic nevi: A systematic review. *Plastic and Reconstructive Surgery, 113*(7), 1968–1974.

STUDY QUESTIONS

1. Piebaldism is an acquired disease of hypopigmentation.
   a. True
   b. False

2. Albinism is a disorder of hypopigmentation secondary to a defect in which of the following?
   a. Melanocyte
   b. Keratinocyte
   c. Lymphocyte
   d. Melanophage

3. Which of the following statements regarding melasma is *false*?
   a. There is increased number and activity of melanocytes.
   b. Hormones may influence the condition.
   c. It is most commonly treated with narrowband UVB.
   d. Common distribution is on the face.

4. Hyperpigmentation of the skin may be caused by which of the following?
   a. Antimalarials
   b. Heavy metals
   c. Infection
   d. Topical tar-containing preparations
   e. A, B, and C
   f. A and C
   g. All of the above

5. First-line treatment for Becker nevus is surgical excision.
   a. True
   b. False

6. Nevus spilus commonly evolves into melanoma.
   a. True
   b. False

7. Congenital dermal melanocytosis occurs rarely on the buttocks of Asian newborns.
   a. True
   b. False

8. Which of the following comprise the follicular occlusion triad?
   a. Psoriasis, hidradenitis, and acne
   b. Hidradenitis suppurativa
   c. Acne conglobata
   d. Dissecting cellulitis
   e. B, C, and D

9. Dermatosis papulosa nigra is:
   a. Most unique to people of African descent
   b. A benign condition
   c. Commonly seen as numerous 1- to 5-mm papules
   d. Cosmetically unacceptable to most individuals
   e. All of the above
   f. A, B, and C

10. Keloids are common in:
    a. Dark-skinned individuals
    b. Individuals who easily sunburn
    c. Light-skinned people of Finland
    d. All of the above

11. The best treatment for pseudofolliculitis is which of the following?
    a. Discontinuing shaving the affected area
    b. Shaving against the direction of the hair growth
    c. Applying shaving cream before shaving
    d. Shaving as close as possible to the skin surface

12. Longitudinal melanonychia:
    a. Reveals melanin deposits in the nail plates
    b. Are striped in appearance in the nail plates
    c. Should include melanoma in the differential diagnosis
    d. All of the above
    e. A and C

13. Clinical features of psoriasis are the same in fair-skinned and dark-skinned individuals.
    a. True
    b. False

Answers to Study Questions: 1.b, 2.a, 3.c, 4.g, 5.b, 6.b, 7.b, 8.e, 9.e, 10.a, 11.a, 12.d, 13.b

Hypersensitivities, Drug Eruptions, Vasculitides, and Miscellaneous Inflammatory Disorders

Cathleen K. Case • *Kelli Turgeon-Daoust*

OBJECTIVES

After studying this chapter, the reader will be able to:

- List the four general types of hypersensitivity reactions.
- Differentiate between immediate- and delayed-type hypersensitivities.
- Understand diseases associated with hypersensitivity reactions.
- Define the major characteristics of small-vessel vasculitis.
- Understand management of adverse drug reactions.
- Describe the spectrum of Stevens-Johnson syndrome/toxic epidermal necrolysis (SJS/TEN) and identify major features of erythema multiforme (EM).

KEY POINTS

- The immune system is designed to protect the host but may fail.
- Assessment and history-taking skills are of paramount importance in the evaluation of a suspected hypersensitivity reaction.
- Avoidance of allergens and irritants, when possible, is the best treatment of urticaria and other hypersensitivity reactions.
- Differential diagnosis of many cutaneous eruptions includes drug reactions.
- Urticarial lesions that last longer than 24 hours or present with purpura should be biopsied to rule out urticarial vasculitis.
- Episode of urticaria lasting more than 6 weeks is considered chronic urticaria. First-line therapy for urticaria is nonsedating H1 antagonist antihistamines.
- Erythema multiforme is a self-limited but potentially recurrent disease, commonly associated with herpes simplex virus infection.
- Erythema nodosum is the most common type of panniculitis and may occur in association with systemic disease such as sarcoidosis or inflammatory bowel disease, drug therapy such as oral contraceptive pill, or other infection; half of cases are idiopathic.
- Cutaneous small-vessel vasculitis, also called leukocytoclastic vasculitis and hypersensitivity vasculitis, is the most common form of small-vessel necrotizing vasculitis. Palpable purpura is characteristic for this disorder.
- The characteristic lesion of pyoderma gangrenosum is a painful ulcer with a rolled or undermined border frequently on the legs; it is neither infectious nor gangrenous.
- Toxic epidermal necrosis is a medical emergency with a high mortality rate.

I. OVERVIEW

There are two opposite sides to immunity: host protection and injury. **The immune response to an antigen is designed to protect the host.** Disorders of the immune system include hypersensitivity, autoimmunity, and immunodeficiency. These response mechanisms produce a wide range of clinical conditions from local reactions to life-threatening diseases. The primary biological effects of the immune response are the humoral (antibody) and cellular recognition and elimination of infectious agents and other foreign antigens. If there is re-exposure to the same antigen in a previously sensitized individual, there may be an exaggerated or "hypersensitivity" reaction. This is a misdirected immune response that results in local tissue injury or systemic manifestations, which may include shock and death. Immune responses that result in tissue injury or other pathophysiologic changes are called allergic/immunopathologic (hypersensitivity) reactions. There are four types of hypersensitivity reactions.

A. Causes of tissue injury

1. Release of vasoactive substances; primary and secondary mediators
2. Phagocytosis or lysis of cells
3. Activation of components of the complement system
4. Release of proteolytic enzymes, cytokines, and other mediators of tissue injury and inflammation from recruited inflammatory cells

TABLE 18-1 Four Types of Hypersensitivity Reaction

Type	Mediators	Mechanism	Response Time	Appearance	Associated Conditions
Type I (immediate, anaphylactic)	IgE, histamine, tryptase, and leukotrienes	IgE, produced in excessive amounts, interacts with mast cells to cause release of histamine and other vasoactive mediators of hypersensitivity	Usually 15–30 min; may have delayed onset of 10–12 h	Wheal and flare	Anaphylaxis, asthma, urticaria, and angioedema
Type II (cytotoxic)	IgM or IgG, complement	Antibody is bound to antigen on cell surface, triggering complement activation, cell lysis, and cytotoxicity	Minutes to hours	Lysis and necrosis	Transfusion reaction, some drug reactions, and drug-induced pemphigus
Type III (immune complex)	Immune complex IgG or IgM	Antigen–antibody immune complexes are deposited in tissue, activating mast cells, neutrophils, and phagocytes and triggering complement cascade	3–10 h	Erythema and edema, and necrosis	Serum sickness, Arthus reaction, vasculitis, and systemic lupus erythematosus
Type IV (delayed/cell mediated)	Antigen-specific T cells, monocyte chemotactic factor, interleukin-2, interferon-gamma, TNF-alpha, and TNF-beta	Activated antigen-specific helper T cells stimulate release of cytokines and chemokines, which attract and activate macrophages, eosinophils, and neutrophils; cytotoxic T cells cause damage directly	1–3 d; up to 4 wk for some reactions	Erythema and induration	Allergic contact dermatitis, tuberculin reaction, granuloma formation secondary to infection and foreign antigens (tuberculosis, leprosy), and fixed drug eruption

B. Hypersensitivity reactions, their mediators, and associated conditions (Table 18-1)

This chapter focuses on urticaria, angioedema, and anaphylaxis, certain drug reactions, cutaneous small-vessel vasculitis (CSVV), and other hypersensitivity syndromes, including:

1. Erythema multiforme (EM)
2. Stevens-Johnson syndrome (SJS)
3. Toxic epidermal necrolysis (TEN)
4. Erythema nodosum (EN)
5. Pyoderma gangrenosum (PG)

URTICARIA, ANGIOEDEMA, AND ANAPHYLAXIS

I. OVERVIEW

Approximately 1 in 5 people will experience urticaria. Urticaria may be more common in atopic individuals and is usually classified as acute or chronic; however, the majority of cases are acute lasting from hours to a few weeks. Chronic urticaria is defined as episodes of urticaria lasting for more than 6 weeks; however, all urticaria begins in an acute phase. Occasionally, acute urticaria is associated with deeper less well-demarcated edema referred to as angioedema.

Allergic angioedema can be associated with anaphylaxis including life-threatening bronchoconstriction and hypotension. The eyelids and lips are most typically affected by angioedema. The cause of acute urticaria may be identified and generally self-limiting; the cause of chronic urticaria may be determined in only 5% to 20% of cases.

A. Definition

1. Urticaria, also called hives or wheals, is a common and distinctive cutaneous reaction pattern involving the superficial dermis. It is usually transient, demonstrating localized edema caused by dilatation and increased permeability of the capillaries and marked by the development of wheals. A wheal or hive is a well-demarcated, erythematous or white, nonpitting, edematous papule or plaque that is usually pruritic. The lesions are polymorphous and often form annular, arciform, or polycyclic plaques (Figures 18-1 and 18-2). The lesions change shape and size during the few hours or days they are present. Urticaria can be acute or chronic, and the physical urticarias depend on an external or exogenous factor. Chronic urticaria is defined as episodes of urticaria lasting for more than 6 weeks; however, all urticaria begins in an acute phase.

2. Angioedema (angioneurotic edema) is a hive-like swelling caused by increased vascular permeability in the subcutaneous tissue of the skin and mucosa and submucosal layers of the respiratory and gastrointestinal (GI) tracts. Hives and angioedema can occur simultaneously and may have the same etiology. Angioedema is usually located on the eyes, as seen in Figure 18-3, and mouth (Figure 18-4) but may also occur on the hands and feet or in the throat. Laryngeal edema does not usually occur with urticaria or simple angioedema. There are multiple syndromes of angioedema including idiopathic, allergic, and medication-induced angioedema; hereditary angioedema (HAE); and acquired angioedema (AAE). The presence or absence of hives is used to characterize the different syndromes of angioedema.

3. Anaphylaxis is a severe, potentially fatal, systemic allergic reaction that occurs suddenly after contact with an allergy-causing substance.

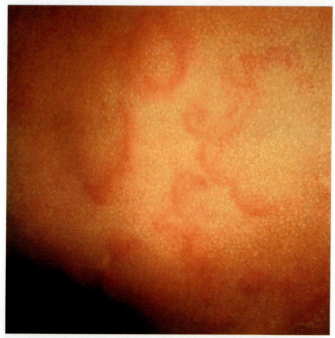

FIGURE 18-1. Large edematous plaques of urticaria. (From Elder, D. E. (2012). *Atlas and synopsis of Lever's histopathology of the skin*. Philadelphia, PA: Wolters Kluwer.)

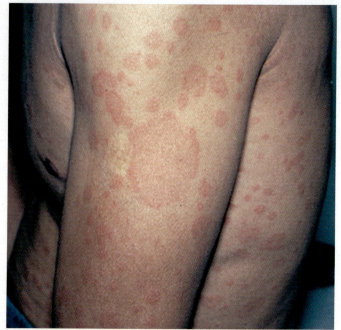

FIGURE 18-2. Typical hives of different sizes. (From Anderson, M. K. (2012). *Foundations of athletic training*. Philadelphia, PA: Wolters Kluwer.)

B. Etiology
  1. Urticaria
     a. Most cases of acute urticaria are IgE-mediated type I hypersensitivity reactions. Circulating antigens such as foods, drugs, or inhalants react with cell membrane–bound IgE to release histamine. IgE antigen on the mast cell surface unites with the antigen of food, drug, stinging insect venom, or pollen and causes an immediate and large release of histamine and other vasoactive mediators from mast cells.
     b. Complement-mediated acute urticaria may be caused by administration of whole blood, plasma, immu-

noglobulins, and drugs or by insect stings. Type III hypersensitivity reactions occur with deposition of insoluble immune complexes in vessel walls (Arthus reactions). The complexes are composed of IgG or IgM, the trapped complexes activate complement, and the process releases histamine from mast cells. A frequent reason for acute urticaria is viral infections of the upper respiratory tract, which increases mast cell reactivity.
     c. Nonimmunologic release of histamine occurs when pharmacologic mediators, such as acetylcholine, opiates, polymyxin B, or strawberries, react directly with

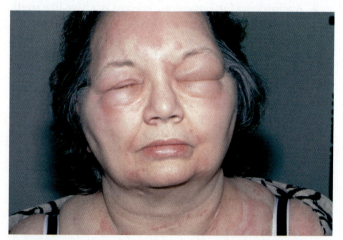

FIGURE 18-3. Urticaria with angioedema around the eyes. (From Goodheart, H. P. (2003). *Goodheart's photoguide of common skin disorders* (2nd ed.). Philadelphia, PA: Lippincott Williams & Wilkins.)

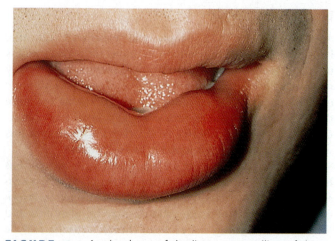

FIGURE 18-4. Angioedema of the lip, tense swelling of the dermis and subcutaneous tissue. (Neville, B., Damm, D., White, D., & Waldron, W. (1991). *Color atlas of clinical oral pathology*. Philadelphia, PA: Lea & Febiger. Used with permission.)

cell membrane–bound mediators to release histamine. Aspirin and other nonsteroidal anti-inflammatory drugs (NSAIDs) can cause nonimmunologic release of histamine; these patients may have a history of allergic rhinitis or asthma. The physical urticarias may be induced by both direct stimulation of cell membrane receptors and immunologic mechanisms.

d. Patients with history of hives lasting more than 6 weeks may be classified as having chronic urticaria. The lesional morphology is similar to acute hives, any skin surface can be affected, and the lesions last less than 24 hours. Angioedema occurs in 50% of cases of chronic urticaria. Chronic urticaria patients are likely to exhibit physical urticaria, is usually nonallergic, and is usually idiopathic. Angioedema associated with chronic urticaria is different from HAE in that it rarely affects the larynx. Table 18-2 displays the clinical classification of urticaria/angioedema.

e. A partial list of the etiologic classification of urticaria is found in Table 18-3.

2. Angioedema

a. Most cases of angioedema are idiopathic. Angioedema will often occur with hives, and angioedema without wheals is seen with drug reactions and C1 inhibitor deficiency.

b. Severe allergic type I immediate hypersensitivity IgE-mediated reactions can cause acute angioedema. Angioedema can occur with other symptoms of anaphylaxis including hypotension and respiratory distress.

c. Drugs such as contrast dyes, NSAIDs, aspirin, indomethacin, and ACE inhibitors can cause angioedema with nonimmunologic mechanism.

d. AAE results from an acquired C1 inhibitor deficiency considered to be an autoimmune disease. HAE is an inherited C1 inhibitor deficiency and results from lack of the functional C1 esterase inhibitor.

3. Anaphylaxis

a. Immediate-type hypersensitivity reactions may occur locally or systemically causing mild symptoms or sudden death from anaphylactic shock. Food allergies, including allergy to tree nuts and peanuts,

TABLE 18-3 Etiologic Classification of Urticaria

Etiology	Examples
Food	Fish, shellfish, nuts, eggs, strawberries, cow's milk, wheat, and yeast
Food additives	Salicylates, benzoates, penicillin, and sulfites
Drugs	Penicillin, aspirin, sulfonamides, and drugs that cause a nonimmunologic release of histamine (morphine, codeine, dextran, polymyxin, curare, quinine)
Infections	Chronic bacterial infections (sinus, dental, urinary tract), fungal infections, viral infections (hepatitis B prodrome, infectious mononucleosis, coxsackie), intestinal worms, and malaria
Inhalants	Pollens, mold spores, animal dander, house dust, and aerosols
Internal disease	Systemic lupus erythematosus, hyperthyroidism, autoimmune thyroid disease, carcinomas, lymphomas, leukocytoclastic vasculitis, polycythemia vera, rheumatic fever, and transfusion reaction
Physical stimuli (physical urticarias)	Listed in Table 18-4
Nonimmunologic contact urticaria	Plants (nettles), animals (caterpillars, jellyfish), and medications (cinnamic aldehyde, dimethyl sulfoxide)
Uncertain mechanism	Ammonium persulfate used in hair bleach, chemicals, foods, textiles, wood, saliva, cosmetics, perfumes, and bacitracin
Skin diseases	Mastocytosis, dermatitis herpetiformis, pemphigoid, and amyloidosis
Hormones	Pregnancy and premenstrual flare (progesterone)
Genetic	Hereditary angioedema, familial cold urticaria, and vibratory urticaria

and crustaceans are common causes of serious anaphylactic reactions. Other common causes include antibiotics, especially penicillins; other drugs and chemicals, including radiographic contrast agents; and hymenoptera stings.

C. Incidence

1. Estimates of the lifetime occurrence of urticaria range from less than 1% to as high as 30% of the population. Hives can occur at any age, is a worldwide disease, and may be more common in atopic patients.

2. Angioedema frequently occurs with acute urticaria, which is more common in children and young adults. Chronic urticaria is more common in women in the third to fifth decades of life; there is no consensus on the prevalence of chronic urticaria.

3. Most cases of angioedema are idiopathic. It can occur at any age but is most common in the 40- to 50-year-old age group, women being more affected than men. Angiotensin-converting enzyme inhibitors (ACEIs) are the number one drug cause of acute angioedema; the incidence may be higher in Black Americans. HAE affects between 1 in 10,000 and 1 in 50,000 persons and begins in late childhood or early adolescence.

4. True incidence of anaphylaxis is unknown; lifetime prevalence is 1% to 2% for the population as a whole.

TABLE 18-2 Clinical Classification of Urticaria

Clinical Class	Duration
Ordinary urticaria (acute and chronic)	3–36 h
Physical urticaria Adrenergic (stress) Aquagenic Cholinergic Cold Delayed pressure Dermatographism Exercise-induced urticaria (anaphylaxis) Solar Vibratory angioedema	30 min to 2 h except delayed pressure urticaria that may last longer than 2 h
Contact urticaria	1–2 h

D. Pathologic processes
1. There are several types of stimuli that cause urticaria, which include immunologic, nonimmunologic, physical, and chemical. Several are listed in Table 18-3.
2. The mast cell is the primary effector cell in urticaria. Release of mast cell mediators causes inflammation and mast cell degranulation that results in the release of histamine and inflammatory mediators, as well as an accumulation and activation of other cells including eosinophils, neutrophils, and, possibly, basophils. Histamine causes endothelial cell contraction that allows vascular fluid to leak between the cells through vessel walls, causing tissue edema and wheal formation.
3. When histamine is injected into the skin, there is vasodilation causing *local erythema*, a *peripheral flare* characterized by erythema beyond the border of local erythema (axon reflex), and a *wheal* produced by leakage of fluid from the postcapillary venules.
4. Angioedema is a hive-like swelling in the subcutaneous tissue of skin, mucosa, and submucosal layers of the respiratory and GI tracts. The reaction is similar to that of urticaria in the upper dermis. Hives and urticaria may have the same etiology and often occur simultaneously.
5. Anaphylaxis can be mediated by *immunologic* (IgE-mediated and non–IgE-mediated [e.g., IgG and immune complex complement–mediated]) and *nonimmunologic* factors, which include events resulting in sudden mast cell and basophil degranulation in the absence of immunoglobulins.
E. Considerations across the life span
1. Urticaria, angioedema, and anaphylaxis can occur at any age.

II. ASSESSMENT

The diagnosis of urticaria is often one of exclusion. It is essential to rule out the presence of serious illnesses of which recurring hives and/or edema can be a symptom. Examples of such illnesses may include hepatitis, hyperthyroidism, lymphomas, lupus, and cancers of the rectum, kidneys, and GI tract.
A. History and physical examination
1. History and physical exams are the most important parts of the initial evaluation and should include an evaluation of the following factors.
   a. Association with any specific substance or activity: drug ingestion or exposure; respiratory infection; food and drink; exposure to pollens and chemicals; physical location of work, travel, hobby, or home; and medications, supplements, or homeopathic compounds.
   b. Appropriate description of the character of the primary lesion in urticaria is important, usually an edematous and erythematous papule or plaque.
   c. Location of the lesions—itchy lesions that come and go, located anywhere on the skin.
   d. Length of response—individual hives do not usually last for more than 24 hours. Note time of onset, appearance, day, year, and season. Duration of

individual lesions: less than 1 hour, physical urticaria and typical hives; less than 24 hours, typical hives; longer than 25 hours, and that burn or resolve with purpura require a biopsy to exclude urticarial vasculitis.
   e. Assessment of previous incidence of symptoms related to common causes of urticaria. Table 18-3 lists possible causes. Drugs are common causes in adults, and viral respiratory or streptococcal infections are common causes in children.
   f. Evaluation of recent exposure to possible allergens.
   g. Assessment of common subtypes of urticaria (Table 18-2).
   h. Evaluate the role that occupation can play in establishing the diagnosis of urticaria.
   i. Differentiation of angioedema from urticaria is of utmost importance related to the life-threatening possibilities associated with angioedema. Urticarial lesions are superficial and widespread, while lesions associated with angioedema are deep, and the eyelids and lips are the areas most typically affected. Urticaria and angioedema frequently occur at the same time. Any patient with recurrent angioedema or abdominal pain without wheals should be evaluated for HAE.
   j. Evaluate for physical urticaria by stroking the arm with a tongue blade to test for dermatographism. This may indicate one of the physical urticarias.
   k. Anaphylaxis almost always involves the skin and/ or mucous membranes with a combination of erythema, urticaria, angioedema, or pruritus. Adults will present with cutaneous and respiratory symptoms and children may show more respiratory symptoms.
B. Skin findings
1. A wheal or hive is a well-demarcated, erythematous or white, nonpitting, edematous papule or plaque that is usually pruritic. The lesions of urticaria change shape and size during the few hours or days they are present. The central area (wheal) can be pale compared to the surrounding erythematous area (flare). Wheals are sharply marginated and predominantly flat topped. Their color varies from light pink to dark red depending on the amount of fluid present between the skin surface and the underlying dilated vascular bed. Wheals frequently have a dimpled surface because of the anchoring effect of hair follicles as fluid fills the papillary dermis surrounding them. The physical urticarias have unique characteristics and are outlined in Table 18-4.
   a. The evolution of urticaria is dynamic and lesions are transient.
   b. Hives result from local capillary vasodilation and dermal edema; the edema is in the superficial dermis.
   c. Lesions vary in size from 2 to 4 mm seen in cholinergic urticaria up to a giant hive that may cover an entire extremity.
   d. Lesions will be round, oval, polycyclic, or incomplete rings. Color may be solid red or white, or white in center with red border. Purpura within individual lesions may indicate urticarial vasculitis.

TABLE 18-4 The Physical Urticarias

Urticaria	Relative Frequency	Precipitant	Local Symptoms	Systemic Symptoms
Symptomatic dermatographism	Most frequent	Stroking skin	Irregular, pruritic wheals	None
Delayed dermatographism	Rare	Stroking skin	Burning, deep swelling	None
Pressure urticaria	Frequent	Pressure	Diffuse, tender swelling	Flulike symptoms
Solar urticaria	Frequent	Various light wavelengths	Pruritic wheals	Wheezing, dizziness, and syncope
Familial cold urticaria	Rare	Change in skin temperature from cold air	Burning wheals	Tremor, headache, arthralgia, and fever
Essential cold urticaria	Frequent	Cold contact	Pruritic wheals	Wheezing and syncope
Heat urticaria	Rare	Heat contact	Pruritic wheals	None
Cholinergic urticaria	Very frequent	General overheating of the body	Papular, pruritic wheals	Syncope, diarrhea, vomiting, salivation, and headaches
Aquagenic urticaria	Rare	Water contact	Papular, pruritic wheals	None reported
Vibratory angioedema	Very rare	Vibrating against skin	Angioedema	None reported
Exercise-induced anaphylaxis	Rare	Exercise; in some cases, ingestion of certain foods	Pruritic wheals	Respiratory distress and hypotension

e. Thicker plaques with fluid in dermis and subcutaneous tissue are considered angioedema.

f. Hives are generally ITCHY; however, intensity may vary.

g. Purpura within a wheal may indicate urticarial vasculitis and will need biopsy.

2. The reaction of angioedema is deeper than wheals and produces more diffuse swelling. The swelling is painful and burning but not pruritic.

   a. Lips, palms, soles, trunk, limbs, and genitalia are commonly affected.

   b. There may be involvement of respiratory or GI tracts producing dyspnea, dysphagia, abdominal pain, and diarrhea.

   c. Angioedema may develop as a result of trauma.

3. The physiologic responses to the release of anaphylaxis mediators include smooth muscle spasm in the respiratory and GI tracts, vasodilation, increased vascular permeability, and stimulation of sensory nerve endings.

   a. These physiologic events lead to some or all of the classic symptoms of anaphylaxis: flushing; urticaria/angioedema; pruritus; bronchospasm; laryngeal edema; abdominal cramping with nausea, vomiting, and diarrhea; and feeling of impending doom.

C. Differential diagnosis

1. Urticarial stage of bullous pemphigoid

2. Dermatitis herpetiformis

3. Drug eruptions

4. Erythema multiforme

5. Papular urticaria

6. Polymorphic eruption of pregnancy

7. Urticaria pigmentosa

8. Urticarial vasculitis

D. Diagnostic tests

1. Complete blood count (CBC) with differential.

2. Liver and thyroid function tests.

3. Urine analysis.

4. Erythrocyte sedimentation rate (ESR).

5. If the history provides evidence that warrants additional tests, consider test for hepatitis A, B, and C; infectious mononucleosis; thyroid antibodies; and antinuclear antibody (ANA).

6. Biopsy for urticarial lesions with purpuric center or for lesions that last for more than 36 hours to evaluate for urticarial vasculitis. Also, biopsy if there is fever, arthralgia, elevated ESR, or petechiae.

7. Sinus x-rays may be considered for evaluation of chronic urticaria if there is a corresponding history.

8. If HAE is suspected, C4 level can be a screening test.

III. COMMON THERAPEUTIC MODALITIES

A. Systemic therapy for urticaria and associated angioedema

1. First-line therapy is (nonsedating) second-generation H1 antagonists to inhibit mast cell mediators.

   a. Cetirizine 10 mg nightly or twice daily

   b. Loratadine 10 mg daily or twice daily

   c. Fexofenadine 120 to 180 mg daily

2. First-line therapy may include first-generation H1 (sedating) antihistamines and/or H2 receptor antagonists if symptoms are not controlled after a week or two of treatment.

   a. Diphenhydramine 10 to 25 mg four times daily.

   b. Hydroxyzine HCl 10 to 25 mg four times daily.

   c. Doxepin 10 to 25 mg nightly.

   d. H2 receptor antagonists include cimetidine 400 mg twice daily, ranitidine 150 mg twice daily, or famotidine 20 mg twice daily.

3. Second-line therapy may include systemic corticosteroid.

   a. Prednisone 0.5 to 1 mg/kg daily for short course may provide relief for severe cases.

4. Third-line therapy may include leukotriene receptor agonists and can be combined with antihistamines.

   a. Montelukast 10 mg daily

   b. Zafirlukast 20 mg twice daily

   c. Zileuton 600 mg four times a day

5. Treatment of choice for angioedema associated with anaphylaxis is epinephrine given intramuscularly (IM) (1:1,000 solution) when intravenous is not available. Diphenhydramine 50 mg can also be given IM. The IM route is better and more quickly absorbed than subcutaneous.

B. Nonpharmacologic interventions
1. Identify and eliminate underlying cause.
   a. Avoid common triggers such as aspirin, NSAIDs, food additives, heat, and alcohol.
   b. Whether urticaria is acute or chronic, consider stopping vitamins, laxatives, antacids, toothpaste, cigarettes, cosmetics and all toiletries, chewing gum, household cleaning solutions, and aerosols.
   c. Chronic hives are not caused by food allergies; however, some individuals find that hives are worsened after eating certain foods. Consider stopping fruits, tomatoes, nuts, eggs, shellfish, chocolate, milk, cheese, bread, diet drinks, and junk food.
2. Avoid eliciting stimuli.
   a. Take cool showers or baths, apply cool compresses (except with cold urticaria), wear loose fitting clothes, and avoid strenuous activity.
   b. Swimming in cold water is the most common cause of severe cold urticaria reaction. Patients should be advised never to jump into a cold body of water, and water activities should be done under supervision.
   c. Strategies to reduce stress can be helpful.

C. Medication therapy monitoring
1. The role of pharmacotherapy is symptom management, and control of pruritus is critical in helping patients find relief.
2. Antihistamine therapy usually starts with nonsedating antihistamines; however, if symptoms are not managed well, sedating antihistamines will be needed.
3. All patients, especially the elderly, should be educated on possible side effects including sedation, dry mouth, urine retention, and dizziness.
4. Start with low dose to monitor tolerance.

D. Other nursing interventions
1. Discuss skin care with patients recommending emollients and bathing not too hot or cold.
2. Emollients with anti-itch properties such as menthol, phenol, and pramoxine can be helpful especially for spot treatment and comfort.
3. Quality-of-life issues for patients with chronic urticaria should be acknowledged and addressed especially around relief of pruritus. Disease management needs to be prompt, and an individual approach is necessary due to the complex nature of urticaria. In addition, the management must be a close working cooperation with the patient.
4. When the cause of acute urticaria is promptly avoided, symptoms resolve rapidly. Reassure patients with acute urticaria that most cases resolve within 6 weeks; patients are often frustrated and fearful especially with chronic urticaria. The evolution from acute to chronic urticaria

is not well understood, and the prognosis for resolution after 6 months is unclear.

E. Complementary alternative medicine
1. Certain foods can act as natural antihistamine:
   a. Foods high in vitamin C such as carrots, mangoes, spinach, and tomatoes.
   b. Foods high in vitamin A such as oranges, lemons, tangerines, limes, and grapefruit.
   c. Pineapples can also be considered as an alternative and natural antihistamine. Bromelain is an enzyme found in high concentration in pineapple. Adding pineapples to daily diet can act as an alternative way to prevent and treat hive outbreaks.

PATIENT EDUCATION
Urticaria, Angioedema, and Anaphylaxis

- Evaluate extensive review of medications, environment exposures, supplements, diet preferences, and medical history. The patient should be an active participant in the search for inducing agents.
- Discuss that physical urticarias are more common than expected and may require provocative tests; delayed urticaria from pressure may occur several hours after the stimulus.
- Instruct patients and family to understand diagnosis.
- Provide handouts and any other literature pertaining to diagnosis to have patient bring home. These are for future reference and to encourage patient to discuss with family for support.
- Educate to prevent future flare-ups and promote treatment compliance. Treatment plan includes avoidance of contributing factors that can aggravate condition.
- Reinforce that antihistamines or other medications may need to be taken for an extended time to prevent further hives or swelling. It is important to not abruptly stop treatment without provider advice.
- Select patients who will need special education on use of EpiPen as prescribed for emergency situations if swelling of the lips, tongue, and face develops.
- Reduce emotional and physical stress as may be helpful to minimize urticarial flares.

IV. HOME CARE AND FOLLOW-UP

Patients with chronic urticaria may need referral to allergist, immunologist, or urticaria specialist if the cause cannot be found and the urticaria is interfering with quality of life. Allergy testing may be helpful for urticaria evaluation, but it is imperative for individuals who have had an anaphylactic episode. In general, patients with urticaria can be cared for on an outpatient basis unless their urticaria is severe and does not respond to antihistamine therapy or if they progress to laryngeal angioedema and/or anaphylactic shock or have comorbidities that require inpatient therapy.

VASCULITIS

I. OVERVIEW

Vasculitis is a nonspecific term that encompasses and a large and heterogeneous group of disorders characterized by inflammation of blood vessels. The process can involve the walls of any size or type of vessel causing damage that results in tissue necrosis. Cutaneous vasculitis may be limited to the skin, there may be secondary systemic involvement, or it may be a cutaneous manifestation of a systemic disease. There is no uniform classification system for vasculitis, although some classify according to the type of cell within the vessel walls (neutrophil, lymphocyte, or histiocyte), the type of circulating immune complexes, and the size and type of primary vessel involved (venule, arteriole, artery, or vein). The International Chapel Hill Consensus Conference of the Nomenclature of Systemic Vasculitides (CHCC2012) recently updated their system that specifies the name that should be used for a specifically defined disease process, used when a patient fulfills a definition. The spectrum of this group of diseases is too large for the context of this text, and therefore, the focus will be on some of the more common vasculitides affecting small vessels. This will include CSVV/leukocytoclastic vasculitis (LCV) and Henoch-Schönlein purpura (HSP).

A. Definition

1. All vessel sizes of venous and arterial systems can be involved. Small vessels include arterioles, capillaries, and postcapillary venules that are found in the superficial and middermis of the skin. Medium-sized vessels include the main visceral arteries and veins, and small arteries and veins within the deep dermis and subcutaneous tissue. Large vessels include the aorta, major branches and corresponding veins, and other named arteries such as the temporal artery.
2. Table 18-5 lists the main vasculitides classified by vessel size.
3. CSVV has in the past been referred to as LCV and hypersensitivity vasculitis and is the most commonly seen form of small-vessel necrotizing vasculitis. The condition may be limited to the skin or may involve different organs.
4. HSP is acute LCV that occurs mainly in children between ages 2 and 10; however, adult cases are reported. HSP is characterized by deposits of IgA immune complexes in venules, capillaries, and arterioles. HSP is the most common systemic vasculitis in children.

B. Etiology

1. Generally, there is hypersensitivity to various antigens including drugs, chemicals, microorganisms, and endogenous antigens. This results in the formation of immune complexes that are deposited in the vessel walls. There are many diseases that may be associated with hypersensitivity vasculitis; however, in many cases, the cause is not determined. These include the following:
   a. Hepatitis B and C virus
   b. Other infections
   c. Drugs
   d. Malignant neoplasm
   e. Connective tissue disease
   f. Rheumatologic disease
   g. Inflammatory bowel disease
2. HSP may be preceded by a streptococcal or viral upper respiratory infection 1 to 3 weeks before the vasculitis presents and tends to occur in the spring. Other infectious agents and drugs have been implicated, but general etiology is unknown.

C. Pathologic process

1. The term LCV describes the histologic picture that is produced when leukocytes fragment during the inflammatory process, leaving nuclear debris or "dust." This is called leukocytoclasis. CSVV, also referred to as hypersensitivity vasculitis and LCV, is the most commonly seen form of small-vessel vasculitis. On histology, there is fibrinoid necrosis of small dermal blood vessels, leukocytoclasis, endothelial swelling, and extravasation of red blood cells.
2. IgA plays a major role in the pathogenesis of HSP. There are increased concentrations of serum IgA, IgA deposits in vessel walls, and renal mesangium. There can be widespread circulating IgA-containing immune complexes in vessel walls of the skin, kidneys, and GI tract, which will lead to systemic symptoms.

D. Incidence

1. CSVV is usually seen over age 16 and HSP usually under the age of 16 but is also reported in adults.
2. If a drug or viral illness has caused the CSVV, patients may only experience one episode. Multiple episodes may occur if associated with a systemic disease such as rheumatoid arthritis or systemic lupus erythematosus.

TABLE 18-5 Classification of Vasculitides Based on Vessel Size

Predominant Caliber of Affected Vessel	Classification	Subclassification
Small	Cutaneous small-vessel vasculitis	Idiopathic Henoch-Schönlein purpura Acute hemorrhagic edema of infancy Erythema elevatum diutinum
Small and medium sized	Secondary	Infections and septic vasculitis Inflammatory disorders (SLE, rheumatoid arthritis, Sjogren syndrome) Drug exposure Neoplasms
	Cryoglobulinemic ANCA associated	Microscopic polyangiitis Wegener granulomatosis Churg-Strauss syndrome
Medium sized	PAN	Systemic form Benign cutaneous form
Large	Temporal arteritis Takayasu arteritis	

ANCA, antinuclear cytoplasmic antibodies; PAN, polyarteritis nodosa; SLE, systemic lupus erythematosus.

3. Adults with HSP usually have no precipitating event, lower frequency of abdominal pain and fever, higher frequency of joint symptoms, and more frequent and severe renal involvement.

E. Considerations across the life span
   1. CSVV is generally seen in adults, and HSP is generally seen in children.

II. ASSESSMENT

A. History and physical examination
   1. Complete review of systems to assess prodromal symptoms of fever, malaise, myalgia, skin pain or pruritus, and abdominal symptoms. Joint symptoms, kidney issues such as frank hematuria, and scrotal swelling in boys with HSP.

B. Skin findings and systemic involvement
   1. Characteristic lesions of cutaneous small-vessel vasculitis are palpable purpura (Figure 18-5). May start asymptomatic and look like cutaneous hemorrhages that become palpable as blood leaks out of damaged vessels, and palpable purpura of vasculitis may be unifocal or bilateral. Ulceration, nodules, urticaria, and livedo reticularis may also be present.
   2. Lesions coalesce and produce large areas of purpura. Hemorrhagic blisters and ulcers indicate more severe vessel inflammation and necrosis. Older lesions may have brownish red color.

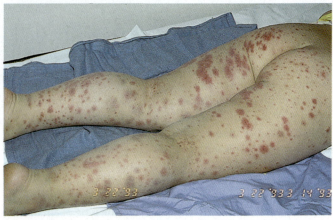

FIGURE 18-6. Palpable purpura in a patient with HSP. Note the dark, necrotizing center of the lesions. (From Fleisher, G. R., Ludwig, S., & Baskin, M. N. (2004). *Atlas of pediatric emergency medicine*. Philadelphia, PA: Lippincott Williams & Wilkins.)

3. Diascopy can be used to evaluate blanchable versus nonblanchable lesions. Press a glass slide over a purpuric papule, the red blood cells in the skin will blanch when not vasculitic. Vasculitic papules with fibrosis, necrosis, and thrombosis will not blanch.
4. There may be a few or numerous purpuric lesions, most commonly located on lower extremities but can be seen in any dependent area. Figure 18-6 shows a patient with HSP on the legs and buttocks.
5. Small lesions itch and are painful; nodules, ulcers, and bullae will be more painful.
6. CSVV systemic manifestations may include the following:
   a. Vasculitis of the kidneys causing microscopic hematuria and proteinuria; necrotizing glomerulonephritis may lead to chronic renal insufficiency.
   b. Peripheral neuropathy with paresthesia or hypoesthesia.
   c. Vasculitis of bowel will cause abdominal pain, nausea, vomiting, diarrhea, and melena.
   d. Pulmonary vasculitis may be seen as nodule or infiltrate on chest film or with cough, shortness of breath, and hemoptysis.
   e. Joint swelling, erythema, and pain.
   f. Arrhythmias and congestive heart failure can be seen with myocardial angiitis.
7. Systemic manifestations of HSP include the following:
   a. GI symptoms of colicky abdominal pain, nausea, vomiting, GI bleeding, diarrhea, and blood in stool. GI symptoms may precede skin disease.
   b. Arthralgia from periarticular edema involves the ankles, knees, and dorsum of hands and feet.
   c. Nephritis occurs in 20% to 50% of children, and onset may be acute or delayed for weeks or months. Microscopic hematuria is a frequent feature, and gross hematuria occurs less frequently. Heavy proteinuria at onset of disease requires close and long-term follow-up; renal disease can reappear after recovery.
   d. Acute scrotal swelling may be the only presenting feature of HSP vasculitis in a young boy and may mimic testicular torsion or incarcerated hernia.

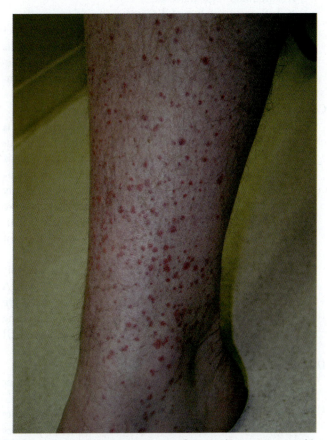

FIGURE 18-5. Palpable purpura of CSVV. (From Dr. Barankin Dermatology Collection.)

C. Differential diagnosis
1. Arthropod bites
2. Erythema multiforme
3. Morbilliform drug eruption with hemorrhage
4. Cellulitis
5. Thrombosis from hypercoagulable state
6. Over anticoagulation with warfarin or heparin
7. Livedoid vasculopathy
8. Urticaria
9. Pigmented purpura
10. Pyogenic granuloma
11. Panniculitis
12. Infection (Rocky Mountain spotted fever, subacute bacterial endocarditis, viral infections)
13. Sepsis
14. Cholesterol emboli

D. Diagnostic tests
1. Initial diagnostic test should be punch or excisional skin biopsy of new lesion preferable 24 to 48 hours old being sure to collect subcutaneous tissue to evaluate for larger involved vessels. Additional biopsy for direct immunofluorescence is needed to identify immunoglobulins and complement in the blood vessels; IgA may be found in HSP.
2. Workup will be determined by positive findings on review of systems and physical exam.
3. CBC with differential abnormalities may lead to investigation of infection, malignancy, or other underlying disease.
4. ESR and C-reactive protein are nonspecific inflammatory markers and are frequently elevated; may be more helpful for monitoring disease progress.
5. Electrolytes, blood urea nitrogen, and creatinine may reflect kidney involvement.
6. Urinalysis with microscopy to evaluate hematuria and proteinuria.
7. Abnormal liver function tests may indicate liver disease, infection, or malignancy.
8. Chest x-ray, cardiac workup, and stool guaiac considered based on exam.

III. COMMON THERAPEUTIC MODALITIES

A. Systemic therapy
1. Initial therapy for CSVV and HSP is aimed at identifying and removing the offending antigen (drug, chemical, or infection) and no other treatment may be necessary. Class I or II topical corticosteroids are usually very helpful for CSVV. NSAIDs are used for myalgia, arthralgia, fever, and persistent lesions. Prednisone may be necessary for ulcerated lesions and other systemic symptoms; slow taper is recommended to avoid rebound.
2. Second-line systemic therapy may include colchicine or dapsone.

B. Local therapy and other medical interventions
1. Supportive care includes rest with leg elevation and local wound care to any skin ulcerations.
2. Supportive medical care as indicated for systemic involvement. Monitor for secondarily infected lesions and treat with topical or systemic antibiotics as warranted.

3. Compression therapy with Unna boots; once edema has decreased, elastic compression stocking can be used in combination with leg elevation to prevent recurrence.

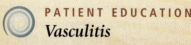

PATIENT EDUCATION
Vasculitis

- Instruct patients and family to understand diagnosis.
- Provide handouts and any other literature pertaining to diagnosis to have patient bring home. These are for future reference and to encourage patient to discuss with family for support.

IV. HOME CARE AND FOLLOW-UP

A. Continuity of care concerns
1. Children with HSP exhibiting abdominal pain and evidence of nephritis need appropriate and timely referrals to specialists. Those with renal involvement will need follow-up for at least 3 months monitoring blood pressure and urinalysis; females should be monitored for the same during any pregnancy.
2. If not healing:
   a. Re-evaluate for infection.
   b. Check patient compliance.
   c. Consider change in current treatment plan.
3. If healing:
   a. Continue to monitor care closely, approximately every 2 months.
   b. Continue to educate patient on compliance and prevention.

CUTANEOUS DRUG REACTIONS

I. OVERVIEW

A cutaneous reaction may be caused by a chemical substance or combination of substances that are ingested, injected, inhaled, inserted, instilled, or topically applied to the skin or mucous membranes and is among the most frequently observed reactions. Adverse reactions may result from overdose, accumulation, pharmacologic side effect, drug–drug interactions, idiosyncrasy, microbiologic imbalance, exacerbation of existing latent or overt disease, hypersensitivity, autoimmune-like reaction, teratogenic effect, interaction of the drug and sunlight or other light sources, or other unknown mechanisms. Drug reactions are common; data on incidence differ. The most common causative agents are aspirin, penicillin, sulfa, and blood products.

A. Definition
1. An adverse cutaneous reaction caused by a drug is any undesirable change in the structure or function of the skin, its appendages, or mucous membranes.

B. Etiology
1. Cutaneous drug eruptions/rashes are among the most common complications of drug therapy. They can occur in many forms and can mimic many other dermatoses.

2. Any cutaneous reaction that occurs within 2 weeks of starting a medication should be considered possibly drug induced.

C. Pathologic process

1. Immunologic mechanism: Common cutaneous drug eruptions are hypersensitivity reactions with an underlying immunologic basis. Hypersensitivity drug reactions may be grouped according to the classification outlined in Table 18-1. When drug-specific IgE antibodies bind to the corresponding mast cell or basophil surface receptor, vasoactive mediators are released causing immediate-type reaction. This is seen clinically as pruritus, erythema, urticaria, angioedema, or anaphylaxis.

2. Non–immunologic-mediated drug reactions account for the majority of all drug reactions. Some features include:

   a. Accumulation: blue-gray discoloration of nails and skin (argyria) can occur with the use of silver nitrate nasal sprays.

   b. Adverse effects are normal but unwanted effects of a drug such as hair loss associated with several chemotherapeutic agents.

   c. Direct release of mast cell mediators is dose dependent and does not involve antibodies. Aspirin, NSAIDs, radiographic contrast material, alcohol, opiates, cimetidine, hydralazine, atropine, and vancomycin are some drugs that can cause release of several mast cell mediators.

   d. Idiosyncratic reactions may occur such as seen in certain patients with infectious mononucleosis who develop rash when given ampicillin.

   e. Imbalance of endogenous flora may occur as seen in candidiasis occurring with antibiotic therapy.

   f. Intolerance may occur in patients with altered metabolism. Individuals who have difficulty metabolizing the enzyme N-acetyltransferase are at risk of developing drug-induced lupus from procainamide.

   g. Overdose is considered an exaggerated response to an increased dose of a medication; increased doses of anticoagulants may cause purpura.

D. Incidence

1. Drug eruptions occur in approximately 2% to 5% of hospitalized patients and more than 1% of outpatients. Hospitalized patients are frequently on multiple medications.

E. Considerations across the life span

1. There is no correlation between development of adverse drug reaction and patient age, diagnosis, or survival. Adverse cutaneous reactions are more prevalent in women than in men and in elderly patients.

II. ASSESSMENT

A. History and physical examination

1. Determine the primary lesion and distribution. Morphology of the rash might give clue to causative agent.

2. When did it start? Is there pruritus? Interval of drug introduction and onset of eruption?

3. Note that some drugs cause itching, burning, and pain without rash.

4. Always suspect drug if hives are present.

5. Other constitutional symptoms: fever, chills, arthralgia, myalgia, tachycardia, palpitations, and hypotension.

6. Involvement of palms, soles, and mucous membranes.

7. Petechiae or nonpalpable purpura on lower extremities.

8. Palpable purpura that does not blanch on diascopy might suggest vasculitis.

9. Review complete medication list, including over-the-counter drugs and supplements.

10. Any history of previous adverse reactions to drugs.

11. Any concurrent infections, metabolic disorders, or is patient immunocompromised?

B. Specific skin changes/clinical presentation

1. Clinical patterns and the most frequently causal drugs are listed in Table 18-6. Some of the drug eruption presentations are discussed below; EM minor and major and SJS/TEN are discussed in separate section of this chapter.

2. Urticaria: hives can be induced by most drugs; aspirin, penicillin, and blood products are the most frequent causes. Drug-induced urticaria caused by anaphylactic and accelerated reactions (immunologic histamine release), nonimmunologic histamine release, and serum sickness.

   a. Anaphylactic immunoglobulin E–dependent reactions are immediate (in minutes) or accelerated (hours).

   b. Serum sickness (circulating immune complex disease) has urticaria that may occur 4 to 21 days after drug ingestion and hives fade in less than 24 hours.

   c. Nonimmunologic histamine reactions can occur in minutes. The drug or agent may exert a direct action on the mast cell (morphine, codeine, polymyxin B, lobster, strawberries).

3. Exanthem: maculopapular eruptions are the most frequent of all cutaneous reactions and are often indistinguishable from viral exanthem.

   a. Onset occurs 7 to 10 days after starting drug and may present after drug is stopped. Usually fades in 7 to 10 days, on occasion even if the drug continues.

   b. Maculopapular eruption, red macules and papules, coalescing in generalized distribution often spares the face (Figure 18-7). Pruritus is common. Palms, soles, and mucous membranes may be involved.

4. Exfoliative erythroderma reactions are potentially life threatening. There is generalized redness and desquamation.

5. Fixed drug eruptions

   a. Single or multiple, round, sharply demarcated, dusky red papules or plaques appear soon after drug exposure and reappear in same site each time drug is taken. The area may blister then erode, brown pigmentation forms with healing, and itching or burning may precede or occur with the lesions (Figure 18-8).

TABLE 18-6 Drug Reactions and Some of the Drugs That Cause Them[a]

Type of Reaction	Causative Agents
Maculopapular (exanthematous) eruptions	Ampicillin, barbiturates, gentamicin, gold salts, isoniazid, phenothiazines, phenylbutazone, phenytoin, quinidine, sulfonamides, thiazides, thiouracil, and trimethoprim–sulfamethoxazole (in patients with AIDS)
Anaphylactic reactions	Aspirin, penicillin, radiographic dye, and animal-derived sera
Serum sickness	Aspirin, penicillin, streptomycin, sulfonamides, and thiouracils
Acneiform (pustular) eruptions	Bromides, hormones (androgens, corticosteroids, oral contraceptives), iodides, isoniazid, lithium, and phenytoin
Alopecia	Allopurinol, anticoagulants, antithyroid drugs, chemotherapy agents, colchicine, hypocholesteremic drugs, indomethacin, levodopa, oral contraceptives, propranolol, retinoids, thallium, and vitamin A
Erythema nodosum	Iodides, oral contraceptives, sulfonamides
Exfoliative erythroderma	Allopurinol, arsenicals, barbiturates, captopril, cefoxitin, chloroquine, cimetidine, gold salts, hydantoins, isoniazid, lithium, mercurial diuretics, para-aminosalicylic acid, sulfonamides, and sulfonylureas
Fixed drug eruptions	Aspirin, barbiturates, methaqualone, phenazones, phenolphthalein, phenylbutazone, sulfonamides, tetracyclines, trimethoprim–sulfamethoxazole, and many others reported
Erythema multiforme-like eruptions	Allopurinol, barbiturates, carbamazepine, hydantoins, minoxidil, nitrofurantoin, nonsteroidal anti-inflammatory agents, penicillin, phenolphthalein, phenothiazines, rifampin, sulfonamides, sulfonylureas, and sulindac
Lupus-like eruptions	Antitumor necrosis factor-α agents, carbamazepine, chlorpromazine, hydralazine, isoniazid, methyldopa, minocycline, procainamide, propylthiouracil, quinidine, and sulfasalazine
Photosensitivity	Amiodarone, carbamazepine, chlorpropamide, doxycycline (less with tetracycline and minocycline), furosemide, griseofulvin, lomefloxacin, methotrexate, nalidixic acid, naproxen, phenothiazines, piroxicam, psoralens, quinine, sulfonamides, thiazides, and tolbutamide
Skin pigmentation	ACTH (brown as in Addison disease), amiodarone (slate gray), anticancer drugs, antimalarials (blue-gray or yellow), arsenic (brown, diffuse, macular), bleomycin (brown, patchy, linear), cyclophosphamide (nails), doxorubicin (nails), chlorpromazine (slate gray in sun-exposed areas), clofazimine (red), heavy metals (silver, gold, bismuth, mercury), minocycline (patchy or diffuse blue-black), oral contraceptives (chloasma, brown), psoralens, and rifampin—high dose (red man syndrome)
Vesicles and blisters	Barbiturates (pressure areas), bromides, captopril (pemphigus-like), cephalosporins (pemphigus-like), clonidine (cicatricial pemphigoid-like), furosemide (phototoxic), iodides, naproxen (like porphyria cutanea tarda), penicillamine (pemphigus foliaceous-like), phenothiazines, piroxicam, and sulfonamides
Chemotherapy-induced acral erythema	Bleomycin, cyclophosphamide, cytosine, doxorubicin, fluorouracil, hydroxyurea, mercaptopurine, methotrexate, and mitotane
Stevens-Johnson syndrome/ toxic epidermal necrolysis	Allopurinol, aminopenicillins, antiretroviral drugs, barbiturates, carbamazepine, lamotrigine, phenylbutazone, phenytoin, piroxicam, sulfadiazine, sulfasalazine, trimethoprim–sulfamethoxazole, and many others reported
Vasculitis	Anti-TNF agents, COX-2 inhibitors, GCSF, leukotriene inhibitors, NSAIDs, penicillins, propylthiouracil/other antithyroid agents, quinolones, serum, and streptokinase

ACTH, adrenocorticotropic hormone; AIDS, acquired immunodeficiency syndrome; COX, cyclooxygenase; GCSF, granulocyte colony–stimulating factor; NSAIDs, nonsteroidal anti-inflammatory drugs; TNF, tumor necrosis factor.
[a]Not a complete list.

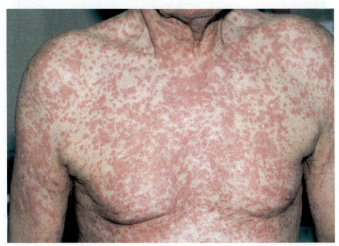

FIGURE 18-7. Exanthematous reaction to penicillin. (From Goodheart, H. P. (2003). *Goodheart's photoguide of common skin disorders* (2nd ed.). Philadelphia, PA: Lippincott Williams & Wilkins.)

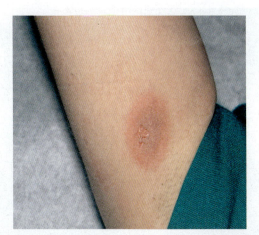

FIGURE 18-8. Fixed drug eruption. An oval lesion occurred at the identical site where it had occurred previously. In both episodes, the rash emerged after this patient ingested a sulfonamide antibiotic. Note the eroded blister in the center of the lesion. (From Goodheart, H. P. (2003). *Goodheart's photoguide of common skin disorders* (2nd ed.). Philadelphia, PA: Lippincott Williams & Wilkins.)

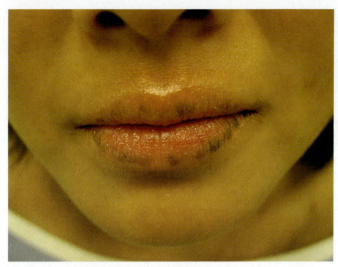

FIGURE 18-9. Drug-induced hyperpigmentation of the lips secondary to minocycline. (From Dr. Barankin Dermatology Collection.)

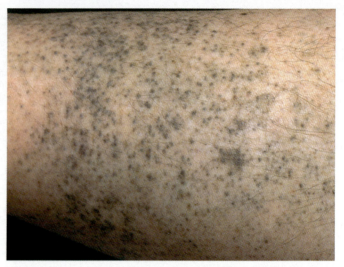

FIGURE 18-10. Punctate hyperpigmentation secondary to minocycline. (From Craft, N., Taylor, E., Tumeh, P. C., Fox, L. P., Goldsmith, L. A., Papier, A., …, Rosenblum, M. (2010). *VisualDx: Essential adult dermatology*. Philadelphia, PA: Wolters Kluwer.)

b. Lesions can occur on any part of the skin or mucous membrane: lips, hands, genitalia (especially glans penis), and oral mucosa.

6. Drug-induced hyperpigmentation
   a. Drugs and chemicals may increase production of melanin causing pigment incontinence or hyperpigmentation caused by deposition (Table 18-6; Figures 18-9 and 18-10).

7. Lichenoid drug eruptions
   a. Clinically and histologically, this eruption resembles lichen planus with multiple, flat-topped, violaceous, pruritic papules, and oral lesions may be present (Figure 18-11). Lesions heal with brown pigmentation.
   b. Latent period can be 3 weeks to 3 years from beginning of administration and the eruption.

8. Photosensitivity drug eruptions
   a. Systemic and topical medications can induce photosensitivity.
   b. Phototoxic reactions are related to concentration of drug and can occur in anyone. Rash occurs within a few hours of drug exposure, resembles an exaggerated sunburn, confined to sun-exposed areas, can occur on first administration, and will subside when drug is stopped (amiodarone, ciprofloxacin, doxycycline, furosemide, lomefloxacin, 8-methoxypsoralen, naproxen, tetracycline, topical tar, and thiazides) (Figure 18-12).
   c. Photoallergic reaction is less common, not related to concentration, and may spread to areas not exposed to sun (possible autosensitization); reaction can

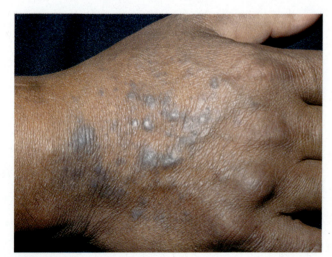

FIGURE 18-11. Lichen planus drug eruption induced by quinine. (From Lugo-Somolinos, A., Lee, I., McKinley-Grant, L., Goldsmith, L. A., Papier, A., Adigun, C. G., …, Fredeking, A. (2011). *VisualDx: Essential dermatology in pigmented skin*. Philadelphia, PA: Wolters Kluwer.)

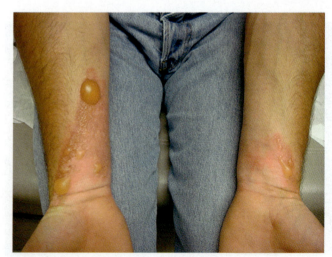

FIGURE 18-12. Topical drug-induced (8-methoxypsoralen) phototoxic eruption. (From Goodheart, H. P. (2010). *Goodheart's same-site differential diagnosis: A rapid method of diagnosing and treating common skin disorders*. Philadelphia, PA: Wolters Kluwer.)

persist for years even without further drug exposure (griseofulvin, ketoprofen, piroxicam, quinidine, quinine, quinolones, sulfonamides).

d. Onycholysis may occur with photosensitivity to tetracyclines, psoralens, and fluoroquinolones.

9. Small-vessel vasculitis

a. Any drug can evoke vasculitis in a predisposed patient.

b. Small-vessel vasculitis, palpable purpura, is most often seen on the lower legs; kidneys and joints may be involved.

10. Chemotherapy-induced acral erythema

a. This palmoplantar reaction is characterized by symmetric, well-demarcated, painful erythema of the palms and soles. Tingling on the skin is followed in a few days by symmetric, painful, well-defined swelling and erythema and may progress to desquamation or blisters.

b. Treatment is supportive and may require modification of the chemotherapy dose schedule.

11. Acute generalized exanthematous pustulosis (AGEP)

a. AGEP is characterized by small superficial pustules covering most of the body (Figure 18-13).

b. Antibacterial agents (penicillin) is the most common cause.

c. Occurs within 5 days of ingestion of the drug and usually resolves within 15 days.

d. Fever, leukocytosis, and ill-appearing patient is common; desquamation occurs.

C. Differential diagnosis

1. Viral exanthem

2. Infection

3. Collagen vascular disease

4. Primary skin conditions

5. Neoplasia

D. Diagnostic tests

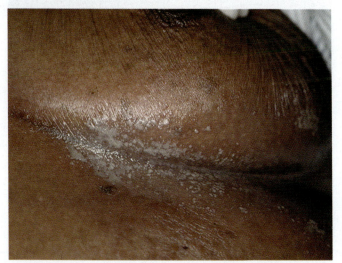

FIGURE 18-13. Multiple small opaque pustules are characteristic of AGEP. (From Lugo-Somolinos, A., Lee, I., McKinley-Grant, L., Goldsmith, L. A., Papier, A., Adigun, C. G., ..., Fredeking, A. (2011). *VisualDx: Essential dermatology in pigmented skin*. Philadelphia, PA: Wolters Kluwer.)

1. Skin biopsy has nonspecific histology but may rule out other diseases.

2. Drug levels may be helpful for comatose patient or overdose.

3. Patch test if considering contact dermatitis.

4. Referral for allergy testing if indicated with urticarial reaction.

5. Blood tests will be determined by the differential diagnosis.

PATIENT EDUCATION
Cutaneous Drug Reactions

- Educate patients on allergies and/or adverse reactions to medications and the importance of communicating the information with provider.

- Review warnings about any related cross-reacting drugs and risk of family members for patients who have had severe reactions.

- Educate patient on signs and symptoms of adverse reactions, and stress the importance of stopping drugs under supervision of provider, which may possibly be causing cutaneous reactions (rash).

- Promote proper hygiene and skin care to reduce chance of infection.

III. COMMON THERAPEUTIC MODALITIES

A. Interventions

1. Stop offending drug.

2. Provide symptomatic relief with cool compresses.

3. Topical corticosteroid creams are helpful for rash and itching.

4. Oral prednisone may be indicated with extensive eruption for 7- to 10-day course.

ERYTHEMA MULTIFORME AND STEVENS-JOHNSON SYNDROME/ TOXIC EPIDERMAL NECROLYSIS

I. OVERVIEW

EM is a distinct disorder with different clinical signs, epidemiology, and precipitating factors than SJS and toxic epidermal necrolysis (TEN). SJS and TEN are considered variants of the same entity within a spectrum of adverse drug reactions.

A proposed classification system divides the spectrum of these reactive skin disorders into five categories but does not account for differences in etiology. EM minor is not included in this spectrum, with little or no mucosal involvement and no systemic involvement:

A. EM major: detachment of less than 10% of body surface area (BSA) plus localized target lesions

B. SJS: detachment of less than 10% of BSA plus widespread erythematous or purpuric macules or flat atypical lesions

C. Overlapping SJS/TEN: detachment between 10% and 30% of BSA plus widespread erythematous or purpuric macules or atypical target-like annular patches

D. TEN with spots: detachment of greater than 30% BSA plus widespread erythematous or purpuric macules or atypical target lesions

E. TEN without spots: detachment in large epidermal sheets greater than 10% BSA without purpuric macules or target lesions

ERYTHEMA MULTIFORME

A. Definition

EM is an acute, self-limiting skin disease with an abrupt onset of papular "target" lesions. Papular lesions may be typical with three separate zones or atypical with only two different zones and poorly defined border. EM minor has mostly typical papular target lesions with little or no mucosal involvement and no systemic symptoms. EM major will have typical and may have atypical papular target lesions with severe mucosal involvement and systemic symptoms. Generally, EM is self-limited but may be recurrent. The most common precipitating factor is herpes simplex virus (HSV) infection.

B. Etiology

The most common precipitating factor is HSV infection; there may be other preceding infectious agents or rarely drug exposure. *Mycoplasma pneumoniae* infection is an important cause of EM, especially in children. Drugs that have been implicated in EM include NSAIDs, sulfonamides, antiepileptics, and antibiotics; drug etiology is less than 10% of cases; and infection represents approximately 90% of cases with HSV being the most common.

C. Pathology

EM is thought to be a mucocutaneous manifestation of a distinct skin-directed cytotoxic immune response to drug antigen, infection most commonly HSV, and in certain predisposed individuals. Immune complex formation and subsequent deposition in the cutaneous microvasculature play a role in the pathogenesis of EM.

D. Incidence

The annual incidence of EM is unknown. It is predominantly seen in young adults and very common during childhood. There is a slight male preponderance.

I. ASSESSMENT

A. History and physical examination

1. Clinical history to include acute onset, self-limiting or episodic course, signs and symptoms of associated infections such as HSV (Figure 18-14) or pneumonia, and history of new medications.

2. Clue to diagnosis includes targetoid lesions, raised atypical papules, or mucosal involvement.

3. Symptoms may include itching and burning skin, swelling of hands and feet, and pain with mucosal erosions.

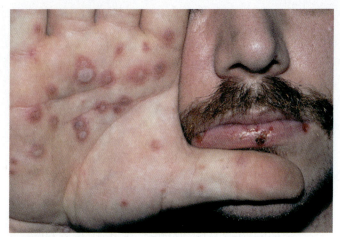

FIGURE 18-14. Erythema multiforme. This patient has a recurrent herpes simplex virus infection. Note the drying crust of the herpetic "cold sore" on his lower lip and the target-like lesions on his palm. (From Goodheart, H. P. (2003). *Goodheart's photoguide of common skin disorders* (2nd ed.). Philadelphia, PA: Lippincott Williams & Wilkins.)

B. Clinical findings

1. EM with mucosal involvement may have prodromal symptoms of fever, malaise, or myalgias.

2. Target lesions and papules are dusky red maculopapules that appear in symmetric pattern on palms and soles, dorsum of hands and feet, and extensor arms and legs that spread in centripetal manner. Trunk, face, or neck may be involved in more severe cases.

3. Classic target or "iris" lesion results from centrifugal spread of red macule or papule that becomes cyanotic, purpuric, or vesicular in the center with outer zone of erythema; there may be a middle zone of

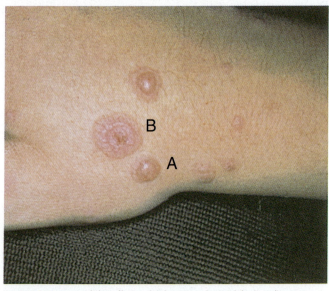

FIGURE 18-15. (**A**) Bulla and (**B**) target (or iris) lesion (in erythema multiforme). (From Bickley, L. S., & Szilagyi, P. (2003). *Bates' guide to physical examination and history taking* (8th ed.). Philadelphia, PA: Lippincott Williams & Wilkins.)

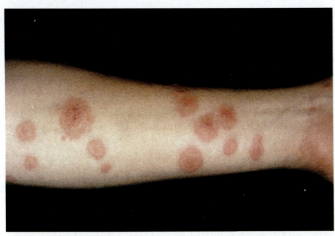

FIGURE 18-16. Erythema multiforme (type II hypersensitivity). (Reproduced with permission from Roche Laboratories. Sauer, G. C., & Hall, J. C. (1996). *Manual of skin diseases* (7th ed.). Philadelphia, PA: Lippincott-Raven.)

pale edema. Target lesions evolve over 24 to 48 hours, appear in crops, and resolve in 1 to 2 weeks (Figures 18-15 and 18-16).
4. Atypical EM may be partially formed targets, round, edematous papules with only two zones, poorly defined border, annular, or polycyclic.
5. Bullae and erosions may form in the oral cavity; most common sites are lips and buccal mucosa. Genital and ocular involvement is less frequent.
6. Subsets of patients may experience recurrent EM over many years or persistent EM that is prolonged and uninterrupted occurrence of lesions.

C. Differential diagnosis
1. Urticaria
2. Stevens-Johnson syndrome
3. Fixed drug eruption
4. Pemphigoid or pemphigus
5. Sweet syndrome
6. Polymorphous light eruption
7. Urticarial vasculitis

D. Diagnostic tests
1. Laboratory findings are not specific with EM. Increased ESR, white blood cell count, and liver enzymes may be seen in severe cases.
2. Skin biopsy for hematoxylin and eosin stain with direct immunofluorescence to rule out autoimmune blistering disease when diagnosis in question.

II. COMMON THERAPEUTIC MODALITIES

A. Therapy
1. Most patients with EM do not require treatment.
2. Widespread EM may be treated with systemic corticosteroids, and prednisone should be given 40 to 80 mg/day until lesions resolve and dose tapered; this approach is controversial.
3. Recurrent HSV-associated EM can be prevented with suppressive therapy: oral acyclovir 200 mg two or three

times a day or 400 mg twice daily; valacyclovir 500 mg daily, and famciclovir 125 mg twice daily.
4. Eroded skin or blisters can be treated with topical antibiotics or antibiotics for symptomatic improvement.
5. Oral lesions can be symptomatically treated with the following:
   a. Mixture of kaolin, viscous lidocaine, and diphenhydramine elixir may help discomfort of oral lesions.
   b. Half-strength aqueous hydrogen peroxide (1.5%) mouthwash three to five times a day for cleansing.
   c. Dyclone solution, viscous lidocaine, or a mixture of kaopectate in elixir of diphenhydramine can be applied directly to oral lesions for discomfort.
   d. Chloraseptic mouthwash may be helpful for relief of discomfort and cleansing.

 PATIENT EDUCATION
Erythema Multiforme

- Educate the patient about erythema multiforme and specific symptoms and treatment to promote adherence to the treatment plan.
- Stress the importance of avoiding any identified triggers or agents to decrease the risk of recurrence.

STEVENS-JOHNSON SYNDROME

A. Definition
   SJS and TEN have been considered the most severe forms of EM in the past. It has been proposed that EM major is distinct from SJS and TEN on the basis of clinical criteria. EM is characterized by typical target lesions, most often postinfectious disorder and most commonly HSV, and is often recurrent but with low morbidity. The SJS/TEN spectrum is characterized by widespread blisters and purpuric macules; usually a severe drug-induced reaction with high morbidity, SJS involves a relatively smaller percentage of BSA when compared to TEN; TEN has highest morbidity and a worse prognosis. The categorization of EM, SJS, and TEN remains a topic of controversy, and there are differing opinions of the classification of EM major and SJS as well as SJS and TEN. Currently, EM is considered to be a separate condition distinct from SJS and TEN. SJS and TEN have been unified within a spectrum of the same entity based on similar clinical and histologic features with variable severity in epidermal detachment.
1. SJS is a vesiculobullous disease of the skin, mouth, eyes, and genitals.
   a. Cutaneous findings are preceded by upper respiratory symptoms.
   b. SJS requires involvement of two or more mucosal surfaces with less than 10% BSA of cutaneous erythematous or purpuric macules or flat atypical lesions (Figure 18-17).
2. TEN presents with symptoms similar to SJS mucous membrane disease and progresses to diffuse,

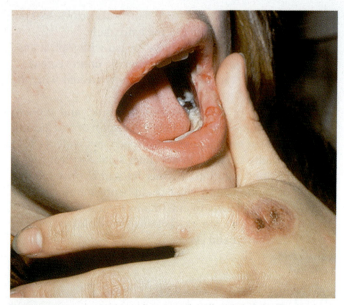

FIGURE 18-17. Patient diagnosed with SJS has bullous lesions on lips and buccal mucosa and targetoid lesions on the hand. (From Goodheart, H. P. (2003). *Goodheart's photoguide of common skin disorders* (2nd ed.). Philadelphia, PA: Lippincott Williams & Wilkins.)

generalized detachment of the epidermis through the dermoepidermal junction.

   a. TEN requires greater than 30% BSA involvement with epidermal detachment.

   b. TEN may or may not have purpuric macules or target lesions.

   c. TEN is a systemic disease involving ophthalmic, pulmonary, genitourinary, and GI systems, in addition to the skin, and results in high death rate.

  3. Overlapping SJS/TEN has between 10% and 30% of BSA with widespread erythematous or purpuric macules or atypical target-like annular patches.

B. Etiology

  1. Drugs are implicated in approximately 50% of cases of SJS and over 95% of cases of TEN.

  2. Patients at greater risk include those who are immunocompromised with a thousandfold increase in those with human immunodeficiency virus (HIV).

  3. The most frequently implicated drugs include allopurinol, antibiotics (chloramphenicol, macrolides, penicillin, quinolones, sulfonamides, sulfasalazine, cephalosporins), anticonvulsants (carbamazepine, lamotrigine, phenobarbital, phenytoin, valproate), and NSAIDs.

  4. TEN reaction is independent of drug dosage; seen frequently with conditions requiring simultaneous drug treatment for infections and pain.

  5. TEN may be linked to an inherited defect in the detoxification of drug metabolites.

C. Pathologic Process

  1. Skin biopsy in SJS shows full-thickness epidermal necrosis with little dermal change; biopsy can distinguish TEN from staphylococcal scalded skin syndrome

(SSSS); direct immunofluorescence will rule out autoimmune blistering disease.

  2. The marked skin sloughing in TEN may be due to increased keratinocyte programmed cell death (apoptosis), subepidermal blister formation, and keratinocyte necrosis; cytotoxic T cells may contribute to the pathogenesis of blister formation by causing degeneration of drug-altered keratinocytes.

D. Incidence

  1. SJS and TEN have annual incidence of 1.2 to 6 and 0.4 to 1.2 million persons, respectively; death rate for SJS is 1% to 5% and 34% to 40% for TEN.

  2. SJS can occur in all ages but is more common in children and young adults; TEN occurs in all age groups and is more frequent in women and the elderly.

E. Considerations across the life span

  1. Treatment considerations for children are the same as for adults.

I. ASSESSMENT

A. History and physical examination

  1. Initial symptoms for SJS include fever, stinging eyes, and pain with swallowing that precedes skin manifestations by 1 to 3 days. Prodromal symptoms for TEN include fever and upper respiratory infection symptoms including headache and sore throat. Clinical history of symptom timeline and medication history is important.

  2. Patients with HIV and certain autoimmune conditions such as systemic lupus erythematosus may be at greater risk for TEN.

  3. SJS/TEN are conditions preceded by fever, malaise, cough, and abdominal pain. Uncomplicated SJS resolves in 1 month, and recurrence is uncommon unless there is re-exposure to causative drug.

  4. Poor outcome predictors for TEN include old age, widespread bullae, neutropenia, and impaired renal function.

B. Clinical findings

  1. Skin lesions in SJS can develop abruptly, are flat patches and macules, atypical target morphology, purpuric macules with dusky center, on the trunk and extremities. The palms and soles may be early sites. SJS lesions are more centrally distributed on the face and trunk.

  2. SJS will begin with upper respiratory symptoms, fever, chills, cough, rhinitis, and sore throat. Within 2 weeks, the mucosal erosions and rash develop.

  3. Initially, patients with TEN will have diffuse, warm erythema with dusky gray macules and epidermal necrosis. This spreads over wide areas starting on the trunk and progressing to the neck, face, mucosa, and extremities. The skin becomes painful, and with mild pressure of the thumb, the skin wrinkles and slides laterally, and the skin splits at the dermal–epidermal junction. This is Nikolsky sign and is considered to be a life-threatening sign (Figure 18-18). Mucous membranes develop very painful erosions.

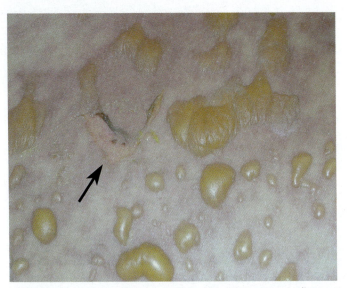

FIGURE 18-18. Bullae on patient with TEN; *arrow* indicates Nikolsky sign. (From Mulholland, M. W., Lillemoe, K. D., Doherty, G. M., Maier, R. V., Simeone, D. M., & Upchurch, G. R. (2006). *Greenfield's surgery: Scientific principles and practice* (4th ed.). Philadelphia, PA: Lippincott Williams & Wilkins.)

4. In TEN, bullae and erosions may appear on the conjunctiva and mucous membranes of the nose, mouth, anus, vulvovaginal region, and urethral meatus; lesions spread symmetrically from the face and trunk to the extremities. SJS will also have oral, genital, and perianal mucosa bullae and erosions. Figure 18-19 shows diffuse trunk involvement.
5. Corneal ulcerations occur with SJS; severe eye involvement in TEN is a frequent feature.
6. Life-threatening pulmonary involvement may occur secondary to involvement of bronchial epithelium in TEN. Septicemia and gram-negative pneumonia are the most common causes of death.
7. SJS/TEN can affect pulmonary, GI, central nervous, and renal systems.

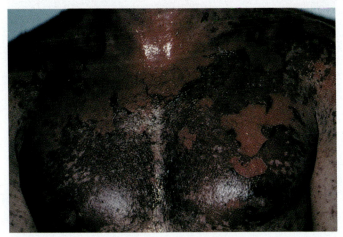

FIGURE 18-19. Toxic epidermal necrolysis has resulted from treatment with nevirapine. (From Goodheart, H. P. (2003). *Goodheart's photoguide of common skin disorders* (2nd ed.). Philadelphia, PA: Lippincott Williams & Wilkins.)

C. Differential diagnosis
  1. For SJS: anticonvulsant hypersensitivity syndrome, paraneoplastic pemphigus, pemphigus vulgaris, and SSSS
  2. For TEN: SSSS, graft versus host disease (GVHD), staphylococcal toxic shock syndrome, drug-induced linear immunoglobulin A dermatosis (linear IgA), AGEP, drug reaction with eosinophilia and systemic symptoms (DRESS), and generalized morbilliform drug eruption
D. Diagnostic tests
  1. Laboratory testing is not necessary; viral culture can confirm or rule out herpes. There may be elevated ESR, leukocytosis, eosinophilia, and elevated AST and ALT.
  2. Skin biopsy can be helpful when diagnosis is uncertain.

II. COMMON THERAPEUTIC MODALITIES

A. Systemic therapy
  1. Identify and treat source of infection, withdraw suspected drug, and maintain fluid, electrolyte, and nutritional balance. Minimize time between onset of cutaneous symptoms and arrival at appropriate specialty unit for care is crucial for improving potential for survival.
  2. The role of systemic corticosteroids is controversial for SJS/TEN, and there is no consensus.
  3. Intravenous immunoglobulin G (IVIG) used to improve survival if administered early in the course of TEN has been proposed; however, evidence for decreasing mortality has been inconclusive.
  4. Other immunosuppressives such as cyclosporine or cyclophosphamide may be considered for TEN.
B. Topical therapy/supportive skin care
  1. Extensive epidermal damage requires timely supportive care focused on maintenance and reconstruction of the barrier function of the skin, fluid balance, prevention of ocular damage, monitoring, and treatment of infection. This will be best in a burn unit or comparable intensive care setting.
  2. Products used for coverage of denuded skin include paraffin gauze, porcine xenografts, and human allografts.
  3. Newer products include Biobrane, a skin substitute made of synthetic bilaminar membrane, and Aquacel Ag, a moisture-retentive hydrofiber dressing that releases silver within the dressing.
  4. Ocular damage can be prevented or minimized by continual lubrication of the eye and topical antibiotic use. Corticosteroid eyedrops can minimize inflammation.
  5. Oral care is outlined under EM.

III. HOME CARE AND FOLLOW-UP

A. If there has been oral mucosal involvement, assess nutritional status related to difficulty swallowing, review signs of dehydration, and educate patients and families about nutrition and fluid/electrolyte balance.
B. An ophthalmologist should be consulted if there is any eye involvement.
C. Immediate hospitalization and fluid resuscitation will be required for TEN.
D. Long-term sequelae of SJS and mostly TEN include effects from scarring such as contracture of joints; corneal scarring can lead to blindness.

PYODERMA GANGRENOSUM

I. OVERVIEW

The primary role of inflammation is to deliver neutrophils and other leukocytes to a site of injury and activate the cells to perform their protective function against infection; neutrophils are the first to arrive at sites of inflammation. PG is one of several neutrophilic dermatoses that often occurs in patients with underlying inflammatory or malignant disease, including Crohn disease, ulcerative colitis, rheumatoid arthritis, myelodysplasia, or multiple myeloma. Neutrophilic dermatoses are considered possible manifestations of a potentially multisystemic neutrophilic disease. Sweet syndrome and erythema elevatum diutinum are also within the spectrum, and PG will be discussed here.

A. Definition
   1. PG is uncommon, chronic and recurrent, noninfectious, inflammatory, neutrophilic skin disease characterized by ulcerative lesions that enlarge rapidly, usually on the legs, and are painful; lesions may begin spontaneously or secondary to trauma.
   2. PG is not infectious or gangrenous.
   3. Enlargement of the lesion (pathergy) with trauma is characteristic of PG.

B. Etiology
   1. Commonly associated with inflammatory bowel disease, ulcerative colitis, Crohn disease, and rheumatoid arthritis.
   2. There is less common association with chronic active hepatitis, a monoclonal gammopathy, myelodysplasia, myeloid leukemia, multiple myeloma, and solid organ tumors.
   3. Approximately 50% of PG cases occur in association with ulcerative colitis; in 40% to 50% of patients, no associated disease is found; there is recent favor given to the presence of an underlying immunologic abnormality in patients with PG.

C. Pathologic process
   1. Generally, the pathology is nonspecific especially if the lesions are partially treated or minimally inflamed.
   2. Early lesions have a neutrophilic vascular reaction; active, untreated expanding lesions have neutrophilic infiltrate and often features of LCV.
   3. Fully developed ulcers have marked tissue necrosis.

D. Incidence
   1. PG is a global disease and affects individuals between 20 and 50 years of age, most commonly women.
   2. Approximately 4% of cases occur in children and infants.

II. ASSESSMENT

A. History and physical examination
   1. Thorough history and physical examination, any symptoms of an associated disease (inflammatory bowel or arthritis), and review of medications
   2. Description and measurement of lesions noted: painful ulcer, rapid progression of ulceration, type of lesion preceding ulcer (papule, pustule, vesicle), and pathergy
   3. Character of lesions: tenderness, necrosis, irregular violaceous border, undermined, and rolled edges

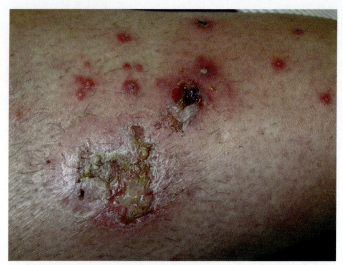

FIGURE 18-20. Pyoderma gangrenosum, early pustules, and ulcerations on the shin. (From Goroll, A. H., & Mulley, A. G. (2009). *Primary care medicine*. Philadelphia, PA: Wolters Kluwer.)

B. Skin findings
   1. Initial lesions are tender papulopustule with surrounding erythematous or violaceous induration, an erythematous nodule, and/or a bulla on erythematous base (Figure 18-20).
   2. Generally painful, occur most often on lower legs especially pretibial region, but can occur anywhere including mucous membranes and peristomal.
   3. Lesions then ulcerate with necrosis that is shallow or deep with purulent base; loss of tissue may expose tendons and muscles. Edges are rolled, elevated and inflamed, gunmetal-colored border that extends centrifugally (Figures 18-21 and 18-22).
   4. Number of lesions varies from one to many, size 3 to 10 cm, and they may coalesce.

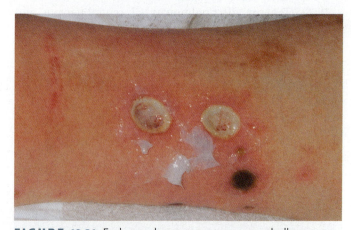

FIGURE 18-21. Early pyoderma gangrenosum: shallow ulcerations on an erythematous, indurated base with a tendency to coalesce. The border extends centrifugally and is irregular; it becomes undermined and overhanging in fully developed lesions. (From Berg, D., & Worzala, K. (2006). *Atlas of adult physical diagnosis*. Philadelphia, PA: Lippincott Williams & Wilkins.)

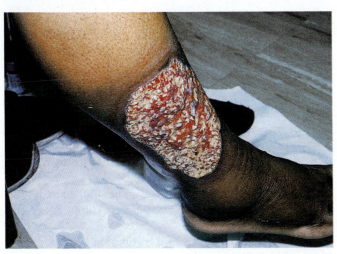

FIGURE 18-22. Large ulceration of pyoderma gangrenosum healing with crater-like scar. (From Goodheart, H. P. (2003). *Goodheart's photoguide of common skin disorders* (2nd ed.). Philadelphia, PA: Lippincott Williams & Wilkins.)

C. Differential diagnosis
  1. Sweet syndrome
  2. Systemic vasculitis
  3. Behçet disease
  4. Cellulitis
  5. Insect bite reaction
  6. Infections
  7. Cutaneous T- and B-cell lymphomas
D. Diagnostic tests
  1. Histology analysis of PG is not always diagnostic; however, sterile biopsy of active skin lesion with depth to include subcutaneous fat evaluation is recommended.
  2. Tissue may be needed for cultures (bacterial, mycobacterial, fungal, and viral).
  3. Diagnosis relies on clinical, historical, and pathologic correlation and exclusion of other conditions that produce ulcerations.
  4. Studies to evaluate for underlying causative conditions: GI tract studies, hematologic evaluation, chest x-ray, and urinalysis.

III. COMMON THERAPEUTIC MODALITIES

A. Systemic therapy
  1. Initial and primary goal of treatment is to reduce the inflammatory process of the wound in order to promote healing and control pain. Control of the underlying disease is done simultaneously.
  2. No specific therapy is uniformly effective for patients with PG.
  3. Systemic oral or intravenous steroids are given at high doses to quickly suppress the immune response in rapidly advancing disease. Often, combined local and systemic corticosteroid therapy is utilized.
  4. Adjunctive systemic therapy is needed for extensive disease using other immunosuppressants, which may also reduce recurrences, that is, cyclosporine, mycophenolate

mofetil, and azathioprine. Infliximab may be indicated in patient with concomitant Crohn disease.
  5. The nature and intensity of treatment approach depend on the extent of lesions and if they are expanding, underlying disorder, medical status of the patient, and risk of treatment; hospitalization may be required for severe cases.
  6. Oral antibiotics including sulfonamides, minocycline, and dapsone have been used with some success in limited disease.
  7. Other therapies include hyperbaric oxygen.
B. Topical therapy
  1. Superpotent topical corticosteroids may be used for limited disease.
  2. Intralesional corticosteroids can be used for small lesions being careful not to injure the skin.
  3. Topical tacrolimus ointment 0.1% or pimecrolimus cream 1% may be effective for mild or early skin lesions.
  4. Care must be taken not to traumatize or injure the skin, and local wet dressings with Burrow solution may be used for local care.
C. Surgical considerations
  1. Surgery should be avoided if possible due to pathergy phenomenon that can occur with surgical manipulation or grafting. This could result in wound enlargement or development of PG at a harvest site.

PATIENT EDUCATION
Pyoderma Gangrenosum

- Instruct patients and family to understand diagnosis.
- Discuss proper hygiene and daily inspections of skin necessary, reporting any skin barrier defects to health care provider immediately. Injury or trauma to skin can provoke new ulcers to form. Specifically:
  ○ Proper nail and foot care. Avoid walking barefoot and avoid any activity resulting in trauma to affected areas; stress importance of appropriate fitting shoes.
  ○ Rest and elevation are recommended; however, maintain range of motion and complete activities as tolerated.
- Provide handouts and any other literature pertaining to diagnosis to have patient bring home. These are for future reference and to encourage patient to discuss with family for support.
- Promote the importance of treatment compliance to promote wound healing, and lifelong therapy may be needed to prevent recurrence.

IV. HOME CARE AND FOLLOW-UP

A. Continuity of care.
B. Multiple methods of wound care are available, and care must be given to prevent pathergy.
C. Patients may need referrals to specialists for management of systemic illness including gastroenterology, rheumatology, oncology, or plastic surgery if indicated.

D. PG patients should receive follow-up care on a regular basis to maintain drug therapy and to access patient compliance. Wound care may be needed regularly along with regular measurements of lesion(s) to ensure proper wound healing is taking place.

ERYTHEMA NODOSUM

I. OVERVIEW

EN is a nodular erythematous eruption that usually presents on the extensor surfaces of the extremities. EN is a hypersensitivity reaction to a variety of antigenic stimuli, may be associated with certain diseases, and also is seen in drug therapies; more than half of cases are idiopathic.

A. Definition
1. EN is a panniculitis (inflammation of subcutaneous adipose tissue).

B. Etiology
1. EN is a hypersensitivity reaction to a variety of antigenic stimuli and may occur in association with several systemic diseases, drug therapies, or infection; half of cases are idiopathic.
2. Most common cause in children is streptococcal infection and noninfectious inflammatory diseases.
3. In adults, the most common cause is streptococcal infection and sarcoidosis. EN may occur in up to 39% of cases of sarcoidosis.
4. Coccidioidomycosis is the most common cause of EN in the West and Southwest United States.
5. Inflammatory bowel disease may trigger EN.
6. Sulfonamides, bromides, and oral contraceptives may cause EN.

C. Pathologic process
1. Tissue samples need to be deep enough to adequately evaluate the subcutaneous fat. Tissue shows granulomatous inflammation and fibrosis in the septa of the subcutaneous fat, features of a septal panniculitis.

D. Incidence
1. Peak incidence between ages of 18 and 34 years.
2. Female-to-male ratio is 5:1.
3. EN may occur in children and adults over 70 years. Age distribution will vary with geographic location and etiology.
4. Most cases of EN resolve without sequelae; however, rarely, EN can persist for months or years.

II. ASSESSMENT

A. History and physical examination
1. Most pertinent physical findings are limited to skin and joints.
2. There may be prodromal symptoms of fatigue and malaise or symptoms of upper respiratory tract infection; these may precede skin eruption by several weeks.
3. Pulmonary hilar adenopathy may develop in EN cases with diverse causes.
4. The possibility of an underlying primary tuberculous infection should not be overlooked.

B. Skin findings
1. Characteristic lesions are red, node-like swellings over the shins, usually both legs are involved as seen in Figures 18-23 and 18-24.
2. Lesions may occur on the extensor surface of forearms, thighs, and trunk.
3. Lesions may vary in size from 2 to 6 cm, usually oval in shape.
4. Initially, lesions are tense, hard, and painful.
5. Color changes from bright red to bluish or livid and gradually fades to yellowish hue.
6. The overlying skin will desquamate; individual lesions last approximately 2 weeks, but new lesions present for 3 to 6 weeks.
7. Ankle edema with leg pain is common.

C. Nonskin findings
1. Clinical picture usually of nonspecific illness possibly with low-grade fever, malaise, cough, headache, arthralgias, and arthritis.
2. Arthralgia occurring in more than 50% of EN cases may precede skin eruptions by 2 to 8 weeks. Joint symptoms may last for up to 2 years but resolve without destructive joint changes. Ankles, knees, and wrist are affected most commonly.
3. Bilateral hilar adenopathy may be associated with sarcoidosis; unilateral changes may occur with malignancy or infection.

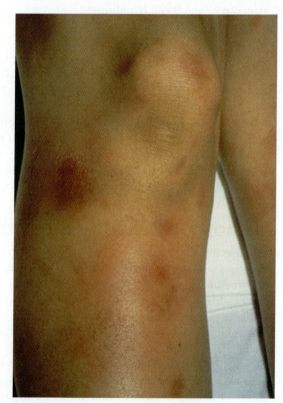

FIGURE 18-23. Erythema nodosum. These are acute red, tender nodules. (From Goodheart, H. P. (2003). *Goodheart's photoguide of common skin disorders* (2nd ed.). Philadelphia, PA: Lippincott Williams & Wilkins.)

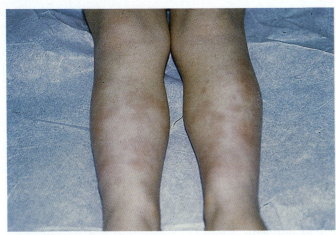

FIGURE 18-24. Erythema nodosum. Tender erythematous nodules on extensor aspects of lower legs. (Courtesy of George A. Datto, III, MD.)

D. Differential diagnosis
   1. Urticaria
   2. Insect bites
   3. Cellulitis
   4. Superficial and deep thrombophlebitis
   5. Minor trauma
   6. Vasculitis
   7. Other forms of panniculitis
E. Diagnostic tests
   1. Throat culture to exclude group A beta-hemolytic streptococcal infection.
   2. Antistreptolysin (ASO) titer and ESR.
   3. Chest x-ray.
   4. Laboratory evaluation should be guided by history and physical examination.
   5. Deep skin biopsy to evaluate subcutaneous fat will be helpful in patients with atypical lesions.
   6. Stool cultures in patients with GI symptoms to exclude infection by *Yersinia*, *Salmonella*, and *Campylobacter* organisms.

III. COMMON THERAPEUTIC MODALITIES

A. Systemic therapy
   1. NSAIDs are the mainstay of treatment for symptom relief.
   2. Potassium iodide may be helpful for chronic recurrent EN or very painful involved lesions.
   3. Colchicine has been used in some refractory cases with improvement.
   4. Associated diseases and infections should be identified and treated, and precipitating drugs should be discontinued.
B. Local therapy
   1. Rest and elevation of legs.
   2. Cool wet compresses and gradient support stockings or bandages may help decrease edema and discomfort.

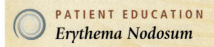

PATIENT EDUCATION
Erythema Nodosum

- Instruct patients and family to understand diagnosis.
- Restrict patient mobility during acute phase if pain and swelling are significant.

IV. HOME CARE AND FOLLOW-UP

A. Continuity of care concerns
   1. Bed rest and decreased activity are encouraged during the active phase.
   2. The course of EN is self-limited, and the condition is benign.

BIBLIOGRAPHY

Arndt, K. A., & Hsu, J. T. S. (2007). *Manual of dermatologic therapeutics* (7th ed.). Philadelphia, PA: Wolters Kluwer/Lippincott Williams & Wilkins.

Aurelian, L., Ono, F., & Burnett, J. (2003). Herpes simplex virus (HSV)-associated erythema multiforme (HAEM): A viral disease with an autoimmune component. *Dermatology Online Journal, 9*(1), 1.

Chung, L., Kea, B., & Fiorentino, D. F. (2008). Cutaneous vasculitis. In J. L. Bolognia, J. L. Jorizzo, & R. P. Rapini (Eds.), *Dermatology* (2nd ed., pp. 347–367). Spain: Mosby Elsevier.

Fiorentino, D. F. (2003). Cutaneous vasculitis. *Journal of the American Academy of Dermatology, 48*(3), 311–340.

French, L. E., & Prius, C. (2008). Erythema multiforme, Stevens-Johnson syndrome, and toxic epidermal necrolysis. In J. L. Bolognia, J. L. Jorizzo, & R. P. Rapini (Eds.), *Dermatology* (2nd ed., pp. 287–291). Spain: Mosby Elsevier.

Ghaffar, A. (2010). Immunology—Chapter 17. Hypersensitivity reactions. In: *Microbiology and immunology on-line*. University of South Carolina. http://pathmicro.med.sc.edu/ghaffar/hyper00.htm

Grattan, C. E. H., & Black, A. K. (2008). Urticaria and angioedema. In J. L. Bolognia, J. L. Jorizzo, & R. P. Rapini (Eds.), *Dermatology* (2nd ed., pp. 261–276). Spain: Mosby Elsevier.

Grattan, C. E. H., Sabroe, R. A., & Greaves, M. W. (2002). Chronic urticaria. *Journal of the American Academy of Dermatology, 46*(5), 645–647.

Habif, T. P. (2010). *Clinical dermatology: A color guide to diagnosis and therapy* (5th ed.). Philadelphia, PA: Mosby.

Habif, T. P., Campbell, J. L., Chapman, M. S., Dinulos, J. G., & Sug, K. A. (2011). *Skin disease: Diagnosis & treatment* (3rd ed.). Philadelphia, PA: Elsevier Saunders.

Jennette, J. C., Falk, R. J., Bacon, P. A., Basu, N., Cid, M. C., Ferrario, F., ..., Watts RA. (2013). 2012 Revised International Chapel Hill Consensus Conference Nomenclature of Vasculitides. *Arthritis and Rheumatism, 65*(1), 1–11.

Mellors, R. C. (2006). Hypersensitivity reactions: Tissue injury initiated by immune responses. In: *Immunopathology*. http://www.medpath.info/MainContent/Immunopathology/Immuno_02.html

Patterson, J. W. (2008). Panniculitis. In J. L. Bolognia, J. L. Jorizzo, & R. P. Rapini (Eds.), *Dermatology* (2nd ed., pp. 1511–1535). Spain: Mosby Elsevier.

Pite, H., Wedi, B., Bornego, L. M., Kapp, A., & Raap, U. (2013). Management of childhood urticaria: Current knowledge and practical recommendations. *Acta Dermato-Vereneologica, 93.* http://www.medicaljournals.se/acta/content/?doi=10.2340/00015555-1573&html=1

Scharma, P., Sharma, S., Baltaro, R., & Hurley, J. (2011). Systemic vasculitis. *American Family Physicians, 83*(5), 556–565.

Schwartz, R. A., McDonough, P. H. & Lee, B. W. (2013). Toxic epidermal necrolysis. Part I. Introduction, history, classification, clinical features, systemic manifestations, etiology, and immunopathogenesis. *Journal of the American Academy of Dermatology, 45*(2), 173–186.

Schwartz, R. A., McDonough, P. H. & Lee, B. W. (2013). Toxic epidermal necrolysis. Part II. Prognosis, sequelae, diagnosis, differential diagnosis, prevention, and treatment. *Journal of the American Academy of Dermatology, 45*(2), 187–204.

Schwarzen, K., Werchniak, A. E. & Ko, C. J. (Eds.). (2009). In D. M. Elston (Series Ed.), *Requisites in dermatology: General dermatology.* Philadelphia, PA: Saunders Elsevier.

Sokumbi, O., & Wetter, D. A. (2012). Clinical features, diagnosis, and treatment of erythema multiforme: A review for the practicing dermatologist. *International Journal of Dermatology, 51*, 889–902.

Zuberbier, T. (2012). A summary of the New International EAACI/GA²LEN/EDF/WAO Guidelines in urticaria. *World Allergy Organization Journal, 5*, S1–S5.

STUDY QUESTIONS

1. Characteristic of the primary lesion in urticaria is an edematous papule or plaque called:
   a. Lesion
   b. Mass
   c. Wheal
   d. Whelp

2. Which of the following drugs may produce photosensitivity diseases?
   a. Doxycycline
   b. Furosemide
   c. HCTZ
   d. All of the above

3. Morbilliform reactions are:
   a. Exanthems
   b. Shaking syndrome, much like Parkinson disease
   c. Most commonly produced by ampicillin
   d. A and C
   e. All of the above

4. Chronic urticaria is defined as episodes lasting more than:
   a. 6 weeks
   b. 4 weeks
   c. 2 weeks
   d. 3 weeks

5. Which of the following statements regarding causes of angioedema is *true*?
   a. Angioedema may have idiopathic causes.
   b. Edema may cause angioedema.
   c. Angioedema may be medication induced.
   d. A and C.

6. Common causes of anaphylactic reactions include:
   a. Peanuts
   b. Antibiotics
   c. Trees
   d. A and C

7. Cutaneous reactions may be caused by a chemical substance that is:
   a. Ingested
   b. Injected
   c. Inhaled
   d. All of the above

8. Which of the following drug may cause acute generalized exanthematous pustulosis (AGEP)?
   a. Antiviral agents
   b. Antibacterial agents (penicillin)
   c. Topical steroids
   d. Diuretic agents

9. Which of the following is the most common cause of erythema multiforme?
   a. Herpes simplex virus
   b. Rubella
   c. Herpes zoster
   d. Parvovirus

10. Primary treatment for urticaria includes:
    a. Cetirizine
    b. Loratadine
    c. Fexofenadine
    d. Doxepin
    e. A, B, and C
    f. All of the above

11. Management of adverse drug reactions includes:
    a. Discontinuing the offending drug
    b. Orally administered antihistamine
    c. Orally administered prednisone for severe reactions
    d. Topical symptom management
    e. A and B
    f. All of the above

Answers to Study Questions: 1.c, 2.d, 3.d, 4.a, 5.d, 6.d, 7.d, 8.b, 9.a, 10.f, 11.f

Connective Tissue Disorders

Theresa Coyner • Karen Congelio • Katrina Nice Masterson

OVERVIEW

Connective tissue disorders (collagen vascular disease) are defined as a group of acquired disorders that have the commonality of immunologic and inflammatory changes in small blood vessels and connective tissue. Common features may include arthritis, skin lesions, iritis and episcleritis, pericarditis, pleuritis, subcutaneous nodules, myocarditis, vasculitis, and nephritis. Lupus, scleroderma, and myositis will be discussed in this chapter.

I. LUPUS ERYTHEMATOSIS

A. Definition: Lupus is a chronic autoimmune disease resulting in inflammation and tissue damage. The name "lupus," Latin for wolf, was coined in the 10th century possibly because the lesions resembled wolf bites.

B. Etiology

1. The exact cause of lupus is unknown; however, current research points to interrelated immunologic, environmental, hormonal, and genetic factors.

2. Of the babies born with neonatal lupus erythematosus (NLE), 98% were reported to have anti-Ro antibodies and approximately one third with La antibodies. These IgG antibodies pass from the placenta to the fetus.

3. Recent studies are looking at chromosome 1 for a genetic link; however, only 10% of lupus patients will have a close relative with lupus. About 5% of children born to individuals with lupus will develop the disease.

4. Often called a "woman's disease," lupus strikes women 10 to 15 times more frequently than men and occurs most often during childbearing years.

5. Although the disease occurs worldwide, it is most prevalent in persons with African, American Indian, and Asian origins.

C. Symptoms

1. Arthralgia
2. Fever greater than 100°F
3. Arthritis
4. Prolonged or extreme fatigue
5. Skin rashes
6. Anemia
7. Kidney involvement
8. Pleurisy
9. Butterfly-shaped (malar) rash across the cheeks and nose
10. Less frequent occurring symptoms include photosensitivity, hair loss, mouth or nose ulcers, abnormal blood clotting problems, Raynaud phenomenon, and seizures.

D. Types of lupus

1. Cutaneous lupus erythematosus has many different types including:

a. Chronic cutaneous lupus erythematosus (CCLE)

(1) The most common form of CCLE is discoid lupus erythematosus (DLE).

(a) DLE lesions are often erythematous, scaly, and thickened and may produce scarring or discoloration of the skin; usually painless and nonpruritic.

(b) *Localized DLE*: lesions limited to the head (possible alopecia), ears, and neck (Figures 19-1 and 19-2).

(c) *Generalized DLE*: lesions present anywhere on skin.

(d) Long-standing lesions are at risk for skin cancer.

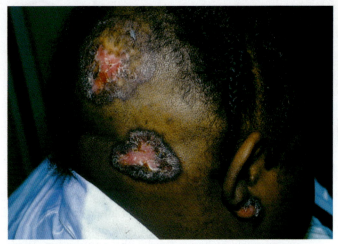

FIGURE 19-1. Chronic cutaneous lupus erythematosus (CCLE) causing scarring alopecia. (From Goodheart, H. P. (2003). *Goodheart's photoguide of common skin disorders* (2nd ed.). Philadelphia, PA: Lippincott Williams & Wilkins.)

(2) Hypertrophic (thickened) or verrucous (wart-like) lupus erythematosus (LE)

(3) Lupus profundus: DLE lesions occurring in conjunction with firm lumps in the fatty tissue (panniculitis) (Figure 19-3)

(4) Mucosal DLE: lesions that occur in mucous membranes of the mouth, nose, and eyes

(5) Chilblain lupus: lesions consisting of red to purplish papules that usually occur on the toes and fingers

b. Subacute cutaneous lupus erythematosus (SCLE)

(1) Papulosquamous: erythematous plaques

   (a) May resemble psoriasis

   (b) Most common on sun-exposed areas of the arms, shoulders, neck, and trunk; face less frequently involved

(2) Erythemic annular lesions with no scale (LE tumidus)

(3) Both forms are photosensitive to natural and artificial light.

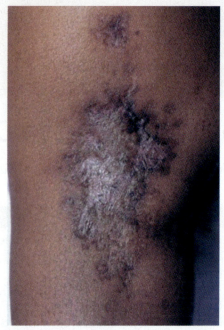

FIGURE 19-3. Lupus profundus (lupus panniculitis). (From Elder, D. E. (2012). *Atlas and synopsis of Lever's histopathology of the skin*. Philadelphia, PA: Wolters Kluwer.)

(4) Lesions usually do not scar but may cause discoloration of skin.

c. Acute cutaneous lupus erythematosus (ACLE)

(1) Produces flat erythemic areas resembling sunburn, which can be transient, lasting several days to weeks (Figure 19-4).

(2) *Localized ACLE* involves both cheeks and nose presenting as a butterfly-shaped malar rash.

(3) *Generalized ACLE* presents with a maculopapular eruption representing a photosensitive dermatitis.

2. Systemic lupus erythematosus (SLE) attacks multiple systems in the body, which may include the skin (classic butterfly-shaped malar rash most common), liver,

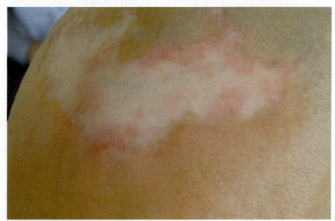

FIGURE 19-2. Discoid lupus erythematosus (DLE). (From Edward, S., & Yung, A. (2011). *Essential dermatopathology*. Philadelphia, PA: Wolters Kluwer.)

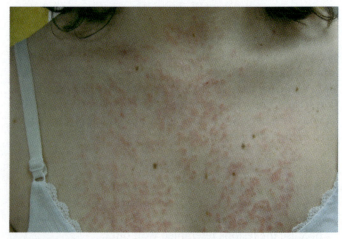

FIGURE 19-4. Acute cutaneous lupus erythematosus (ACLE) maculopapular eruption in a photosensitive pattern. (From Knight, L. (2013). *Medical terminology: An illustrated guide*. Philadelphia, PA: Wolters Kluwer.)

joints, lungs, blood vessels, heart, kidneys, liver, brain, and nervous system. SLE can have significant morbidity and potential mortality when associated with acute lupus erythematous as a manifestation (Box 19-1).

3. Drug-induced lupus may develop after taking certain medications. Symptoms usually resolve weeks to months after discontinuation of the drug (Figure 19-5).

4. Neonatal lupus erythematosus
   a. NLE is rare.
   b. Occurs in neonates with transplacentally acquired maternal anti-Ro (SS-A) and/or anti-La (SS-B) antibodies.
   c. Manifestations may include:
      (1) Congenital heart block
      (2) Cutaneous lesions
      (3) Liver disease
      (4) Thrombocytopenia

E. Lupus as a disease continuum
   1. CCLE is seen as the mild end of the spectrum with only localized lesions.
   2. SCLE presents with mild SLE.
   3. Active SLE with internal organ involvement (possible death), with or without skin lesions, is at the far end of the disease spectrum.

F. Diagnosis
   1. A complete history and physical should be performed, including a full-skin assessment.
   2. Currently, there is no single definitive laboratory test for lupus.

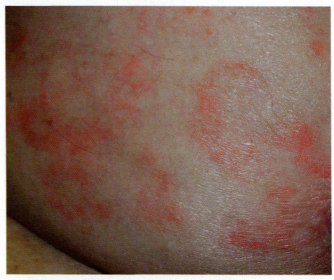

FIGURE 19-5. Drug-induced cutaneous lupus. (From Elder, D. E. (2014). *Lever's histopathology of the skin*. Philadelphia, PA: Wolters Kluwer.)

3. Lupus symptoms can mimic other illnesses and are often vague and transient, resulting in misdiagnosing and underdiagnosing of lupus.

4. The American College of Rheumatology and the Systemic Lupus International Collaborating Clinics issued a list of criteria to assist the practitioner in diagnosing SLE and to establish consistency for epidemiologic surveys (Box 19-1).

G. Pregnancy and lupus
   1. There is no reason why a woman with lupus should not become pregnant, unless she has organ involvement.
   2. There is risk of disease activity during and 3 to 4 weeks after pregnancy; therefore, she should be monitored closely.
   3. Many persons with lupus have antiphospholipid antibodies, which affect coagulation factors and are associated with miscarriage.

H. Diagnostic testing may include:
   1. CBC with differential.
   2. Platelet count.
   3. Erythrocyte sedimentation rate.
   4. Serum electrophoresis.
   5. Antinuclear antibodies (ANA) and LE cell tests.
   6. Anti–double-stranded deoxyribonucleic acid (anti-dsDNA) antibody: this is the most specific test for lupus and correlates with disease activity.
   7. Urine studies.
   8. C3 and C4 serum studies
   9. Chest x-rays.
   10. Skin biopsy for H&E. If not definitive, skin biopsy for direct immunofluorescence.
   11. Lupus anticoagulant and anticardiolipin tests.

I. Treatment
   1. Prevention is key to minimizing symptoms, reducing inflammation, and maintaining normal bodily functions.
      a. Avoid sun exposure/wear sunscreen to prevent rashes.

Box 19-1. **Criteria for the Diagnosis of Systemic Lupus Erythematosus**

Patient must meet four of the following criteria, including at least one immunologic criterion and at least one clinical criterion; or the patient has biopsy-proven nephritis compatible with systemic lupus in the presence of either antinuclear antibody or anti-double-stranded deoxyribonucleic acid.

Clinical criteria
Oral lesions
Nonscarring alopecia
Synovitis of the joints
Serositis of the lining around organs
Renal involvement
Neurological involvement
Hemolytic anemia
Leukopenia
Thrombocytopenia

Immunologic criteria
Elevated antinuclear antibodies
Elevated anti-double-stranded deoxyribonucleic acid
Anti-Smith antibodies
Antiphospholipid antibodies
Low complement
Direct Coombs (antiglobulin) test in the absence of hemolytic anemia

Adapted from Petri, M., Orbai, A. M., Alarcon, G. S., Gordon, C., Merrill, J. T., Fortin, P. R., ..., Magder, L. S. (2012). Derivation and validation of systemic lupus international collaborating clinics classification criteria for systemic lupus erythematosus. *Arthritis and Rheumatology*, 64(8), 2677–2686.

   b. Exercise regularly to prevent muscle weakness and fatigue.
   c. Participate in support groups and/or counseling to reduce stress.
   d. Eliminate negative habits, such as smoking, drinking, etc.
   e. Avoid artificial light sources, such as tanning beds.
2. Treatment is individualized and based upon presenting symptoms.
3. Treatments may include:
   a. Nonsteroidal anti-inflammatory drugs (NSAIDs).
   b. Acetaminophen.
   c. Corticosteroids (topical, systemic, or intralesional). Ultrapotent topical corticosteroids may be indicated even on the face.
   d. Topical immunomodulators such as pimecrolimus and tacrolimus.
   e. Antimalarials.
      (1) Hydroxychloroquine sulfate. Usual dose 200 mg one to two times daily. Dosage generally should not exceed 6.5 mg/kg/daily.
      (2) Chloroquine phosphate. Usual dose is 250 mg one to two times daily.
      (3) Quinacrine hydrochloride. Usual dose is 100 mg one to two times daily.
      (4) All antimalarials may cause eye toxicities. Patients should have eye examinations by optometrist/ophthalmologist every 6 months.
4. Extensive or persistent cutaneous disease
   a. Oral prednisone, oral retinoids, methotrexate, thalidomide, and azathioprine have all been utilized.
5. Systemic disease will be treated by rheumatology.
   a. Prednisone, azathioprine, mycophenolate mofetil, cyclophosphamide, cyclosporine, interferon, leflunomide, TNF alpha inhibitors, CD4 monoclonal antibodies, and bone marrow transplant have all been utilized.
6. Specific treatment for systemic disease involving organ may include antihypertensive medications, dietary changes to reduce hypertension, anticoagulants, and dialysis and or kidney transplant for renal failure.

PATIENT EDUCATION
Lupus Erythematosus

- Provide a comprehensive explanation of the disease process.
- Discuss medication side effects and report these to the provider.
- Acknowledge emotional stress and provide support.
- Provide patient and families with resources for education and support (Box 19-2).
- Encourage good nutrition to promote healing and well-being.
- Reinforce the need for routine skin evaluations and follow for disease process.

Box 19-2. Resources for Patients with Connective Tissue Disorders

American Autoimmune and Related Diseases

22100 Gratiot Avenue
Eastpointe, MI 48021
Phone: 586-776-3900
Toll Free: 800-598-4618
Email: aarda@aarda.org
www.aarda.org

American Skin Association, Inc.

6 East 43th Street, 28th Floor
New York, NY 10117
(800)499-SKIN fax (212)889-4959
Email: info@americanskin.org
www.americanskin.org

Inflammatory Skin Disease Institute

Inflammatory Skin Disorders
PO Box 1074, Newport News, VA 23601
(800)484-6800 ext.6321 fax (757)595-1842

Lupus Foundation of America, Inc.

9302 N. Meridian Street, Suite 203, Indianapolis
IN 46260
(317)-225-4000
www.lupus.org

National Institute of Arthritis, Musculoskeletal and Skin Diseases
Information Clearinghouse
National Institutes of Health

1 AMS Circle, Bethesda, MD 20892-3675
Phone: 301-495-4484
Toll free: 877-226-4267
Fax: 301-718-6366
Email: NIAMSinfo@mail.nih.gov
www.niams.nih.gov

National Organization for Rare Disorders

National Organization for Rare Disorders National
Headquarters
55 Kenosia Avenue
Danbury, CT 06810
Phone: 203-744-0100
http://rarediseases.org

Scleroderma Foundation

300 Rosewood Drive, Suite 105, Danvers, MA 01923
(800)-722-HOPE (4673)
Email: sfinfo@scleroderma.org
www.scleroderma.org

Scleroderma Research Foundation

220 Montgomery Street, Suite 1411, San Francisco,
CA 94104
(800)-441-CURE (2873)
www.srfcure.org

Myositis Association of America

1737 King Street, Suite 600
Alexandria, VA 22314
www.myositis.org

II. SCLERODERMA (SYSTEMIC SCLEROSIS)

A. Definition: Scleroderma (which literally means "hard skin") is a chronic, often progressive autoimmune disease, which can cause thickening and tightening of the skin by excessive collagen production. Scleroderma widely varies in severity; in some cases, internal organs such as the lungs, heart, kidneys, esophagus, and GI tract are seriously damaged.

B. Etiology and incidence
   1. The exact cause(s) of scleroderma is/are unknown, but multiple genetic and environmental factors likely do play a part in determining the risk of developing systemic scleroderma.
   2. Most patients do not have a family member with the disease.
   3. Females are affected 4:1 over males.
   4. *Localized* scleroderma is more common in children, whereas *systemic* scleroderma occurs more in adults.

C. Classifications of scleroderma
   1. Localized scleroderma
      a. Affects the collagen-producing cells in limited skin areas and usually spares the internal organs and blood vessels
      b. Occurs as patches of thickened skin: *morphea* (*see special note below*) or as *linear* scleroderma, a line of thickened skin that may extend down an arm or leg. If the line occurs on the forehead, it is called *en coup de sabre* ("cut of the saber") (Figure 19-6).
      c. Affects children more often than adults

      d. Topical treatment may consist of topical corticosteroids, topical immunomodulators, phototherapy, and pulse dye lasers.
      e. Systemic treatment for persistent and extensive lesions may include methotrexate either alone or with a combination of systemic steroids and phototherapy.
      f. *Special note*: Morphea is a mild, mostly benign, and self-limiting disease of the skin with less than a 1% chance of progressing to scleroderma. It is important to use proper terminology and not frighten patients/parents with the term scleroderma unless appropriately diagnosed by the practitioner.
   2. Systemic scleroderma (also called progressive systemic sclerosis)
      a. The immune system causes damage to small blood vessels and the collagen-producing cells throughout the body.
      b. The small blood vessels in the hands/fingers narrow or completely close, often causing slow healing and/or spontaneous ulcerations.
      c. Patients are often cold sensitive.
      d. 95% of patients with systemic scleroderma suffer from Raynaud phenomenon (intermittent attacks of ischemia of the extremities of the body, especially the fingers, toes, ears, and nose, characterized by severe blanching, cyanosis, redness, numbness, tingling, burning, and often pain).
      e. Scar tissue (scleroses) may occur in one or more organs including the heart, lung, skin, kidneys, or GI tract.

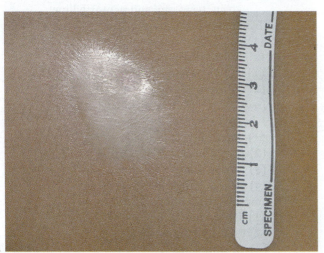

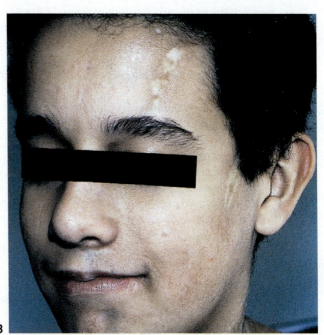

FIGURE 19-6. A: Morphea: well-demarcated white plaque. (From Goodheart, H. P. (2003). *Goodheart's photoguide of common skin disorders* (2nd ed.). Philadelphia, PA: Lippincott Williams & Wilkins.) **B:** Linear morphea: "coup de sabre" lesion. (From Lugo-Somolinos, A., Lee, I., McKinley-Grant, L., Goldsmith, L. A., Papier, A., Adigun, C. G., …, Fredeking, A. (2011). *VisualDx: Essential dermatology in pigmented skin*. Philadelphia, PA: Wolters Kluwer.)

    f. Systemic scleroderma is divided into two forms:
      (1) *Limited scleroderma* (often referred to as the CREST form): calcinosis (calcium deposits in the skin), Raynaud phenomenon (see above), esophageal dysfunction (acid in the esophagus—heartburn), sclerodactyly (tight, thick skin of the fingers), and telangiectasias (multiple, small, punctate macules that are particularly prominent on the face and hands).
      (2) *Diffuse scleroderma* has significantly greater organ involvement.
  3. Scleroderma-related disorders
    a. Scleroderma occurs in patients with other autoimmune disorders and may be referred to as an "overlap syndrome."
    b. Some studies suggest that exposure to various drugs (e.g., bleomycin) and chemicals can cause lesions similar to those seen in scleroderma. Often, these skin changes are indistinguishable from those of systemic sclerosis, and the exposure may be unknown to the patient.

D. Diagnosis of scleroderma
  1. Medical history
    a. A detailed history of signs/symptoms during general systems review that prompted medical services may indicate progression and severity of disease process.
    b. Question patient as to possible exposure to drugs or chemicals.
  2. Physical exam
    a. Full-skin exam: see above for detailed cutaneous manifestations of each category of scleroderma
      (1) Approximately 98% of patients will present with hardening or thickening of the skin of the fingers.
      (2) Raynaud phenomenon is present in 95% of patients.
    b. Systemic manifestations identified by a complete physical exam may include:
      (1) Gastrointestinal
        (a) Decreased motility/absorption
        (b) Esophageal dysphagia, reflux, and/or strictures
      (2) Pulmonary fibrosis
        (a) Decreased pulmonary function, vital capacity
        (b) Pulmonary hypertension
        (c) Dyspnea and decreased breath sounds
      (3) Renal vascular involvement: hypertension, insufficiency, or failure
      (4) Cardiovascular
        (a) Cardiac fibrosis with possible arrhythmias/myocardial infarction
        (b) Pericarditis
      (5) Musculoskeletal
        (a) Arthralgias
        (b) Myalgias

  3. Skin biopsy
    a. Confirms diagnosis of morphea
  4. Laboratory and radiologic tests for systemic scleroderma
    a. Complete blood count
    b. Urinalysis
    c. Renal function tests
    d. Chest radiograph
    e. Pulmonary function tests
    f. Barium swallow
    g. Antinuclear antibody test
      (1) Nucleolar staining is associated with mixed connective tissue disease.
      (2) Anticentromere staining is associated with CREST syndrome.
      (3) A positive Scl-70 antibody indicates diffuse scleroderma.

E. Treatment
  1. There is no cure for scleroderma; treatment plans are individualized to each patient's type and severity of symptoms.
  2. Medications are prescribed according to treatment goals:
    a. Control high blood pressure
      (1) ACE inhibitors
      (2) Angiotensin II inhibitors
      (3) Others: clonidine, prazosin
    b. Relieve pericarditis
      (1) NSAIDs
      (2) Corticosteroids
    c. Reduce joint and tendon pain
      (1) NSAIDs
      (2) Analgesics
      (3) Corticosteroids
    d. Prevent Raynaud phenomenon
      (1) Calcium channel blockers
      (2) Others: nitroglycerine ointment, prazosin, doxazosin, terazosin, and pentoxifylline
    e. Treat small bowel dysfunction
      (1) Broad-spectrum antibiotics
    f. Relieve constipation
      (1) Bulking agents
      (2) Softening agent
      (3) Others: lactulose, bisacodyl
    g. Prevent heartburn
      (1) Antacids
      (2) H_2 blockers
      (3) Proton pump inhibitors
      (4) Others: sucralfate, cisapride
    h. Improve swallowing difficulties
      (1) H_2 blockers
      (2) Proton pump inhibitor
      (3) GI stimulants
    i. Treat digital ulcerations
      (1) Oral/topical antibiotics
      (2) Recommendations from wound care specialist

j. Reduce skin itching
  (1) Skin lotions/emollients
  (2) Note: diphenhydramine not recommended as it may increase symptoms of dry eyes and dry mouth
k. Relieve dry mouth: saliva substitute
l. Relieve dry eyes: artificial tears/lubricants
m. Treat reactive depression
  (1) SSRIs
  (2) Tricyclic antidepressants
  (3) Others: bupropion, venlafaxine, and trazodone
3. Disease modifiers
  a. At present, there are no FDA-approved drugs to modify the course of scleroderma; however, there are several drugs currently under study.
  b. Currently, methotrexate, cyclosporin, as well as chemotherapy and immunosuppressants are being used to impair the immune and inflammatory response.
  c. Interferons (alpha and gamma) have been used to suppress collagen production, but there is no conclusive study to prove effectiveness.
  d. D-penicillamine is used to weaken collagen; however, studies done have been unable to prove effectiveness.

PATIENT EDUCATION
Scleroderma

- Provide education to both family and patient regarding medication protocols and possible side effects.
- Provide resources for education and support (Box 19-2).
- Continue to assess the patient for disease progression and emphasize the need for skin exams and follow-up.

III. INFLAMMATORY MYOPATHIES

A. Definition: Inflammatory myopathies are a group of muscle diseases characterized by inflammation of connective tissue and muscle fibers that can cause extensive necrosis and destruction of the muscle fibers. They are believed to be autoimmune disorders. The inflammatory myopathies are dermatomyositis (DM), juvenile dermatomyositis (JDMS), polymyositis (PM), and inclusion body myositis (IBM).
B. Etiology and incidence
  1. Inflammatory myopathies have been designated as autoimmune diseases because of the presence of autoantibodies in the serum of those affected.
  2. Prevalence rates are approximately 6 per 1,000,000 persons.
  3. Occurs in all ethnic groups
  4. PM and DM affect females 2:1 over males.
  5. PM rarely affects people under the age of 20.
  6. IBM symptoms usually begin after age 50 and occur in males more frequently than females.

C. Classifications and descriptions of inflammatory myopathies
  1. Dermatomyositis
    a. Easily recognized by distinctive rash: a patchy, dusky, reddish, or lilac rash on the eyelids with periorbital edema (heliotrope), cheeks, and bridge of nose. Gottron papules, small (<1 cm), flat, smooth, reddish/purplish papules found over joints such as knuckles, fingers, elbows, knees, and medial malleoli. Presence of Gottron papules is of diagnostic significance between DM and LE. Erythema of the hands in LE spares the joints (Figure 19-7).
    b. May also include several of the following signs/symptoms:
      (1) Proximal muscle weakness/pain usually follows rash and typically develops over a period of weeks.
      (2) Nail fold changes demonstrating ragged edges with telangiectasias
      (3) Poikiloderma of the scalp with pruritus
      (4) Elevated serum CK-MM and oral aldolase levels
      (5) Polyarthralgia/polyarthritis
      (6) Positive histidyl tRNA synthetase antibody
      (7) Raynaud phenomenon
      (8) Signs of systemic inflammation (fever: >37°C axillary, elevated CRP)
      (9) Myogenic EMG changes
      (10) Muscle biopsy reveals necrosis, inflammation, and degradation.
      (11) Skin biopsy reveals interface dermatitis with mucin.
      (12) Calcinosis cutis may occur in juvenile individuals.
      (13) Possible malignancy: malignant neoplasms in older individuals.
  2. Polymyositis (PM)
    a. Similar presentation as DM, but without characteristic rash
    b. Symmetrical muscle weakness, joint pain, difficulty in swallowing, fever, fatigue, and weight loss. Muscle weakness can begin slowly or suddenly and may worsen for weeks or months.
    c. Difficulty swallowing is common.
  3. Inclusion body myositis (IBM)
    a. Very similar in presentation to PM
    b. Only definitive test is muscle biopsy.
    c. Duration of illness greater than 6 months
    d. Age of onset greater than 30 years old
    e. Affects proximal and distal muscles of arms and legs
    f. Patient will exhibit one or more of the following:
      (1) Finger flex or weakness
      (2) Wrist flex or greater than wrist extension or weakness
      (3) Quadriceps muscle weakness
    g. Serum CK-MM less than 12 times normal

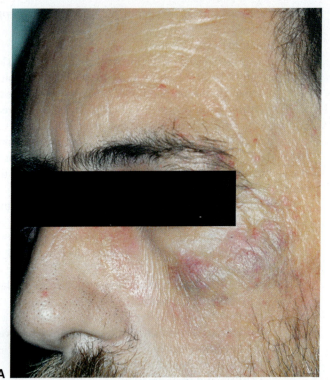
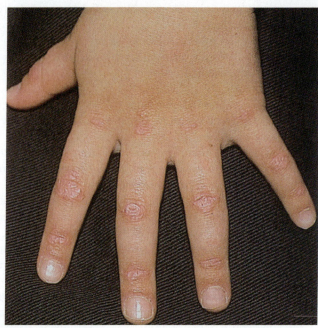

FIGURE 19-7. A: Heliotrope rash in dermatomyositis. **B:** Gottron papules erupting over the joints of extensor surfaces on the hands and fingers. (From Berg, D., & Worzala, K. (2006). *Atlas of adult physical diagnosis*. Philadelphia, PA: Lippincott Williams & Wilkins, with permission.)

4. Juvenile dermatomyositis
   a. Juvenile idiopathic inflammatory myopathy (JIIM) or JDMS usually presents as dermatomyositis (JDMS) with the distinctive heliotrope rash (see DM above).
   b. Proximal muscle weakness usually follows rash.
   c. Dysphagia and dysphonia (hoarseness) are common.
   d. Muscle pain occurs in approximately 50% of children.
   e. Abdominal pain and arthralgia can occur.
   f. Calcinosis cutis
5. DM sine myositis (amyopathic dermatomyositis)
   a. Variant of DM
   b. No muscle involvement
   c. Classic heliotrope rash is present.
   d. Increased incidence of malignancy is possible.
D. Treatment
   1. There is no known cure for inflammatory myopathies.
   2. High doses of immunosuppressants and/or steroids have been effective for many patients. Prednisone is most commonly used at 1 mg/kg/d with a slow taper over many months.
   3. Intravenous immunoglobulins (IVIg) have proven effective for those patients not responding to immunosuppressants.

4. Numerous new drugs are currently being studied.
5. Physical therapy is strongly recommended to maintain mobility.
6. Referral to nutritional therapist is recommended for dysphagia and nutritional assessment.
7. Topical steroids for lesions
8. Analgesics PRN for pain
9. Protection from ultraviolet light
10. Referral to internal medicine for age appropriate malignancy screenings and treatment if malignancies are identified.
11. Evaluate and treat for possible depression

PATIENT EDUCATION
Inflammatory Myopathies

- Evaluate and treat any pain on a routine basis.
- Provide a supportive environment.
- Assess for dysphagia at each patient encounter.
- Educate patient and family regarding medication side effects and reporting to provider any changes in condition.

BIBLIOGRAPHY

Callen, J. P., & Camisa, C. (2013). Antimalarial agents. In S. E. Wolverston (Ed.), *Comprehensive dermatologic drug therapy* (3rd ed., pp. 241–251). Philadelphia, PA: Saunders Elsevier.

Connolly, M. K. (2012). Systemic sclerosis (scleroderma) and related disorders. In J. L. Bolognia, J. L. Jorizzo, & J. V. Schaffer (Eds.), *Dermatology* (3rd ed., pp. 643–656). St. Louis, MO: Mosby Elsevier.

Fett, N. (2013). Morphea (localized scleroderma). *JAMA Dermatology, 149*(9), 1124.

Garza, R. M., & Jacobe, H. T. (2014). Morphea. In M. G. Lebwohl, W. R. Heymann, J. Berth-Jones, & I. Coulson (Eds.), *Treatment of skin diseases* (4th ed., pp. 183–187). Philadelphia, PA: Saunders Elsevier.

Gatto, M., Kiss, E., Naparstek, Y., & Doria, A. (2014). In/off label use of biologic therapy in systemic lupus erythematosus. *BMC Medicine, 12*, 30.

Habif, T. P. (2010). Connective tissue diseases. In T. P. Habif (Ed.), *Clinical dermatology* (5th ed., pp. 671–709). St. Louis, MO: Mosby Elsevier.

Hachulla, E., & Launay, D. (2011). Diagnosis and classification of systemic sclerosis. *Clinical Reviews in Allergy and Immunology, 40*(2), 78–83.

Jacobe, H. T., Sontheimer, R. D., & Saxton-Daniels, S. (2012). Autoantibodies encountered in patients with autoimmune connective tissue diseases. In J. L. Bolognia, J. L. Jorizzo, & J. V. Schaffer (Eds.), *Dermatology* (3rd ed., pp. 603–614). St. Louis, MO: Mosby Elsevier.

Jorrizzo, J. L., & Vleugels, R. A. (2012). Dermatomyositis. In J. L. Bolognia, J. L. Jorizzo, & J. V. Schaffer (Eds.), *Dermatology* (3rd ed., pp. 631–642). St. Louis, MO: Mosby Elsevier.

Lahouti, A. H., & Christopher-Stine, L. (2015). Polymyositis and dermatomyositis: Novel insights into the pathogenesis and potential therapeutic targets. *Discovery Medicine, 107*, 463–470.

Lee, L. A., & Werth, V. P. (2012). Lupus erythematosus. In J. L. Bolognia, J. L. Jorizzo, & J. V. Schaffer (Eds.), *Dermatology* (3rd ed., pp. 615–630). St. Louis, MO: Mosby Elsevier.

Li, S. C., Torok, K. S., Pope, E., Dedeoglu, F., Hong, S., Jacobe, H. T., …, Fuhlbrigge, R. C. (2012). Development of consensus treatment plans for juvenile localized scleroderma: A roadmap toward comparative effectiveness studies in juvenile localized scleroderma. *Arthritis Care and Research, 64*(8), 1175–1185.

Lin, J. H., & Dutz, J. P. (2007). Pathophysiology of cutaneous lupus erythematosus. *Clinical Reviews in Allergy and Immunology, 33*(1–2), 85–106.

Maverakis, E., Patel, F., Kronenberg, D. G., Chung, L., Hummers, L. K., Duong, C., …, Gershwin, M. E. (2014). International consensus criteria for the diagnosis of Raynaud's phenomenon. *Journal of Autoimmunity, 48–49*, 60–65.

Olsen, N. J., Yousif, M., Mutwally, A., Cory, M., Elmagboul, N., & Karp, D. R. (2013). Organ damage in high-risk patients with systemic and incomplete lupus syndromes. *Rheumatology International, 10*, 2585–2590.

Petri, M., Orbai, A. M., Alarcon, G. S., Gordon, C., Merrill, J. T., Fortin, P. R., …, Magder, L. S. (2012). Derivation and validation of systemic lupus international collaborating clinics classification criteria for systemic lupus erythematosus. *Arthritis and Rheumatism, 64*(8), 2677–2686.

Pope, J. E., & Jonson, S. R. (2015). New classification for systemic scleroderma. *Rheumatology Diseases Clinics of North America, 3*, 383–398.

Röcken, M., & Kaman G. (2012). Morphea and lichen sclerosis. In J. L. Bolognia, J. L. Jorizzo, & J. V. Schaffer (Eds.), *Dermatology* (3rd ed., pp. 657–670). St. Louis, MO: Mosby Elsevier.

Sartori-Valinotti, J. C., Tollefson, M. M., & Reed, A. M. (2013). Updates on morphea: Role of vascular injury and advances in treatment. *Autoimmune Diseases*, article ID: 467808. doi: 10.1155/2013/467808

Thiers, B. H. (2014). Discoid lupus erythematosus. In M. G. Lebwohl, W. R. Heymann, J. Berth-Jones, & I. Coulson (Eds.), *Treatment of skin diseases* (4th ed., pp. 193–194). Philadelphia, PA: Saunders Elsevier.

Vleugels, R. A., & Callen, J. P. (2014). Dermatomyositis. In M. G. Lebwohl, W. R. Heymann, J. Berth-Jones, & I. Coulson (Eds.), *Treatment of skin diseases* (4th ed., pp. 183–187). Philadelphia, PA: Saunders Elsevier.

Zaglout, S. S., Marraki, N. A. Y., & Goodfield, M. J. D. (2014). Scleroderma. In M. G. Lebwohl, W. R. Heymann, J. Berth-Jones, & I. Coulson (Eds.), *Treatment of skin diseases* (4th ed., pp. 703–706). Philadelphia, PA: Saunders Elsevier.

STUDY QUESTIONS

1. All of the following statements about lupus are true *except:*
   a. The exact cause of lupus is unknown.
   b. Lupus is often called a "woman's disease."
   c. Rash is a common symptom.
   d. Currently, there is no single test that can diagnose lupus.
   e. Sun exposure/ultraviolet light will help to eliminate skin lesions.

2. The ratio of lupus in women to men is:
   a. 3:1
   b. 5:1
   c. 9:1
   d. 15:1

3. Morphea is:
   a. Just another name for scleroderma
   b. A term to refer to discoid lesions associated with cutaneous lupus
   c. A skin disease with a less than 1% chance of progressing to systemic scleroderma
   d. A form of inflammatory myopathy, which typically occurs in adult men
   e. A severe form of Raynaud phenomenon

4. Which of the following terms is *not* part of the CREST acronym?
   a. Calcinosis
   b. Raynaud phenomenon
   c. Esophageal dysfunction
   d. Sclerodactyly
   e. Trigeminal

5. Which of the following diseases is associated with a heliotrope rash?
   a. Inclusion body myositis (IBM)
   b. Systemic lupus erythematosus (SLE)
   c. Systemic scleroderma
   d. Dermatomyositis (DM)
   e. Acne vulgaris

6. Malignancies associated with dermatomyositis are more common in which of the following populations?
   a. Older adult patients.
   b. Juvenile patients.
   c. It does not occur in any type of patient with dermatomyositis.
   d. Its occurrence is equal between older adults and juvenile patients.

7. Which of the following medications are used in the treatment of SLE?
   a. Anti-inflammatory drugs.
   b. Corticosteroids.
   c. Antimalarials.
   d. Cytotoxic or immunosuppressive drugs.
   e. All of the above are used to treat SLE.

8. Raynaud phenomenon can best be described as which of the following?
   a. A syndrome in which mothers with SLE pass along the genetic trait for lupus
   b. Intermittent attacks of ischemia of the extremities of the body, especially the fingers, toes, ears, and nose
   c. An inflammation involving a spinal nerve root, resulting in pain and hyperesthesia
   d. Discoid-shaped plaques that occur on the trunk in patients suffering from inflammatory diseases
   e. A condition of abnormally increased muscle tone or strength

9. A patient is suspected of having an autoimmune connective tissue disorder. A clinical sign of erythema on the dorsal hands and fingers that *spares* the joints is associated with which of the following?
   a. Dermatomyositis
   b. Scleroderma
   c. Morphea
   d. Lupus erythematosus

10. The inflammatory myopathies include all of the following *except:*
    a. Coccidioidomycosis
    b. Inclusion body myositis
    c. Dermatomyositis
    d. Polymyositis
    e. Juvenile dermatomyositis

Answers to Study Questions: 1.c, 2.c, 3.c, 4.e, 5.d, 6.a, 7.e, 8.b, 9.d, 10.a

Bullous and Vesicular Diseases

Constance L. Hayes

OBJECTIVES

After studying this chapter, the reader will be able to:

- Distinguish between the different disease processes of pemphigus vulgaris, bullous pemphigoid, epidermolysis bullosa, epidermolysis bullosa acquisita, and dermatitis herpetiformis.
- Describe the tools available to make the diagnosis of pemphigus vulgaris, bullous pemphigoid, epidermolysis bullosa, epidermolysis bullosa acquisita, and dermatitis herpetiformis.
- Define the therapeutic interventions used in treating pemphigus vulgaris, bullous pemphigoid, epidermolysis bullosa, epidermolysis bullosa acquisita, and dermatitis herpetiformis.
- Identify the nursing interventions that assist in providing optimal care to patients.
- Discuss the health maintenance important to patient/families with bullous/vesicular diseases.

KEY POINTS

- Bullous and vesicular skin diseases can be acute but are primarily chronic blister-forming diseases. A genetic defect or immunological event causes a break in continuity within the epidermis or epidermal junction.
- Topical treatments, drug therapies, and specific diagnostics are the cornerstone for health care management in bullous diseases.
- Assessment for skin and systemic infections is imperative in all phases of care with impaired skin integrity.
- Close monitoring of drug therapies for side effects and nutritional needs for growth/skin repair of the patient is essential.
- Lesion biopsies, direct immunoflourescent studies, and blood studies are indicated for accurate diagnosis and treatment plans.
- *Pemphigus vulgaris* is an autoimmune "intraepidermal" reaction against connections between epidermal cells. It has two distinct forms: *P. vulgaris*, the most common and severe with flaccid, fragile vesicles/bullae, which scab and heal without scaring, and *P. foliaceus*, less severe, superficial vesicles and crusted erosions that are absent in the mucosal areas.
- Bullous pemphigoid is an autoimmune "subepidermal" reaction against epithelial cell attachments to the basement membrane and presents with subepidermal,

intact, tense bullae that are less fragile and less severe than the group of ruptured, scabbed *P. vulgaris* bullae.
- The "onion skin" approach describes a system to classify existing and newly identified genes and clinical phenotypes of inherited epidermal bullosa diseases.
- Dermatitis herpetiformis is "virtually always" associated with celiac disease.
- A multidisciplinary team of health care professions are needed to develop a workable comprehensive and optimal skin care plan for the patient and family.

PEMPHIGUS VULGARIS

I. OVERVIEW

A. Definition: Acute or chronic Pemphigus vulgaris (PV) is a rare, yet, serious bullous, autoimmune intradermal disease of the skin and mucous membranes caused by autoantibodies against the connections between cells in the epidermis.

B. Etiology
   1. PV is due to autoimmune antibodies (IgG) against plakoglobin and desmogleins (desmoglein-1 and desmoglein-3—Dsg1, Dsg3), which are glycoproteins that help connect skin cells together. These are found in skin and mucous membrane keratinocytes at the spot desmosome location.
      a. Dsg3 is more involved with mucous membrane disease.
   2. Spot desmosomes, containing the desmogleins are found at the intracellular junctions in the stratum spinosum. In PV the desmogleins, Dsg1 and Dsg3, are not able to connect keratinocyte squamous cells together.
   3. A genetic association has been proven through immunogenetics.
   4. Additionally, various drugs may induce PV: antibiotics (penicillins, cephalosporin, rifampin), thiol drugs (captopril, enalapril, lisinopril, piroxicam, penicillamine), and pyrazolone derivatives (phenylbutazone, oxyphenbutazone).

C. Pathophysiology
   1. Dsg1 and Dsg3 are glycoproteins in the desmosome of the keratocyte that "glue connecting skin cells" together. In PV, circulating IgG autoantibodies bind to the cell surface of keratinocytes in the lower part of the

epidermis and prevent Dsg3 specifically from providing its function of cell-to-cell adhesion.

2. These autoantibodies affect the spot desmosomes by disrupting and preventing connections between keratinocyte squamous cells of the epidermis, causing large, flaccid, superficial and fragile, intraepidermal bullae that rupture easily and scab.

3. Two variants of this disease are pemphigus vegetans (PVe) (a thickened verrucous-like change), which carries Dsg3 glycoprotein only, and pemphigus foliaceus (PF) (a more superficial variant), which carries Dsg1 glycoprotein only (Figure 20-1).

4. PV bullae are quite fragile and superficial as the roof consists of a thin portion of the upper epidermis that when dessicated leaves painful erosions with scabs that heal without scarring.

5. Painful oral erosions typically precede the skin blisters in PV by weeks or months.

6. PV is characterized by acute exacerbations and remissions, oftentimes requiring lifelong therapy. Severe cases can result in secondary infection and fluid loss.

7. Immunoflourescent biopsy indicates an *intraepidermal* pattern with a lacy outline of individual epidermal cells as autoantibodies bind to the junctions between the cells.

8. PF is less common and less severe with superficial vesicles that have crusted erosions, which are absent in the mucosal areas.

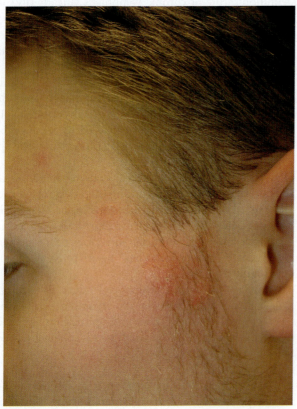

FIGURE 20-1. Pemphigus foliaceus, preauricular lesions. (Image provided by Stedman's.)

D. Incidence
1. Usually occurs in 40- to 60-year-old persons; more common in people of Jewish, Mediterranean, and Indian decent
2. Equal incidence in males and in females
3. PV is the most common and most severe type.

E. Considerations across the lifespan
1. PV in pregnancy, otherwise known as pemphigoid gestationis (PG), is remarkably rare; yet, it is associated with increased risk of stillbirths, infant death, and intrauterine growth restriction (IUGR). As an autoimmune subepidermal blistering disease, there is a genetic susceptibility and hormonal influence from pregnancy, parturition, and oral contraceptives that are implicated in its etiology.
2. Neonatal PV may afflict up to 2% to 4% of infants born to mothers with PV; it is thought to occur from passive transplacental transfer of maternal antidesmoglein IgG antibodies to the fetus, which resolves with a few weeks of birth.

II. ASSESSMENT

A. History and physical examination
1. Vesicles and bullae are flaccid, easily ruptured, and weeping and arise on normal or erythematous skin. Subsequent erosions can bleed easily. Crusts may form and can affect any skin surface including the scalp.
2. The arrangement is randomly scattered, but there is a high propensity for oral mucosa; esophageal or vulvar involvement may occur.
3. Nikolsky sign is positive: Dislodging of the epidermis occurs with the application of lateral finger pressure where a vesicle is located, which leads to an extension of the vesicle and/or removal of epidermis (erosion). (This test is no longer used since it is nonspecific and because it creates an additional lesion.)

B. Specific skin changes
1. PV manifests with superficial erosions and flaccid weeping blistering or bullous lesions, 1 to 3 cm, that rupture easily, leaving denuded areas that crust.
2. Bullae may form from normal-looking skin or an erythematous base, with a predilection for seborrheic skin areas—face, midchest, and upper back.
3. Mucous membranes may involve mouth, vaginal, perianal, and conjunctiva. Site of first lesions may be oral mucosa, occurring in 50% to 70% with PV (Figure 20-2).
4. Symptoms of burning and/or pain occur in affected areas. Conjunctival involvement, which is rare, manifests with photophobia, irritation, and pain.
5. Patients may experience weakness, malaise, and weight loss especially if there is prolonged oral mucosal involvement.

C. Differential diagnosis
1. Include most bullous presentations: bullous pemphigoid, epidermolysis bullosa acquisita (EBA), dermatitis herpetiformis (DH), erythema multiforme, Grover

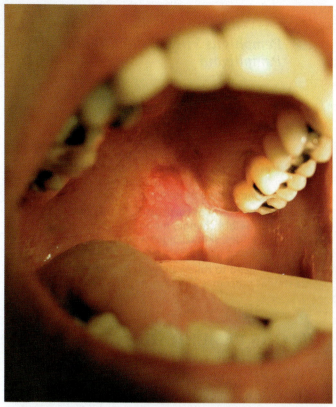

FIGURE 20-2. Pemphigus vulgaris. The first lesions may be in the oral mucosa. (From Dr. Barankin Dermatology Collection.)

disease, Hailey-Hailey disease, Darier disease, pemphigus erythematous, and pemphigus foliaceus.
2. Similar immune disorders: linear IgA dermatosis and IgA pemphigus.

D. Diagnostic tests
1. Biopsy the edge of an early small bulla or, if not present, the margin of a larger bulla or erosion for histopathological light microscopy. There is a loss of intercellular cohesion (acantholysis) in the desmosomes of the keratinocytes near the bottom of the epidermis.
2. Direct immunofluorescence (DIF) testing is performed on a perilesional skin biopsy to detect IgG antibodies against Dsg1 and Dsg3; a lace-like pattern outlining individual cells develops where autoantibodies bind at the junctions between cells.
3. Enzyme-linked immunosorbent assay (ELISA) can help detect autoantibodies to Dsg1 and Dsg3 and is helpful to direct therapy (medication dosing) as it usually correlates with activity of the disease.
4. Complete blood counts (CBC) for leukocytosis, albumin, and electrolyte panels for disease management of potential infections, electrolyte, and protein losses/imbalance.
5. Prior to initiating corticosteroid or immunosuppressive therapies, secure chest x-ray, serum glucose, tuberculin skin test, and CBC.
6. In PV, significant esophageal symptoms or even strictures may occur, which would necessitate endoscopy and/or biopsy.

III. COMMON THERAPEUTIC MODALITIES

A. Systemic therapy
1. Systemic corticosteroids for blister suppression are the principal method of treatment with oral starting doses of 0.5 to 1.0 mg/kg. The dose may be doubled until remission is achieved.
2. Intravenous immunoglobulin (IVIG) has been used as second-line therapy where oral medication approaches were ineffective, are contraindicated (as in pregnancy), or had caused significant side effects.
3. Azathioprine immuno-suppressant 1 to 3 mg/kg/d, immunosuppressant may help during pregnancy when trying to minimize systemic steroid therapy for severe cases.

B. Local or topical therapy
1. Topical corticosteroids (both as creams or ointments on the skin and gel or liquid for mucosal lesions) can be beneficial for pruritic and erythematous areas.
2. Intralesional steroids may be used for resistant localized lesions.
3. Topical antibiotic creams or ointments such as silver sulfadiazine or mupirocin for blisters or erosions.
4. Medicated baths (e.g., potassium permanganate [$KMNO_4$] or oilated oatmeal) and/or wet dressings (aluminum subacetate, $KMNO_4$, or Domeboro solution) are useful for their antibacterial and cleansing effects, change every 2 hours.

C. Medical intervention
1. Primary goal for treatments: Reduce autoantibody synthesis by immune system.
2. Immediate start of high-dose systemic corticosteroids with tapering after good clinical response over several months. Adding immunomodulators or antimetabolites can help prevent significant steroid side effects.
3. In widespread disease, electrolytes of sodium, chloride, calcium may decrease while potassium increases. Secure electrolyte panel.
4. Patients with significant impetiginization of the eroded areas may show an increased WBC count. Secure CBC and check platelets with certain drug therapies.
5. Patients treated with systemic corticosteroids or biological immunomodulators should be placed on calcium and vitamin D, screened annually for tuberculosis/HIV, have comprehensive blood work and blood pressures every six months for close monitoring.
6. Patients with severe cases may require hospitalization on an inpatient dermatology unit or burn unit. Plasmapheresis can be used in conjunction with corticosteroids for more rapid control in extremely severe cases.

D. Medication—drug therapy
1. Immunosuppressants such as methotrexate, 20 to 50 mg per week; cyclophosphamide orally 1 to 3 mg/kg/d; or cyclosporine are generally used for remission induction or as an adjunct to steroid therapy.
2. Biologic immune response modifiers, like rituximab or mycophenolate mofetil, help reduce autoantibody synthesis and can be added to systemic steroid therapy.

3. Alternatives to immunosuppressives include diamino-diphenylsulfone, tetracycline, or minocycline, which are used alone or in combination with high-dose steroids.

4. Less frequently, antimalarial drugs such as chloroquine, hydroxychloroquine, or a combination of both are used.

E. Diet management

1. Support nutritious diet to replace protein and fluid losses from erosions. Full liquid or mechanical soft diets in acute phases with oral lesions are helpful.

2. High-protein liquid nutritional supplements are easily ingested until ulcers heal.

3. Provide topical anesthetic (viscous lidocaine) as an oral rinse prior to meals, in 4.

4. Use sponge swabs for oral hygiene when soft bristle toothbrushes are not tolerated.

F. Surgical interventions. None noted.

G. Supportive skin care

1. Continuous wet dressings, changed every 2 to 3 hours, prevent the dressing from drying/adhering to the skin and are preferred over "wet-to-dry" dressings.

2. Apply creams or ointments to dressings rather than eroded skin to reduce pain when changing dressings; may switch to body temperature lotions or dusting powder if creams or ointments are not tolerated

3. Refrain from using any tape that may exacerbate bullae formation.

4. Maintain body temperature with warm wet dressings, wrap quickly with towels.

H. Other nursing interventions

1. Explain need to monitor progress on latent infection reactivation or current infection exacerbation.

2. Assess patient/family's financial ability to provide balanced diet and supplements and proper skin care supplies with dressings and creams.

3. Assess patient/family's understanding and motivation to perform recommended treatments with available home bathing facilities.

I. Complimentary alternative medicine (consult primary provider before use)

1. Swedish bitters liquid may relieve tongue blisters by diluting 1 tablespoon in a glass of water or herbal tea swish/gargle prior to eating and as needed.

2. Soap wart (natural plant, *saponaria officinalis*): Cleanse blistered skin with soap wart solution of 1 teaspoon soap wart to 1 cup tepid water; drying naturally helps eliminate toxins.

IV. HOME CARE CONSIDERATIONS

A. Continuity of care concerns

1. Develop an achievable care plan with the patient/family for regular follow-ups and emphasize need to comply with all provisions of the treatment regimen.

2. Identify if the patient is able to care for self or identify a caregiver.

3. Call patients routinely during the acute phase to assess and prevent complications.

4. Provide contact numbers of provider(s) for patient inquiries and a 24-hour telephone number for emergencies.

PATIENT EDUCATION
Pemphigus Vulgaris and Bullous Pemphigoid

- Teach proper aseptic skin care techniques with patient/family members to avoid potential skin infections and allow for return demonstration opportunities.

- Explain the need to avoid individuals with infectious processes (flu, colds, coughs, skin infections, like herpes simplex lesions) especially since most therapies involve some degree of immunosuppression.

- Review side effects of corticosteroid therapies (GI bleed, weight change, mood swings, acne, bone density changes, skin changes with overuse, and steroid-induced diabetes).

- Reinforce need to follow up with providers to assess treatment outcomes and prevent infections.

BULLOUS PEMPHIGOID

I. OVERVIEW

A. Definition. Bullous pemphigoid (BP) is an uncommon, autoimmune, subepidermal blistering disease that mainly afflicts the elderly.

B. Etiology

1. BP is due to antibodies directed against the basement membrane zone of the epidermis (the "foundation" of the skin), creating subepidermal, mostly intact and less fragile, tense bullae than PV.

2. Drug reactions may induce BP: furosemide, penicillin, captopril, B-blockers, sulfonamides, terbinafine, penicillamine, NSAIDs, and potassium iodide.

C. Pathophysiology

1. Autoantibodies in BP, IgG, and, in some cases, IgA mediate tissue-destructive proteases, BPA1 and BPA2, against "hemidesmosomes" (intracellular junctions which attach epithelial cells to the dermis basement membrane).

2. BP can be self-limiting and may go into remission 2 to 6 years after onset.

3. Immunoflourescent findings include a line at the BSE of the epidermis (not the lace-like pattern outlining epidermal cells as seen in PV).

4. Variants of BP are:

a. Localized—usually limited to lower extremities and responds well to treatment; may progress to generalized disease.

b. Benign mucosal pemphigoid—synonym for cicatricial pemphigoid or scarring pemphigoid; recurring bullae either on a mucous membrane or on the skin near an orifice; and has the tendency to scar.

D. Incidence

1. Rarely seen in children, BP usually presents in adults over the age of 60 to 70 years.

2. Estimated incidence is 7 to 14 per 100,000 per year, afflicting men more than women by 2:1 in some studies.

II. ASSESSMENT

A. History and physical examination
   1. Presents as a chronic blistering eruption on an inflammatory or urticarial base.
   2. Manifests with tense, intact, serum-filled bullae on normal and erythematous skin that rupture easily—but less fragile than PV bullae.
   3. Urticarial plaques and papules can precede bullae formation by months.
   4. The distribution is generalized or localized; small oral ulcers occur infrequently.
   5. The sites of predilection are generally flexural and include axillae, medial aspects of thighs and groin, flexor aspects of forearms, and lower legs.
   6. Remissions in most adults occur within 5 years, more rapidly in children.

B. Specific skin/nail changes (Figure 20-3)
   1. Begins as a hive-like preblistering rash where pruritus and nonspecific eczematous or papular lesions can precede the bullae.
   2. Pruritic fixed urticarial plaques and tense bullae can be seen together; when the latter rupture, erosions can occur.
   3. Oral lesions involved in 10% to 35%, much less common than PV.
   4. Nail dystrophy associated with BV includes hyperkeratosis, shedding, hemorrhage, and horizontal ridging.

C. Differential diagnosis
   1. Dermatitis-herpetiformis (DH), drug-induced bullous disorder, epidermolysis bullosa (EB), EBA, erythema multiforme, and linear IgA dermatosis. At the beginning or presentation, erythema multiforme, fixed drug reaction, impetigo, or viral (varicella in adults) rash may resemble DH.

D. Diagnostic tests
   1. Biopsy of a skin lesion shows subepidermal blister with inflammation and edema. The blisters usually contain a mixture of eosinophils and polymorphonuclear leukocytes.

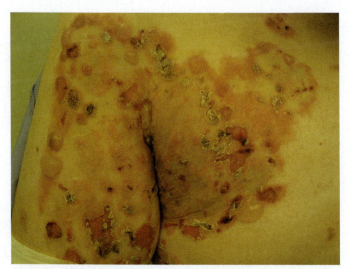

FIGURE 20-3. Bullous pemphigoid on the chest and arm. (From Dr. Barankin Dermatology Collection.)

   2. Direct immunofluorescence biopsy of perilesional skin shows immunoreactants at the basement membrane in a fine line (in contrast to the lacy pattern outlining epidermal cells found in PV).
   3. In 70% of patients, circulating antibasement membrane IgG antibodies are detected by indirect immunofluorescence. Antibody titers typically do not correlate with the course of the disease.

III. COMMON THERAPEUTIC MODALITIES

A. Systemic therapy
   1. Systemic corticosteroids, starting at 50 to 100 mg/day, are usually given orally until clear and in lower doses than used in PV unless the disease is severe. Then, pulse IV steroids with immunosuppressives and/or immunomodular therapies are indicated.
   2. Severe and refractory cases may require immunomodulators, immunosuppressive drug treatments, and possible IV immunoglobulin therapy or plasmapheresis.

B. Local or topical therapy
   1. Topical treatment is the same as for PV.
   2. Intralesional corticosteroids may be beneficial in localized lesions.

C. Medical intervention
   1. Treatment goals are primarily to arrest blistering by reducing autoantibody synthesis in the immune system, decrease itching, protect the skin from further inflammation, and prevent infection.
   2. Team approach with dermatologist, primary care provider, and nursing care is important to monitor disease progression.
   3. Those treated with systemic corticosteroids should be placed on calcium and vitamin D, screened annually for tuberculosis, and closely monitored for blood pressures and serum glucose levels.
   4. Admission to an inpatient dermatology unit or burn unit may be indicated in severe cases.

D. Medication—drug therapy
   1. Very potent topical steroids are indicated, safe and effective in BP.
   2. Nicotinamide (vitamin B_3, niacin) in association with minocycline, doxycycline, or tetracycline may be used when corticosteroids are contraindicated.
   3. Erythromycins, penicillins, dapsone, sulfonamides, or methotrexate 2.5 to 10 mg orally per week
   4. Topical immunomodulators, like tacrolimus, may be helpful in mild cases or local.

E. Diet management
   1. Provide balanced diet high in vitamin C and B complex, protein, and fluids to replace protein and fluid losses from erosions.

F. No surgical interventions

G. Supportive skin care
   1. Provide care as outlined for PV.

H. Other nursing interventions. Provide care as outlined for PV.

I. Complimentary alternative medicine. Follow care as outlined for PV.

IV. HOME CARE CONSIDERATIONS

A. Continuity of care concerns. Follow care guidelines as in PV.

B. Patient teaching. Follow PV guidelines.

EPIDERMOLYSIS BULLOSA

I. OVERVIEW

A. Definition. EB is a group of heterogeneous, inheritable disorders characterized by abnormal mechanical fragility of the skin and mucosa membranes.

B. Etiology

1. The cause of EB is due to distinct mutations in 10 different genes encoding skin structure proteins such that proper attachment of the epidermis to the dermis does not occur.

2. The classification system for hereditary EB was updated in 2014 to maintain the four major types with many subtypes defined by inheritance patterns, histology, and gene mutations so as to provide a starting point to identify EBA.

3. EB acquisita (EBA) represents a similar disorder acquired (thus, "acquisita") later in life. EBA is an autoimmune condition, where antibodies are directed against type VII collagen.

C. Pathophysiology

1. At birth or during infancy, patients with EB present with blisters at sites of minor trauma or may appear spontaneously. Patients with EBA have similar manifestations later in life.

2. Depending on the specific type, the patient may only occasionally have blisters with little effect on health or lifestyle. Those patients with severe types have widespread cutaneous and mucosal blisters, which can be fatal.

3. The bullae may be nonscarring or scarring. The disorder has been compared to a chronic burn.

4. The most common complications are chronic iron deficiency anemia, malnutrition, growth retardation, and respiratory, GI, and GU blisters and erosions.

D. Incidence

1. Estimates range from 1 in 50,000 to 1 in 100,000 births for types of EB presenting at birth or early childhood when child starts to crawl, walk, and run or when young adult becomes more physically active.

2. Equal incidence in males and in females.

II. ASSESSMENT

A. History and physical examination

1. Classification of EB is based on the pattern of inheritance and ultrastructural level of blistering. There are over several dozen subtypes of gene mutations.

2. Four major classifications.

   a. EB simplex: (1) localized or (2) generalized; both afflict epidermis basal layer and are autosomal dominant.

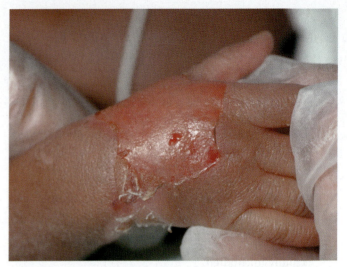

FIGURE 20-4. Large erosion after blistering in Bart syndrome, a type of epidermolysis bullosa. (From Lugo-Somolinos, A., et al. (2011). *VisualDx: Essential dermatology in pigmented skin.* Philadelphia, PA: Wolters Kluwer.)

   b. Junctional EB (JEB): (1) lethal or (2) nonlethal; both are autosomal recessive.

   c. Dystrophic EB (DEB): (1) dominant or (2) recessive; both afflict the dermis and follow its named genetic pattern.

   d. Kindler syndrome is mixed in its location and is autosomal recessive.

B. Cutaneous involvement (Figures 20-4, 20-5, and 20-6)

1. EB simplex, localized, has the most superficial mild blistering, mainly on hands and feet, rarely mucosa involvement, and blisters heal without scaring unless secondary infection occurs.

2. Recessive JEB (RJEB) exhibits a wide range of severity: Common to all subtypes of RJEB are oral involvement, atrophy at sites of repeated injury, nail dystrophy, and dysplastic enamel.

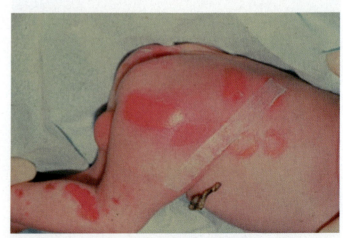

FIGURE 20-5. Epidermolysis bullosa congenita. (From Dr. Barankin Dermatology Collection.)

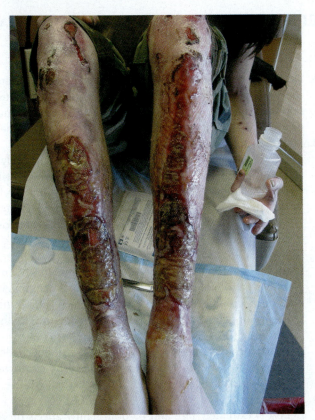

FIGURE 20-6. Dominant dystrophic epidermolysis bullosa of legs. (Image provided by Stedman's.)

3. Dominant DEB exhibits repeated blistering–scarring (cigarette paper–like), milia, enamel defects, and dystrophic nails.
4. Recessive dystrophic EB (RDEB) usually presents at birth with generalized blistering and erosions, involves multiple extracutaneous and deformity sites, and has increased risk to develop invasive cutaneous squamous cell carcinoma in areas of chronic erosions. RDEB with high mortality exhibit "Mitten" deformities (hand and feet) and severe respiratory/gastrointestinal tract scarring.
5. Kindler syndrome is autosomal recessive EB—exhibits poikiloderma, blisters in trauma areas, mucosal inflammation, photosensitivity, stenosis, and dental problems.
6. Nikolsky sign is positive.

C. Differential diagnoses
1. Bullous impetigo, staphylococcal scalded skin syndrome, autoimmune blistering disorders of infancy, and epidermolytic ichthyosis.

D. Diagnostic tests
1. Biopsy of a fresh blister (<24 hours old) for routine histology, direct immunofluorescence (to rule out other immunobullous diseases), and electron microscopy
2. Immunochemistry of basement membrane zone antigens to detect some forms of junctional EB
3. A positive family history is helpful in establishing the diagnosis but will be negative in patients with types caused by a new mutation and in patients with recessive

forms who are born to unaffected parents carrying the disease.
4. Prenatal diagnosis has been successfully performed on fetuses at risk for all major forms of EB. Diagnosis is made via skin biopsy obtained through fetoscopy from a fetus at risk—DNA is analyzed for characteristic abnormalities of EB.

III. COMMON THERAPEUTIC MODALITIES

A. Systemic therapy
1. Corticosteroids orally; psoralens in combination with UVA irradiation, vitamin E, cyclosporine, antimalarials, and retinoids may be beneficial to promote healing.

B. Local or topical therapy
1. Cleansing areas of blistering and erosions with saline or water and gentle debridement; covering wounds with nonadherent dressings.
2. Rotate antibiotic ointments for skin infections taking care not to treat prophylactically.
3. Other useful topical agents are silver sulfadiazine and fusidic acid. Nonadhering dressings or Vaseline-impregnated gauze secured by roller gauze will decrease trauma to the affected body part. Only the involved area should be treated.

C. Medical intervention
1. EB care is mainly supportive: avoid trauma, manage blisters, and wound care (padding soft clothing, no adhesive use).
2. Multidisciplinary team helps coordinate care and monitor for complications.
3. Supportive treatment includes optimal nutritional management with all patients but especially those patients with oral lesions, esophageal scarring, and gastric outlet obstruction.
4. Premedication with mild analgesics such as acetaminophen may be useful for young patients prior to bathing and wound care.
5. Older children and adults with recessive DEB must have periodic full-body skin exams with biopsy of nonhealing ulcers to exclude invasive squamous cell cancers.

D. Medication—drug therapy
1. Topical agents to provide healing and wound infection as described above.
2. An allogenic composite cultured skin can be used to treat hands and donor sites in patients with RDEB.

E. Diet management
1. Provide written plan of what constitutes a healthy diet to enhance child growth.
2. Encourage foods high in iron (meats, vegetables, fruits), combining these with vitamin C foods/liquids to aid iron absorption. Refrain from drinking tea that binds iron when ingested together.

F. Supportive skin care
1. Daily wound care is a major challenge for the EB patient and caregiver. Rotating topical antibiotics will decrease emergence of resistant bacterial strains and decrease incidence of developing a contact sensitivity.

2. Lance to drain blisters by placing small window at its base can relieve pressure and promote healing, while judicious oral antibiotic use avoids chronic treatment.

G. Other nursing interventions
   1. Nursing care must include interventions targeted to pain, nutrition, high risk for infections due to trauma-related blistering, and impaired skin integrity.
   2. Include child in the teaching process, with information provided geared to the child's developmental level.
   3. Premedicate with mild analgesia 45 minutes prior to bathing and wound care.
   4. Well-lubricated gloves help prevent trauma to fragile skin during skin care.

H. Complimentary alternative medicine
   1. An oral solution of viscous lidocaine/Mylanta/Benadryl (magic mouthwash) prior to eating may reduce pain.
   2. St. John's Wort tea leave oral solution rinse can sooth mouth blisters.

IV. HOME CARE CONSIDERATIONS (FOLLOW PV GUIDELINES)

A. Continuity of care concerns
   1. Same care concerns as PV.
   2. Referral to a multidisciplinary team of a grief counselor, dietician, geneticist, social worker, physical therapist, and home nurse as specified by disease severity.
   3. Referral to Dystrophic EB Research Association (DEBRA) is helpful as an information clearinghouse for the patient and caregiver.

PATIENT EDUCATION

Epidermolysis Bullosa and Epidermolysis Bullosa Acquisita

- Identify and demonstrate techniques whereby parents can feed infants/toddlers minimizing skin trauma and promote nurturing and healing.
- Teach medication/relaxation techniques to help diminish pain in bathing/dressing change; distraction is helpful for young children.
- Discuss aseptic technique with strict handwashing in patient care to prevent skin infection.
- Patients with EBA may experience partial remissions with periods of exacerbation, yet most can live a normal lifespan with proper care and treatment. Consider genetic testing for clients of childbearing age for future family planning.
- Primary goals of care are to stop and prevent blistering, scarring, and complications by minimizing physical trauma to skin surfaces.

EPIDERMOLYSIS BULLOSA ACQUISITA

I. OVERVIEW

A. Definition: Epidermolysis Bullosa Acquisita (EBA) is a rare, chronic subepidermal autoimmune blistering disease of the skin and mucous membranes associated with autoimmunity to type VII collagen in the basement membrane zone.

B. Etiology
   1. EBA results from an acquired dysfunction of the body's immune system, which attacks its own anchoring fibrils in the subepidermis with antibodies (IgG and rarely IgA) that cause blisters to form after mechanical trauma. In a few cases, drug therapy is a cause, and in most cases, the cause is unknown.

C. Pathophysiology
   1. In EBA, autoimmune antibodies (IgG mainly) bind with type VII collagen, the major structural component of anchoring fibrils, that prevents the anchoring fibrils in the upper dermis to adhese the epidermis to the dermis.
   2. Four types have been identified: (a) classic mechanobullous, (b) bullous pemphigoid-like, (c) cicatricial pemphigoid-like, and (d) IgA bullous dermatosis-like.

D. Incidence
   1. EBA is extremely rare and predominantly affects those in 4th to 5th decade of life but can occur in any age.
   2. Black Americans of African descent have higher EBA when shown to have a genetic marker, HLA-DRB1.
   3. Male: female ratio is not known; yet, the incidence is 1 in 4 million people.

II. ASSESSMENT

A. History and physical examination
   1. Classification of EBA is based on the pattern of inflammatory versus noninflammatory presentations and location of blistering.
   2. Diagnosis is by clinical findings, routine histology, direct immunofluorescence, indirect immunofluorescence, and split-skin direct immunofluorescence testing.
   3. Other health problems commonly experienced by patients with EBA are Crohn disease, multiple myeloma, amyloidosis, and systemic lupus erythematosus.

B. Specific skin changes
   1. In the classic mechanobullous presentation, noninflammatory blisters arise in sites of friction or in the trauma-prone skin areas of the trunk, elbows, knees, toes, and sacrum that heal with *significant* scarring and milia (Figure 20-7).
   2. With the bullous pemphigoid-like presentation, widespread inflammatory vesiculobullous subepidermal blistering involves erythema or urticarial lesions of the trunk, skin folds, and extremities that heal with *minimal* scar and milia.
   3. Cicatricial pemphigoid-like presentation has a predilection for mucous membranes where erosions and scaring occur (mouth, esophagus, conjunctiva, anus, and vagina).

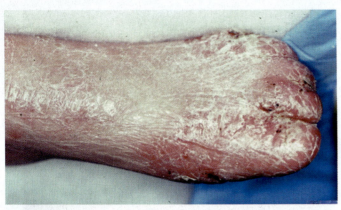

FIGURE 20-7. Epidermolysis bulllosa acquisita: erythematous shiny plaques with scarring over extensor surfaces—a consistent finding. (Courtesy of Dr. J. Timothy J. Wright.)

  4. Vesicles arranged in an annular fashion characterize the IgA bullous dermatosis-like presentation.
C. Differential diagnoses
  1. Porphyria cutanea tarda, pseudoporphyria, bullous pemphigoid, bullous systemic lupus, and mucous membrane pemphigoid.
  2. Bullous systemic lupus erythematosus (SLE) contains the same autoantibodies (IgG) to type II collagen, but also to "laminas 5 and 6," differentiating it from EBA.
D. Diagnostic tests
  1. Skin biopsy of a fresh blister (<24 hours old) for routine histology, electron microscopy, and serum for direct and indirect IgG and IgA class autoantibodies.
  2. Direct immunofluorescence (DIF) of a perilesional or vesicle margin where immune deposits are typically located on the dermal side of the cleavage can help distinguish EBA from bullous pemphigoid (BP).

III. COMMON THERAPEUTIC MODALITIES

A. Systemic therapy
  1. Systemic corticosteroids orally with either mycophenolate mofetil or dapsone or both can be used as a corticosteroid-sparing plan of treatment.
  2. Intravenous immunoglobulin (IVIG) treatment has shown blister reduction and healing.
B. Local or topical therapy
  1. Gently cleaning of blistered areas with saline and water without friction and then applying nonadherent dressings containing Vaseline may be beneficial.
  2. Topical agents are silver sulfadiazine, followed by nonadhering dressings, or Vaseline-impregnated gauze secured by roller gauze will decrease trauma to the affected body part.
C. Medical intervention
  1. Treatment is mainly supportive: Avoid trauma, manage blisters, and wound care (padding soft clothing, no adhesive use) as the noninflammatory subset is usually resistant to conventional medical therapies.

  2. Multidisciplinary teams benefit patients by monitoring for early complications and coordinate care between dermatologist, primary care providers, dentists, and family members.
  3. Supportive treatment includes optimal nutritional management with all patients, but especially those patients with oral lesions, esophageal scarring, and mucous membrane involvement.
  4. Premedication with mild analgesics prior to bathing and wound care is recommended.
  5. Plasmapheresis and photopheresis have shown good results as well as extracorporeal photochemotherapy use in a few cases with refractory disease.
D. Medication—drug therapy
  1. Topical agents to provide healing and wound infection (as described above)
  2. Colchicine or cyclosporine may have benefit to reduce blister formation.
  3. Rituximab, a monoclonal antibody against B-cell–specific targets, has been effectively used in EBA.
E. Diet management
  1. Same as PV
F. Supportive skin care
  1. Daily wound care is a major challenge for the EBA patient and caregiver.
  2. Apply lubricants to the skin to keep moist and prevent friction.
  3. For open blisters, use sterile nonstick bandages with an antibiotic ointment on the bandage—wrap with gauze to prevent tape-adhesive reaction with the skin.
G. Other nursing interventions
  1. Provide care with the primary goals to avoid direct physical trauma to skin surfaces, to stop blistering and scarring, to promote healing, and to prevent complications:
   a. Apply mittens during sleep to prevent scratching.
   b. Keep rooms at even temperature to prevent sweating and overheating.
   c. Use simple, soft clothing to dress children and use sheepskin on hard surfaces such as car seats.
  2. Referral to a multidisciplinary team to include dermatologist, dentist, dietician, ophthalmologist, social worker, physical therapist, and home health nurse depending on severity of disease.
  3. Consider genetic counseling to childbearing clients for family planning.
H. Complimentary alternative medicine. May follow PV guidelines.

IV. HOME CARE CONSIDERATIONS

A. Continuity of care concerns
  1. Referral to a multidisciplinary team to include dermatologist, dentist, dietician, geneticist, ophthalmologist, social worker, physical therapist, and home health nurse depending on severity of disease
  2. Follow care guidelines as in PV.

DERMATITIS HERPETIFORMIS

I. OVERVIEW

A. Definition: DH is a chronic, pruritic, autoimmune bullous disease that is a cutaneous manifestation of gluten sensitivity and celiac disease.

B. Etiology.
  1. DH is considered to have a genetic component within families sensitive to gluten protein (wheat, rye, barley) and those with celiac disease.
  2. The course of DH is usually lifelong, but general health is not usually directly affected. DH is neither caused by nor related to the herpes virus.

C. Pathophysiology.
  1. Autoantibodies (IgA) are produced in the gut lining against gluten protein that reacts in the dermis causing neutrophils and eosinophils to invade the dermis.
  2. The main autoantigen of DH is epidermal transglutaminase (eTG) with cross-reactions to gluten protein, forming IgA antibodies. The IgA/eTG complexes are found deposited in the dermis to cause the lesions of DH.
  3. Iodine is required for the IgA/eTG reaction, so people with DH should avoid iodized salt.
  4. Gluten-sensitive enteropathies (GSE) occur in nearly 90% of patients with DH.
  5. The IgA/eTG deposits can disappear after long-term (10 years) avoidance of gluten and reduce the appearance of rash with DH.

D. Incidence and considerations across the lifespan
  1. DH is most common in men, is more common in the descendants of the North European population, and is uncommon in blacks.
  2. The mean age of onset is in the 4th decade and may occur in children or the elderly.

II. ASSESSMENT

A. History and physical examination
  1. The grouped erythematous, tense, papulovesicles with clear fluid may be hard to see intact since the pruritic eruption is often rapidly excoriated by the patient.
  2. Primary sites include scalp, posterior shoulders, sacral region, buttocks, knees, and extensor areas near the elbows.
  3. Assess for abdominal pain, bloating, loose stools, and fatigue with GI system.
  4. Associated diseases include sarcoidosis, vitiligo, autoimmune thyroid disease (up to 50%), insulin-dependent diabetes, lupus erythematosus, alopecia areata, and Sjögren syndrome.

B. Specific skin changes
  1. DH eruptions can be bullous, papular, papulovesicular, or urticarial and grouped, symmetrical, or erythematous patches; all types of lesions can be present on the same patient (Figure 20-8).

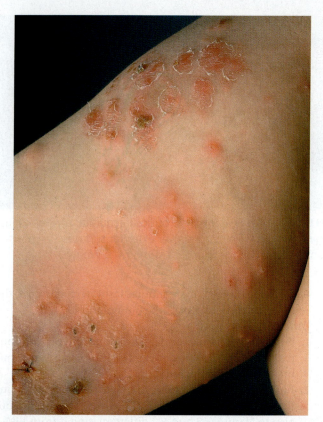

FIGURE 20-8. Dermatitis herpetiformis with small erosions, erythematous plaques, and annular scale. (From Craft, N., et al. (2010). *VisualDx: Essential adult dermatology*. Philadelphia, PA: Wolters Kluwer.)

C. Nonspecific skin changes
  1. Intense burning or itching sensations may precede the arrival of blisters in the skin.
  2. Rarely does the rash appear in mucous membranes other than the mouth and lips.

D. Differential diagnoses include drug reactions, contact dermatitis, dyshidrosis, scabies, and varicella.

E. Diagnostic tests
  1. Diagnosis usually requires at least one punch biopsy of a new red papular lesion that has not blistered.
  2. Direct immunofluorescence studies can be taken from the area adjacent to the lesion (about 1 cm from a lesion).
  3. Serologic studies can detect circulating IgA antiendomysial, antireticulum, and antigliadin antibodies (for celiac disease), gliadin assay (IgA and IgG), and deamidated gliadin peptide antibody—tTG (IgA). Anti-eTG or transglutaminase 3 (TG3) provides higher sensitivity and specificity.
  4. A lymphoma workup to include small bowel biopsy may be done due to the increased incidence in DH patients.
  5. Monitor and/or test for associated diseases including thyroid and diabetes disease.

III. COMMON THERAPEUTIC MODALITIES

A. Systemic therapy

1. Dapsone (contraindicated in sulfa allergy) is a oral therapy of choice for DH; it has anti-inflammatory and immunomodular effects most likely from its blockade of myeloperoxidase and not as an antibacterial agent.

2. When dapsone is not tolerated, other treatments not as efficacious may be used, like colchicine, nicotinamide, tetracycline, sulfapyridine, lymecycline, or sulfamethoxypyridazine.

B. Local or topical therapy

1. Dapsone cream may be applied to blistered areas or ultrapotent topical steroids.

2. Cool compresses; or caladryl lotion for drying and anesthetic for painful vesicles

C. Medical intervention

1. Illness, stress, and variations in diet provoke exacerbations.

2. A gluten-free diet, which is difficult for patients to follow, does improve the clinical condition and thus reduces the required dose of medication.

D. Medication—drug therapy

1. Dapsone is very effective for patients with DH. Pruritus is sometimes relieved within hours of the initial dose. Adjust dose to the lowest amount that provides acceptable relief, and monitoring leukocyte count and hemoglobin is critical.

2. Close monitoring of potential side effects of dapsone is also essential. Peripheral motor neuropathy is one of the most serious side effects. Symptoms slowly improve over months after dapsone is discontinued.

3. Antihistamines may be used for intense pruritus.

E. Diet management

1. Gluten-free diet—no wheat, rye, and barley in diet. Complete gluten elimination is curative, yet relief takes months; iron and multivitamin should be supplemented.

2. Avoiding gluten long term (10 years) can reduce DH rash and IgA/eTG deposits.

F. Surgical interventions—gastroenterology consults for possible lymphomas

G. Supportive skin care. Follow care guidelines as in PV.

H. Other nursing interventions

1. Bathe with tepid water and mild soaps, and pat skin dry avoiding rubbing skin.

2. Monitor for impetiginous skin infections due to intense pruritus and itching.

3. Assist client's responses to questions from others concerning lesions and contagion—as DH lesions are not contagious, instead result from an autoimmune reaction.

IV. HOME CARE CONSIDERATIONS

A. Continuity of care concerns

1. Multidiscipline approach to include dermatologist, dietician, health educators, rheumatologist, and gastroenterologist can help identify and address gluten-sensitive enteropathies.

2. Celiac Disease Foundation and the Gluten Intolerance Group can give added support and dietary advice.

B. Patient education. Refer to PV patient education guidelines.

PATIENT EDUCATION

Dermatitis Herpetiformis

- Stress gluten diet restrictions as DH is "virtually always" associated with celiac disease.
- Reiterate DH lesions are not contagious but result from autoimmune gluten sensitives.
- Be alert to secondary skin infections due to intense itching—such as impetigo.
- Be aware of and report symptoms of other autoimmune disease associated with DH: thyroid, diabetes, lupus erythematosus, alopecia areata, and Sjögren syndrome.

BIBLIOGRAPHY

Bolognia, J. L., Schaffer, J. V., Duncan, K. O., & Ko, C. J. (2014). *Dermatology essentials*. Philadelphia, PA: Elsevier-Saunders.

Bolotin, D., & Petronic-Rosic, V. (2011). Dermatitis herpetiformis. Part 1. Epidemiology, pathogenesis, and clinical presentation. *Journal of the American Academy of Dermatology, 64*(6), 1017–1024. doi: 10.1016/j.jaad.2010.09.777

Bolotin, D., & Petronic-Rosic, V. (2011). Dermatitis herpetiformis. Part II. Diagnosis, prognosis, and management. *Journal of the American Academy of Dermatology, 64*(6), 1027–1033. doi: 10.1016/j.jaad.2010.09.776

Callen, J. P., & Jorizzo, J. L. (2009). *Dermatological signs of internal disease* (4th ed.). Philadelphia, PA: Elsevier-Saunders.

Chen, M., Kim, G. H., Prakash, L., & Woodley, D. T. (2012). Epidermolysis bullosa acquisita: Autoimmunity to anchoring fibril collagen. *Autoimmunity, 45*(1): 91–101. doi: 10.3109/08916934.2011.606450

Fine, J.-D., Bruckner-Tuderman, L., Eady, R. A., Bauer, E. A., Bauer, J. W.., Has, C., … Zambruno, G. (2014). Inherited epidermolysis bullosa: Updated recommendations on diagnosis and classification. *Journal of the American Academy of Dermatology, 70*(6), 1103–1126. doi: 10.1016/j.jaad.2014.01.903

Fitzpatrick, J. E., & Morelli, J. G. (2011). *Dermatology secrets plus* (4th ed.). Philadelphia, PA: Elsevier-Saunders.

Gürcan, H. M., & Ahmed, A. R. (2011). Current concepts in the treatment of epidermolysis bullosa acquisita. *Expert Opinion on Pharmacotherapy, 12*(8), 1259–1268. doi: 10.1517/14656566.2011.549127

Kroumpouzos, G. (2014). *Text atlas of obstetric dermatology*. Philadelphia, PA: Wolters Kluwer/Lippincott Williams & Wilkins.

Labib R. Zakka, L. R., Shetty, S. S., and Ahmed, A. R. (2012). Rituximab in the treatment of pemphigus vulgaris. *Dermatology and Therapy, 2*(17), 1–13. doi: 10.1007/s13555-012-0017-3

Lebwohl, M. G., Heymann, W. R., Berth-Jones, J., & Coulson, I. (2014). *Treatment of skin disease: Comprehensive therapeutic strategies* (4th ed.). Philadelphia, PA: Elsevier-Saunders.

Samadi, S., Khadivzadeh, T., Emami, A., Moosavi, N. S., Tafaghodi, M., & Behnam, H. R. (2010). The effect of Hypericum perforatum (St. John's Wort) on the wound healing and scar of cesarean. *Journal of Alternative and Complementary Medicine, 16*(1), 113–117. doi: 10.1089/acm.2009.0317

Wolff, K., Johnson, R. A., & Saavedra, A. P. (2013). *Fitzpatrick's color atlas and synopsis of clinical dermatology* (7th ed.). New York, NY: McGraw-Hill.

Wong, R., Prajapati, V., & Barankin, B. (2013). Can you identify this condition? Dermacase: Bullous pemphigoid. *Canadian Family Physician, 59*(9), 963–965.

STUDY QUESTIONS

1. Bullous and vesicular skin diseases can be acute but are primarily chronic blister-forming diseases.
   a. True
   b. False

2. Close monitoring of which of the following for side effects is needed for growth/skin repair of the patient with bullous and vesicular disease?
   a. Topical treatments
   b. Drug regimens
   c. Nutritional needs
   d. All of the above

3. Adhering to a gluten-free diet and refraining from iodine salt use may reduce dose of oral medication in which of the following diseases?
   a. Bullous pemphigoid
   b. Epidermolysis bullosa
   c. Dermatitis herpetiformis
   d. Pemphigus vulgaris

4. Which of the following is an acquired autoimmune disorder that resembles an inherited bullous disease?
   a. Epidermolysis bullosa
   b. Dermatitis herpetiformis
   c. Pemphigus foliaceus
   d. Epidermolysis bullosa acquisita

5. The site of the first lesion in pemphigus vulgaris is most commonly the:
   a. knee.
   b. conjunctiva.
   c. oral mucosa.
   d. all of the above.

6. Which of the following is the most common form of pemphigus?
   a. Pemphigus vegetans
   b. Pemphigus foliaceus
   c. Pemphigus erythematosus
   d. Pemphigus vulgaris

7. Lesions such as bullae, vesicles, and erosions may be present in:
   a. bullous pemphigoid.
   b. pemphigus vulgaris.
   c. epidermolysis bullosa.
   d. epidermolysis bullosa acquisita.
   e. all of the above.

8. Which of the following is found most often in infancy?
   a. BP
   b. Pemphigus vulgaris
   c. Dermatitis herpetiformis
   d. Epidermolysis bullosa

9. Nikolsky sign:
   a. is pathognomonic for pemphigus vulgaris.
   b. is defined as dislodging of the epidermis with lateral pressure placed on the skin.
   c. is often used as a diagnostic test since it is cost-effective.
   d. usually does not result in cutaneous erosion.

10. Monitoring for squamous cell skin cancers must be part of the medical plan in patients with which of the following conditions?
    a. Dermatitis herpetiformis
    b. Dystrophic epidermolysis bullosa
    c. Epidermolysis bullosa aquisita
    d. Kindler syndrome

Answers to Study Questions: 1.a, 2.d, 3.c, 4.d, 5.c, 6.d, 7.e, 8.d, 9.b, 10.b

CHAPTER 21

Cutaneous Manifestations of Systemic Disease

Constance L. Hayes

OBJECTIVES

After studying this chapter, the reader will be able to:

- Describe at least five systemic disorders demonstrating significant cutaneous signs and symptoms.
- Identify the cutaneous signs and symptoms common to leukemia/lymphoma.
- Discuss the potential skin alterations in the patient with sarcoidosis, hypothyroidism, hyperthyroidism, Behçet disease, graft versus host disease, and diabetes mellitus.
- List at least five cutaneous signs of possible internal malignancy.
- Discuss education needs for patients with cutaneous lesions related to systemic disease.
- Identify common therapeutic modalities for systemic illnesses with cutaneous manifestations.

KEY POINTS

- The skin is fundamentally related and integrated with all body systems and functions.
- Cutaneous signs and symptoms may be the first indication of a systemic illness.
- Dermatology nursing care for patients with systemic illness presents unique challenges requiring a multidisciplinary approach.
- Skin changes may precede, follow, or have a parallel course with suspected internal malignancies.
- Patients with suspected systemic illness and concurrent skin signs and symptoms require a comprehensive multisystem assessment and relevant diagnostic workup.
- Lymphomas exhibit lymphadenopathy with very firm, rubbery lymph nodes.
- Nonblanching petechial rashes of acute leukemia have a slower onset associated with anemia, lymphadenopathy, and hepatosplenomegaly when compared to viral or bacterial causes.
- Low iodine levels and exposures to goiter-causing agents such as bromide, fluoride, and chlorine need to be investigated in autoimmune thyroiditis.

- Even when thyroid-stimulating hormone, T_4 and T_3, levels are normal, evaluate individuals with elevated lipid levels and hypothyroid symptoms by checking thyroid antibodies and adding low-dose thyroid hormone replacement to abate symptoms.
- Thyroid dermopathy or localized myxedema is an uncommon manifestation of an autoimmune thyroid disease (Grave disease) seen mostly in the pretibial region (formerly known as pretibial myxedema) but can be found elsewhere. Thyroid dermopathy is nearly always associated with thyroid ophthalmopathy.
- Weight loss to a normal body mass index level (18.5 to 24.9 pounds) improves glucose metabolism and reduces cutaneous lesions and metabolic sequelae associated with diabetes mellitus.
- All cutaneous sarcoidosis lesions demonstrate an "apple-jelly" semitranslucent yellow–brown color when blanched under a glass slide.

INTERNAL MALIGNANCY: LEUKEMIA/LYMPHOMA

I. OVERVIEW

A. Definition: Cutaneous lesions may develop with internal hematopoietic and lymphoid malignancies, which are classified by dominant cell type, cell maturity, and duration from onset to death (acute vs. chronic). Leukemia classifications describe the type of white blood cell (WBC) multiplying while lymphomas develop from lymph node, spleen, or other organ lymphocytes. Some classifications include the following:

1. *Acute myelomonocytic* involves monocytosis in the peripheral blood.
2. *Monocytic leukemia* affects the reticuloendothelial (macrophage) system with an excess of phagocytic cells, macrophages, and monocytes in connective tissues that overrun the blood and accumulate in the lymph nodes and spleen.

3. *Acute lymphocytic leukemias* exhibit lymphoblast proliferation and enlarged lymphoid tissues, while *aleukemic leukemias* have no abnormal cells in the blood.
4. *Acute myeloblastic leukemia* has a proliferation of immature myeloblasts in tissues, organs, and blood; frequently, it is associated with Sweet's syndrome (SS).
5. *Chronic hairy cell leukemia* shows hairy cells in reticuloendothelial organs/blood.
6. *Non-Hodgkin lymphoma* represents multiple cytologic classifications, other than *Hodgkin disease*, of either nodular or diffuse tumor pattern.
B. Etiology. Unknown for both leukemias and lymphomas; however, some studies may indicate a possible genetic, environmental, or viral link.
C. Pathophysiology
   1. Leukemia is characterized by neoplasia of the WBC in the bone marrow, interfering with normal blood cell maturation and resulting in anemia, decreased platelet production, and granulocytopenia.
   2. Non-Hodgkin lymphomas show an abnormal proliferation of various cell types—histiocytic, lymphocytic, or mixed. Malignant cells may spread to lymph nodes, bone marrow, liver, spleen, and gastrointestinal (GI) tract.
   3. Tumor cells may directly invade the skin manifesting as papules, macules, flat or infiltrated plaques, nodules, or ulcerative skin lesions.
   4. As an indirect result of the malignancy, skin lesions may manifest as pallor (anemia), excoriations (pruritus), petechiae (thrombocytopenia), and opportunistic infections such as severe candidiasis (with neutropenia).
D. Incidence
   1. Leukemia accounts for 3.1% of all new US cancers and has an annual prevalence reported at 9 per 100,000.
   2. Non-Hodgkin's Lymphoma (NHL) is a broad spectrum of lymphomas. It is three times more common than Hodgkin lymphoma. The majority of cutaneous lymphomas are of T-cell origin due to their function in the skin and lymphoid tissues.
E. Considerations across the life span
   1. Acute leukemia is most common in children, while chronic leukemia is more common in adults in the third to sixth decade of life.
   2. Non-Hodgkin lymphoma is most common in the fifth and sixth decades of life and it accounts for 7.0% of all childhood cancers.

II. ASSESSMENT

A. History and physical examination
   1. A careful review of systems is essential to determine constitutional symptoms such as headaches, fatigue, fever, malaise, easy bruising, hemorrhages, bone or joint pain, and nutritional deficits (anorexia and weight loss with lymphomas with added nausea, vomiting, and diarrhea in leukemias).

2. Skin examination from leukemias and lymphomas may demonstrate both specific and nonspecific lesions.
3. Common physical examination findings may be hepatomegaly, splenomegaly, painless lymphadenopathy (lymphomas or leukemias), and musculoskeletal- or neurological-related pain and weakness (headaches, visual changes, vertigo, tinnitus in leukemia and pain/paresthesias/paralysis of affected nerve pathways) (Figure 21-1).
4. Clinical hematologic abnormalities include anemias, thrombocytopenia, local/systemic infections (respiratory and skin with leukemias), and opportunistic infections.
B. Specific skin changes
   1. Most common are rubbery, erythematous/purplish papules, plaques, or nodules, randomly distributed and/or found in mucous membranes. Less common are flesh-colored lesions (Figures 21-2 through 21-6).
   2. Least common are lesions similar in appearance to mycosis fungoides (flat plaques, arciform papules, and ulcerated nodules or tumors, most pruritic in plaque stages) (Figures 21-7 through 21-10).
   3. Early skin changes are most common in acute myelomonocytic and monocytic leukemia and include infiltrated, hyperplastic, friable gingiva, bruising or petechiae, and slow healing of cuts.
   4. Aleukemic leukemia cutis presents in the skin as erythematous papules or nodules in the absence of malignant cells in the peripheral blood; Leder stain is the key to diagnosis.
C. Nonspecific skin changes
   1. Skin and mucous membrane findings attributable to cytopenia include pallor, purpura, gingival bleeding, oral ulcerations, and recurring skin infections.
   2. Skin changes in which the pathogenesis is unknown include acute febrile neutrophilic dermatosis (Sweet's syndrome), atypical pyoderma gangrenosum, generalized pruritus, vasculitis, acquired ichthyosis, vesicular disease, and xanthomas.
D. Differential diagnosis
   1. Differentials include viral, bacterial, and fungal infections seen in tuberculosis, cat-scratch fever, sarcoidosis, dermatomyositis, lymphogranuloma venereum, mononucleosis-type syndromes, human immunodeficiency virus (HIV) infection, Kaposi sarcoma, secondary syphilis, serum sickness, and Kawasaki disease.
   2. Pseudolymphomas of the skin may manifest as insect infestations or bites, lymphomatoid papulosis, drug-induced pseudolymphoma, actinic reticulosis.
E. Diagnostic tests
   1. General diagnostic tests include CBC with differential; HIV; rapid plasma reagin (RPR); hepatitis B surface antigen (HBsAg); antinuclear antigen (ANA); mononucleosis serology; purified protein derivative (PPD) skin test; metabolic panel with lipid profile; x-rays/scans of the chest, abdomen, and bone; and, when indicated, lymph node and/or bone marrow biopsy.

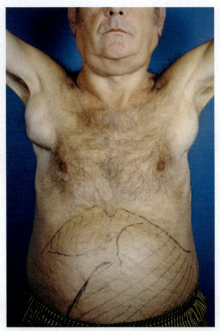

FIGURE 21-1. Massive lymphadenopathy in a patient with chronic lymphocytic leukemia. (From Tkachuk, D. C., & Hirschman, J. V. (2007). *Wintrobe's atlas of clinical hematology* (p. 154, Fig. 5.1). Philadelphia, PA: Lippincott Williams & Wilkins.)

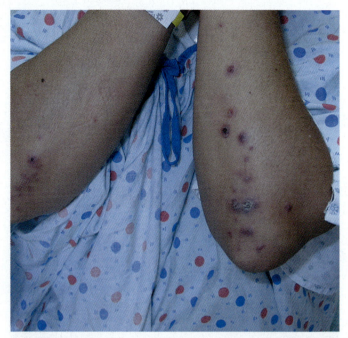

FIGURE 21-2. Lymphoma/leukemia—purple/red plaques and papules of leukemia cutis—extensor area of arms. (Image provided by Stedman's.)

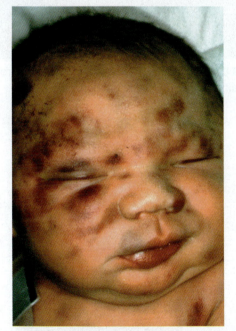

FIGURE 21-3. Leukemia cutis in an infant with congenital leukemia. (From Arceci, R., & Weinstein, H. (2005). Neoplasia in the neonate and young infant. In G. B. Avery, (Ed.). *Neonatology: Pathophysiology and management of the newborn*. Philadelphia, PA: JB Lippincott, with permission.)

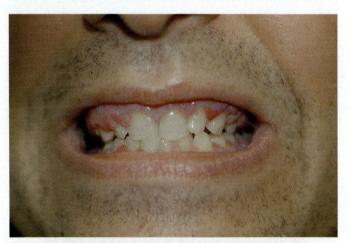

FIGURE 21-4. Gingival infiltration of leukemic cells in a patient with acute myeloid leukemia. (From Greer, J. P., Foerster, J., Rodgers, G. M., Paraskevas, F., Glader, B., Arber, D. A., & Means Jr, R. T. (2009). *Wintrobe's clinical hematology* (12th ed., p. 1680, Fig. 72.8). Philadelphia, PA: Lippincott Williams & Wilkins.)

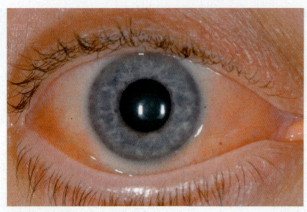

FIGURE 21-5. Ocular involvement in a 60-year-old man with chronic lymphocytic leukemia. (From Shields, J. A., & Shields, C. L. (2015). *Eyelid, conjunctival, and orbital tumors: An atlas and textbook*. Philadelphia, PA: Wolters Kluwer.)

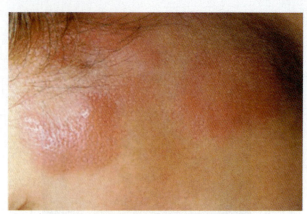

FIGURE 21-6. Cutaneous B-cell lymphoma. Asymptomatic erythematous lavender plaques and tumors on the face and scalp. (From Elder, D. E. (2012). *Atlas and synopsis of lever's histopathology of the skin*. Philadelphia, PA: Wolters Kluwer.)

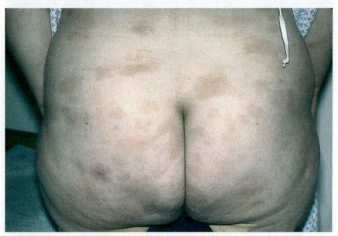

FIGURE 21-7. Cutaneous T-cell lymphoma. Note "smudgy patches." (Reproduced with permission from Goodheart, H. G. (2009). *Photoguide to common skin disorders: Diagnosis and management* (3rd ed.). Philadelphia, PA: Lippincott Williams & Wilkins.)

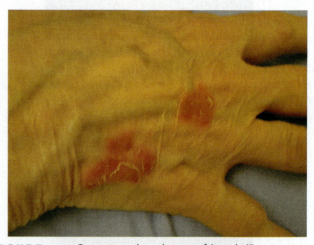

FIGURE 21-8. Cutaneous lymphoma of hand. (From Dr. Barankin Dermatology Collection.)

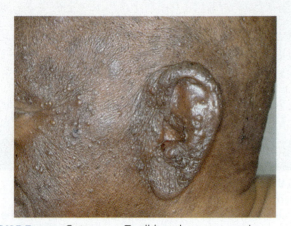

FIGURE 21-9. Cutaneous T-cell lymphoma: mycosis fungoides with follicular papules and plaques on face. (From Lugo-Somolinos, A., Lee, I., McKinley-Grant, L., Goldsmith, L. A., Papier, A., Adigun, C. G., …, Fredeking, A. (2011). *VisualDx: Essential dermatology in pigmented skin*. Philadelphia, PA: Wolters Kluwer.)

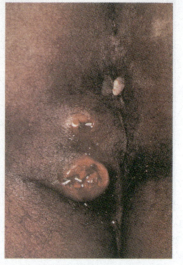

FIGURE 21-10. Large non-Hodgkin rectal lymphoma eroding through the perianal skin. (From Corman, M. (2012). *Corman's colon and rectal surgery*. Philadelphia, PA: Wolters Kluwer.)

2. Skin biopsy will demonstrate specific type of malignant cell but must be correlated with the history, physical exam, and other diagnostic data.

III. COMMON THERAPEUTIC MODALITIES

A. Systemic therapies include multiple modalities—chemotherapy, radiation, immunotherapy, and bone marrow transplant.
   1. Supportive systemic therapies possible are antibiotic prophylaxis, blood/platelet transfusions, and/or use of bone marrow growth factors (erythropoietin, granulo-cyte-macrophage colony-stimulating factor [GM-CSF]).
B. Local therapies utilized are skin radiation therapy (SRT) to specific lesions or intralesional corticosteroid injections.
   1. Supportive management includes topicals for pruritus, oral ulceration or bleeding, and emollients and moisturizers after showering for xerosis.
C. Medical interventions treat primary and secondary disease
   1. Clinically assess and monitor supportive blood/platelet replacement transfusions when needed.
   2. Monitor skin lesions, blood, urine, and pulmonary systems for potential sources of infection; when indicated, obtain appropriate wound, body fluid, or skin cultures for suspected infections.
D. Medication/drug therapy use and monitoring when indicated
   1. Add supportive therapy with antibiotic prophylaxis or treatment of infection.
   2. Bone marrow growth factors (erythropoietin or human GM-CSF) to treat anemias and prevent fatigue/malaise.
   3. Apply topical anesthetic creams to manage possible oral ulcerations.
   4. Administer nonaspirin antipyretic or apply cooling blanket for fever.
E. Diet management
   1. Promote adequate fluid intake, multivitamin use, and well-balanced diet and add high-protein foods when skin breakdown is evident.
   2. Encourage daily intake of vitamin B complex, to include B_6, B_{12}, and folate, supplementation due to high bone marrow turnover with leukemias.
   3. Encourage frequent, small feedings of soft nonspicy, nonacidic foods when oral ulcerations are present.
   4. Cooled foods may be better tolerated until ulcerations resolve.
F. Surgical intervention
   1. Selective splenectomy may be utilized to manage chronic lymphocytic leukemia.
G. Supportive skin care
   1. Maintain mobility and body positioning to promote skin integrity and prevent skin breakdown.
   2. Use nondeodorant, mild skin cleansing agent.
   3. Apply emollients to lips to prevent chapping, dryness, bleeding, or pain.
   4. Lubricate skin with cream- or ointment-based skin care product after bathing.
   5. If incontinent, keep skin clean and dry and use barrier ointment to prevent chaffing, breakdown, and candida organism overgrowth.

6. Assess and treat opportunistic skin infections like candidiasis or herpes infections.
H. Other nursing interventions
   1. Maintain good pulmonary toilet to prevent respiratory illness.
   2. Maintain healthy oral cavity; identify oral ulcers or lesions for topical treatments.
   3. Prevent constipation or bladder infections with effective bowel/bladder elimination plans.
   4. If neutropenic or during acute exacerbation, consider reverse isolation to protect patient from infection.
   5. Avoid any unnecessary invasive procedures such as venipunctures, injections, and urethral catheterizations.
I. Complementary alternative medicine
   1. Arsenic trioxide (intra-venous) is an FDA-approved treatment for acute promyelocytic leukemia.
   2. Follow diets that may decrease inflammation within the body such as antiyeast diets, low glycemic diet, and reduced or gluten-free diets.
   3. Supplement diets to enhance immune responses against tumor growths with vitamin E, which enhances T-cell–mediated immune function, and vitamin D to help regulate the immune system response by suppressing T-cell proliferation and modulate macrophage functions.

IV. HOME CARE CONSIDERATIONS

A. Continuity of care concerns
   1. The home may need to be adapted for the patient's health needs.
   2. Assistance with activities of daily living may be required during treatment or recuperation periods.
   3. Home care nurses are beneficial in monitoring patient status and providing ongoing emotional support and physician liaison services.

PATIENT EDUCATION
Leukemias and Lymphomas

- Provide patient and family members with education on means to avoid possible infectious agents or persons with obvious communicable illnesses such as upper respiratory infections/pneumonia, flu symptoms, or contact with herpes simplex lesions.

CUTANEOUS SIGNS OF SYSTEMIC MALIGNANCY: PARANEOPLASTIC DERMATOSES

I. OVERVIEW

A. Definition. Paraneoplastic dermatoses are a heterogeneous group of cutaneous nonmalignant skin disorders (papulosquamous, erythematous, bullous, and others) that may develop in relation to distant tumors, systemic neoplasms, or their metastases. Early recognition of these dermatoses can direct diagnostic workups for associated malignant neoplasms or tumors.

B. Etiology

1. A wide range of cutaneous signs have become associated with particular cancers—lung, liver, gastrointestinal, ovarian, breast, pancreas, renal–bladder, leukemias, and lymphoma being the most common.

2. Curth postulates, used for several decades, are criteria to associate a dermatosis and malignancy:

   a. The malignancy and skin disorder have a concurrent onset and run a parallel course.

   b. Treatment success of the cancer resolves the skin disorder and a remission of the malignancy shows cutaneous disorder return.

   c. The characteristic cutaneous eruptions are specific to the tumor cell or site causing them.

   d. The malignancy and the skin disorder should be demonstrably associated supported by sound case–control studies.

C. Pathophysiology

1. Pathogenesis is unclear but may be due to tumor or neoplasm secretions affecting cutaneous structures or a "cross-reaction" to skin structures by host defense antibodies directed at the tumor or neoplasm.

D. Incidence

1. Paraneoplastic symptoms/syndromes are found in nearly 20% of cancer patients, often being unrecognized.

2. Nearly three in four cancers in patients with assumed paraneoplastic syndromes can be identified with history, physical, and sex-/age-appropriate cancer screens.

3. Recognition of these relatively unusual paraneoplastic dermatoses can lead to early diagnosis of an associated cancer with potential for better outcomes.

E. For common paraneoplastic dermatoses findings, signs, and associated neoplasias, refer to Table 21-1 and Figures 21-11 through 21-26.

TABLE 21-1 Skin Lesions Associated with Possible Systemic Neoplasia

Lesion	Description	Associated Malignancy	Comment
Acanthosis nigricans (AN)—type I associated with malignancies (Figure 21-11) Acanthosis palmaris (AP) (tripe palms)	Gray-, brown-, or black velvety–textured hyperpigmented plaques found in a symmetric distribution. Common on the face, neck, nipples, and folds of axillae, groin, knees, elbows, waist, umbilicus, and anus. Thickened, velvety palms with dermatoglyphics pronounced.	Mostly adenocarcinoma (stomach 60%) and common in the lung, breast, and Gastro-intestinal/Genito-urinary (GI/GU) tracts. Lung cancer most common when AP only involved; gastric cancer when AP associated with AN.	Rare type of AN, most common in older adults, with no racial predilection, associated with weight loss and quick onset. Rule out other endocrinopathies, familial tendency, or obesity/insulin resistance. AP: 95% occur with cancers; 77% seen with benign AN types.
Acrokeratosis paraneoplastica (Bazex syndrome)—nongenetic type (Figures 21-12 and 21-13)	Violaceous erythema, scaling, and psoriasiform plaques over acral areas. Starts with fingers, toes, nose, and ear helices and then spreads to nails that exhibit longitudinal and horizontal nail ridging with painful paronychia with absence of infection. May see palmoplantar keratoderma with honeycomb appearance.	Upper airway and upper GI tract are the most common, usually as squamous cell carcinoma. Course of skin changes often parallels course of malignancy.	Rare skin condition, psoriasis-like scaling. More common in males than females. May spread to scalp, extremities, or trunk areas.
Carcinoid syndrome	Flushed, erythematous skin occurring in face, head, neck, chest, and epigastric areas from minutes to hours. Recurrent flushing develops telangiectasia and persistent redness. May see scaling in areas of sun-exposed skin (like pellagra).	Carcinoid tumors excrete excess hormones once metastasized to the liver; as an example, hyper-serotonemia (serotonin hormone secretion) is a common one.	Symptoms of this serotonin syndrome are flushing, diarrhea, abdominal pain, muscle spasms, shivering, tremors, agitation, confusion, heart palpitations, and low blood pressure. Serotonin tumor marker in urine for diagnosis: 5-hydroxyindole acetic acid (5-HI).
Dermatomyositis (Figures 21-14 through 21-16)	Inflammatory myopathy. Heliotrope—periorbital macular, violaceous erythematous rash and edema. Periungual telangiectasia with nail fold overgrowth. Gottron papules on knuckles and phalangeal joints. Diffuse scalp scaling/pruritus. Photo distributed poikiloderma of shoulders, anterior neck, and chest.	Associated with ovarian, lung, colorectal, pancreatic, and nasopharynx carcinoma and with non-Hodgkin lymphoma in Caucasians.	Course is not parallel with skin changes. Malignancy is commonly associated with rapid-onset diabetes mellitus, grossly elevated ESR or creatinine kinase, and lack of Raynaud phenomenon; seen frequently in fifth and sixth decades of life.
Erythema gyratum repens (Figure 21-17)	Gyrate serpiginous erythematous bands—6- to 8-cm rings of irregular shapes—across skin form scales of a "wood grain pattern."	Variable sites and types of malignancies—none specific.	Skin course parallel to neoplasm. Requires extensive evaluation to determine site. Occurs in all ages and genders equally.

TABLE 21-1 (*Continued*)

Lesion	Description	Associated Malignancy	Comment
Exfoliative erythroderma (Figure 21-18)	Extensive erythema, scaling, and edema. Dull scarlet color with small, laminated scales that exfoliate profusely. Vesicles and pustules are usually absent.	Cutaneous T-cell or systemic lymphomas, Hodgkin disease, or leukemias. Rare in B-cell lymphoma. Solid tumor association also reported	Concurrent course of skin and tumor burden
Florid cutaneous papillomatosis (FCP) (Figures 21-19 and 21-20)	Numerous warty small papules and larger nodules on the trunk, upper surface of hands, and extremities can spread to face. Pruritus may occur.	Gastric adenocarcinoma most common; others include GU/GI cancers, lung, and non-Hodgkin lymphoma.	FCP has rapid onset, is always associated with internal malignancy, and presents before or at the time of diagnosis. Often occurs simultaneously with AN or Leser-Trélat syndrome. Biopsy so as to distinguish from virus.
Hypertrichosis lanuginosa (malignant down)	Sudden growth of profuse, soft, nonpigmented, fine, downy, hair in a generalized distribution or localized to the face on an adult without signs of virilization. In time, these hairs may become coarser.	Associated with varied sites and cell types. Most common are lung, colon, or breast cancers.	Malignancy often discovered at time of skin change. Must evaluate for neoplastic growth in patients without cause for sudden hair growth (medication or endocrine abnormality).
Migratory thrombophlebitis (also known as Trousseau syndrome)	Inflamed, reddened, recurrent superficial thrombophlebitis affecting veins or arterioles of the neck, chest, abdomen, and legs/feet.	Pancreas, lung, and prostate adenocarcinomas are common—nearly 50% with this syndrome have an underlying cancer.	Blood clotting imbalance thought to be due to chronic, low-grade, intravascular coagulopathy. Secure an abdominal CT scan.
Necrolytic migratory erythema (NME), also known as glucagon syndrome (GS)	Bullous, ring-shaped red blisters that erode, crust, brown markings. Itchy and painful. Glossitis, angular chelitis, cracked dry lips, and nail ridging are common.	Pancreas, slow-growing cancerous tumor of alpha cells that secrete glucagon hormone	Is rare, afflicts adults over age 50. Secure CT of pancreas. Symptoms clear once cancer cleared. Can metastasize, decreasing treatment benefits
Paget disease (PD) of the breast (Figure 21-21)	Unilateral, sharply marginated, erythematous, eczematous plaque affecting nipple. Increased growth may spread to areola and beyond.	Occurs in conjunction with adenocarcinoma of the breast	Considered a malignant infiltrate rather than a paraneoplastic sign and most likely due to migration of malignant cells
Extramammary Paget disease (EMPD; Figure 21-22)	Erythematous, well-demarcated, plaques involving any region of male or female genitalia. Intense pruritus common; hyper- or hypopigmentation lesions of several centimeters size	Genitourinary cancers. Other associated distant cancers can include breast, colon, liver, kidney, gall bladder, or skin.	Much less common than PD; multifocal lesions possible, afflicts adults in sixth and seventh decade of life. Penal–scrotal EMPD is not common in black populations.
Paraneoplastic pemphigus	Bullous lesions. Painful erosive mucosal lesions may appear lichenoid and lips may crust. Skin lesions appear as erythematous macules, lichenoid, erythema multiforme–like, and flaccid bullae.	Thymomas (benign and malignant), non-Hodgkin lymphoma, chronic lymphocytic leukemia, Castleman tumor, and sarcoma	Review chest x-ray carefully for evidence of a thymoma. Bronchiolitis obliterans is a common complication. Course of skin disorder does not parallel the malignancy.
Pityriasis rotunda (PR) type 1	Round or oval, sharply defined, pigmented patches with dry ichthyosis-like scaling that mainly occurs on the trunk, arms, and legs. Fewer than 30 hyperpigmented lesions in PR type 1	Most often occurs with liver and stomach cancer; others include chronic myeloid leukemia, squamous cell carcinoma, and multiple myeloma	Type 1 associated with malignancy in Black, Asian, or Italian patients older than 60 years. Comprehensive workup needed to assess malignancy
Porphyria cutanea tarda (PCT; Figures 21-23 and 21-24)	Hyperpigmentation of sun-exposed areas, hypertrichosis and, less commonly, intact noninflammatory vesicles/bullae that rupture easily	Hepatic tumors	Requires careful liver, iron, and ferritin evaluations. Onset most common in midlife. Associated with viral and alcoholic hepatitis
Sudden-onset multiple seborrheic keratosis (Figure 21-25)	Raised papules or plaques with "stuck-on" appearance. Lesion surface is usually wart-like.	Intra-abdominal adenocarcinoma	May occur simultaneously with AN. Known as sign of Leser-Trélat syndrome
Sweet's syndrome - an acute febrile neutrophilic dermatosis; (Figure 21-26)	Sharply marginated, tender, raised, erythematous plaques, 2–10 cm diameter. Typically involve face, neck, trunk, and extremities with burning but not pruritic sensation	Myelogenous leukemia or plasma cell dyscrasia; underlying solid tumors are rare—but are mainly GU, breast (in women), and gastrointestinal (in men).	Associated with fever and anemia, course parallels that of the leukemia. Solitary or ulcerative lesions are frequently associated with malignancies.

CT, computed tomography; GI, gastrointestinal; GU, genitourinary

Data from Bolongnia, Shaffer, Duncan, Ko (2014); James, Berger, Elson (2011); Lebwohl, Heymann, Berth-Jones, Coulson (2014).

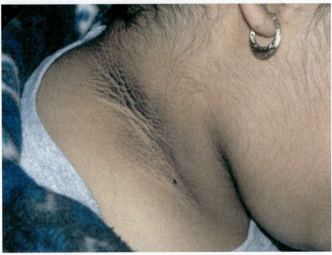

FIGURE 21-11. Acanthosis nigricans. (From Goodheart, H. P. (2003). *Goodheart's photoguide of common skin disorders* (2nd ed.). Philadelphia, PA: Lippincott Williams & Wilkins.)

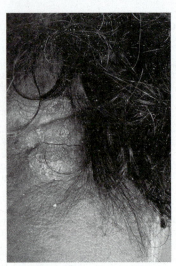

FIGURE 21-12. Bazex syndrome with psoriasiform dermatitis. (From NYU Langone Medical Center, Ronald O. Perelman Department of Dermatology slide collection.)

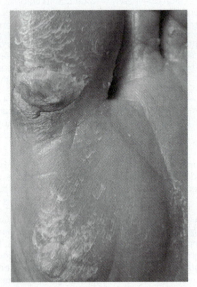

FIGURE 21-13. Bazex syndrome; foot involvement. (From NYU Langone Medical Center, Ronald O. Perelman Department of Dermatology slide collection.)

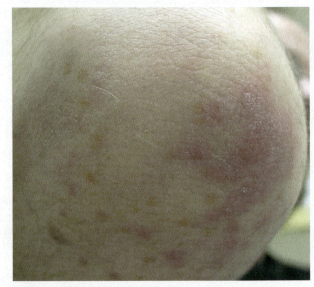

FIGURE 21-14. Dermatomyositis: Gottron sign. (From Dr. Barankin Dermatology Collection.)

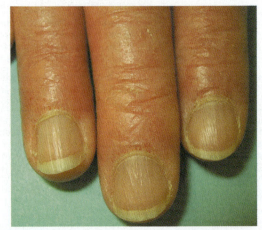

FIGURE 21-15. Dermatomyositis: nail fold with dilated capillary loops. (Image provided by Stedman's.)

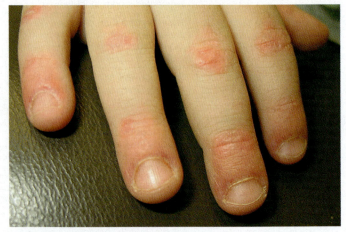

FIGURE 21-16. Juvenile dermatomyositis: hand. (From Dr. Barankin Dermatology Collection.)

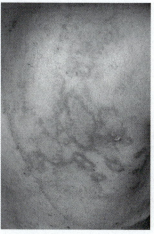

FIGURE 21-17. Erythema gyratum repens. (From NYU Langone Medical Center, Ronald O. Perelman Department of Dermatology slide collection.)

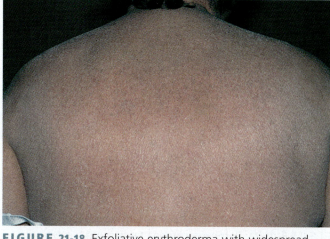

FIGURE 21-18. Exfoliative erythroderma with widespread erythema and scaling. (From Goodheart, H. P. (2003). *Goodheart's photoguide of common skin disorders* (2nd ed.). Philadelphia, PA: Lippincott Williams & Wilkins.)

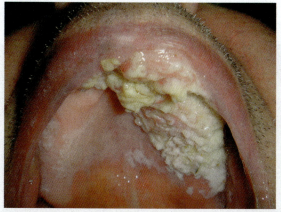

FIGURE 21-19. Oral florid papillomatosis (squamous cell carcinoma). (From Goodheart, H. P. (2010). *Goodheart's same-site differential diagnosis: A rapid method of diagnosing and treating common skin disorders*. Philadelphia, PA: Wolters Kluwer.)

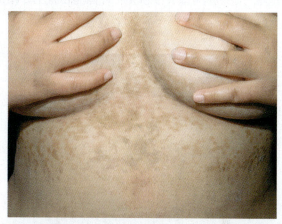

FIGURE 21-20. Cutaneous papillomatosis: confluent and reticulated on the trunk with hyperpigmented papules surrounding islands of normal skin. (From Craft, N., Taylor, E., Tumeh, P. C., Fox, L. P., Goldsmith, L. A., Papier, A., ..., Rosenblum, M. (2010). *VisualDx: Essential adult dermatology*. Philadelphia, PA: Wolters Kluwer.)

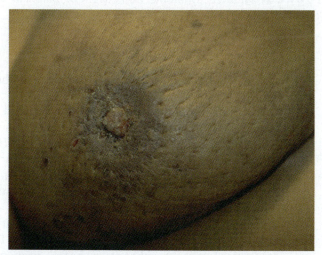

FIGURE 21-21. Paget nipple. Ulceration of nipple with progression onto areola. (From Harris, J. R., Lippman, M. E., & Osborne, C. K. (2014). *Diseases of the breast* (5th ed.). Philadelphia, PA: Wolters Kluwer.)

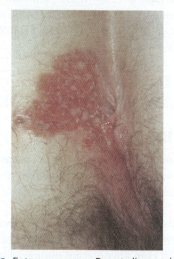

FIGURE 21-22. Extramammary Paget disease has caused an irregular but well-marginated erythematous erosive patch with slightly indurated edges in this patient. (Courtesy of Arnold Medved, MD.)

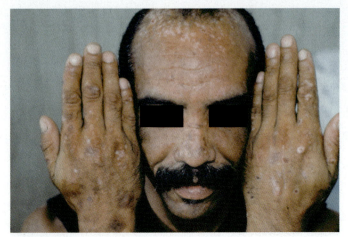

FIGURE 21-23. Porphyria cutanea tarda (note blisters on hands and frontal forehead; also characteristic excess hair on lateral cheeks). (From Goodheart, H. P. (2010). *Goodheart's same-site differential diagnosis: A rapid method of diagnosing and treating common skin disorders*. Philadelphia, PA: Wolters Kluwer.)

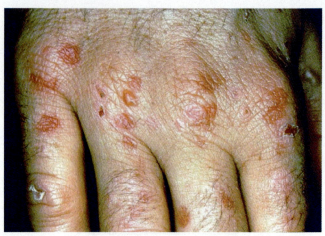

FIGURE 21-24. Skin eruptions in a patient with porphyria cutanea tarda. (From Ferrier, D. R. (2013). *Lippincott illustrated reviews: Biochemistry*. Philadelphia, PA: Wolters Kluwer.)

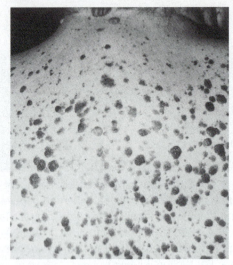

FIGURE 21-25. Sign of Leser–Trélat. Note that multiple seborrheic keratoses *per se* do not have the same significance as this sign. (Photograph courtesy of Dr. Cliff Dasco of California, with permission.)

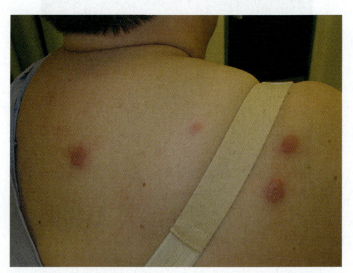

FIGURE 21-26. Sweet syndrome: back. (From Dr. Barankin Dermatology Collection.)

METABOLIC/NUTRITIONAL DISORDERS: HYPOTHYROIDISM

I. OVERVIEW

A. Definition: metabolic disorder with decreased production of free thyroid hormone involving systemic and cutaneous manifestations

B. Etiology

1. Primary hypothyroidism is due to a defect in the thyroid gland itself resulting in reduced thyroid hormone (T_3, T_4) production even after normal pituitary stimulation.

    a. Autoimmune process (chronic: Hashimoto thyroiditis)—is most common cause in areas of world with sufficient amounts of elemental iodine, like the United States

    b. Transient thyroiditis (subacute, silent, postpartum)

    c. Congenital (cretinism)

    d. Iatrogenic (surgical/radiotherapy ablation or neck radiation exposure)

    e. Drugs (lithium, interferon alfa, amiodarone, rifampin, phenytoin, carbamazepine, phenobarbital, sulfisoxazole, betaroxime, bexarotene)

    f. Dietary deficiencies (iodine) or excessive dietary intake of goitrogens (substances that inhibit T_4 production) such as cabbage, soybeans, peanuts, peaches, peas, spinach, and strawberries

2. Secondary hypothyroidism is attributed to pituitary failure to secrete thyroid-stimulating hormone (TSH)—hypopituitarism.
   a. Pituitary tumor or pituitary failure (Sheehan syndrome) is a rare cause for secondary hypothyroidism.
   b. Traumatic brain injury or radiation therapy to brain, head, and neck.
3. Tertiary hypothyroidism results from a malfunction of the hypothalamus to secrete thyroid-releasing hormone (TRH).
   a. Tumor of the hypothalamus
   b. Radiation to the brain
   c. Infiltrative granulomatous disease like amyloidosis or sarcoidosis

C. Pathophysiology
   1. Deficiency of circulating thyroxine (T_4) and triiodothyronine (T_3) decreases basal metabolism and oxygen consumption in tissues.
   2. Severe hypothyroidism results in the deposition of hydrophilic mucopolysaccharides in interstitial skin tissues (myxedema).
   3. Thyroid gland becomes atrophied and fibrotic.

D. Incidence
   1. More common after age 65; more common in women than men, 10:1 ratio.
   2. About 95% have primary form of disease and about 5% of cases result from pituitary/hypothalamic dysfunction.

E. Considerations across the life span
   1. Primary hypothyroidism most common in third to sixth decade of life.
   2. Fetal or infantile hypothyroidism affecting physical or mental development is termed cretinism. Early detection and treatment are often preventative.
   3. Risk factors: family history of autoimmune disorder (Graves, Hashimoto disease), advancing age, autoimmune endocrine disorders (diabetes mellitus [DM], type 1), pulmonary hypertension, Down syndrome, and Turner syndrome.
   4. Detection in the elderly is more difficult since the signs and symptoms develop slowly and can be attributed to arteriosclerotic manifestations.

II. ASSESSMENT

A. History and physical
   1. A thorough history is essential to determine the presence of nonspecific, early symptoms such as excessive fatigue, somnolence, lethargy, and deepening voice.
   2. Allow extra time for the patient to assimilate questions and formulate a response since mental functioning may be slowed. Facial expressions are often dull and flat with macroglossia and swollen lips preventing clear speech.
   3. Assess for nonpitting, interstitial edema (found in myxedema) and cold intolerance.

B. Skin, hair, and nail changes
   1. Skin changes
      a. Skin texture is coarse, dry, and scaly exhibiting increased skin creases with potential to develop an acquired ichthyosis vulgaris and palmoplantar keratoderma.
      b. Skin is cold, pale, appearing swollen, and boggy with nonpitting edematous (myxedema) areas that are waxy due to the deposition of hydrophilic mucopolysaccharides.
      c. Palms and soles are hypohidrotic and hyperkeratotic with a yellow tint.
      d. Ivory or yellow cast to skin is due to improper metabolism of beta carotene in the liver. Eruptive and/or tuberous xanthomas are common due to hyperlipidemia.
      e. Easy bruising with capillary fragility resulting in ecchymosis and purpura may be seen as well as telangiectasias on arms and fingertips.
      f. Increased incidence of vitiligo is reported.
   2. Hair has slow growth (increase in telogen [resting] phase) that appears dull, coarse, and brittle with classic thinning of the outer third of eyebrows and increase of alopecia areata; and often, a loss of pubic, axillary, and facial hair occurs.
   3. Nails are thin, brittle, slow to grow, and longitudinally or transversely striated, with rare occurrence of onycholysis.

C. Systemic manifestations are multisystem and generally related to decreased metabolic state and myxedematous involvement of body tissues.
   1. Early symptoms include fatigue, lethargy, somnolence, and cold intolerance.
   2. General signs and symptoms include slow heart rate, anemia, impaired wound healing, constipation, decreased appetite, weight gain, paresthesias of hands or feet, slurred speech/hoarseness, myalgias/arthralgias, slowed muscle movement and reflexes, headaches, apathy, and forgetfulness.
   3. Reproductive effects for women include menorrhagia, infertility, and decreased libido and for men include decreased libido and impotence.

D. Differential diagnosis
   1. Depression, Alzheimer disease, anemia, and fibromyalgia
   2. Cutaneous symptoms: scleroderma, vitamin deficiencies, anorexia, and menopause

E. Diagnostic tests include serology, radiology, and skin biopsies.
   1. Thyroid function studies, antithyroid antibody titer, and calcitonin levels assess potential sources for disease.
      a. TSH is elevated in primary hypothyroidism.
      b. TSH is low or nondetected in pituitary failure.
   2. Thyroid scan and radioactive iodine (RAI) uptake can assess for cold or hot nodules to identify thyroid cancers.
   3. Skin biopsy the suspected lesions to verify myxedema.

III. COMMON THERAPEUTIC MODALITIES

A. Systemic therapies: Identify thyroid hormone replacements as synthetic or natural.
   1. Levothyroxine sodium or liothyronine sodium are synthetic drug replacements for T_4 and T_3, respectively, whereas, natural desiccated pig thyroid (*Armor*) contains pig T_3, T_4, and calcitonin hormones as possible replacement choices.
   2. Thyroid replacement will reverse the skin findings of hypothyroidism.
B. Local/topical therapies can address dry, pruritic skin common in hypothyroidism.
   1. Apply hydrating emollients to dry skin frequently, especially after bathing.
   2. Avoid excessive bathing and use gentle cleansing agent.
   3. Apply antipruritic creams containing oatmeal or aloe vera.
C. Medical interventions
   1. Assess for therapeutic responses to medications at routine intervals.
   2. Monitor and treat potential sequelae: pericardial or pleural effusions, cardiac dilatation, bradycardia due to mucopolysaccharide deposits, carpal tunnel, or other entrapment syndromes due to impaired muscle function.
D. Medications
   1. Avoid drugs with potential drug–thyroid hormone–producing interactions, such as aluminum and magnesium antacids, iron-containing compounds, or cholesterol-binding agents.
   2. Replacement hormones may be synthetic or natural desiccated pig thyroid.
E. Dietary management if applicable
   1. Ensure a proper diet containing iodine (important in thyroid hormone formation), high fiber, and low-fat foods and avoidance of excessive goitrogenic foods that inhibit iodine metabolism and thyroid hormone production. Goitrogenic foods include crucifers (broccoli, kale, spinach, cauliflower, and radishes), fruits such as strawberries and peaches, as well as peanuts and soy-based foods.
   2. Take thyroid hormone replacements on empty stomach 30 to 60 minutes before meals or 3 hours afterward to avoid drug–food interactions.
F. Surgical excision considered for large goiters or those nonresponsive to treatment
G. Supportive skin care is considered for patients with hypothyroidism.
   1. Assess routinely for skin breakdown, especially over bony prominences such as elbows, spine, sacrum, coccyx, and any other potential pressure points.
   2. Provide passive range of motion, frequent repositioning, and elevation of dependent extremities to decrease edema and promote venous return as needed by patient status. Specialty beds may be indicated for immobile patients.
   3. Avoid bruising or skin injury.
H. Other nursing interventions
   1. Evaluate for pruritus of xerosis, chelitis, and ulcers on dependent extremities, which may be seen in hypothyroidism.

2. Encourage patients to obtain periodic thyroid hormone levels to ensure adequate response to hormone replacement treatment.
I. Complementary alternatives
   1. Follow hypothyroid diets that allow for adequate iodine intake without excessive goitrogenic foods. Use iodized salt when cooking.
   2. Selenium is essential to transform T_4 to its active form, T_3; adding whole grains, nuts, seeds, and seafood can provide this needed element.

IV. HOME CARE CONSIDERATIONS

A. Continuity of care
   1. The patient must be monitored for adherence to medication and diet regime and potential side effects of either hypo- or hyperthyroidism.
   2. Enlist family members to promote physical activity and healthy diets for elderly individuals who may live alone and need long-term medication monitoring.

METABOLIC/NUTRITIONAL DISORDERS: HYPERTHYROIDISM

I. OVERVIEW

A. Definition: metabolic disorder with increased production of free thyroid hormone involving systemic and cutaneous manifestations
B. Etiology
   1. Hyperthyroidism (thyrotoxicosis) results when tissues are exposed to high levels of thyroid hormones (T_3, T_4), usually due to hyperactivity of the thyroid gland.
      a. Autoimmune process (Grave disease)—must be evaluated with antithyroid peroxidase (TPO) antibodies involved in iodine metabolism and for thyroglobulin (TG) antibodies
      b. Toxic multinodular goiter (TMNG, *Parry or Plummer disease*)
      c. Thyroid adenoma
      d. Thyroiditis (lymphocytic and subacute postpartum)
      e. Iatrogenic: excessive intake of thyroxine- or iodine-containing medications
C. Pathophysiology
   1. Excess of circulating thyroxine (T_4) and triiodothyronine (T_3) increases basal metabolism and oxygen consumption in tissues.
   2. An increase in sympathetic nervous system activity results in classic symptoms of fine motor tremors, weight loss, muscle wasting, tachycardia, palpitations, high cardiac output, nervousness, fatigue, restless, emotional lability, insomnia, excess sweating, heat intolerance, oligomenorrhea, and exophthalmos.
   3. Thyroid gland may become hypertrophied.
D. Incidence
   1. Graves disease, the most common form of hyperthyroidism, is more common in Whites and Asians with lower incidence in African Americans; it is more common in women than men in 7:1 ratio.

2. TMNG accounts for 5% of all hyperthyroid cases in the United States.

3. Struma ovarii, a rare tumor, contain thyroid cells within the ovaries that oversecrete thyroid hormone from the ovaries.

E. Considerations across the life span

1. Graves disease has a peak age between 20 and 30. In contrast, TMNG primarily affects those greater than 40 years of age.

2. Risk factor: family history of autoimmune disorder (Graves or Hashimoto diseases).

3. Thyroid storm (crisis) is a severe life-threatening form of thyrotoxicosis with symptoms of high fever, tachycardia, congestive heart failure, agitation, and delirium that requires rapid diagnosis and management.

II. ASSESSMENT

A. History and physical

1. Secure a thorough history to determine nonspecific or early symptoms; pregnancy and viruses may trigger thyroiditis; and any use of medications may cause hyperthyroid—such as iodine or amiodarone therapy.

2. Physical manifestations of Graves disease include exophthalmos or proptosis with vision changes, acropachy with finger clubbing, diffuse goiter, and/or dermopathy with pretibial myxedema (PTM) lesions developing within 1 to 2 years after diagnosis or sooner.

3. Assess for weight loss; nonpitting, interstitial edema (found in myxedema); atrial fibrillation; systolic murmurs; fatigue; weakness; nervousness; and labile emotions.

B. Skin, hair, and nail changes

1. Overall, skin texture is fine, velvety, and smooth with increased warmth and moisture due to heat intolerance and increased sweating. Facial flushing may be seen.

2. Urticaria and dermatographism are common symptoms as are palmar erythema and soft tissue swelling of hands and feet. Vitiligo is associated with autoimmune disorders—Graves disease and Hashimoto thyroiditis being the most frequent.

3. Hair changes manifest as a fine texture with thinning and mild, diffuse alopecia with an increase in alopecia areata.

4. Nails may have clubbing; are brittle, thin, and striated either longitudinally or transversely causing free edges to break easily; or assume a scoop-shovel appearance.

C. Cutaneous involvement related to hypermetabolic state

1. Thyroid dermopathy, previously known as PTM, begins as pink, skin-colored, or purple–brown lesions that are bilateral, localized, nonpitting edematous infiltrates of glycosaminoglycans (hyaluronic acid and chondroitin sulfates) causing a peau d'orange appearance with prominent follicular openings (Figure 21-27).

2. These nodules or plaques of thickened skin favor the shins and may develop into grotesque verrucous lesions of the anterior/lateral areas of lower legs and dorsal of feet and may appear 1 to 2 years, or sooner, after thyroid treatments or occasionally develop into elephantiasis. Educate client that thyroid dermopathy lesions

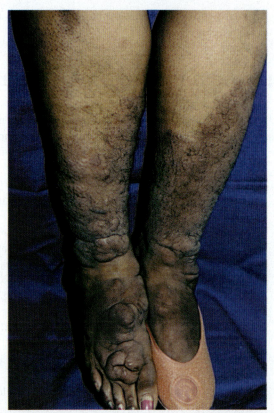

FIGURE 21-27. Pretibial myxedema lesion. This patient is hyperthyroid. Note the red–brown plaques on her shins and the dorsum of her right foot. (From Goodheart, H. P. (2003). *Goodheart's photoguide of common skin disorders* (2nd ed.). Philadelphia, PA: Lippincott Williams & Wilkins.)

may appear 1 to 2 years, or sooner, *after* hyperthyroidism has been treated.

3. Lesions may be found over shoulders, arms, head, and neck; likewise, they may clear spontaneously in several years without any lesional treatment.

4. Skin pigmentation changes can occur as an increase in vitiligo, hyperpigmented melasma of cheeks, a generalized bronze appearance, or melanoderma.

D. Differential diagnosis

1. Cutaneous disease: actinic lichen planus, chloasma of pregnancy, Addison disease, stasis dermatitis, amyloidosis lichen, and insect bites

2. Anxiety, arrhythmias, menopause, pheochromocytoma, postpartum thyroiditis, thyroid malignancy, neurofibromas, and diabetes mellitus type 1 or 2 (DM-T1 or DM-T2)

E. Diagnostic tests

1. Thyroid function studies, antithyroid antibody titer, and calcitonin level

   a. TSH is markedly suppressed in patients with hyperthyroidism, except those with a TSH-secreting pituitary adenoma.

   b. Free T_3, T_4, and calcitonin (found in the cells of thyroid gland) are elevated.

   c. Anti-TSH antibodies are often associated with Graves disease.

2. Twenty-four–hour radioiodine scan may help to identify etiology.
3. Secure a skin biopsy to verify myxedema.

III. COMMON THERAPEUTIC MODALITIES

A. Systemic therapies
   1. Antithyroid drugs, propylthiouracil (PTU), and methimazole inhibit the use of iodine in thyroid hormone synthesis by the thyroid gland. PTU also blocks conversion of T_4 to T_3 in the tissues.
   2. *Plasmapheresis* may improve severe myxedema (thyroid dermopathy); use has been shown effective in combination with rituximab.

B. Local/topical therapies
   1. High-potency topical corticosteroids, alone or under occlusion, to significant myxedematous skin lesions for 2 months is the mainstay of treatment.
   2. Inject intralesional corticosteroids 3 to 5 mg/mL for smaller lesions.
   3. Compression bandages combined with above therapies may be helpful.
   4. Complete decongestive physiotherapy shows promise with elephantiasis form of PTM.
   5. Apply hydrating eye drops to prevent corneal ulceration from exophthalmos that prevents lid closures.

C. Medical interventions
   1. RAI to eradicate excess thyroid gland nodules. Pregnancy is an absolute contraindication for RAI ablation of the thyroid gland.
   2. Monitor and treat potential sequelae of thyroid storm with fluid replacements, beta-adrenergic blocking drugs to decrease T_4 effects on heart muscle, and glucocorticoids to correct adrenal insufficiency from stress of thyrotoxicosis.
   3. Pretibial ultrasound and/or digital infrared thermal imaging to measure skin thickness to assess treatment response of myxedema lesions.

D. Medications
   1. Avoid drugs with aspirin, which increases levels of free T_3, and avoid amiodarone, a common antiarrhythmic drug rich in iodine, known to increase T_4 and lower T_3 synthesis.
   2. Pentoxifylline, a methylxanthine analog, may reduce extent of myxedematous lesions; use concomitantly with topical/intralesional corticosteroids.
   3. Intralesional weekly injections of octreotide, a somatostatin analog, decrease hyaluronic acid within dermopathy lesions but are costly and need more randomized controlled studies before it can be recommended as treatment.
   4. Low-dose oral glucocorticoids (prednisone, 5 mg/day) may be beneficial.

E. Dietary management if applicable
   1. Ensure proper diet, calorie intake, to prevent weight loss and avoidance of excessive goitrogenic foods; may schedule to eat six to eight small meals daily.

F. Surgical interventions
   1. Surgical excision of part or all of thyroid gland (less frequently used than medication).
   2. Surgical excision of pretibial lesions was effective in only a few cases, as a high risk of recurrence from the scarring makes this an infrequent modality.

G. Supportive skin care
   1. Goals of skin treatment include long-term effects of pretibial thyroid dermopathy to prevent decreased range of motion or foot drop with nerve entrapment.
   2. Assess routinely for skin breakdown at sites of dermopathy.

H. Other nursing interventions
   1. Monitor treatment outcomes collaborating with a multiteam approach to include primary care, endocrinologist, dermatologist, and nursing personnel.
   2. Provide passive range of motion, frequent repositioning, and elevation of dependent extremities to decrease edema and promote venous return as needed by patient status. Specialty beds may be indicated for immobile patients.
   3. Monitor for adverse effects of prolonged topical corticosteroid therapy, such as atrophy, ecchymosis, and telangiectasias.

I. Complementary alternatives
   1. Refrain from eating kelp, iodine-containing foods, or salts.
   2. Acupuncture in conjunction with traditional therapies can help ease symptoms of hyperthyroidism to calm one's anxiety.

IV. HOME CARE CONSIDERATIONS

A. Continuity of care
   1. The patient must be monitored long term for adherence to medication, diet regime, potential side effects of either hyper- or hypothyroidism during therapy, and regular ophthalmology evaluations.
   2. Encourage consistent and frequent provider visits to obtain periodic thyroid hormone levels to ensure adequate response to treatments.

PATIENT EDUCATION
Hypothyroidism and Hyperthyroidism

- Enlist the patient's participation in knowledge of thyroid disease(s) as in informed consumer and to report symptoms or outcomes with specific treatments.
- Reinforce the chronicity of this disease with need for replacement hormones, even if thyroid dermopathy occurs or subsides.
- Inform the clients with Grave disease that they may experience ophthalmopathy, finger clubbing, and/or dermopathy together, separately, or not at all.

METABOLIC/NUTRITIONAL DISORDERS: DIABETES MELLITUS

I. OVERVIEW

A. Definition. System-wide metabolic disorder involving altered insulin utilization or production with resultant abnormalities in metabolism of dietary nutrients.

B. Etiology is still being researched, yet current theories include genetic, autoimmune, dysregulation of pancreatic hormones, and/or environmental factors (obesity, stress).

C. Pathophysiology

1. Type I diabetes mellitus (DM) primarily involves decreased or absent insulin production within the pancreas.

2. Type II diabetes mellitus (DM) involves one or more factors including too much or too little insulin production, diminished responsiveness of tissues to the available insulin, abnormal glucose regulation within the liver, as well as glucagon in the pancreas.

3. Miscellaneous causes (small percentage of total cases): genetic effects of mitochondrial DNA and B-cell functions, pancreatic diseases (cystic fibrosis or hemochromatosis), acromegaly or Cushing syndrome, toxins, and drug induced (glucocorticoids, β-blockers, protease inhibitors, therapeutic niacin doses).

4. The complications related to DM primarily affect the heart, kidneys, and eyes due to micro- and macroangiopathy. Neuropathy and skin alterations are also common complications.

D. Incidence

1. Existing and new case numbers are increasing in the United States.

2. 25.8 million people (8.3% of population) in the United States are afflicted as of 2010 statistics.

3. Every 9 out of 10 adults with diabetes are type II.

4. Type I DM accounts for less than 10% of all US DM cases.

5. Nearly half of all new-onset diabetes in children has been type II, thought to be in relation to childhood obesity epidemic reported since early 1990s.

6. Trends in incidence demonstrate minority (American Indian, Hispanics, and Asians), and elderly populations are disproportionately affected.

E. Considerations across the life span

1. Type II is commonly associated with adults older than 40 but may occur at any age. Up to one third of adults greater than 65 years of age have impaired glucose tolerance.

2. Type I is more common in children and young adults but may occur at any age.

II. ASSESSMENT

A. History and physical examination to include a system-wide approach, determining family/patient history, coping and compliance skills, general state of health, and potential or actual complications

B. Systemic involvement

1. Prurigo pigmentosa—pruritic urticarial papules or papulovesicles with reticular violaceous pigmentation that erupt on nape of neck, back, or chest may be associated with diabetic ketoacidosis. DM control helps resolve lesions.

2. Carotenoderma—diffuse orange–yellow discoloration mainly on palms/soles related to increased carotene blood levels.

3. Polycystic ovarian syndrome—strongly linked with insulin resistance and glucose intolerance associated with type II DM. Treatment with insulin sensitizers helps reduce symptoms of menstrual irregularities, hirsutism, acne, and cystic ovaries.

4. Scleredema, a connective tissue disorder, with dermal induration of skin on posterior neck and upper back, may progress to lungs and cardiac arrhythmias.

5. Vascular changes—ulcerations and gangrenous digits are the results of microangiopathy.

6. Acral erythema—erysipelas-like blanching erythema of the hand or feet

C. Cutaneous skin manifestations of DM include many types.

1. Rubeosis is a chronic flushing of face and neck, also found on the extremities.

2. Diabetic dermopathy initially develops as a cluster of red papules that later coalesce into hyperpigmented, atrophic patches on lower extremities (Figure 21-28).

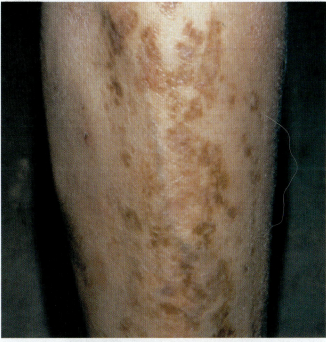

FIGURE 21-28. Diabetic dermopathy. Small, brownish, atrophic, scarred, hyperpigmented plaques are seen. (From Goodheart, H. P. (2003). *Goodheart's photoguide of common skin disorders* (2nd ed.). Philadelphia, PA: Lippincott Williams & Wilkins.)

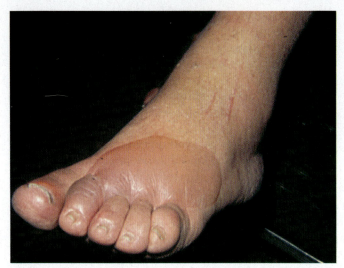

FIGURE 21-29. Diabetic bullous disease. Large, tense blister on dorsum of foot. (From Goodheart, H. P. (2003). *Goodheart's photoguide of common skin disorders* (2nd ed.). Philadelphia, PA: Lippincott Williams & Wilkins.)

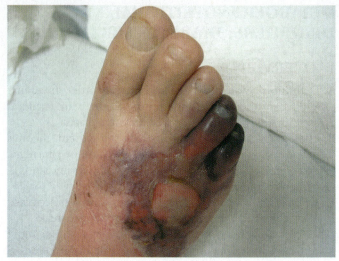

FIGURE 21-30. Diabetes mellitus. Diabetic foot digit necrosis and broken bullae dorsum of foot. (From Dr. Barankin Dermatology Collection.)

3. Bullosis diabeticorum is nonscarring, tense bullae more common to the lower extremities (Figures 21-29 and 21-30).
4. Necrobiosis lipoidica diabeticorum is a yellow–brown, well-circumscribed patch with erythematous borders on lower extremities that may ulcerate (Figures 21-31 and 21-32).
5. Acanthosis nigricans hyperpigmentation is a velvety thickening in intertriginous areas (Figure 21-11).
6. Xanthomas are small, yellow–red papules (Figure 21-33).

7. Skin infections can occur as candida, tinea pedis, and mucormycosis (acute periorbital swelling and rhinorrhea due to fungal *Phycomycetes* infection, with potential for cerebral involvement and death).
8. Hemochromatosis presents as a bronze skin tone.
9. Sclerotic skin, most common on hands and over joints, can limit mobility.
10. Perforating folliculitis are keratotic papules and nodules with central plug or excoriation seen in 5% to 10% of patients on renal dialysis with diabetes.
11. Lipodystrophy is localized lesions at insulin injection sites.
12. Vitiligo is a depigmented macular patch occurring in diabetic patients.
13. Poor glucose control can lead to neurotrophic ulcers and muscle atrophy.

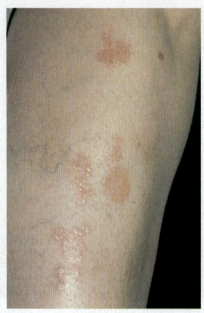

FIGURE 21-31. Necrobiosis lipoidica diabeticorum—early lesion consist of yellow–red plaques. (From Goodheart, H. P. (2003). *Goodheart's photoguide of common skin disorders* (2nd ed.). Philadelphia, PA: Lippincott Williams & Wilkins.)

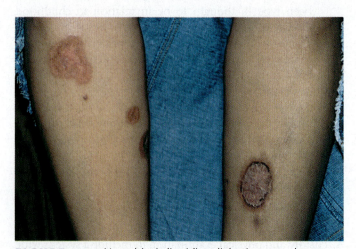

FIGURE 21-32. Necrobiosis lipoidica diabeticorum—late lesion of epidermal atrophy and telangiectasias tend to occur. (From Goodheart, H. P. (2003). *Goodheart's photoguide of common skin disorders* (2nd ed.). Philadelphia, PA: Lippincott Williams & Wilkins.)

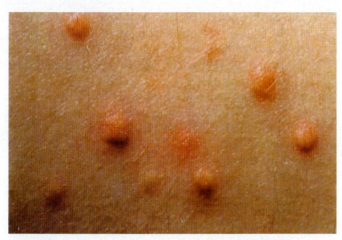

FIGURE 21-33. Diabetes mellitus. Eruptive xanthomas: multiple yellow–red papules–nodules, frequently with an opaque center. Testing may reveal markedly elevated triglycerides. (From Elder, D. E. (2012). *Atlas and synopsis of Lever's histopathology of the skin*. Philadelphia, PA: Wolters Kluwer.)

D. Differential diagnosis
   1. Hyperglycemia: nondiabetic glycosuria, hyperglycemia secondary to other causes than diabetes, pancreatic tumors, cystic fibrosis, and Cushing syndrome
   2. Cutaneous: Lyme disease, syphilis, amyloidosis, multiple sclerosis, lead/heavy metal poisoning, multiple myeloma, and vitamin B deficiency
E. Diagnostic tests
   1. Type I and type II diagnostic tests include fasting blood glucose, postprandial blood sugar, glycosylated hemoglobin, blood urea nitrogen and creatinine, electrolytes, lipid profile, thyroid panels, complete urinalysis with periodic microalbuminuria, and complete eye, foot, and neurologic exam.
   2. Skin biopsy may be required if skin lesion in question is related to diabetic changes or complications.

III. COMMON THERAPEUTIC MODALITIES

A. Systemic therapy
   1. Continuous subcutaneous insulin infusion by insulin pump (not for all patients, who need to test blood sugar levels six to eight times daily, time eating and physical activities to prevent hypoglycemia) controls blood sugars to normal and reduces or prevents skin manifestations.
   2. Incretin—Regulating-based analogs given by injection to control glucagon-like peptide-1 (GLP-1) with GLP-1 agonists or dipeptidyl peptidase-4 (DPP-4) can help lower blood sugar production and prevent cutaneous outcomes.
B. Local or topical therapy—dependent on cutaneous presentations
   1. Acanthosis nigricans: Apply topical tretinoin and 12% ammonium lactate cream.
   2. Necrobiosis lipoidica: Use intralesional or topical corticosteroids under occlusion.
   3. Hydrating emollients can prevent dry, cracked skin and possible infection.
   4. Treat perforating folliculitis with tretinoin, tazarotene gel, ultraviolet B (UVB), and narrowband UVB; if not improved, may use psoralen plus ultraviolet light of long A wavelength (PUVA) and oral retinoid as second line.
   5. Bullosis diabeticorum can be treated with clobetasol propionate 0.05%.
C. Medical interventions—mainly to prevent hyperglycemia and promote proper glucose metabolism for healthy skin growth.
   1. Manage diet and exercise activities to maintain glucose–insulin control: Blood sugars between 80 and 100 mg/dL helps decrease inflammation within the body associated with diabetes.
   2. Regular, frequent medical assessments of endocrinopathy (glucose, lipids, thyroid, cardiac, kidney, liver functions) are needed to prevent DM sequelae.
   3. Biopsy skin necrobiosis lipoidica to exclude sarcoidosis or squamous cell cancer.
D. Medication therapies
   1. Insulin, oral hypoglycemic agents, and incretin-based therapies are used to control blood sugar and prevent hyper/hypoglycemia.
   2. Perforating folliculitis may use allopurinol, isotretinoin, PUVA, or acitretin as second-line therapy when not improved with topicals.
   3. Bullosis diabeticorum can be treated with systemic corticosteroids, tetracycline and nicotinamide, or possibly minocycline, and if needed, azathioprine, mycophenolate mofetil, or methotrexate, as second-line therapy.
E. Diet management
   1. Nutritious daily diet recommended by the American Diabetes Association to control glucose throughout the day in conjunction with regular active exercise
F. Surgical interventions—considerations to manage ulcer complications
G. Supportive skin care
   1. Stress the importance of meticulous skin care to prevent diabetic ulcerations and potential infectious complications.
   2. Avoid skin injuries, scratching, and dryness. Skin should be kept well-lubricated and hydrated.
H. Other nursing interventions
   1. Monitor for signs of altered tissue perfusion such as changes in vital signs, delayed capillary refill, and dusky or deep red color to lower extremities.
   2. Encourage active range of motion or perform passive range of motion to improve circulation to extremities and active exercise with walking and gentle stretching with frequent rest periods as needed.
   3. Assess for loss of skin integrity, especially at bony prominences and feet.
   4. Instruct the patient on means to avoid trauma to skin, especially the feet and lower extremities. Encourage daily practice of skin and foot inspection.

I. Complementary alternatives
1. Magnesium intake (as almonds, nuts, potatoes, lentils, brown rice, avocados, and greens like spinach and peas) improves glucose tolerance as it helps insulin secretion and glucose regulation for type 1 and type 2 diabetic patients. Magnesium also helps regulate triglycerides and LDL cholesterol.
2. Vitamin D_3 taken with foods high in magnesium can increase absorption.
3. The spice cinnamon improves insulin function and curbs appetites.

IV. HOME CARE CONSIDERATIONS

A. Continuity of care
1. Regular follow-up is essential to health maintenance and preventing complications.
2. Good personal hygiene is essential with emphasis on foot care.
3. Medical alert cards, bracelets, and necklaces are crucial to identifying diabetics within the home and community.

PATIENT EDUCATION
Diabetes Mellitus

- Disease pathology education and support systems are keys to success management.
- Self-management is ideal with support group or diabetes education classes to include family members supporting continuing education and key to the successful management of diabetes for some patients.
- Avoid activities or clothing that impairs circulation (girdles, tight shoes, crossing legs, standing or sitting for long periods, constrictive clothing, cold temperatures, and cigarette smoking).
- Stress need to monitor changes in circulatory status and reporting changes or onset of pain, nonhealing ulcer, paresthesias, or injuries—especially lower extremities.

NEUROLOGIC DISORDERS: NEUROFIBROMATOSIS (VON RECKLINGHAUSEN DISEASE)

I. OVERVIEW

A. Definition: heterogeneous group of disorders (eight subtypes identified) with multiple benign nerve sheath tumors and characteristic skin findings.
B. Etiology
1. In 50% of cases, it is related to an inherited, autosomal dominant trait.
2. Thirty to fifty percent of cases are considered new mutations.
C. Pathophysiology
1. The cutaneous neurofibromatosis (NF) lesions originate from Schwann cells of the peripheral nervous system. Proliferations of perineural fibroblasts produce tumor-like growths.

2. The genetic defect has been localized to chromosome 17 for NF type 1 (von Recklinghausen disease) and is characterized by at least two of the following:
   a. Six or more café au lait macules—tan to dark brown uniform pigmented
   b. Axillary or inguinal freckling
   c. At least two neurofibromas or one plexiform neurofibroma
   d. Optic glioma
   e. Lisch nodules (yellow–brown smooth nodules within the iris)
   f. Thinning of long bone cortex or sphenoid bone dysplasia
   g. First-degree relative meeting at least two of the above criteria
3. Type 2 disease is linked to chromosome 22 and is characterized by bilateral acoustic neuromas and less skin involvement.
4. Type 3 disease (formerly called mixed type) is characterized by multiple intracranial tumors, paraspinal neurofibromas, neurofibromas primarily of the palms, and café au lait spots.
5. Type 4 (coined variant NF) includes the range of phenotypes that don't neatly fit elsewhere and are placed in this category.
6. Type 5, also called segmental type, is typified by café au lait spots or neurofibromas limited to a single unilateral or dermatomal area.
7. Type 6 is familial, characterized by multiple café au lait spots without neurofibromas (rare).
8. Type 7 includes the presentation of neurofibromas, after the age of 20, without other cutaneous changes (rare).
9. Type 8 is for all other atypical cases of NF not fulfilling any other specified criteria. Type 4 and type 8 cases are often interchanged.
D. Incidence of neurofibromatosis
1. Type 1 occurs in 1 out of 3,000 live births; type 2 occurs in about 1 out of 40,000; and prevalence for types 3 to 8 is considered uncommon or rare. There is no sex or racial predilection.
E. Considerations across the life span include youth to adulthood
1. Often manifests in childhood: By age 8, 97% of National Institutes for Health (NIH) diagnostic criteria for NF1 are met.
2. Juvenile xanthogranulomas (JXG): most resolve by age 6 with slight skin pigmentation.
3. Lesions become more extensive and cosmetically disfiguring during adulthood.
4. Malignant tumors (sarcomas) may develop in up to 5% of lesions over time.

II. ASSESSMENT

A. History and physical exam
1. Cutaneous findings are usually the presenting signs of NF.
2. Clinician should assess for familial history and one or more oral/skin/optic findings. Oral manifestations can be found in nearly 72% of NF1 patients.

3. Regular developmental assessment of children must include head circumference and blood pressures.

B. Systemic manifestations
   1. Systemic involvement is variable in incidence, extent, and severity.
   2. Central nervous system involvement may include optic nerve gliomas (most common), acoustic neuromas, meningiomas, intellectual deficiencies, speech impediments, and possible macrocephaly.
   3. Musculoskeletal changes seen can be pseudarthrosis and kyphoscoliosis.
   4. GI visceral tumors (leiomyomas, neurofibromas) are common and symptoms of constipation, obstruction, intussusception, and hemorrhage are related to tumor involvement.
   5. Hypertension in adults may indicate pheochromocytomas. Hypertension in children may indicate renal artery stenosis.

C. Cutaneous involvement—skin changes (Figure 21-34)
   1. Café au lait spots (hyperpigmented macules) are characteristic of this disease.
   2. Axillary freckling is most common (Crowe sign), but inguinal or inframammary freckling is also seen—usually present by 4 to 6 years of age.
   3. Soft cutaneous and subcutaneous tumors that invaginate when palpated (button-holing sign)—begin to appear around puberty
      a. Tumors are sessile or pedunculated.
      b. Large drooping masses that develop along a nerve (plexiform neuromas) may develop in about 20% of NF1 patients.
   4. JXG—pink to yellow–brown papule/nodule; typically develops in first 3 years of life
   5. Lisch nodules are asymptomatic iris hamartomas, which occur in 90% of NF1 patients over the age of 6.
   6. Glomus tumors of fingers and toes are solitary, painful papules or nodules found in nail beds.
   7. Distribution is generalized but commonly spares the palms and soles.

D. Differential diagnosis
   1. Brain stem gliomas, dermal nevi and papillomas, low-grade astrocytoma, and meningioma must be considered.

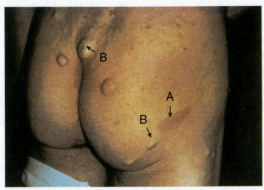

FIGURE 21-34. Neurofibromatosis: patch known as café au lait spot (**A**) and nodules (**B**) are seen—a combination typical of neurofibromatosis. (From Sauer, G. C. (1985). *Manual of skin diseases* (5th ed.). Philadelphia, PA: JB Lippincott.)

E. Diagnostic tests
   1. Skin biopsy demonstrates a well-circumscribed dermal tumor.
   2. Plexiform neurofibromas are highly diagnostic for NF1.
   3. Multisystem evaluation for diagnosis by clinical criteria, genetic testing, and disease progression or disease complications is recommended.

III. COMMON THERAPEUTIC MODALITIES

A. Systemic therapy
   1. For local aggressive tumors, systemic steroids or chemotherapy may be possible.

B. Local/topical therapy
   1. Possible to use CO_2 laser treatment for local removal of tumors.

C. Medical interventions
   1. Genetic counseling is advised, with first-degree relatives being screened for cutaneous and ophthalmologic signs of neurofibromas.
   2. Symptomatic treatment of neurological, gastrointestinal, and musculoskeletal symptoms may be offered.
   3. Conduct annual eye exams to assess for gliomas up to age 8 and then every 2 years.
   4. Plan radiotherapy after malignant tumor resection (schwannoma arising from NF1).
   5. Use MRI (brain, optic nerves, spinal cord) for focal or abnormal neurologic signs.

D. Medication therapies
   1. Chemotherapy is controversial.
   2. New angiogenesis inhibitors and anti-inflammatory agents that inhibit cell growth and induce apoptosis are in clinical trials for potential future use.

E. Surgical interventions
   1. Biopsy and surgical excision of fast-growing lesions are recommended, not only for cosmetics but also for threat of malignant degeneration in 2% of patients.
   2. Surgical excision is also recommended for lesions with cosmetic or functional concerns.

F. Supportive skin care
   1. Postsurgical wound care when tumors are excised or removed by laser.

G. Other nursing interventions
   1. Instruct on preoperative expectations for lesion excisions to include diagnostic studies, preop restrictions, and expectations during or after procedure.
   2. Discuss postoperative pain control plan and wound care and instruct on signs and symptoms of infection. Provide with emergency/follow-up phone numbers.

IV. HOME CARE CONSIDERATIONS

A. Continuity of care
   1. Assess the ability to understand and comply with pre- and postoperative instructions and care within the patient's cognitive and physical abilities.
   2. Assess the need to involve social services in view of chronicity of disease requiring multiple procedures over the life span.

LYMPHORETICULAR DISORDERS: SARCOIDOSIS

I. OVERVIEW

A. Definition: an inflammatory, granulomatous, multisystem disorder primarily affecting the lungs, liver, lymph nodes, spleen, skin, glandular tissues, and eyes.

B. Etiology is unknown but may be related to a variety of infectious agents in genetically predisposed individuals or exposure to certain drugs.

C. Pathophysiology

1. Lymphoreticular disorder is characterized by several abnormal immune-related functions causing granulomas (small lumps of immune cells that microscopically look like grains of sugar or sand, depositing in the skin, lungs, and lymph nodes).
   a. Impaired delayed hypersensitivity
   b. Imbalanced CD4/CD8 ratio
   c. Hyperreactivity of B cells
   d. Increased production of circulating immune complexes

2. In the presence of a causative antigen, an abnormal immune response among T lymphocytes and macrophages/monocytes is initiated and sarcoidal granulomas ultimately develop in targeted tissues.

D. Incidence

1. Ranges from 11 to 40 per 100,000 people in the United States
2. Fourteen times more common in African Americans than Caucasians
3. Disease is worldwide but is most common in Scandinavia.
4. In black populations, the male to female ratio is approximately 1:2.
5. Cutaneous sarcoidosis occurs in 20% to 35% of patients with sarcoidosis and may be its first sign predating knowledge of other organ systems involved.

E. Considerations across the life span

1. Onset is most common during ages 20 to 40.
2. Sarcoidosis may regress spontaneously within 1 to 2 years.

II. ASSESSMENT

A. History and physical exam
1. Up to one third of patients are asymptomatic; diagnosis is often incidentally made with chest x-ray demonstrating hilar adenopathy and pulmonary fibrosis.
2. Patients should be questioned regarding systemic symptoms such as fatigue, weight loss, fever, malaise, and weakness.

B. Systemic involvement
1. Respiratory involvement (most common) includes hilar adenopathy and pulmonary parenchymal disease. Symptoms may include dyspnea, dry cough, hemoptysis, or pneumothorax.
2. Ocular involvement, affecting 25% to 50% of patients, most commonly results in uveitis. Symptoms may include conjunctival injection, photophobia, and tearing.
3. Lymph node and splenic involvement occurs in about 30% of patients. Lymphadenopathy and splenomegaly are often asymptomatic for the patient.
4. Bone involvement occurs in 10% to 15% of patients, manifesting with cystic bone lesions. Patients complain of arthralgias and demonstrate arthritic changes. The wrists, knees, and ankles are most commonly affected.
5. Neurologic involvement occurs in 5% to 15% of patients with systemic involvement. This most commonly manifests as optic nerve disease, facial nerve palsy, meningitis, and cerebral granulomas.
6. Hepatic involvement may occur in about 20% of patients but rarely produces functional difficulties. Liver function tests may be elevated.
7. Cardiac involvement is considered common, yet often asymptomatic. It may result in congestive heart failure, arrhythmia, or conduction defects.
8. Other involvement may include granulomatous changes in kidneys, endocrine glands, stomach, bone marrow, spinal cord, and gonads.

C. Cutaneous manifestations
1. Most common specific cutaneous lesions are 0.2 to 5.0 mm papules of red, violaceous, yellow–brown, brown, hyper-/hypopigmented, or skin color that are common in a symmetric pattern on the head and neck (Figure 21-35).
2. When blanched under a glass slide, all cutaneous sarcoidosis lesions demonstrate an "apple-jelly" semitranslucent yellow–brown color. Scalp lesions may cause scarring alopecia.
3. The second most common specific skin lesions are plaques in an annular, polycyclic, or serpiginous pattern with the same coloration as above whereby the surface can be smooth or scaly and common on extremities, trunk, or buttocks.
   a. *Lupus pernio* refers to violaceous, soft, doughy infiltrations on the nose, cheeks, neck, or earlobes found symmetrically and are telangiectatic (Figure 21-36).
   b. Scar sarcoidosis involves the infiltration of old scars with granulomatous lesions.

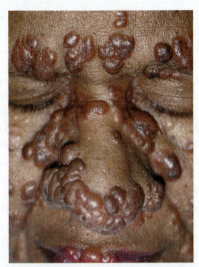

FIGURE 21-35. Cutaneous sarcoidoisis. (From Lugo-Somolinos, A., Lee, I., McKinley-Grant, L., Goldsmith, L. A., Papier, A., Adigun, C. G., …, Fredeking, A. (2011). *VisualDx: Essential dermatology in pigmented skin*. Philadelphia, PA: Wolters Kluwer.)

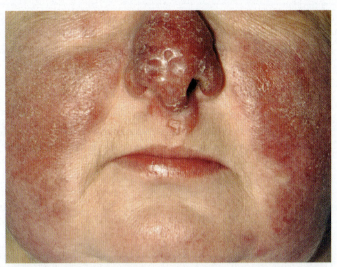

FIGURE 21-36. Sarcoidosis: lupus pernio with infiltration and atrophy of the nose. (From Craft, N., Taylor, E., Tumeh, P. C., Fox, L. P., Goldsmith, L. A., Papier, A., …, Rosenblum, M. (2010). *VisualDx: Essential adult dermatology*. Philadelphia, PA: Wolters Kluwer.)

4. The most common nonspecific lesions are erythema nodosum characterized by firm, red, subcutaneous nodules most commonly found on the anterior tibial surface. Less common nonspecific cutaneous lesions present as acquired ichthyosis, calcinosis cutis, nail clubbing, and erythema multiforme.
5. Cystic lesions can occur in phalangeal bones known as osteitis cystica.
D. Differential diagnosis of cutaneous sarcoidosis includes granuloma annulare, syphilis, cutaneous T-cell lymphoma, lymphoma cutis, lupus erythematosus, tinea fungal/bacterial infections, inflammatory morphea, and cutaneous tuberculosis.
E. Diagnostic tests
1. Pulmonary function testing should include CXR and MRI—brain scan.
2. Skin biopsy demonstrates noncaseating epithelioid cell tubercles.
3. Tissue biopsy when organ involvement is suspected (lung, lymph node, liver, conjunctival, bone marrow, muscle, mediastinum).
4. Laboratory tests may reveal elevated sedimentation rate, elevated gamma globulins, hypercalcemia, and increased levels of angiotensin-converting enzyme.

III. COMMON THERAPEUTIC MODALITIES

A. Systemic therapies
1. Systemic corticosteroids are indicated for unresponsive/progressive ocular, pulmonary, neurologic, hypercalcemia, functional endocrine abnormalities, symptomatic cardiac involvement, or disfiguring skin manifestations. Care must be taken during the tapering process to avoid systemic disease flare-ups.

2. Immunomodulators (infliximab or adalimumab)—inhibiting tumor necrosis factors—can be of use with methotrexate.
B. Local or topical therapies
1. High-potency topical corticosteroids may be helpful. If no effect in 4 weeks, intralesional steroids are indicated for its direct delivery into the dermis.
2. CO_2 laser, pulsed-dye laser, PUVA, cryosurgery, photodynamic therapy for cutaneous lesions
3. Intralesional chloroquine may also be considered.
C. Medical interventions
1. Treatments goals: Prevent organ damage, reduce symptoms, and promote high quality of life. Pulmonary, cardiac, ophthalmology, renal, neurology, and dermatology multidisciplinary approach to management is best.
D. Medications
1. Antimalarial agents (hydroxychloroquine sulfate or chloroquine phosphate) may be helpful in cutaneous sarcoid.
2. Methotrexate, azathioprine, chlorambucil, thalidomide, isotretinoin, leflunomide, and apremilast may be utilized.
E. Surgical interventions
1. Biopsy and surgical excision of lesions are recommended for cosmesis or identifying malignant lesions.
F. Supportive skin care
1. Postsurgical wound care when tumors are excised or removed by laser.
2. Apply antipruritic creams to prevent itching.
G. Other nursing interventions
1. Assess for sarcoid-associated systemic cancers: 40% to 60% of patients with sarcoidosis are more likely to develop malignancy such as lymphomas, Hodgkin disease, and leukemias, as well as nonmelanoma skin cancers.

H. Complementary alternatives
   1. Melatonin may be an effective therapeutic alternative in chronic sarcoidosis with resistance or contraindications to steroids.

IV. HOME CARE CONSIDERATIONS

A. Continuity of care
   1. Assess the need for social service involvement.
   2. Ensure appropriate follow-up care with multidisciplinary health members as appropriate.

PATIENT EDUCATION
Sarcoidosis

- Impart how this disease causes inflammation as tiny clumps of cells, known as granulomas, most often in lung, lymph nodes, eyes, skin, and other organs. Treatment goals are to prevent organ damage with early diagnosis, treatment, and monitoring.
- Patients may have varying degrees of this disease. Minor forms exhibit few symptoms and disappear within a few years; moderate forms may have remissions and flares; whereas severe forms slowly worsen over several years and can result in permanent organ scarring.

GRAFT VERSUS HOST DISEASE

I. OVERVIEW

A. Definition: a multiorgan disorder commonly associated with allogeneic bone marrow (BMT) or hematopoietic cell transplantation (HSCT) that results when host tissues are identified as foreign by the donor (graft) cells or organ. Graft versus host reaction (GVHR) is an expression of graft versus host disease (GVHD) in a specific organ. Acute cutaneous GVHR is the most frequent GVHR occurring 10 to 30 days after BMT. Chronic cutaneous GVHR occurs more than 60 days after allogeneic BMT; it presents with lichenoid and sclerodermal characteristics.

B. Etiology
   1. Immunologic reaction by immunocompetent graft T lymphocytes in an immunocompromised host who is unable to reject the graft (donor cells) causes multiorgan failure.
   2. Less frequent GVHD include nonirradiated blood product transfusions to immunocompromised host, in organ transplantation, and in maternal–fetal transmission to an immunodeficient neonate.

C. Pathophysiology
   1. The host (recipient) of HSCT or BMT expresses tissue antigens not present in the donor (graft) cells, which are recognized as foreign by the donor T lymphocytes. When the host is not able to reject the transplanted (graft) cells, cytokines (IL-2, TNF-α, INF-γ) develop and cause tissue destruction.
   2. Transplanted solid organs have lymphoid tissue allowing the grafts to act in the same manner as mini-BMT: immunological cell reactions causing GVHD.
   3. Chronic GVHD develops autoantibodies and cutaneous sclerosis, which mimic autoimmune connective tissue diseases resulting in lichenoid and sclerodermoid presentations.

D. Incidence
   1. Acute GVHD occurs in 25% to 40% of HSCT, usually within 4 to 6 weeks.
   2. Chronic GVHD occurs in approximately 50% to 80% of HSCT who have had acute GVHD, as a progression of acute GVHD, as a recurrence from a disease-free time, or in the absence of acute GVHD history.
   3. The mortality rate in organ transplant is 75% to 90% due to sepsis, pneumonia, renal failure, or intestinal bleeding.

II. ASSESSMENT

Refer to Table 21-2 and Figures 21-37 through 21-42.

TABLE 21-2 Graft Versus Host Disease

	Acute GVHD (aGVHD)	Chronic GVHD Lichenoid	Chronic GVHD Sclerodermoid
Type and Definition	Immunologic reaction by T-cell lymphocytes in the donated (graft) cells to the host tissue that occurs within 100 days of transfer of immunocompetent donated cells (graft) to an immunocompetent host (most common during a bone marrow, stem cell, or solid organ transplant).	Same as a GVHD but usually occurs at least 60–100 days after the transplant. Classification is based more on clinical presentation rather than time of onset, as chronic GVHD can occur early on in the disease. Timelines are discouraged.	As with chronic lichenoid, but usually occurs after 60–100 days of transplant. Classification is based more on clinical presentation due to the fact that chronic GVHD can present early in the disease and timelines are discouraged.
Etiology/ Pathology	More severe reactions and incidence linked to allogeneic (between two people) mismatch of donor marrow or solid organ, older age, and type of preparation for transplant. Skin change is usually the most common and earliest effect seen, occurring within 100 days of transplant, but typically is seen in first 10–30 days. Progression of disease occurs over several weeks; liver/GI tracts are usually involved.	Manifestation of faulty regulation of host immune system. Usually precedes chronic sclerodermoid, but there is much overlap among GVHD presentations. A graft vs. tumor effect (whereby donated T cells attack malignant cells as well as host cells) decreases incidence of relapse.	Manifestation of faulty regulation of host immune system with scleroderma symptoms. A graft vs. tumor effect decreases incidence of relapse.

TABLE 21-2 *(Continued)*

	Acute GVHD (aGVHD)	Chronic GVHD Lichenoid	Chronic GVHD Sclerodermoid
Diagnosis	Based on onset of clinical lesions, clinical picture, and differential diagnosis. Exclusion of TEN, drug eruption, viral exanthem, and transient acantholytic dermatosis. Histopathology may show basal vacuolization, necrotic epidermal/dermal lymphocytes separation, and subepidermal cleft formation.	Clinical symptoms and history: Skin lesions resemble lichen planus, especially in oral area. Histopathology commonly involves acanthosis, ortho-ridges, basal vacuolization, necrotic epidermal cells, and melanophages in upper dermis.	Clinical symptoms and history: Abnormal LFTs, eosinophilia, autoantibody formation, hypergammaglobulinemia. Histopathology involves thick collagen bundles with loss of interstices, eccrine coil entrapment, loss of pilosebaceous anatomy, and lacrimal/salivary gland lymphocyte infiltration.
Skin Changes	Erythema or perifollicular or maculopapular rash commonly starts on pinna, palms, and soles and progresses to trunk and extremities (Figures 21-37 and 21-38). In acute GVHD, eyes and mucous membranes are less commonly affected. Stages of skin involvement: Stage 1: <25% Stage 2: >25% Stage 3: Erythroderma Stage 4: Vesicles and bullae (life-threatening).	Lichen planus–like with red to purple irregular-shaped papules on flexor surfaces. White, lacy patches on oral mucosa. Skin lesions resolve with postinflammatory hyperpigmentation and thickening. Dry eyes and visual changes may occur as eye and mucous membranes are more commonly involved in the chronic stage.	Resembles scleroderma with plaques of shiny, atrophic, thickened skin and hyper-/hypopigmentation (Figures 21-39 through 21-42). Erosions due to skin ischemia. Alopecia, nail dystrophy, and recurrent bacterial skin infections. In some, the skin may be normal, but the underlying tissue (fascia) is hard.
Systemic Symptoms	Ill appearing with fever, diarrhea, abdominal pain or cramps, nausea/vomiting, elevated liver function tests, hepatomegaly, +/– jaundice, and possibly dry or irritated eyes.	As with acute GVHD, the skin, gut, liver, or mouth can be affected. More likely, joint contractures, neuropathy, and lung inflammation. Nutritional deficits.	Widespread disease may lead to joint contractures, fasciitis, general wasting, esophagitis, sicca symptoms (dry mouth and eyes), and pulmonary fibrosis.
Treatment	*Premedications (prevention)*: Tacrolimus (FK506), methotrexate, or cyclosporine. Pretransplant depletion of T lymphocytes in donor-grafted marrow and use of non-CMV donor cells. *Skin directed*: Topical steroids and PUVA. *Systemic treatment (stages 2–4)*: Systemic steroids, tacrolimus, monoclonal antibodies, cyclosporine, antithymocyte globulins (ATG).	*Systemic*: Combinations of steroids, cyclosporine, azathioprine, mycophenolate mofetil, and thalidomide. Anti-Tac interleukin-2 antibody investigational use. May require chronic antibiotic prophylaxis. *Photochemotherapy*: PUVA and/or photophoresis may be helpful.	Systemic and photo chemotherapies as noted for chronic GVHD lichenoid. The sclerodermatous form of chronic GVHD is most refractory to standard treatments. Etretinate, a synthetic retinoid, can be helpful in these cases. May require chronic antibiotic prophylaxis. Pentoxifylline (Trental, Pentoxil) has active anti-inflammatory properties against TNF-α that may be helpful for chronic skin ulcers or erosions.
Nursing Care/ Comments	High risk for sepsis and severe fluid and electrolyte disturbances. Nutritional and fluid management, intensive skin care, and management of pain with analgesics are essential. Patient/family education and support.	Common cause of death is severe systemic infections. Periodic bacterial and fungal cultures needed. Intense skin, eye, and oral care with pain control. Needs outpatient occupational and physical therapy and nutrition.	See comments for chronic GVHD lichenoid.

LFTs, liver function tests; TENS, toxic epidermal necrolysis syndrome.
Data from Bolgnia, J. L., Schaffer, J. V., Duncan, K. O., & Ko, C. J. (2014). *Dermatology essentials.* Philadelphia, PA: Elsevier-Saunders; James, W. D., Berger, T. G., Elston, D. M. (2011). *Diseases of the skin: Clinical dermatology* (11th ed.). Philladelphia, PA: Elsevier; Lebwohl, M. G., Heymann, W. R., Berth-Jones, J., & Coulson, I. (2014). *Treatment of skin disease: Comprehensive therapeutic strategies* (4th ed.). Philadelphia, PA: Elsevier-Saunders.

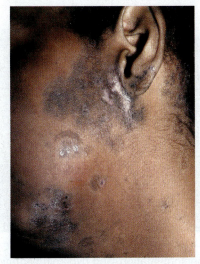

FIGURE 21-37. Atrophy and hyperpigmentation on cheek and ear in graft versus host disease. (From Lugo-Somolinos, A., Lee, I., McKinley-Grant, L., Goldsmith, L. A., Papier, A., Adigun, C. G., …, Fredeking, A. (2011). *VisualDx: Essential dermatology in pigmented skin.* Philadelphia, PA: Wolters Kluwer.)

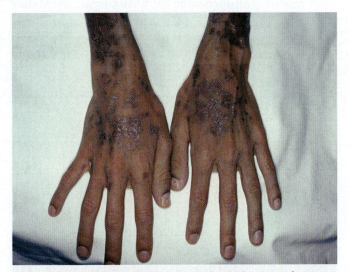

FIGURE 21-38. Symmetrical lichenoid papules in graft versus host disease. (From Lugo-Somolinos, A., Lee, I., McKinley-Grant, L., Goldsmith, L. A., Papier, A., Adigun, C. G., …, Fredeking, A. (2011). *VisualDx: Essential dermatology in pigmented skin.* Philadelphia, PA: Wolters Kluwer.)

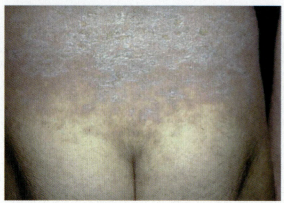

FIGURE 21-39. Lichenoid chronic graft versus host disease: lumbar region with flat-topped, violaceous papules; shiny and lacy white pattern to surface. Confluent in some areas with hypertrophic plaques. (Courtesy of T. L. Diepgen and G. Yihune, Dermatology Online Atlas [http://www.dermis.net/doia].)

BEHCET DISEASE

I. OVERVIEW

A. Definition: chronic multisystem mucocutaneous tissue disorder characterized by a triad of oral, genital, and eye ulcerations as well as systemic inflammation of vasculitis (Figure 21-43).

B. Etiology/pathophysiology: Etiology is unknown.
1. Related to abnormalities in humoral and cellular immunity with antimucosal antibodies present in serum.
2. Cell-mediated hypersensitivity linked to aphthous ulcers, characterized by erratic exacerbations.
3. May be genetic-inherited component in susceptible individuals (HLA-B5 and HLA-B51 gene). In the United States and Europe, there is no consistent HLA association.

C. Incidence
1. Evident worldwide but more prevalent in "Silk Road" regions of Mediterranean basin, Asia, Japan, and Middle

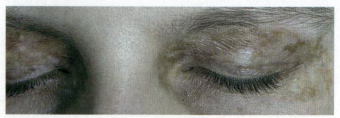

FIGURE 21-40. Chronic graft versus host disease. Scleroderma-like, irregular-shaped, macular lesions with atrophy of dermal and subcutaneous tissues giving paper-thin, easily wrinkled, shiny appearance. (Courtesy of T. L. Diepgen and G. Yihune, Dermatology Online Atlas [http://www.dermis.net/doia].)

East. In the United States, prevalence is 5 in 100,000 people.
2. Disease triad more frequently found in men for Mideast and Asian countries. In the United States and Western Europe, it is more common in women.

D. Considerations across the life span.
1. All ages are affected, but more common in third and fourth decades of life.

II. ASSESSMENT

A. History and physical exam
1. Assess for incidence of trauma-induced lesions (pathergy).
2. Typical course starts with aphthous stomatitis and genital ulceration accompanied by systemic symptoms.
3. Repeated bacterial (streptococcal) or viral (herpes simplex) infections may be linked as causative trigger.
4. Encourage patients to keep log of where and when symptoms occur to assist in diagnosis and treatment as signs and symptoms may not be present at time of clinician examination. Photographs are also helpful.

B. Systemic involvement may include joints, gastrointestinal, renal, cardiac, and eyes.
1. Arthralgias, asymmetrical synovitis, or noninflammatory large joint effusions

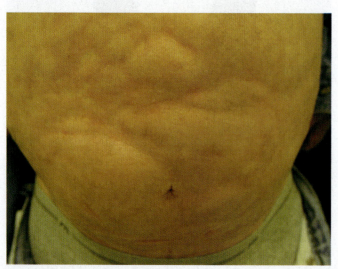

FIGURE 21-41. Chronic graft versus host disease. Sclerodermoid changes to abdomen. (From Dr. Barankin Dermatology Collection.)

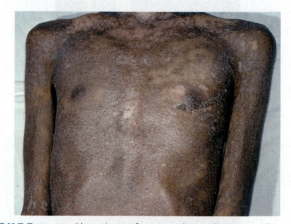

FIGURE 21-42. Chronic graft versus host disease with sclerosis, hypopigmentation, and hyperpigmentation. (From Lugo-Somolinos, A., Lee, I., McKinley-Grant, L., Goldsmith, L. A., Papier, A., Adigun, C. G., ..., Fredeking, A. (2011). *VisualDx: Essential dermatology in pigmented skin.* Philadelphia, PA: Wolters Kluwer.)

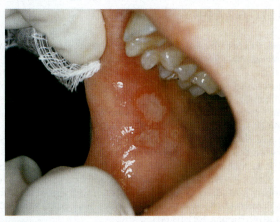

FIGURE 21-43. Behcet oral aphthous ulcer. (From Neville, B. W., Damm, D. D., & White, D. K. (1998). *Color atlas of clinical oral pathology* (2nd ed.). Baltimore, MD: Lippincott Williams & Wilkins.)

2. Cardiac vessel disease of superior or inferior vena cava, superficial and deep thrombophlebitis, and phlebitis of retinal veins and dural sinuses may occur.
3. Gastrointestinal ulceration or perforations can accompany oral stomatitis.
4. Central nervous system onset may be delayed occurring in 25% of patients that may involve meningoencephalitis (headaches, stiff neck, and poor coordination) and psychosis.
5. Lung involvement with artery aneurysm development and/or pleuritis
6. Renal function abnormalities as glomerulonephritis may occur.

C. Cutaneous involvement
1. Aphthous lesions begin as vesicles or pustules and generally heal with scar tissue while deeper lesions begin as submucosal or dermal nodules that heal by scar formation (Figure 21-43).
2. Three typical ulcerative presentations commonly seen on lips, gums, cheeks, and tongue with severe cases also affecting the pharynx and soft palate
   a. Superficial, gray erosions (similar to canker sores)
   b. Deeply punched-out erosions (similar to periadenitis mucosa necrotica recurrens—Sutton disease)
   c. Superficial, herpetiform punctate erosions (rare)
3. Other mucosal involvement may include the esophagus, stomach, intestine, and anus, further complicated by perforation.
4. Eye involvement is the most common cause of morbidity and usually presents unilaterally as iritis or uveitis, scleritis, glaucoma, cataracts, and hypopyon (uncommon hallmark) but eventually progresses to bilateral disease followed by blindness with vitreous hemorrhage and optic neuritis
5. Erythematous pustules, papules, and/or erythema nodosum–like lesions (most common and can ulcerate) may present on legs, torso, and face, which may be trauma induced (pathergy).

D. Differential diagnosis includes aphthous stomatitis, erythema nodosum, erythema multiforme, acute febrile neutrophilic dermatosis, panniculitis, nodular or pustular acne, herpes simplex, acute lupus erythematosus, furunculosis, folliculitis, pyoderma gangrenosum, Sweet disease, Crohn disease, and Reiter syndrome.

E. Diagnosis is based on clinical criteria as a triad of oral ulcerations accompanied by any two manifestations listed below in 1 to 4. (No lab test exists.)
1. Genital ulcers (men: scrotum; women: vulva)
2. Eye lesions
3. Skin lesions
4. Positive testing for pathergy: trauma-induced papule greater than 2 mm within 48 hours following 20- to 22-gauge needle prick (most common in Mediterranean and Middle East).
5. Histology is nonspecific but vasculitis is present, and there is commonly a majority of helper-inducer T cells over T-suppressor cytotoxic cells.

III. COMMON THERAPEUTIC MODALITIES

A. Systemic therapy
1. Systemic steroids are a mainstay of therapy and are often used in combination with other therapies.
2. Anti-TNF therapies have been used successfully: rebamipide, etanercept, and infliximab (note: prior screen for latent tuberculosis infection must be done).

B. Local or topical therapy
1. Topical and intralesional corticosteroids are main treatments.
2. Topicals to accelerate healing and decrease pain may include viscous lidocaine, sucralfate, topical tacrolimus, or tetracycline suspension.

C. Medical interventions
1. Multidisciplinary approach must include dermatologist, rheumatologist, urologist, gynecologist, ophthalmologist, gastroenterologist, and neurologist.
2. Lab testing needed are herpes viral cultures, vitamin levels, HLA-B27, and urinalysis.

D. Medications
1. Nonsteroidal anti-inflammatory drugs include levamisole, colchicine, dapsone, and sulfapyridine and may be helpful for mucosal and/or arthritic symptoms.
2. Immunomodulators include thalidomide for mucosal involvement (cautious use due to its teratogenic effects) and interferon-alpha 2A and 2B.
3. Immunosuppressants may include azathioprine, cyclosporine, and FK506, which may be used for eye and CNS involvement, cyclophosphamide and chlorambucil (alkylating agents), and methotrexate.
4. Anticoagulants for thrombosis may be necessary.

E. Diet management
1. Encourage a bland diet with soft foods. Avoid spicy and acidic foods/beverages.
2. Encourage fluid intake of 3 to 4 L/day if medical condition permits.
3. Offer frequent, small feedings with cool/cold foods being more soothing.

F. Surgical intervention may be needed for eye, gastrointestinal, or cardiac involvement.

G. Supportive skin care
   1. Use topical steroids, anesthetics, and antibiotics for skin and mucosal lesions.

H. Other nursing interventions
   1. Assist with coordination of multidisciplinary approach and ensure good communication among all health care team members.
   2. Assess for depression and need for individual/family counseling related to stressors of living with a chronic illness.
   3. Assess the pain level and provide adequate pain control measures.

IV. CONTINUITY OF CARE

A. Provide education on diagnosis and local/systemic treatment.

B. Encourage involvement with national/community support systems and information sources such as the American Behcet's Disease Association (ABDA), Arthritis Foundation, and National Arthritis and Musculoskeletal and Skin Diseases Information Clearinghouse (NAMSIC).

PATIENT EDUCATION
Behcet Disease

- Enlist patient's participation in knowledge of Behcet disease as in informed consumer, reporting symptoms or outcomes with specific treatments.

- Reinforce the variability of this disease as it is an autoinflammatory disorder often causing a pustular vasculitis with chronic relapses of oral, genital, eye, or extremity lesions.

BIBLIOGRAPHY

Bolgnia, J. L., Schaffer, J. V., Duncan, K. O., & Ko, C. J. (2014). *Dermatology essential.* Philadelphia, PA: Elsevier-Saunders.

Braverman, L. E., & Coope, D. (2013). *Werner & Ingbar's The thyroid: A fundamental and clinical text* (10th ed.). Philadelphia, PA: Lippincott Williams & Wilkins.

Callen, J. P., & Jorizzo, J. L. (2009). *Dermatological signs of internal disease* (4th ed.). Philadelphia, PA: Elsevier-Saunders.

Deng, A., & Song, D. (2011). Multipoint subcutaneous injection of long-acting glucocorticoid as a cure for pretibial myxedema. *Thyroid, 21*(1), 83–85.

Fazzi, P. I., Manni, E., Cristofani, R., Cei, G., Piazza, S., Calabrese, R., …, Carpi, A. (2012). Thalidomide for improving cutaneous and pulmonary sarcoidosis in patients resistant or with contraindications to corticosteroids. *Biomedicine and Pharmacotherapy, 66*(4), 300–307. doi: 10.1016/j.biopha.2012.03.005

Garber, J. R., Cobin, R. H., Gharib, H., Hennessey, J. V., Klein, I., Mechanick, J. I., …, Woeber, K. A. (2012). American Association of Clinical Endocrinologists and American Thyroid Association Task Force on Hypothyroidism in Adults. Clinical practice guidelines for hypothyroidism in adults: Cosponsored by the American Association of Clinical Endocrinologists and the American Thyroid Association. *Endocrine Practice, 18*(6), 988–1028.

Ghalayani, P., Zahra, S., & Sardari, F. (2012). Neurofibromatosis type I (von Recklinghausen's disease): A family case report and literature review. *Dental Research Journal, 9*(4), 483–488.

James, W. D., Berger, T. G., Elston, D. M. (2011). *Diseases of the skin: Clinical dermatology* (11th ed.). Philadelphia, PA: Elsevier.

Lebwohl, M. G., Heymann, W. R., Berth-Jones, J., & Coulson, I. (2014). *Treatment of skin disease: Comprehensive therapeutic strategies* (4th ed.). Philadelphia, PA: Elsevier-Saunders.

Takasu, N., Higa, H., & Knjou, Y. (2010). Treatment of pretibial myxedema (PTM) with topical steroid ointment application with sealing cover in Grave's patients. *Internal Medicine, 49*(7), 665–669.

Wolff, K., Johnson, R. A., & Saavedra, A. P. (2013). *Fitzpatrick's color atlas and synopsis of clinical dermatology* (7th ed.). New York, NY: McGraw-Hill.

Wu, P. A., & Cowen, E. W. (2012). Cutaneous graft-versus-host-disease: Clinical considerations and management. *Current Problems in Dermatology, 43*, 101–115. doi: 10.1159/000335270

Zang, H. L., & Wu, J. (2010). Role of vitamin D in immune responses and autoimmune diseases with emphasis on its role in multiple sclerosis. *Neuroscience Bulletin, 26*(6), 445–454.

STUDY QUESTIONS

1. Neurofibromatosis (von Recklinghausen disease) may show cutaneous involvement as:
   a. Plexiform neuromas (large masses of skin along nerves)
   b. Crowe sign (axillary freckling)
   c. Multiple café au lait spots
   d. All of the above

2. Lupus pernio involves violaceous, telangiectatic papules, which are found symmetrically on the face and neck in:
   a. Hypothyroidism
   b. Sarcoidosis
   c. Behcet disease
   d. Neurofibromatosis

3. Differential diagnoses of skin lesions typically seen in acute graft versus host disease (GVHD) include:
   a. TENS (toxic epidermal necrolysis syndrome)
   b. Drug eruption
   c. Viral exanthems
   d. All of the above

4. Which of the following statements regarding Behcet disease is *true*?
   a. In the United States and Europe, it is most common in women.
   b. It is related to humoral and cellular immunity, yet the cause is unknown.
   c. Lesions originate from Schwann cells of peripheral nervous system.
   d. All of the above.

5. Acanthosis nigricans, xanthomas, rubeosis, and hemochromatosis may be found in which of the following systemic diseases?
   a. Sarcoidosis
   b. Hyperthyroidism
   c. Diabetes mellitus
   d. Hypothyroidism
   e. Neurofibromatosis

6. Which of the following statements regarding the sign of Leser–Trélat is *false*?
   a. It may occur with acanthosis nigricans simultaneously.
   b. It is associated with intra-abdominal carcinoma.
   c. It is associated with hepatic tumors.
   d. It is the sudden onset of multiple seborrheic keratotic lesions.

7. Which of the following statements regarding the characteristics of hypothyroidism is *false*?
   a. Hair loss pattern includes the outer third of the eyebrows.
   b. Nails are thin, brittle, and striated longitudinally or transversely.
   c. Bruising and telangiectasias can be found on arms, fingertips, and legs due to capillary fragility.
   d. Thyroid dermopathy or pretibial myxedema can occur.

8. Chronic GVHD includes all of the following characteristic lesions *except*:
   a. Erythematous macular rash on pinnae, palms, or soles.
   b. Hyperpigmented or hypopigmented thickened skin.
   c. Lichenoid or sclerodermoid.
   d. White lacy patches on oral mucosa.

9. Medical management for lymphomas and/or leukemias may include:
   a. Blood/platelet transfusions
   b. Intralesional corticosteroid injections
   c. Radiation therapy to individual lesions
   d. All of the above

10. Which of the following statements regarding the characteristics of Trousseau syndrome is *false*?
    a. It is associated with pancreatic or prostate cancer.
    b. Patients exhibit tender erythematous, serpiginous bands like "wood grain" patterns.
    c. Patients exhibit superficial thrombophlebitis of neck, chest, abdomen, and lower extremity veins.
    d. It may be related to chronic intravascular coagulopathy.

Answers to Study Questions: 1.d, 2.b, 3.d, 4.b, 5.c, 6.c, 7.d, 8.a, 9.d, 10.b

Hair and Nails

Kim B. Sanders

NORMAL HAIR

I. OVERVIEW

A. Hair is a keratin structure of the epidermis and a specialized skin appendage. The physiologic functions include insulation, esthetic and cosmetic display, tactile perception, thermoregulation, and protection from UV light.

B. Embryonic development
   1. First follicles form at about 9 weeks of gestation, mainly in the eyebrows, upper lip, and chin. Remainder develop at 4 to 5 months of gestation.
   2. Epidermal cells progressively penetrate downward into the maturing dermis, passing through "germ," "peg," and "bulbous peg" stages of development.
   3. No hair follicles form after birth.

C. Anatomy
   1. The hair shaft is organized into seven longitudinal regions, beginning from the epidermis (Figure 22-1).
      a. Hair canal region—present only during fetal development and extends from the skin surface to the level of the epidermal–dermal junction
      b. Infundibulum—funnel-shaped top of follicular canal. Extends to opening of the sebaceous duct
      c. Sebaceous gland area
      d. Isthmus—located between the entry of sebaceous duct and insertion of arrector pili muscle
      e. Area of the bulge—site of the insertion of the arrector pili muscle
      f. Lower follicle—extends from the area of the bulge to the top of the hair bulb
      g. Hair bulb—is the deepest part of the hair follicle and surrounds the dermal papilla
   2. Cross section of hair follicle reveals a series of cellular compartments (Figure 22-2).
      a. A cellular basement membrane ("glassy membrane"). Surrounds entire follicle
      b. Outer root sheath—most peripheral of cellular components
      c. Inner root sheath—comprised of three separate layers. From outermost to innermost:
         (1) Henle layer
         (2) Huxley layer
         (3) Cuticle
      d. Hair shaft—also comprised of three separate layers. From outermost to innermost:
         (1) Cuticle—the outside portion. Consists of overlapping cell layers arranged like shingles, which protect the hair shaft.
         (2) Cortex—the bulk of the hair shaft. "Cigar-shaped" cells, which synthesize and accumulate proteins while in the lower regions of the hair shaft.

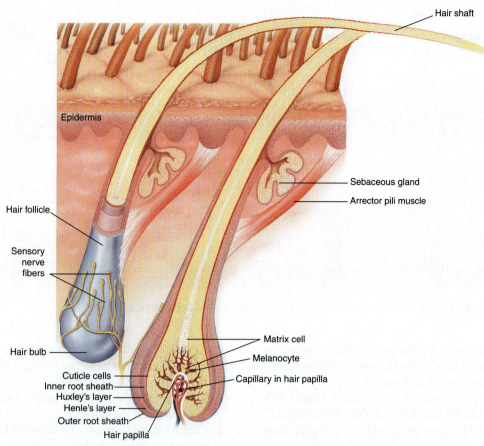

FIGURE 22-1. Schematic drawing showing anatomy of the hair follicle. (From Schalock, P. C., et al. (2010). *Lippincott's primary care dermatology*. Philadelphia, PA: Wolters Kluwer. Asset provided by Anatomical Chart Co.)

(3) Medulla—present only in large terminal hairs. May be discontinuous.

D. Hair growth
1. Hair growth is cyclical, and follicles grow in a repeated three-part cycle. Each follicle functions as an independent unit (Figure 22-3).
   a. Anagen—actively growing hair. Can be subdivided into six stages. For scalp hair, lasts 2 to 7 years.

Hair

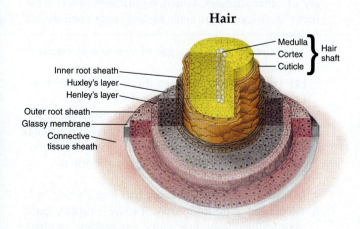

FIGURE 22-2. Cross-section of a hair follicle. (From Anatomical Chart Company, 2004.)

b. Catagen—metabolic processes associated with hair growth gradually decreasing. The hair follicle regresses. Can be subdivided into eight stages. Lasts approximately 2 to 3 weeks regardless of site and follicle type.
c. Telogen—the resting phase. Existing hair will never grow longer. Lasts 3 months for scalp hairs. Hairs have a club-shaped proximal end, which will be shed from the follicle during the telogen-to-anagen transition called exogen.
2. Length of growth cycle varies according to body site with a general relationship of increasing hair length to a longer growth cycle.
3. Genetic programs determine normal growth parameters for hair on different anatomical locations; for example, eyelash hairs remain short while scalp hair grows much longer.
4. Hormones influence hair growth. Androgens influence pubic, axillary, beard, trunk, and extremity hair as well as lead to hair loss in susceptible individuals. Estrogens tend to prolong the telogen phase and delay the anagen phase.

E. Distribution of hair
1. Covers entire body except palms, soles, interspaces of the digits, and portions of the genitalia.

Hair Growth Cyle

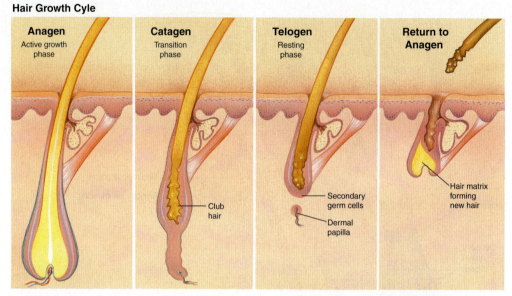

FIGURE 22-3. The hair growth cycle. (From Anatomical Chart Company, 2004.)

2. Greatest density on scalp, numbering 100,000 in people with brown/black hair. Is about 20% greater in natural blondes and 20% less in redheads.
3. At any given time, 85% to 90% of hairs are in anagen, 10% to 15% are in telogen, and less than 1% are in catagen.
4. Normal hair shedding ranges from 50 to 100 scalp hairs per day.

F. Types of hair
1. Hairs are classified into four groups according to texture and length.
   a. Lanugo hairs—soft, fine, lightly pigmented hair. Found in utero on fetal skin. These are shed between 32nd and 36th weeks of gestation.
   b. Vellus hairs—fine, short hair with little pigment. Replace lanugo hairs. Found on all parts of body except palms, soles, parts of genitalia, and periungual areas.
   c. Indeterminate hairs—fall between vellus and terminal hairs in size.
   d. Terminal hairs—thicker, longer, coarser hair. Frequently has a central medulla and is pigmented. Found only on scalp, eyebrows, and eyelashes in children. Androgen production at puberty stimulates conversion from small to large terminal hairs in scalp, beard (males), axillary, and pubic regions.
2. Any one hair follicle can give rise to different types of hair within its lifetime; for example, during puberty, former vellus hairs become terminal hairs in the beard, scalp, pubic, and axillary regions.

G. Hair pigmentation
1. Melanocytes located in the hair bulb of the follicle produce pigment.
2. Pigment is most prominent in the cortex of the hair shaft.
3. Any follicle can produce two types of pigment, although usually only one type at any time is found.
   a. Eumelanin—pigment found in brown or black hairs
   b. Pheomelanin—pigment found in red or blonde hairs

4. Generally, pigment is not found in the hair shaft during the early stages of new hair formation and in the proximal portion of telogen hairs.
5. Color intensity is generally proportional to the amount of pigment in the fiber.
6. Graying hair is a result of a decreased number of melanocytes in the hair bulb.

H. Morphology of hair
1. Four categories: straight, spiral, helical, and wavy.
2. Caucasians are the hairiest and may contain any of these categories.
3. Asian hair is straight due to straight follicles with lower portions oriented vertically to the skin surface.
4. Hair in blacks is spiraled due to curved follicles with lower portions almost horizontal to the skin surface.

II. ASSESSMENT

A. History and physical examination
1. Patient history—cause may be associated with a variety of other diseases, which significantly affect treatment decisions. Pertinent history may include the following:
   a. Hair change duration, age of onset, and extent of involvement including:
      (1) Distinguishing between thinning and shedding
      (2) Loss or gain, diffuse or focal
      (3) Areas of hair loss, scarring or nonscarring
      (4) Increase or decrease in amount of hair lost per day
      (5) Change in color or texture
      (6) Distribution of hair, normal or abnormal
      (7) Gradual or sudden onset
      (8) Symmetric or asymmetric hair loss
   b. Associated symptoms may include pruritus, pain, skin lesions, fever, pregnancy, psychologic or physiologic stress, or presence of systemic disease.
   c. Current medications and supplements

d. Exposure to environmental or occupational toxins or chemicals

e. Nutritional status

f. Current and past treatment and response

2. Physical examination—inspect hair for texture, color, quality, and distribution.

B. Diagnostic tests: when the diagnosis is not clinically evident, the following tests may be indicated.

1. Hair pull test
2. Microscopic examination of the hair
3. Hair counts
4. Biopsy
5. KOH preparation
6. Fungal culture
7. Immune, endocrine, and other laboratory studies, if indicated

PATIENT EDUCATION
Hair Loss Disorders

- Apply sunscreens (SPF > 15) and wear hat/scarf when sun exposure is expected or when outside.
- Limit shampooing, combing, and brushing hair as much as possible.
- Use cream rinse or conditioner after shampooing.
- Avoid vigorous rubbing with a towel, rough combing, and brushing especially when hair is wet.
- Use wide-toothed combs and brushes with smooth tips.
- Avoid hairstyles that pull tightly on the hair and should be alternated with looser hairstyles.

HAIR DISORDERS: ALOPECIA AREATA

I. OVERVIEW

A. Definition: nonscarring alopecia with rapid and complete loss of hair in round patches. Usually involves the scalp, beard, eyebrows, and eyelashes. Chronic and relapsing.

B. Etiology

1. Cause unknown but likely a hair-specific autoimmune disease

C. Pathophysiology

1. Telogen and dystrophic hairs with irregular shapes and fractured ends are removed in hair pull tests.
2. Dystrophic hairs fracture forming "explanation point" hairs found at the edges of hairless patches.
3. Lymphatic infiltrate found around affected hair bulb and lower one third of follicle.
4. Hair cycle is disrupted and an increased number of terminal catagen and telogen hairs are present.
5. Normal total number of hair follicles.
6. Inflammatory insult to matrix causes tapering of hair shaft.

D. Clinical features

1. Classic presentation is a well-defined round or oval patch of total hair loss on the scalp. There are three less common subtypes:

a. Alopecia totalis—loss of all terminal scalp hairs
b. Alopecia universalis—loss of all scalp and body hair
c. Ophiasis—band of alopecia around the temporal and occipital scalp

2. Paresthesia or pruritus may accompany hair loss in some patients.
3. Disease activity may be insidious or rapid.
4. Scarring is not present, unless disease is long standing.
5. Nail findings may include pitting, thin or brittle fingernails and toenails, and longitudinal ridging.
6. With regrowth, the hairs may initially be gray or white, but eventually repigment.

E. Incidence

1. Affects males and females equally.
2. Occurs in both children and adults. However, 50% of cases occur before age 20.

II. ASSESSMENT

A. See Normal Hair, Assessment.

B. If prompted by symptoms, investigate possible disease associations such as:

1. Atopy (atopic dermatitis, allergic rhinitis, or asthma)
2. Autoimmune diseases such as thyroid disease, vitiligo, inflammatory bowel disease, or polyendocrinopathy
3. Emotional distress

III. COMMON THERAPEUTIC MODALITIES

A. Medical interventions

1. Intralesional corticosteroid injections, particularly on scalp or eyebrows. About 66% of patients will experience some growth.

a. Inject involved area with dilute triamcinolone acetonide suspension up to 10 mg/mL (scalp) or 3 to 5 mg/mL (eyebrows) using a 27- or 30-gauge needle.
b. Reinject at 4- to 6-week intervals. Discontinue after 3 months if no growth present.
c. Thinning of regrowth may occur after 3 to 6 months and can be reinjected as necessary.
d. Spontaneous regrowth may occur 3 to 6 months after injection.

2. Potent topical steroids. Short white or finely pigmented hairs develop within 3 to 4 months if treatment is successful.
3. Systemic (oral or IV) corticosteroids can be considered. However, they should not be used for long periods of time due to risk of side effects.
4. Contact sensitizers such as squaric acid dibutylester or diphencyprone

a. Patients are first sensitized to the agent with a 2% concentration in acetone.
b. After 1 week, a 0.001% solution is applied to all affected areas on one side of the scalp. This is repeated weekly.

c. Concentration is titrated up according to previous weeks reaction. Goal reaction is to maintain low-grade erythema, with or without scaling and pruritus, for 2 to 3 days after application.

d. Regrowth consisting of white or finely pigmented hairs develop within 3 to 4 months, if successful.

e. If no growth in 3 to 4 months, consider another therapy.

5. Topical anthralin
   a. Apply lowest concentration to affected area daily.
   b. If no hair growth, concentration may be increased to 1.0%. Apply to affected area 20 to 30 minutes daily.

6. Topical minoxidil
   a. Positive results seen in only a small percentage of patients.
   b. May take up to 4 months to see regrowth.
   c. Will keep working only as long as used.
   d. New hair may be lost when drug is discontinued.

7. Other topical irritants, such as tazarotene or azelaic acid, may be of limited benefit.

8. Light therapy
   a. Psoralens, topical or systemic, with ultraviolet A. Successful in only a small percentage of patients.
   b. Excimer laser—focal narrow band UVB.
   c. Photodynamic therapy.

9. Other compounds with limited studies, but some reported benefit, include isoprinosine, total glucosides of paeony capsules, topical garlic gel (in combination with topical steroids), and aromatherapy.

10. Oral antidepressants.

B. Surgical interventions: none

PATIENT EDUCATION
Alopecia

- Direct patients to the National Alopecia Areata Foundation Web site, www.naaf.com, for information on support groups, wigs/hair prostheses, and research.

ANDROGENIC ALOPECIA

I. OVERVIEW

A. Definition: androgenic alopecia is the most common cause of thinning hair. There are two types, male pattern (common baldness) and female pattern hair loss.

B. Etiology
   1. Inherited condition from either parent

C. Pathophysiology
   1. Regression depends on androgen production with normal serum androgen levels found.
   2. Process is progressive beginning with hair shedding, followed by smaller hair shaft diameter "miniaturization," shortening of anagen, and lengthening of telogen growth phases.
   3. Total number of hair follicles nearly normal (about 35 per 4-mm plug).

TABLE 22-1 Classification of Male Androgenic Alopecia

Type	Clinical Features
I	Normal frontotemporal hairline.
II	Symmetric triangular areas of recession in the frontoparietal regions. Hair also lost along midfrontal scalp border.
II-A[a]	Anterior hairline high on forehead.
III	Deep frontotemporal recession. Minimal extent of hair loss considered to represent baldness. Vertex type—hair is lost chiefly at the vertex with or without frontal recession.
III-A[a]	Alopecic area extends to middle crown area.
IV	Deep frontal and frontotemporal recession in association with hair loss at the vertex.
IV-A[a]	Alopecia extends past midcrown of scalp with posterior thinning.
V	The separation from recessed frontal and frontoparietal alopecia to the vertex area of alopecia now narrower and more sparse than in type IV.
V-A[a]	Area of alopecia not entirely to vertex. Most advanced stage of type A variant.
VI	Frontotemporal and vertex areas of alopecia now confluent. Area of alopecia has extended laterally and posteriorly.
VII	Most severe male pattern baldness with only a narrow horseshoe-shaped band of hair remaining.

[a]Type A variant: Major criteria must be present: anterior hairline recedes posteriorly with no midfrontal island of hair; no concomitant thinning at the vertex. Minor criteria common but not necessary: sparse hairs persist in alopecic area; wreath of remaining temporal and occipital hair wider and higher than in non-A variant.

Adapted from Norwood, O. T. (1975). Male pattern baldness: Classification and incidence. *Southern Medical Journal, 68*(11), 1359–1365.

4. Reduced number of terminal hairs.
5. Increased number of vellus hairs.
6. Increased telogen count when compared with uninvolved scalp.

D. Clinical features
   1. Occurs most commonly in late adolescence or in early 20s.
   2. Patterns of male androgenic alopecia (Table 22-1, Figure 22-4).
      a. Hamilton classification system
      b. Norwood classification system
   3. Ludwig classification system used to describe female androgenic alopecia (Table 22-2, Figure 22-5).

II. ASSESSMENT

A. See Normal Hair, Assessment.

B. Rule out reversible causes of telogen effluvium as these can worsen preexisting alopecia.
   1. Women should be tested for iron deficiency.
   2. Consider testing for thyroid disease and androgen excess as indicated by symptoms.

III. COMMON THERAPEUTIC MODALITIES

A. Medical interventions
   1. Topical minoxidil 5%. Apply to scalp twice daily in men and daily in women.
      a. Shedding may be noticed with the first few months of application.

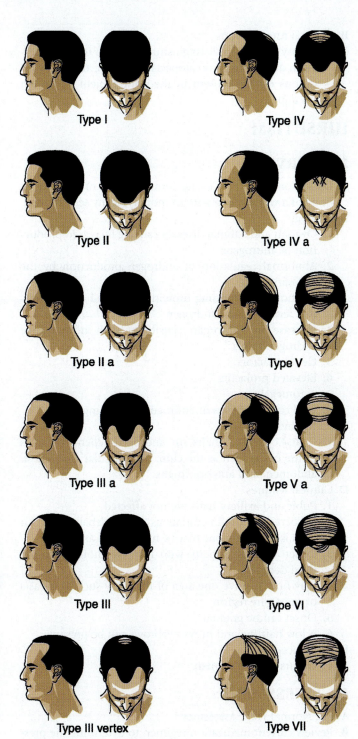

FIGURE 22-4. Norwood-Hamilton classification of male androgenetic alopecia. (From Schalock, P. C., et al. (2010). *Lippincott's primary care dermatology*. Philadelphia, PA: Wolters Kluwer.)

b. May take 4 months to notice an improvement.
c. Will keep working only as long as it is used. New hair is lost when drug is stopped.
d. Can cause facial hair growth in females.
2. Finasteride (Propecia), 1 mg taken daily, acts as a specific competitive inhibitor of steroid type II 5-alpha-reductase.
3. Spironolactone, 50 to 200 mg taken daily, acts as a aldosterone antagonist, for use in women.

TABLE 22-2 Ludwig Classification of Female Androgenic Alopecia

Type	Clinical Features
I	Mild decrease in hair density on the crown; hairs in this area become thinner, shorter, and less pigmented; frontal hairline is retained.
II	Moderate decrease in hair density on the crown; frontal hairline is still retained.
III	Extensive decrease in hair density on the crown; sparse frontal hairline.

B. Surgical interventions
   1. Hair transplant

TELOGEN EFFLUVIUM

I. OVERVIEW

A. Definition: increased shedding of normal telogen hairs in response to a change of health, emotional, or nutritional status
B. Etiology
   1. Most common type of hair loss associated with medications, systemic illness, postsurgery, or severe psychologic stress (Box 22-1)
   2. Usually acute. Chronic form commonly associated with medications, and in many cases, there is no discernible cause.
C. Pathophysiology
   1. Hair shedding starts approximately 3 months after the precipitating event.
D. Clinical features
   1. Hair loss in handfuls. More than the expected 50 to 100 hairs per day.
   2. Telogen hairs characteristic with a depigmented blub at the end.
   3. Hair loss occurs diffusely over the scalp.
   4. Duration of hair loss approximately 3 months with acute disease.
   5. Complete regrowth is expected.
E. Incidence
   1. Occurs in men and women; however, women more likely to experience this condition due to correlation with hormonal changes and the postpartum period.

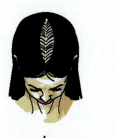
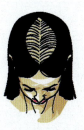
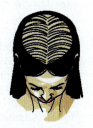

I   II   III

FIGURE 22-5. Patterns of female androgenic alopecia. (From Schalock, P. C., et al. (2010). *Lippincott's primary care dermatology*. Philadelphia, PA: Wolters Kluwer.)

Box 22-1. Possible Causes of Telogen Effluvium

Childbirth
Acute blood loss
Poor nutrition
High fever
Surgery
Severe psychological stress
Hypothyroidism
Severe infection
Medications

II. ASSESSMENT

A. See Normal Hair, Assessment.
B. Review current medications (Box 22-2).
C. Consider laboratory tests for thyroid function, chemistries, ferritin, and hematocrit.
D. Consider biopsy if lasting longer than 6 months.

III. COMMON THERAPEUTIC MODALITIES

A. Medical interventions
1. Stop offending medication, if applicable.
2. Investigate inciting event. If discovered, reassure patient that the shedding should stop after approximately 3 months.
3. Iron supplementation if deficient

Box 22-2. Substances Reported to Cause (or Possibly Cause) Telogen Hair Loss

Allopurinol
ACE inhibitors
Androgens
Anticoagulants
Antithyroid agents
Benzimidazoles
Beta-blockers
Bromocriptine
Carbamazepine
Cimetidine
Clofibrate
Colchicine
Fluconazole
Gold
Immunoglobulin
Interferon alpha and gamma
Ketoconazole
Levodopa
Methotrexate
Methysergide
Minoxidil
Oral contraception
Proguanil
Psychotropic medications
Pyridostigmine bromide
Oral retinoids
Sodium valproate
Sulfasalazine
Excess vitamin A

Adapted from Olsen, E. A. (2003). *Disorders of hair growth, diagnosis and treatment* (2nd ed.). New York, NY: McGraw-Hill Companies, Inc.

B. Surgical interventions
1. Biopsy helpful in distinguishing between telogen effluvium and androgenic alopecia. However, the two conditions can be present in the same patient and often overlap.

HIRSUTISM

I. OVERVIEW

A. Definition: growth of coarse terminal hairs on the face or body of a woman in a pattern more typically seen in men.
B. Etiology
1. Ovarian and adrenal diseases causing increased production of androgens
2. Abnormal regulation of androgen production by the pituitary gland
3. Sex hormone–binding proteins depressed despite normal levels of total androgen
4. Increase in end-organ sensitivity with normal free androgen levels
5. Genetic factors
6. Elevated prolactin
7. Acromegaly
8. Oral contraceptives or androgen-containing drugs
C. Pathophysiology
1. Coarse, terminal hairs on androgen-dependent areas of the body, such as the chin, periauricular area, chest, abdomen, and anterior thighs
D. Clinical features
1. Pubic and axillary hairs are not affected.
2. Major racial and ethnic variations occur with hair growth, so what is normal in one may be hirsutism in another.
3. Onset often at puberty with increases noted into the third decade.
4. May only involve one area of the body such as breasts or mustache region.
5. Onset can be gradual.
6. A low hairline and heavy eyebrows can be present.
E. Incidence
1. Occurs only in women

II. ASSESSMENT

A. See Normal Hair, Assessment.
B. Review current medication regimen to determine the presence of drugs reported to cause hirsutism (Box 22-3).

Box 22-3. Drugs Reported to Cause Hirsutism

Anabolic steroids
Corticosteroids
Cyclosporin
Diazoxide
Minoxidil
Psychogenic drugs
Phenothiazine
Phenytoin
Testosterone

C. Evaluate for acanthosis nigricans, acne, and obesity.

D. Obtain laboratory tests for free and total testosterone levels, dehydroepiandrosterone sulfate (DHEAS), the luteinizing hormone/follicle-stimulating hormone ratio (LH/FSH), and prolactin. Repeat to confirm diagnosis.

E. Normal menstrual history is consistent with nonendocrine cause.

F. Ultrasound and computed tomography (CT) if screening suggests underlying disease.

III. COMMON THERAPEUTIC MODALITIES

A. Medical interventions
1. Oral contraceptive pills for androgen suppression.
2. Prednisone, 5 mg/day, or dexamethasone, 0.5 mg/day, to suppress pituitary–adrenals if indicated.
3. Cyproterone acetate, 50 to 100 mg/day, from the 5th to 15th days of menses. Not available in the United States.
4. Antiandrogens such as spironolactone, flutamide, and finasteride.
5. Bromocriptine to decrease prolactin, if indicated.

B. Surgical interventions
1. Surgery may be required for ovarian and adrenal tumors, as well as some pituitary tumors.

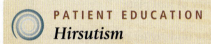

PATIENT EDUCATION
Hirsutism

- Physical methods such as plucking, waxing, chemical depilation, and shaving produce temporary removal of unwanted hair.
- Hair bleaching with hydrogen peroxide will make unwanted hair less obvious.
- Electrolysis or laser hair removal can produce permanent removal of hair.
- Eflornithine hydrochloride cream slows the hair growth cycle.

TRICHOTILLOMANIA

I. OVERVIEW

A. Definition: a form of alopecia resulting from repetitive pulling, plucking, and breaking of one's own hair

B. Etiology
1. Attributed to a variety of psychodynamic conflicts
2. Ultimate cause unclear

C. Pathophysiology
1. Total number of hairs, both terminal and vellus, normal
2. Incomplete, disrupted follicular anatomy
3. Many empty distorted follicles, often with pigment casts
4. No significant peribulbar inflammation

D. Clinical features
1. May involve single or multiple areas of the scalp, particularly the frontal, parietal, or occipital regions, with remainder of scalp normal.
2. Involvement of eyebrows and eyelashes may be seen in 25% of affected patients.
3. Alopecic patches are often unilateral, occurring on the same side at the patient's dominant hand, are variable in size, and often have bizarre shapes and irregular borders.
4. Telogen hairs missing and anagen hairs twisted and broken at various lengths in involved sites.
5. Texture and color of broken hairs unaffected.
6. Pruritus uncommon although some patients complain of itching and may have excoriations.
7. Teenage and adult patients with more severe disease usually deny touching their hair and rarely admit to the self-induced nature of their hair loss.

E. Incidence
1. Two thirds of affected patients are children, adolescents, and young adults.
2. Boys outnumber girls by 3 to 2, but females predominate in the older age groups.

II. ASSESSMENT

A. See Normal Hair, Assessment.

B. Biopsy from involved area reveals:
1. Decreased number of telogen follicles and an increased number of catagen follicles
2. Normal follicles found among involuted, damaged, or empty follicles
3. Presence of pigmented casts, usually in the isthmus or infundibular area, representing clumps of melanin and keratinaceous debris

III. COMMON THERAPEUTIC MODALITIES

A. Medical interventions
1. Discuss the problem frankly with patient and/or parents of an affected child.
2. Perform "hair window" by occluding a clipped area in a location that the patient cannot see. Removal of the occlusion in 1 to 3 weeks should show proportional 1 cm per month hair growth.
3. Arrange psychiatric consultation for psychotherapy, behavior modification therapy, and antidepressant medication including desipramine, clomipramine, or fluoxetine.

B. Surgical interventions: none

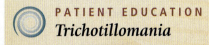

PATIENT EDUCATION
Trichotillomania

- Identify and avoid factors that provoke emotional trauma, stress, anxiety, and fear.

NORMAL NAILS

I. OVERVIEW

A. Definition: the nail covers the upper surface of each finger and toe and acts as a protective covering to the end of each digit. Nails serve as scratching organs, assist in grasping small objects, and have an increasingly important esthetic and cosmetic purpose.

B. Embryonic development
  1. 9 weeks: proximal, lateral, and distal groves of the nail field first appear.
  2. 12 weeks: future nail bed has both granular and horny layers. Vessel formation is present.
  3. 18 weeks: nail bed loses granular zone.
  4. 20 weeks: matrix cells exhibit adult keratinization.

C. Anatomy: the nail unit consists of components, which form, cover, support, anchor, and frame the nail plate (Figure 22-6).
  1. Nail matrix
    a. Most proximal portion of the nail bed extending to the lunula.
    b. Situated above the middle part of the distal phalanx.
    c. Major function is to produce the nail plate.
  2. Nail plate
    a. Major visible part of the nail arising from matrix.
    b. Usually flat and rectangular in shape.
    c. Fingernails approximately 0.5 mm thick in females and 0.6 mm thick in males. Toenails approximately 1.4 mm thick in females and 1.6 mm thick in males.
    d. Distal plate thickness can be ranked thumb, index, middle, ring, and little finger.
    e. Length of matrix determines thickness of nail plate.

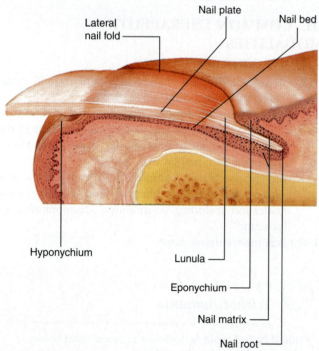

Lateral nail fold
Nail plate
Nail bed
Hyponychium
Lunula
Eponychium
Nail matrix
Nail root

FIGURE 22-6. Structures of the normal nail. (From Anatomical Chart Company, 2004.)

3. Proximal nail fold.
  a. An extension of the skin on the surface of fingers and toes. Becomes a fold and lies superficial to matrix
  b. Contains two layers
    (1) Cuticle or superficial layer
      (a) Adheres and moves a short distance on the surface of nail plate before being shed normally
      (b) Can be seen from the exterior
      (c) Provides a protective seal along nail plate
    (2) Ventral or deep layer is continuous with the matrix epithelium.
4. Lunula
  a. White, crescent-shaped area extending from under the proximal nail fold, seen in some but not all nails.
  b. Is the most distal and visible portion of matrix.
  c. Determines shape of free edge of nail plate.
  d. There are several hypotheses as to why the lunula is white in color.
  e. Marks the end of nail matrix and is the site of mitosis and nail growth.
5. Nail bed
  a. Supports entire nail plate
  b. Extends from lunula to hyponychium
  c. Has longitudinal ridges that fit in a tongue and groove fashion with dermal ridges, which are responsible for striations observed on surface of nail plate
  d. Normal pink color due to enriched vascular network and transparency of nail plate
6. Dermis
  a. Is limited by the underlying phalanx with no subcutaneous tissue
  b. Dermal ridges fit into the parallel and longitudinal groves of epidermal layers and contain the fine capillaries of the nail bed.
7. Hyponychium
  a. Creates a waterproof barrier where the nail plate lifts off the nail bed
  b. Initial site of invasion by dermatophytes in distal subungual onychomycosis
8. Onychodermal band
  a. Darker pink band beneath nail plate proximal to plate separation from hyponychium
  b. Can be more prominent in patients with chronic systemic disease

D. Nail growth
  1. Rate
    a. Controlled by turnover rate of cells in nail matrix.
    b. Fingernail rate approximately 0.1 mm/day or 3 mm/month; toenail rate 1/2 to 1/3 fingernail rate.
    c. Growth greater in the second and third decades with a slight decline thereafter.
    d. Many factors increase and decrease growth rate (Table 22-3).
  2. Thickness
    a. Determined by size of basal cell population in nail matrix.
    b. An increase in matrix length leads to an increase in the thickness of nail.

TABLE 22-3 Factors That Influence Nail Growth Rate

Increase	Decrease
Daytime	Nighttime
Summer	Cold climates
Pregnancy	Starvation/poor nutrition
Young age	Advanced age
Hyperthyroidism	Severe infections
Medications	Onychomycosis
Psoriasis	Medications
	Immobilization

II. ASSESSMENT

A. History and physical examination
1. Patient history
   a. Detailed history is important and should include attention to the evolution of the problem, topical substance exposure, medical, family, and medication histories.
   b. Determine whether underlying systemic disease, recent physical or psychological stress, physical trauma, or exposure to topical agents is present.
   c. Explore any relationship to exposure to drugs, environmental hazards, chemicals, or toxins, or prolonged immersion in water.
   d. Ask about nail grooming techniques, work, and hobbies.
2. Physical examination
   a. Remove polish or lacquer when present.
   b. Always inspect all 20 nails.
   c. Examine with digits relaxed and not pressed against any surface.
   d. Adequate lighting is essential.
   e. Usually, fingernails provide more subtle information than toenails.
   f. Assess color, shape, adherence to nail bed, and presence of lesions.
   g. Note whether nails are soft, hard, brittle, peeling, pitted, splitting, ridged, or thickened.
   h. Examine skin, hair, and mucous membranes for additional evidence of disease.
   i. Perform a complete physical examination as indicated.
B. Diagnostic tests: often, the diagnosis is clinically evident. In other cases, the following tests may be indicated.
1. KOH preparation
2. Fungal cultures
3. Bacterial cultures
4. Nail biopsy
5. X-ray
6. Fluorescence with black light
7. Exfoliative cytology
8. Nail composition studies

NAIL DISORDERS: ONYCHOMYCOSIS

I. OVERVIEW

A. Definition: one of the most common fungal infections of the nail unit. Heat, moisture, trauma, tinea pedis, diabetes mellitus, inheritance, aging, and altered immunologic status are predisposing factors.
B. Etiology
1. Commonly caused by dermatophytes. Can also be caused by *Candida* species and nondermatophyte molds.
C. Pathophysiology
1. Organism penetrates the hyponychium or lateral nail fold region.
D. Clinical features
1. More common in toenails than fingernails.
   a. Toenails commonly infected with dermatophytes
   b. Fingernails commonly infected by yeast and nondermatophyte molds
2. Distal subungual onychomycosis most common.
3. Predisposing factors include years of trauma, decreased peripheral circulation, nail plate dystrophy, malalignment of nail folds, immunosuppression, genetic susceptibility, increased age, diabetes, and psoriasis.
4. Early stages associated with yellowish or whitish discoloration of nail.
5. Nails become thickened and lusterless with subungual debris. Nail plate may crumble.
6. Splinter hemorrhages, onycholysis, and isolated white or yellow islands on nail plate may also be present.
E. Incidence
1. Uncommon in prepubertal children

II. ASSESSMENT

A. See Normal Nails, Assessment.
B. Correct diagnosis by KOH, culture, and/or biopsy is extremely important before beginning therapy.

III. COMMON THERAPEUTIC MODALITIES

A. Medical interventions
1. Terbinafine (Lamisil) 250 mg daily for 6 weeks for fingernails and 12 weeks for toenails. Itraconazole (Sporanox) 400 mg daily for 1 week of each month (pulse therapy). Two to three pulses for fingernails and three to four pulses for toenails. Liver functions tests at baseline and midway through therapy for both drugs.
2. Topical antifungal medications such as ciclopirox (Loprox), terbinafine (Lamisil), or clotrimazole (Lotrimin) can be used in combination with oral therapy to help improve chance for successful treatment.
3. Topical nail lacquers
   a. Ciclopirox (Penlac). Success rate of monotherapy 5.5% to 8.5%
   b. Efinaconazole (Jublia). Success rate of monotherapy 15% to 18%
   c. Tavaborole (Kerydin). Success rate of monotherapy 6.5%

4. Debridement of thickened, crumbling nail plate.
5. Chemical debridement, using various combinations of urea or salicylic acid, can help topical solutions or creams penetrate the nail plate more effectively.
B. Surgical interventions
   1. Nail avulsion, although infrequent
   2. Laser and photodynamic therapy

PATIENT EDUCATION
Onychomycosis

- Dry nails and between digits thoroughly after bathing.
- Apply antifungal powder or spray to shoes daily.
- Fit shoes so they fit well and are nonocclusive.
- Treat symptoms of athletes foot immediately.
- Wear absorbent cotton socks.
- Avoid stockings with wool or synthetic fibers.
- Change hand and bath towels frequently and launder in hot water.
- Throw away old shoes, particularly athletic shoes used for exercise.
- Do not walk barefoot in public places.
- Grooming carefully and regularly. Do not use these grooming tools on unaffected nails.
- Do not share nail grooming tools and be sure other household members with symptoms of athletes foot seek treatment.

PARONYCHIA

I. OVERVIEW

A. Definition: common condition characterized by inflammation of the nail folds. May be acute, which is usually infections and affects only one nail, or chronic, which is usually noninfectious and can affect more than one nail.
B. Etiology
   1. Exogenous factors such as trauma (nail biting, overmanicuring) most likely
C. Pathophysiology
   1. *Staphylococcus aureus*, streptococci, and *Pseudomonas* are most common causative organisms in acute conditions.
   2. *Candida* and low-grade bacterial infection can be present in acute or chronic conditions.
   3. Other causes include allergic or irritant contact dermatitis, vesicular or dyshidrotic eczema, psoriasis, and medications.
D. Clinical features
   1. Redness, swelling, and pain of proximal or lateral nail folds.
   2. Occasionally with serous, hemorrhagic, or purulent drainage.
   3. Predisposing factors such as heat, moisture, trauma to nail folds, local dermatitis or psoriasis, local irritants, diabetes mellitus frequently present.
   4. Once a primary infection has occurred in a nail fold, the area is often predisposed to chronic paronychia.

5. Number of fingers involved is associated with chronicity and can be secondary to other skin disorders such as psoriasis or dermatitis.
6. Loss of cuticle common with chronic paronychia.
E. Incidence
   1. More common in women

II. ASSESSMENT

A. See Normal Nails, Assessment.
B. Important to inquire about the nature of the patient's occupation, household activities, hobbies, and manicuring habits.

III. COMMON THERAPEUTIC MODALITIES

A. Medical interventions
   1. Warm saline or Betadine soaks, 10 to 15 minutes two to four times daily until infection clear for 1 to 2 days. Follow soaks with a topical antibiotic ointment such as mupirocin.
   2. Obtain a bacterial culture.
   3. Oral antibiotics.
   4. For chronic disease, consider topical steroids and topical antifungals.
B. Surgical interventions
   1. Consider incision and drainage.
   2. Consider imaging or biopsy to rule out osteomyelitis or malignancy if unresponsive to treatment.

PATIENT EDUCATION
Paronychia

- All wet work must be stopped.
- Limit exposure to predisposing factors (trauma and irritants).
- Avoid nail cosmetics while disorder is healing.
- Avoid manipulating the cuticle.
- Use proper nail care, cutting toenails straight.
- Avoid overmanicuring.

NAIL INVOLVEMENT ASSOCIATED WITH PSORIASIS

I. OVERVIEW

A. Definition: psoriasis is one of many dermatologic disorders that involve the nails. Nail changes can involve any part of the nail unit and cause a variety of clinical and pathological changes.
B. Etiology
   1. Increased proliferation of keratinocytes with increased cell turnover in the epidermis
C. Pathophysiology
   1. Complex disease that is multifactorial with genetic and immune-mediated components.
D. Clinical features
   1. Nail pitting due to small psoriatic lesions in the nail matrix. Most common sign of nail psoriasis.
   2. Salmon patch or "oil drop sign" represents psoriatic lesions of the nail bed.

3. Onycholysis. Detachment of the distal or lateral edges of nail plate from the nail bed due to psoriatic lesions in the hyponychium and distal nail bed.
4. Subungual hyperkeratosis.
5. Nail plate thickening.
6. Nail plate that crumbles easily.
7. Subungual splinter hemorrhages.
8. Paronychia.
9. Nail psoriasis without psoriasis on other parts of the body is rare.
10. Often associated with psoriatic arthritis.

E. Incidence
1. Psoriasis affects approximately 3% of the population.
2. Up to 50% of individuals affected with psoriasis have nail changes.
3. Fingernails affected more often than toenails. Toenail disease is often indistinguishable from onychomycosis.

II. ASSESSMENT

A. See Normal Nails, Assessment.
B. Lesions commonly seen are pits, discoloration, distal or lateral onycholysis, subungual thickening, crumbling, and grooving of the nail plate.

III. COMMON THERAPEUTIC MODALITIES

A. Medical interventions
1. No consistently effective treatment
2. Avoid trauma
3. Intralesional steroids involving triamcinolone acetonide 2.5 mg/mL to 10 mg/mL injections into proximal nail fold every 4 weeks
4. Topical steroids
5. Topical calcipotriene
6. Topical tazarotene
7. Acitretin
8. Methotrexate, cyclosporin, and biologic medications if indicated for additional psoriasis symptoms

B. Surgical interventions: none

PATIENT EDUCATION
Psoriasis and Nails

- Avoid nail irritants.
- Keep nails trimmed.
- Treat psoriasis elsewhere on the body.

BIBLIOGRAPHY

Arndt, K. A., & Hsu, J. T. S. (2007). *Manual of dermatologic therapeutics* (7th ed.). Philadelphia, PA: Lippincott Williams & Wilkins.

Baran, R., de Berker, D. A., Holzberg, M., & Thomas, L. (2012). *Baran & Dawber's diseases of the nails and their management* (4th ed.). West Sussex, UK: Wiley-Blackwell.

Bolognia, J. L., Jorizzo, J. L., & Schaffer, J. V. (2012). *Dermatology* (3rd ed.). Amsterdam, Netherlands: Elsevier Limited.

Cotsarelis, G., & Botchkarev, V. (2012). Biology of hair follicles. In L. A. Goldsmith, S. I. Katz, B. A. Gilchrest, A. S. Paller, D. J. Leffell, & K. Wolff (Eds.), *Fitzpatrick's dermatology in general medicine* (8th ed., pp. 960–972). New York, NY: McGraw-Hill.

Daniel, C. R. (1996). *Diagnosis of onychomycosis and other nail disorders.* Marceline, MO: Walsworth Publishing Co.

Danial, C. R., & Scher, R. K. (1996). The nail. In W. M Sams, & P. J. Lynch (Eds.), *Principles and practice of dermatology* (pp. 767–777). New York, NY: Churchill Livingstone.

Goldstein, A. M., & Wintroub, B. W. (1994). *Adverse cutaneous reactions to medication—A physician's guide.* New York, NY: CoMedica, Inc.

Hamilton, J. B. (1942). Male hormone stimulation is a prerequisite and an incitant in common baldness. *American Journal of Anatomy, 71*, 451–480.

Hill, M. J. (1994). *Skin disorders.* St. Louis, MO: Mosby.

Hordinsky, M., & Donati, A. (2014). Alopecia areata: An evidence-based treatment update. *American Journal of Clinical Dermatology, 15*(3), 231–246.

James, W. D., Berger, T. G., & Elston, D. K. (2011). *Andrew's diseases of the skin: Clinical dermatology* (11th ed.). Amsterdam, Netherlands: Elsevier, Inc.

Ludwig, E. (1977). Classification of the types of androgenic alopecia (common baldness) arising in the female sex. *British Journal of Dermatology, 97*, 249–253.

Meffert, J. *Psoriasis.* Retrieved from http://emedicine.medscape.com/article/1943419-overview

Norwood, O. T. (1975). Male pattern baldness: Classification and incidence. *Southern Medical Journal, 68*(11), 1359–1365.

Olsen, E. A. (2003). *Disorders of hair growth, diagnosis and treatment* (2nd ed.). New York, NY: McGraw-Hill Companies, Inc.

Otberg, N., & Shapiro, J. (2012). Hair growth disorders. In L. A. Goldsmith, S. I. Katz, B. A. Gilchrest, A. S. Paller, D. J. Leffell, & K. Wolff (Eds.), *Fitzpatrick's dermatology in general medicine* (8th ed., pp. 979–1008). New York, NY: McGraw-Hill.

Pariser, D., Elewski, B., Rich, P., & Scher, R. (2013). Update on Onychomycosis: Effective strategies for diagnosis and treatment. *Seminars in Cutaneous Medicine and Surgery, 32*(Suppl 1), No. 2S.

Scher, R. K., & Daniel III, C. R. (2005). *Nails: Diagnosis, therapy, surgery* (3rd ed.). Amsterdam, Netherlands: Elsevier, Inc.

Spindler, J. R., & Data, J. L. (1992). Female androgenic alopecia: A review. *Dermatology Nursing, 4*(2), 93–100.

Tosti, A., & Piraccini, B. M. (2012). Biology of nails and nail disorders. In L. A. Goldsmith, S. I. Katz, B. A. Gilchrest, A. S. Paller, D. J. Leffell, & K. Wolff (Eds.), *Fitzpatrick's dermatology in general medicine* (8th ed., pp. 1009–1030). New York, NY: McGraw-Hill.

Weinberg, S., Prose, N. S., & Kristal, L. (2008). *Color atlas of pediatric dermatology* (4th ed.). New York, NY: McGraw-Hill.

Wolff, K., Johnson, R. A., & Saavedra, A. P. (2013). *Fitzpatrick's color atlas and synopsis of clinical dermatology* (7th ed). New York, NY: McGraw-Hill.

STUDY QUESTIONS

Hair

1. Normal hair shedding is commonly over 200 hairs per day.
   a. True
   b. False

2. How long after an inciting event does telogen effluvium typically start?
   a. 2 weeks
   b. 1 month
   c. 3 months
   d. 1 year

3. Which of the following is the term for the active growth phase of the hair follicle?
   a. Anagen
   b. Catagen
   c. Telogen
   d. Vellus

4. If a young woman has androgenic alopecia, under which of the following circumstances is an endocrinologic evaluation indicated?
   a. Significant acne.
   b. Significant hirsutism.
   c. Trichotillomania.
   d. A and B.
   e. Endocrinologic evaluation is not necessary.

5. Nail changes that may occur with alopecia areata include which of the following?
   a. Pitting
   b. Longitudinal ridging
   c. Onychomycosis
   d. A and B
   e. B and C

6. Eyebrow and eyelash involvement is observed in what percentage of patients with trichotillomania?
   a. 25%
   b. 10%
   c. 50%
   d. Less than 1%

Nails

1. An increase in matrix length leads to an increase in nail thickness.
   a. True
   b. False

2. Which of the following is a predisposing factor for development of onychomycosis?
   a. Malalignment of the nail folds
   b. Genetic susceptibility
   c. Increased age
   d. Immunosuppression
   e. All of the above

3. Which of the following is the nail component responsible for the shape of the free edge of the nail?
   a. Matrix
   b. Hyponychium
   c. Cuticle
   d. Lunula

4. Which of the following is a sign of nail psoriasis?
   a. Nail pitting
   b. Onycholysis
   c. Salmon patches
   d. All of the above

5. Which of the following is the initial site of invasion by dermatophytes in distal subungual onychomycosis?
   a. Nail bed
   b. Hyponychium
   c. Nail matrix
   d. Proximal nail fold

6. Among patients with psoriasis, what percentage will have characteristic nail changes?
   a. 10%
   b. 30%
   c. 50%
   d. 100%

Answers to Study Questions: Hair 1.b, 2.c, 3.a, 4.d, 5.d, 6.a, Nails 1.a, 2.e, 3.d, 4.d, 5.b, 6.c

CHAPTER

23

Wound Healing

Edna Atwater • Penny S. Jones

OBJECTIVES

After studying this chapter, the reader will be able to:

- Define the phases of wound healing.
- Recognize the difference between healing by tissue regeneration versus healing by scarring and wound contraction.
- List three factors that delay the wound healing process.
- Distinguish between intrinsic and extrinsic factors that affect wound healing.
- Identify various wound dressings and treatments and how to use them to optimize healing.
- Differentiate between the more common chronic wounds (pressure, venous, arterial, and neuropathic ulcers).
- Determine the stage of a pressure ulcer.
- Complete a pressure ulcer risk assessment for a specific patient.

KEY POINTS

- The process of wound healing comprises a naturally occurring series of events (cascade) that are dependent on specialized cells.
- Delayed healing or failure to obtain wound closure is usually due to a disruption in the normal cascade of healing.
- The host's status must be optimized to adequately support tissue repair.
- Wound assessment is the first step in facilitating wound healing.
- Determining the causative factors for development of the wound will determine subsequent treatment plans.
- Pressure ulcer risk assessment is utilized to target individualized patient interventions for pressure ulcer prevention.
- Wound management requires a multidisciplinary approach.
- Choosing an appropriate topical dressing and treatment depends on accurate wound assessment.
- Knowledge of dressing materials and their appropriate use is essential in choosing products.

OVERVIEW

Many terms are used to describe wounds. A wound may be defined as any disruption in the integrity and/or function of the skin or deeper structures that results in a structured healing pathway. A wound may be described in terms of the etiology, location, and healing response. Acute wound healing is an orderly process that occurs as interplay of specialized cells, mediators, and microbes. These events begin at the moment of wounding and end with return of integrity though not necessarily function.

I. PHYSIOLOGY OF ACUTE WOUND HEALING

A. Definition: the wound healing process is a series of events, or cascade (Table 23-1), which is dependent on specialized cells and chemical mediators. Wounds heal by one of two methods, regeneration or repair. The depth of damage will determine the type of healing that a wound will undergo. Regeneration is limited to wounds that involve the epidermis and upper layers of the dermis as well as fetal wound healing. Regeneration results in not only return of integrity but also function of the injured tissues. Wound repair is the healing process that is required for deeper wounds with more extensive tissue destruction. After the fetal period, wound repair with scar formation is due to the inflammatory process.

B. Phase I—Inflammation: upon wounding, the body's immediate response is to achieve hemostasis followed immediately by inflammation. The goal of this phase is to control bleeding, to defend the body against invasion by the environment, and to initiate tissue repair. The clinical characteristics of this phase are the classic signs of inflammation: erythema, edema, warmth, and pain. This phase of wound healing may last for 24 to 48 hours but, in some cases, may continue for up to 2 weeks.

1. Hemostasis: upon injury, small vessels near the site constrict for 5 to 10 minutes, and both the intrinsic and extrinsic pathways of the coagulation cascade are activated. Blood is exposed to collagen in the extracellular matrix. Platelets begin to adhere and aggregate at the site of injury. At the same time, they release mediators and additional adhesive proteins, which cause more

355

TABLE 23-1 Wound Healing Cascade

Phase	Description
Inflammatory	Begins with hemostasis and release of growth factors at the time of wounding—platelets are the primary mediator in this phase. Phagocytosis (breakdown of necrotic material)—polymorphonuclear leukocytes and macrophages are the primary mediators in this phase.
Proliferation	Formation of granulation tissue; wound contraction and epithelialization occur in this phase. Fibroblasts, endothelial cells, and keratinocytes are the primary mediators in this phase.
Maturation	Remodeling of scar tissue through collagen synthesis and collagen breakdown Macrophages and fibroblasts are the primary mediators in this phase.

platelets to adhere, resulting in a platelet plug. A fibrin clot is subsequently formed with the conversion of fibrinogen to fibrins. The end result, blood loss, is slowed and/or stopped.

2. Vascular/cellular response: after brief vasoconstriction, the vessels dilate, which allows needed cells and mediators to enter the area. Platelets and mast cells secrete a multitude of mediators designed to facilitate removal of any microbes, necrotic tissue, foreign bodies, and cellular debris. The two most important mediators are platelet-derived growth factor (PDGF) and transforming growth factor beta (TGF-β). PDGF draws in and stimulates polymorphonuclear leukocytes (PMNs), including neutrophils and monocytes. Monocytes are converted to macrophages, the cellular version of garbage disposals. These cells continue the process of microbe and cellular debris removal. The end result is a clean wound that is ready to progress to the next phase. Macrophages also mediate the release of growth factors and chemoattractants that are critical to initiating the next phase of healing.

C. Phase II—Proliferative phase: this phase overlaps the inflammatory phase beginning about the 4th day postwounding and lasts for approximately 15 to 16 days. The goal of the proliferative phase of healing is to restore the barrier function of the skin. The clinical characteristics of this phase are reepithelialization, granulation, and tissue contraction.

1. Dermal reconstitution: the formation of new tissue begins 3 to 4 days after injury, which involves two processes: angiogenesis and collagen synthesis; these processes occur simultaneously and are codependent; wound contraction occurs concurrently with granulation.

   a. Angiogenesis: the process of new blood vessel formation is chemically mediated by vascular endothelial growth factor A (VEGFA) and fibroblast growth factor 2 (FGF-2). As with most healing signals, it is started at the wound edge from the disrupted capillaries.

   b. Collagen synthesis: TGF-β stimulates the macrophages to secrete the cytokines: FGF (fibroblast growth factor), PDGF, tumor necrosis factor alpha (TNF-α), and interleukin-1 (IL-1). TGF-β stimulates fibroblast proliferation and then migration into the fibrin clot. A complex process begins with the formation of new collagen fibers, proteoglycans, and elastin; fibroblast activity is chemically mediated by PDGF and TGF-β, as well as an acidic, low oxygen condition in the wound center. As angiogenesis proceeds, this stimulus is diminished.

2. Reepithelialization: keratinocytes are activated and begin migrating into the wound within 24 hours of injury. In deep dermal wounds, reepithelialization occurs in conjunction with collagen synthesis. Keratinocyte migration, proliferation, and reepithelialization are chemically mediated by the extracellular matrix, matrix metalloproteinase (MMPs), TGF-α, keratinocyte growth factor, and epidermal growth factor.

3. Contraction: in the later stage, macrophages cause fibroblasts to differentiate into myofibroblasts. These contractile cells pull together the wound edges, gradually reducing the size of the defect.

D. Phase III—Maturation phase: overlaps with the proliferative phase and continues for up to a year or longer after the wound has closed; TGF-β, tumor necrosis factor, and FGF-1 play a role in this phase with controlled and timely apoptosis; in full-thickness wounds, collagen is remodeled. Type III collagen is replaced by type I collagen. The goal of the maturation phase is to maximize the tensile strength of the wound and protect the scar from rupture due to mechanical stress. The tensile strength of a healed wound is always less than that of uninjured tissue. This phase is characterized clinically by raised erythematous scar tissue that gradually flattens and no longer blanches when pressure is applied.

Note: Superficial wounds do not scar; deep dermal wounds will scar.

II. FUNCTION OF CELLS IN WOUND HEALING

The cells involved in the wound healing process include platelets, leukocytes, macrophages, fibroblasts, myofibroblasts, and epithelial cells (keratinocytes).

A. Platelets: the smallest cell in the blood is essential for coagulation of blood and maintenance of hemostasis. It becomes active in clot formation when blood becomes exposed to collagen after tissue injury. Platelets release PDGF and TGF-β, which assist in wound repair.

B. Leukocytes: PMNs migrate into the wound space immediately after injury. PMNs are attracted to the wound by chemoattractants produced by platelets, activated clotting factors, and fibrin. The function of these early, short-lived (approximately 4 days) cells is to provide protection from infection and remove cellular debris.

C. Macrophages: the most significant cells in wound healing. They are phagocytic cells that gradually replace leukocytes beginning approximately 4 days after wounding. Macrophages aggressively ingest bacteria and necrotic tissue, produce chemoattractants and growth factors, convert macromolecules into amino acids and sugars necessary for wound healing, and secrete lactate to stimulate collagen synthesis.

D. Fibroblasts: responsible for synthesis of collagen and other connective tissue substances during wound repair. Chemoattractants and growth factors released by platelets and macrophages stimulate fibroblasts to migrate to the wound bed beginning at the end of the inflammatory phase.

E. Myofibroblasts: fibroblasts with characteristics similar to those of smooth muscle cells. Myofibroblasts stimulate wound contraction after they migrate within the wound space.

F. Epithelial cells: keratinocytes proliferate and migrate from wound edges and intact skin appendages to reestablish an epidermal barrier. In partial-thickness (superficial) wounds, epidermal resurfacing begins within 24 hours. In deeper (full-thickness) wounds, dermal repair must take place before epithelial cells can begin to migrate.

III. WOUND CLOSURE

There are three types of wound healing: primary intention, secondary intention, and tertiary or delayed primary intention.

A. Primary intention: a surgically closed wound whether closed with staples, sutures, or glue. The approximation of wound edges minimizes tissue defect and reduces the potential for infection. Typically, these wounds heal quickly with minimal scar formation.

B. Secondary intention: wound is left open and allowed to heal more slowly. They require a longer healing time for granulation tissue to fill the defect. There is higher risk for infection due to absence of protective barrier. Examples of wounds that heal by secondary intention are pressure ulcers and contaminated surgical wounds.

C. Tertiary intention: intentional delayed primary closure. Example of a wound that heals by tertiary intention is contaminated abdominal wound left open to drain following surgery and later approximated when the wound is granulating and free of infection.

IV. ACUTE WOUNDS

Defined as those wounds caused intentionally (surgery) or by trauma (abrasion, burn, laceration). Vasculature is disrupted so hemostasis must occur. In a healthy host, healing proceeds in a timely manner.

A. Etiology.
  1. Mechanical: stab wound, laceration, abrasion, blister, surgical incision, skin tear
  2. Thermal: burns, including sunburn or frostbite
  3. Chemical: a wound intentionally made through the use of a chemical agent (such as a chemical peel) or unintentionally by exposure to a caustic substance (including stool or urine)

V. CHRONIC WOUNDS

Failure of the normal healing process to proceed in an orderly and timely manner can result in a chronic wound; examples include vascular ulcers, neuropathic ulcers, pressure ulcers, malignancy-related wounds (breast cancer, rectal cancer), and treatment-related wounds (IV infiltrate).

1. Vascular ulcers: may be arterial, venous, or mixed arterial and venous. Arterial ulcers are the result of impaired arterial blood flow from an underlying atherosclerotic condition or as a consequence of vasoactive medications. Venous ulcers result from edema and venous hypertension as a result of incompetent lower extremity veins.

2. Neuropathic ulcers: also known as diabetic foot ulcers, these are the result of loss of sensation to the foot (sensory neuropathy), change in the musculature (motor neuropathy), and shunting of blood and loss of the ability to sweat (autonomic neuropathy). This is often but not always precipitated by diabetes. Various medications may also cause peripheral neuropathy.

3. Pressure ulcer: a localized area of tissue necrosis due to pressure that is usually (but not always) over a bony prominence. Shear forces may also contribute to the development of the ulcer but pressure must be a significant factor.

4. Malignancy-related ulcers: may be due to the primary tumor itself or as a consequence of treatment.

5. Treatment-related ulcers: soft tissue infiltration of vasoactive and vesicant agents can result in full-thickness skin loss. Infiltration of calcium has been known to result in ulcers due to the calcium precipitation in the tissues.

VI. PATHOPHYSIOLOGY OF WOUND HEALING

Delayed healing or nonhealing is usually due to some disruption in the normal cascade of healing. Many factors can impair healing. It is imperative that these factors be recognized and addressed to augment the body's natural ability to heal.

A. Negative factors affecting wound healing.
  1. Intrinsic factors (related to patient's general physical or mental condition)
     a. Age: normal skin changes seen with aging affect the skin's function and healing response through decreased wound contraction, decreased tensile strength, and increased metabolic response. Age-related alterations that increase the potential for injury and impair healing include:
        (1) Decreased collagen density
        (2) Increased capillary fragility
        (3) Decreased mechanoreceptors resulting in decreased sensory reception
        (4) Decreased amount/distribution of subcutaneous fat resulting in impaired thermoregulation
        (5) Reduced inflammatory response but proinflammatory environment
        (6) Slower rate of neoangiogenesis and wound contraction
        (7) Fewer fibroblasts and mast cells

(8) Fragmentation of elastin fibers

(9) Insufficient tensile strength (increased potential for wound dehiscence)

(10) Decreased tissue perfusion secondary to vascular disease

(11) Thinning of dermis and basement layer

(12) Increased reactive oxygen species (ROS) with decreased antioxidant activity resulting in a proinflammatory intrinsic environment and ultimately increased apoptosis and aging skin

(13) Reduced keratinocyte proliferation and turnover time

(14) Less acidic surface pH

(15) Flattening of epidermal–dermal junction and decreased adhesion

b. Nutrition: plays a vital role in all aspects of wound healing

(1) Protein: provides the structural component for tissue repair; deficiency results in decreased fibroblast proliferation, reduced collagen synthesis, decreased angiogenesis, and disrupted maturation; slow gain in tensile strength and increased incidence of wound healing abnormalities are associated with protein–energy malnutrition (PEM); PEM effects all phases of wound healing; usual recommended range of protein intake daily for wound healing is 1.25 to 1.5 g/kg but is as high as 2 g/kg/d for patient with multiple wounds in a severe catabolic state. Specific amino acids (arginine and glutamine) may have a beneficial effect, but conclusive studies are not available. Lysine and proline are also known to impact wound healing.

(2) Vitamins

(a) Vitamin A affects collagen cross-linkage, supports epithelial proliferation and migration and dermal angiogenesis, and enhances the immune system. Recommended supplementation ranges for 10,000 to 50,000 IU orally daily for 10 days.

(b) Vitamin B, especially B_1, thiamine, affects enzyme activity, collagen cross-linkage, and immune response.

(c) Vitamin C is necessary for collagen synthesis, immune modulator, and antioxidant. Supplementation to 100 to 200 mg/day may be beneficial for patients with vitamin C deficiency and wounds. Caution is advised with long-term high-dose supplementation.

(d) Vitamin D accelerates wound closure, promotes reepithelialization, and improves tensile strength.

(e) Vitamin E plays a protective role in antioxidant defense.

(3) Carbohydrates: provide energy needed for wound repair; insufficient carbohydrate intake initiates body protein catabolism and increases potential for infection.

(4) Trace elements: zinc stabilizes membrane structure and function, acts as a cofactor in enzyme systems, affects immune response, and inhibits bacterial growth; copper aids in collagen linkage; iron corrects iron deficiency anemia and affects collagen synthesis; magnesium supports collagen synthesis.

c. Medical condition: underlying disease states alter the body's normal response to healing.

(1) Diabetes: associated with vasculopathy, neuropathy, and immunopathy; greater than 100 cytologic factors associated with diabetes that impair wound healing.

(2) Hypotension: vasoconstriction promotes tissue ischemia and decreased nutrient delivery.

(3) Peripheral vascular disease (PVD): tissue perfusion is decreased resulting in hypoxia and diminished nutrients to tissue as well as impaired removal of waste products.

(4) Renal disease—the effect of uremia on wound healing in humans is not well understood; uremia does cause neuropathy and immune dysfunction.

(5) Hematopoietic abnormalities: inadequate numbers of RBCs impair oxygen transport; inadequate platelets delay the healing cascade.

(6) Gastrointestinal disease: inhibits absorption and compromises nutritional status

(7) Cardiopulmonary disease: PaO_2 is decreased contributing to tissue hypoxia.

(8) Cancer: immune response is altered; risk of infection is increased.

(9) Chronic venous insufficiency: incompetent venous valves cause high-pressure venous hypertension and significant edema.

(10) Sickle cell disease: dysmorphic blood cells occlude smaller vessels, resulting in leg ulcers.

d. Infection: defined as bacterial concentrations greater than 10^5 organisms per gram of tissue; highly virulent organisms can cause infection at lower concentrations; important to distinguish between infection, critically colonized, and colonization. Presence of a bacterial biofilm will also delay wound healing.

(1) Signs of local and regional infection (suppressed in immunocompromised patients)

(a) Erythema

(b) Edema

(c) Induration

(d) Pain

(e) Purulent or foul-smelling drainage (depending on topical therapy, this may not be accurate)

(f) Crepitance

(g) Lymphadenopathy

(h) Delayed wound healing

(i) Pale and friable granulation tissue

(j) Wound breakdown

(2) Signs of systemic infection

  (a) Fever/chills

  (b) Elevation of white blood cell (neutrophil) count; increase in number of bands/segs (shift to the left)

  (c) Positive blood/wound cultures

  (d) Sepsis

e. Drugs: particularly important to evaluate patient's medicines when a chronic, nonhealing wound is present; examples of drugs, which may impair healing.

  (1) Corticosteroids: systemic steroids inhibit fibroblast formation and collagen synthesis; topical steroids may have varying effects on epidermal resurfacing and dermal collagen synthesis.

  (2) Anticoagulants: implied effect on healing by preventing hemostasis

  (3) Nonsteroidal anti-inflammatory drugs (NSAIDs): may inhibit inflammatory phase of healing

  (4) Immunosuppressives: azathioprine and prednisone are associated with significant reduction in tensile strength.

  (5) Chemotherapeutic agents: affect on wound healing depends on the specific drug, dose, and time of administration: increase risk of infection (due to decreased WBCs), act on any rapidly dividing cells, alter the function of fibroblasts and myofibroblasts, and impair collagen synthesis and reepithelialization

  (6) Nicotine: causes vasoconstriction whether patch, gum, or lozenge. There are other studies that dispute this. They are likely better than cigarette smoking with its greater than 250 harmful chemicals but nonnicotine measures may be a better smoking cessation option for patients with wounds.

f. Hypoxia: poor tissue oxygenation slows or completely inhibits healing; this is seen in patients with cardiopulmonary disease (decreased PaO_2), PVD, and diabetes; sustained tissue pressure compromises circulation leading to tissue ischemia, hypoxia, and cell death.

g. Stress: impairs healing by altering normal physiologic response; psychological stress, pain, and noise stimulate the sympathetic nervous system releasing vasoactive substances that promote vasoconstriction and alter tissue perfusion.

2. Extrinsic factors

a. Topical antimicrobials/cleansers: inappropriate use of disinfectants and antiseptics (povidone–iodine, hydrogen peroxide, acetic acid, chlorhexidine, and hypochlorite) impairs healing by having cytotoxic effects on fibroblasts.

  (1) Liquid detergents: may retard healing by changing the pH of the wound bed or by cytotoxic action on fibroblasts

  (2) Antiseptic cleansers (acetic acid, Dakin solution, chlorhexidine, povidone–iodine/Betadine, hydrogen peroxide): cytotoxic to fibroblasts

b. Necrotic tissue: prolongs the inflammatory phase of healing, supports microbial growth, delays epithelial cell migration, and provides a physical obstacle to wound contraction

c. Continued tissue trauma: unrelieved pressure and edema lead to progressive tissue hypoxia and cell death; friction destroys epidermal cells and alters the barrier function of the skin; shearing forces angulate blood vessels, causing localized tissue hypoxia and chronic inflammation; excessive moisture leads to tissue maceration and promotes the growth of microorganisms; wound desiccation prolongs inflammation, retards epithelial cell migration, and impairs collagen synthesis.

d. Radiation therapy: dose, frequency, and location of irradiated area in relation to the wound site will have implications for therapy; residual effects of radiation are permanent; irradiated tissue is easily damaged and slower to heal; Radiation therapy impairs healing through:

  (1) Injury to fibroblasts

  (2) Injury to endothelial cells

  (3) Decrease in collagen production

  (4) Destruction of cells in mitosis

  (5) Vascular damage

  (6) Increased risk of infection

  (7) Apoptosis of healthy cells

VII. WOUND CLASSIFICATION

A. National Pressure Ulcer Advisory Panel (NPUAP) and European Pressure Ulcer Advisory Panel (EPUAP) criteria for classification of pressure ulcer. The classification system is for pressure ulcers only and does not apply to leg ulcers or other acute or chronic wounds. The stage/category of a pressure ulcer represents the greatest depth of tissue destruction and remains constant until complete reepithelialization of the ulcer. Pressure ulcers are not backstaged. The final stage/category of a pressure ulcer cannot be determined if necrotic tissue is present and obscuring the wound base.

1. Stage/category I: intact skin with a localized area with nonblanchable redness (Figures 23-1 and 23-2). The area may be painful, firm, warmer, or cooler as compared to the surrounding skin. Stage/category I lesions may be difficult to see in more darkly pigmented skin. The use of cream may assist in distinguishing the subtle color variation due to pressure.

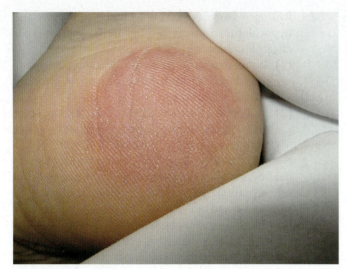

FIGURE 23-1. Stage I pressure ulcer on the heel. (Copyright Duke University, used with permission.)

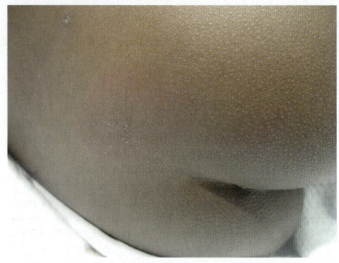

FIGURE 23-2. Stage I pressure ulcer on the sacrum in person of color. (Copyright Duke University, used with permission.)

2. Stage/category II: partial-thickness skin loss involving the epidermis and/or dermis; clinical appearance is a shallow ulcer with a pink wound bed or may be an intact serous-filled blister/bulla (Figures 23-3 and 23-4). There is no slough or eschar. There may be devitalized dermal or epidermal tissue. These lesions are often painful due to exposed dermal nerve endings. Careful consideration required to differentiate and stage II from moisture and/or friction related skin damage.

3. Stage/category III: full-thickness skin loss involving damage or necrosis of subcutaneous tissue that may extend down to, but not through, underlying fascia (Figure 23-5). Actual depth of the ulcer varies with the anatomic location as some areas have a thinner layer of subcutaneous fat than others. Muscle, tendon, and bone are not exposed. There may be undermining and tunneling. Slough or eschar may also be present, but the full depth of the wound is visible.

4. Stage/category IV: full-thickness skin loss with exposed muscle, bone, or supporting structures (Figure 23-6). There may be slough or eschar in the wound bed but the full depth is visible. Undermining and sinus tracts may also be associated with these ulcers.

5. Unstageable: full-thickness skin loss with the base of the wound obscured with necrotic tissue: slough or eschar (Figures 23-7 and 23-8).

6. Suspected deep tissue injury: localized area of purple or maroon intact skin or it may be a blood-filled or purple-based blister/bulla (Figures 23-9 and 23-10). As with stage/category I ulcers, these are difficult to see in darker pigmented skin. As this lesion evolves, it may be reclassified to unstageable, stage/category III or IV. It is unclear what percentage of these ulcers progress to full-thickness skin loss versus resolve without progressing to an open lesion.

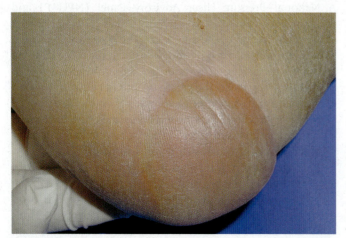

FIGURE 23-3. Stage II pressure ulcer on the heel. (Copyright Duke University, used with permission.)

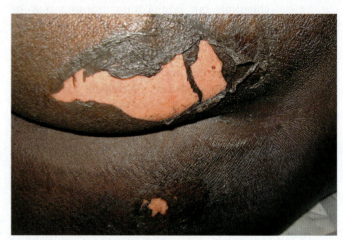

FIGURE 23-4. Stage II pressure ulcer on the buttock in a person of color. (Copyright Duke University, used with permission.)

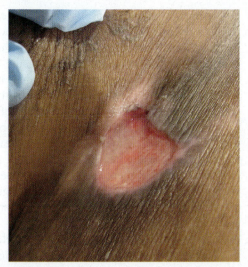

FIGURE 23-5. Stage III pressure ulcer on the sacrum. Note the absence of hair follicles in the wound base. (Copyright Duke University, used with permission.)

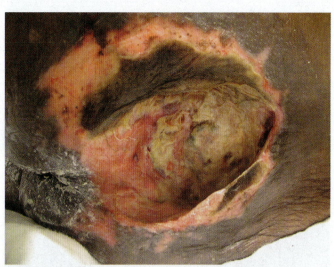

FIGURE 23-6. Stage IV pressure ulcer on the sacrum. If one is able to identify muscle or bone in the wound base, the ulcer is stage IV despite the amount of necrotic tissue. (Copyright Duke University, used with permission.)

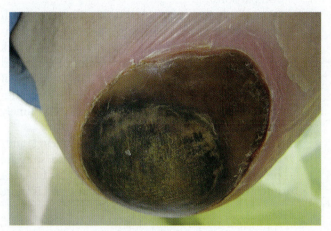

FIGURE 23-7. Unstageable pressure ulcer on the heel. (Copyright Duke University, used with permission.)

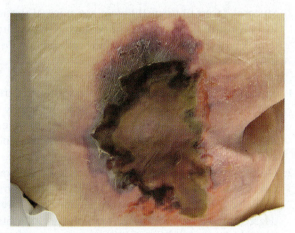

FIGURE 23-8. Unstageable sacral pressure ulcer. This ulcer was very likely a suspected deep tissue injury that is evolving and is now considered unstageable. (Copyright Duke University, used with permission.)

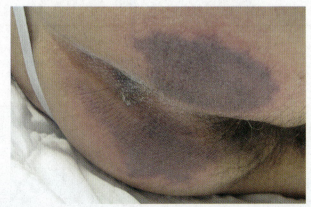

FIGURE 23-9. Suspected deep tissue injury on the buttocks bilaterally. (Copyright Duke University, used with permission.)

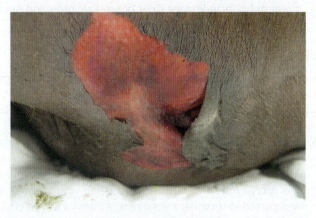

FIGURE 23-10. Evolving suspected deep tissue injury in a person of color. The presence of these ulcers can be missed without close assessment of the skin tone changes. (Copyright Duke University, used with permission.)

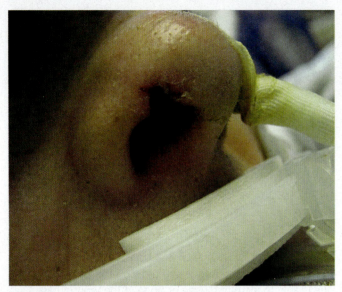

FIGURE 23-11. Mucosal pressure ulcer related to a nasoenteric tube. (Copyright Duke University, used with permission.)

7. Mucosal: layers of tissue different are mucosal surfaces, making use of the above-described staging system problematic; these terms are used for any pressure ulcer on a mucosal surface (Figure 23-11).

B. Classification of wound by tissue depth.

1. Superficial partial thickness: involves the epidermis and upper layers of the dermis; heals primarily by reepithelialization; painful due to exposed nerve endings; examples include abrasion, burn, chemical peel, and skin tear.

2. Deep partial thickness: damage extends to the lower layers of the dermis but does not penetrate the dermis; heals by epithelialization in conjunction with varying degrees of collagen synthesis; examples include burn, dermal biopsy, and deeper skin tear.

3. Full thickness: damage extends through the epidermis and dermis into deeper structures (subcutaneous tissue, fascia, muscle, tendon, or bone); healing occurs primarily by collagen synthesis and soft tissue contraction; examples include stage III or IV pressure ulcer and open postsurgical abdominal wound.

VIII. WOUND ASSESSMENT

A. Anatomic location: provides clues about wound etiology; for example, pressure ulcers commonly occur over bony prominences, venous ulcers often occur on the pretibial area of the calf; skin tears on forearms and legs.

B. Size: wound measurement is a basic parameter of assessment; a healing wound decreases in size over time; interventions should promote a gradual decrease in wound size, except following debridement when wound size can be expected to increase; assessment of size is a way to effectively evaluate efficacy of treatment.

1. Two- or three-dimensional measurement (two-dimensional measurement does not provide information regarding depth of the wound)

a. Linear measurements: measure length of the wound from 12 to 6 o'clock position with 12 o'clock being the head and 6 o'clock the feet. Measure the width at 3 to 9 o'clock position. Measuring the greatest length, width, and depth in cm or mm is not reliably reproducible between providers; gently insert cotton-tipped applicator into deepest area of wound to obtain depth measurement; as much as possible, the patient should be in the same position each time for accurate measurement of full-thickness wounds (soft tissue displacement can alter linear measures). When compared to wound tracing and digital planimetry, there was strong to modest agreement in assessing size (Figure 23-12).

b. Wound tracings: of limited value with electronic medical record; may be useful when wound margins are irregular or poorly demarcated and linear measurement is difficult; use double-layer transparent acetate and permanent marking pen to trace configuration; label clean tracing with date; mark direction of head and foot on tracing for subsequent comparisons.

c. Wound photography: used in conjunction with linear measurement and other assessment parameters; provides visual data to verify change or lack of change in linear dimensions—color of tissue and the condition of the surrounding skin. Concerns of legal issues have been noted; non–health care photos likely in legal proceedings so quality and timely health care photos would be a plus.

d. Digital planimetry: uses an acetate tracing and/or digital photography with the use of a software program to measure the wound area. Can be labor intensive, requires training for accuracy, and is more

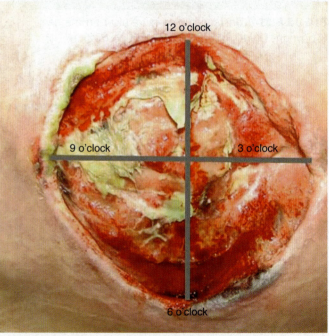

FIGURE 23-12. Wound size. (Copyright Duke University, used with permission.)

costly than use of a disposable ruler for linear measurements. Bien, Anda, and Prokocimer found the ruler measurement to be as reliable as digital planimetry for wound measurements.

2. Volume measurement

a. Wound molds: used to assess the volume of open wounds; biocompatible molding material is poured into open wound and allowed to harden; change in size/weight of mold over time indicates progress; not practical in clinical settings.

b. Fluid instillation: cover wound with transparent film and then instill a known quantity of solution into the wound cavity, filling it to the perimeter; extract fluid with a syringe or suction and record the amount; requires serial measurements; use is limited to deep full-thickness wounds; not practical in clinical settings.

C. Undermining, tracts, or tunneling: evaluate full-thickness (stage III or IV pressure ulcers) wounds carefully for undermining/tracts; undermining most often occurs in wounds as a result of shear; sinus tracts occur generally as a result of dehiscence, infection, or a combination of neuropathy and arterial insufficiency; soft tissue tunneling is common in deep wounds; use a clock face to describe the direction of undermining, tracts, and tunnels; obtain linear measurements when possible. Use a gloved finger or cotton-tipped swab to determine the length (Figure 23-13).

D. Tissue type: accurate assessment of the wound bed leads to appropriate treatment and decreased morbidity. (Note: Viable subcutaneous tissue, fascia, muscle, tendon, and bone may also be visible at the base of deep wounds, especially after surgical debridement.) Quantify the tissue types by percentage of the wound base (Figure 23-14).

1. Epithelial tissue: regrowth of skin from wound edges or skin appendages; initially one cell layer thick, then stratifies; presents clinically as pearly pink wound margins

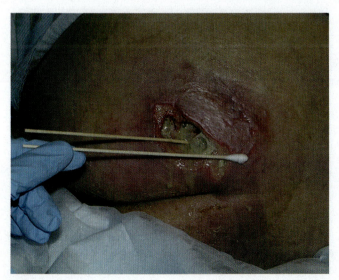

FIGURE 23-13. Measuring amount of undermining with a cotton-tipped swab. (Copyright Duke University, used with permission.)

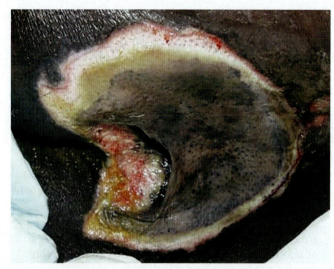

FIGURE 23-14. Quantifying the amount of granulation and eschar slough tissue by percentage: 20% granulation tissue, 80% slough. Quantifying the wound base using colors is acceptable: 20% pink, 20% yellow, 60% black. (Copyright Duke University, used with permission.)

(full-thickness wounds) or fleshy budding of the hair follicles (partial-thickness wounds)

2. Granulation tissue: combination of newly formed blood vessels and collagen deposited into the wound space during the proliferative phase of healing; presents clinically as fleshy granular projections of tissue; healthy granulation is moist and pink to beefy red and has a spongy texture.

3. Eschar: necrotic epidermis and dermis (full-thickness wounds only); delays wound healing by slowing epithelial cell migration and serving as a physical obstacle to wound contraction; acts as a banquet for bacterial growth; presents clinically as thick, dry leathery necrotic tissue attached to the wound surface (e.g., dry gangrene); usually black in color

4. Slough: soft, stringy necrotic tissue that may appear black, gray, yellow, or tan in color; often associated with thick drainage and increased numbers of bacteria

E. Exudate: the amount, viscosity, and color of exudate will vary with the phase of healing, amount and type of necrotic tissue present, and wound dressing.

1. Volume: volume of exudate should decrease as inflammation subsides, necrotic tissue is removed, and infection is controlled; an exception is in the immunocompromised patient where the inflammatory process may be blunted and volume of exudate is altered; volume of apparent exudate increases with use of moisture-retentive dressings for autolytic debridement, osteomyelitis, or spontaneous drainage of a soft tissue abscess; a sudden increase in the volume of exudate may signal impending wound dehiscence in primarily closed wounds; quantify volume of exudate as scant, small, moderate, large, or copious.

2. Color: the color of exudate changes as tissue repair progresses through the various phases of healing; inflammatory wound transudate is initially yellow tinged and watery (serous) as protein-rich transudate leaks from dilated blood vessels; may be blood tinged

(serosanguinous) or show evidence of fresh bleeding (sanguineous); chronic wound exudate changes color (cream, brown, gray, green) with increased proliferation of microorganisms and liquefaction of necrotic tissue.

   3. Consistency: the viscosity of wound exudate changes from a watery consistency (inflammatory transudate) in acute wounds to a purulent consistency in chronic or infected wounds; change in consistency caused by accumulation of blood cells and living or dead organisms.

F. Odor: colonization or infection with certain microorganisms gives the wound a distinct odor (Pseudomonas); a pungent, strong, foul, fecal, or musty odor together with increased erythema, tenderness, and volume of exudate usually suggests infection; some moisture-retentive dressings are also associated with an unpleasant odor in the absence of infection. Quantify odor as mild, moderate, and foul.

G. Condition of periwound skin.

   1. Color: assess for erythema, hypo-/hyperpigmentation, cyanosis, etc.; color changes are more difficult to assess in individuals with darker skin.

   2. Intact: assess for blistering, maceration, dryness/cracking, rashes, denudation, etc.

   3. Signs of active infection: a ring of erythema extending for several centimeters, induration of periwound skin

   4. Directs potential topical therapy: adhesive moisture-retentive dressings not indicated when surrounding skin eroded or denuded (Figure 23-15)

H. Pain response: assess and document the presence of pain or tenderness within or around the wound; may indicate infection, underlying tissue destruction, or vascular insufficiency; absence of pain may indicate nerve destruction.

I. Previous treatment: determine the previous treatment modalities; some treatments may alter wound appearance clinically or retard the healing process; for example, use of topical Neosporin may result in a well-demarcated erythematous rash around the ulcer (Figure 23-16).

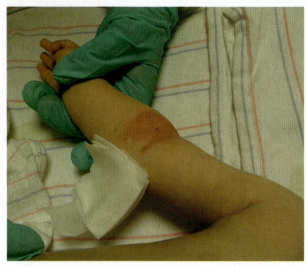

FIGURE 23-16. Contact (allergic) dermatitis to topical treatment. (Copyright Duke University, used with permission.)

J. Infection: bacterial infection negatively affects wound healing; it may either delay the wound healing process or lead to severe morbidity or death; accurate evaluation of bacterial load in a wound is important to treatment planning. Tissue analysis for infection is gold standard but not always possible. As a swab method, the Levine method offers the most reliable and valid method.

   1. Colonization: bacteria present in a wound that has not resulted in a host inflammatory response. May not delay healing.

   2. Critically colonization: an imbalance between the presence of bacteria and wound immune response; often the cause of a stalled wound

   3. Biofilm: are colonies of bacteria that are attached and embedded into the extracellular polymeric substance (EPS). This EPS is a coating that protects the bacteria from destruction by antimicrobials and the host immune response—essentially armor coating for the bacteria (Figure 23-17).

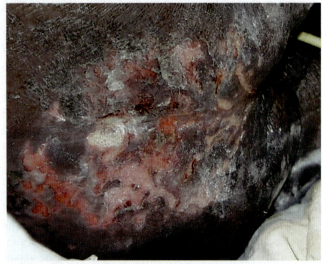

FIGURE 23-15. Unstageable, slough-covered ulcer on the sacrum with significant erosions on the buttocks due to moisture-associated dermatitis. (Copyright Duke University, used with permission.)

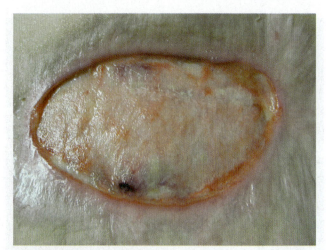

FIGURE 23-17. Pale wound base. There is no evidence of acute infection (foul odor, purulent drainage or surrounding edema, redness, or edema). For this nonhealing postoperative wound, the presence of a biofilm should be suspected. (Copyright Duke University, used with permission.)

K. General health assessment: assess the host—wounds do not exist in a vacuum. It is imperative to assess the status of the host and to correct/optimize any conditions recognized.

1. Age: with normal aging, there is a decrease in the inflammatory response, delayed angiogenesis, decreased collagen synthesis and degradation, slowed epithelialization, and decreased functioning of sebaceous glands; older patients are at higher risk for slow or nonhealing wounds. They are also more likely to have comorbid conditions that impair wound healing.

2. Chronic illness: assess for concomitant medical problems associated with delayed healing: diabetes, COPD, hypertension, ASHD, depression, etc.

3. Medications: assess for medications known to slow/inhibit healing: systemic corticosteroids, anticoagulants, NSAIDs, immunosuppressives, chemotherapeutic agents, and nicotine.

4. Nutritional status: healing may require an increase in calorie intake, vitamins, and trace elements; if a patient is in a state of hypoproteinemia, then healing will be negatively affected.

5. Infection: assess systemic conditions that may increase potential for infection; immune incompetence (interferes with mitosis, protein synthesis, and increases risk of infection). Infection elsewhere in the host will slow wound healing.

6. Psychosocial: assess patient's ability/willingness to be adherent with treatment; assess hygiene; assess support systems/resources available to patient; depression and/or anxiety associated with the wound.

IX. TREATMENT

A. Debridement: the removal of foreign objects, damaged tissue, and cellular debris from the wound surface. The primary objectives of wound debridement are to promote timely progress along the healing continuum from inflammation to proliferation, prevent infection by removing food source for microorganisms, and correct abnormal wound repair.

1. Nonselective debridement: removes devitalized tissue from the wound but may also damage healthy tissue

   a. Wet-to-dry dressings: uses saline and gauze; wet gauze is placed directly onto wound base and allowed to dry before removal; removal mechanically removes anything (health and nonhealthy tissue) that adheres to the gauze from the wound surface; painful to the patient and nonselective (can injure viable tissue); limit use to wounds that contain a large amount of soft necrotic slough or when insoluble debris is not easily removed by rinsing or cleansing; may result in gauze pieces embedded into the wound surface resulting in an increased inflammatory response (Figure 23-18).

   b. Irrigation: uses water or saline to flush the wound and remove superficial nonattached cellular debris; irrigation technique may be forceful (high pressure) or gentle (low pressure); high-pressure irrigation can

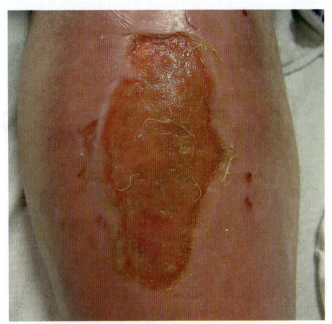

FIGURE 23-18. Gauze embedded in this venous leg ulcer will delay wound healing. (Copyright Duke University, used with permission.)

damage healthy tissue and is not indicated for clean, noninfected wounds, granulating wounds, or superficial wounds.

   c. Hydrotherapy: whirlpool has decreased in use due to infection control issues as well as patient safety. Bedside-pulsed lavage with a single patient use device has been showed to be a safe and effective method of wound irrigation and debridement. It is indicated for debridement of wounds with loosely adherent necrotic tissue and yellow fibrinous or gelatinous exudate, to cleanse wounds of dirt and foreign contaminants; limit to wounds with extensive amounts (>50%) of necrotic tissue; very effective when paired with bedside conservative sharp debridement.

   d. Surgical debridement: use of a scalpel or other instrumentation to dissect and remove necrotic tissue; technique of choice for infected wounds; prepares open wounds for closure; extensive surgical debridement may involve the sacrifice of viable tissue.

   e. Topical agents: Dakin (sodium hypochlorite) solution chemically loosens/removes cellular debris; may be toxic to healthy cells and a chemical irritant to intact skin; not indicated for use on clean superficial wounds.

2. Selective debridement: selectively removes devitalized tissue from the wound without disruption or damage to healthy tissue

   a. Nonionic wound cleansers, surfactants, and sterile normal saline: indicated for cleansing wounds with minimal-to-moderate amounts of slough.

   b. Conservative sharp debridement: requires no anesthesia; can be done on an outpatient basis, bedside, or at home using forceps and scissors; only devitalized tissue is removed.

3. Enzymatic debridement: enzyme preparations applied topically to necrotic tissue to break down targeted substrates; products require moisture for activation; inactivated when exposed to heavy metal ions such as mercury or silver (present in some antiseptics); loose debris should be removed before application.

4. Autolytic debridement: naturally occurring enzymes produced by bacteria and macrophages in wound fluid are used to promote liquefaction of necrotic tissue; autolysis (self-digestion) is promoted by the use of moisture-retentive dressings, which trap fluid next to the wound surface.

5. Maggot therapy: medicinal maggot therapy provides selective debridement by both physical (larvae movement) and chemical (secretes and excretes digestive enzymes) means.

X. CHOOSING THE APPROPRIATE TREATMENT OPTION

Base choice of product on the wound/host assessment, expected outcome of intervention, and cost of treatment.
A. Principles of wound management.
   1. Reduce/eliminate causative factors.
   2. Provide systemic support.
   3. Remove foreign bodies/necrotic tissue.
   4. Choose appropriate topical therapy.
   5. Control bacterial proliferation.
   6. Control drainage.
   7. Curative versus palliation.
B. Goals of wound cleansing/debridement: to remove surface bacteria and other microorganisms and to hasten the removal of devitalized tissue.
C. Goals of topical therapy.
   1. Create an optimum wound healing environment.
   2. Manage exudate.
   3. Obliterate dead space.
   4. Provide insulation.
   5. Protect from trauma.
D. Dressing options.
   1. Semipermeable film dressing: acronyms include moisture vapor-permeable (MVP) dressings, vapor-permeable (VPM), transparent film dressings (TFDs), synthetic adhesive moisture vapor-permeable (SAM) dressings, and polyurethane films (PUFs); retains moisture in wounds with minimal exudate without macerating periwound skin; waterproof; permits oxygen and water vapor to cross the barrier; impermeable to bacteria and contaminants; maintains moist environment; promotes autolysis of necrotic tissue; provides insulation; allows for visualization of the wound; adhesive products may injure new epithelium on removal (avoid use on skin tears); indications include:
      a. Superficial, partial-thickness wounds.
      b. Wounds with minimal necrosis or slough.
      c. Wounds with little or no exudate.
      d. Use as a secondary (cover) dressing.

2. Hydrocolloid dressing: pastes or occlusive adhesive wafers composed of pectinlike material; provides moist environment; promotes autolysis and granulation; insulates wound; impermeable to bacteria and other contaminants; adhesive products may injure new epithelium on removal (avoid use on skin tears); provides moderate absorption; may be used with compression stockings/pumps, wraps, or Unna boot for:
   a. Partial-thickness wounds
   b. Shallow full-thickness wounds
   c. Granulating full-thickness with minimal-to-moderate exudate

3. Foam dressing: wound contact surface is semipermeable or hydrophilic; outer dressing surface is hydrophobic; nonadherent; maintains moist wound environment; promotes autolytic debridement; minimal-to-moderate absorption; protects from trauma; insulates; atraumatic removal; available with and without silver; available with silicone contact layer to promote adhesion and atraumatic removal; indications include:
   a. Partial-thickness wounds with minimal-to-moderate drainage
   b. Full-thickness wounds with depth or dead space; use packing to fill cavity.
   c. May use under compression
   d. To absorb drainage around tubes (trach sites, chest tubes, gastrostomy tubes, etc.)
   e. Atraumatic reduction of hypergranulation tissue (especially useful around pediatric gastrostomy tubes)

4. Calcium alginate/hydrofiber dressing: highly absorbent (can absorb 20 times its weight in wound exudate); conforms to the shape of the wound; must be covered with a secondary dressing; available with and without silver; provides a modest hemostasis effect; available in sheet and ribbon format; indications include:
   a. Partial- and full-thickness wounds with moderate-to-heavy exudate
   b. Wounds with tunneling or sinus tracts
   c. Wounds with moderate-to-small amounts of necrotic tissue
   d. Infected and noninfected wounds
   e. Wounds with small sanguinous ooze (e.g., tumors)

5. Biosynthetic/biologic dressing: skin substitutes; composed of tissue derived from animal or human sources; requires a secondary dressing; indicated for:
   a. Full-thickness wounds
   b. Noninfected wounds

6. Hydrogel dressing: water or glycerin-based amorphous gel, impregnated gauze, or sheet; promotes autolytic debridement; maintains moist environment; limited absorption of exudate; atraumatic removal; refrigerated product provides some pain relief; available with or without silver; most require a secondary dressing; indications include:
   a. Partial- or full-thickness wounds
   b. Deep wounds with minimal exudate

c. Wounds with varying amounts of necrosis or slough

d. Burns or tissue damaged by radiation

7. Composite dressings: combination of two or more dressing materials, moisture-retentive properties; absorptive; provides a bacterial barrier; indications include:

a. Partial-thickness or full-thickness wounds

b. Wounds with moderate-to-heavy exudate

c. Granulating, necrotic, or mixed wounds

8. Gauze dressings: available in many forms—impregnated, nonimpregnated, nonadherent, and nonwoven. Indications include:

a. Mechanical debridement of necrotic tissue and debris (wet-to-dry dressings)

b. Exudating wounds (to wick drainage away from the wound)

c. To fill dead space

d. To deliver topical medications to the wound bed

e. To promote a moist environment for healing

9. Negative pressure wound therapy: a device that applies uniform negative pressure to the wound surface to facilitate granulation tissue growth, increase perfusion, and facilitate removal of surface bacteria and debris. May also be applied to a closed incision to facilitate primary healing:

a. Foam or antibacterial gauze dressings are cut to fit the wound.

b. Dressings are sealed with adhesive occlusive film.

c. A suction catheter is attached to a hole cut into the occlusive film.

d. Continuous or intermittent suction is applied to the closed system at ranges of 80 to 120 mm Hg.

e. Indications include:

(1) Acute, traumatic, and subacute wounds

(2) Grafts and flaps

(3) Nonhealing chronic wounds that have not responded to conventional treatments

(4) Acceleration of granulation tissue formation

(5) To draw wound edges together (large open wounds healing by secondary intention)

(6) Exudate control in heavily draining wounds, including explored fistulas

(7) Reduce periwound tissue edema

f. Contraindications include:

(1) Malignant wounds (unless used for palliative purposes)

(2) Active bleeding

(3) Anticoagulant therapy

(4) Wounds with greater than 30% necrotic tissue

(5) Untreated osteomyelitis

(6) Unexplored sinus tracts or fistulas connecting to organs or body cavities

(7) Placement directly over exposed veins or arteries

10. Collagen/extracellular matrix: stimulates granulation tissue growth; binds with MMPs; available with and without silver; requires a secondary dressing; indications include:

a. Partial- and full-thickness wounds

b. Wounds with minimal or no necrotic tissue

c. Wounds with minimal-to-moderate amount of exudate

d. Wounds affected by radiation therapy

11. Antimicrobial: various materials including cadexomer iodine pad and gel; Manuka honey–containing alginates, gels, and hydrocolloids; silver-containing dressings in various vehicles as noted above; indications include:

a. Infected wounds

b. Critically colonized wounds

c. Chronic nonhealing or stalled wounds

d. Wounds at high risk for infections (immunocompromised host)

12. Growth factors: genetically engineered PDGFs; requires a secondary dressing; indications include neuropathic foot ulcers.

It is extremely important that wound assessment, interventions, and evaluation of response to treatment are documented accurately to allow the clinician to appropriately monitor progress toward healing. If minimal or no wound healing progress noted after 2 weeks, consider full reassessment and modification of topical therapy.

XI. CHRONIC ULCERS

A. Venous ulcers (Figure 23-19).

1. Definition: ulcerations resulting from chronic venous insufficiency

2. Etiology/pathophysiology

a. Dysfunction of the deep venous system (femoral, popliteal, and tibial veins), perforating, or superficial veins causing increased hydrostatic pressure; venous hypertension causes stretching of the vessel walls with leakage of plasma and fibrin into the extravascular space. Fibrin cuffs form around capillaries, preventing diffusion of oxygen and nutrients needed for normal cellular function. Predisposing factors include:

(1) Deep vein thrombosis (DVT)

(2) Valvular incompetence of deep venous system

(3) Postphlebitic syndrome

(4) Congestive heart failure

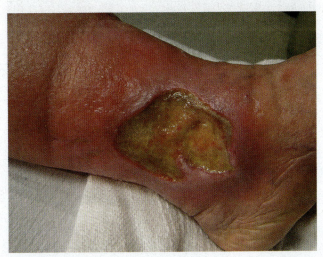

FIGURE 23-19. Venous leg ulcer in the gaiter area of the leg, a typical location. (Copyright Duke University, used with permission.)

(5) Obesity

(6) Pregnancy—multiparity

(7) Superficial vein valve regurgitation

(8) Calf muscle weakness

3. Events related to venous disease

a. Increased hydrostatic pressure

b. Venous hypertension

c. Edema

d. Dermal ulceration

4. Contributing factors

a. Malnutrition

b. Hypoalbuminemia

c. Immobility

d. Trauma

e. Genetics

f. Sedentary lifestyle

5. Clinical characteristics

a. Stasis dermatitis: brown discoloration and scaling of the skin in the gaiter (sock) area of the lower extremities. Increased venous hypertension leads to chronic edema and rupture of dermal capillaries with deposition of hemosiderin, an iron-containing pigment, in the dermis (Figure 23-20).

b. Ulcerations have a predilection for area proximal to the medial malleolus.

c. Lipodermatosclerosis: induration of skin and subcutaneous tissue

d. Painful, pitting edema

e. Dull, constant pain, which improves on elevation

f. Ulcers may have sharply demarcated or poorly defined borders and may be deep or superficial.

g. Pedal pulses usually palpable though may be difficult to feel with extensive edema

h. With removal of crust, a moist, granulating base will be revealed though it may have a thin fibrin covering.

6. Incidence

a. Affects 1% of the general population and 3.5% of persons over 65

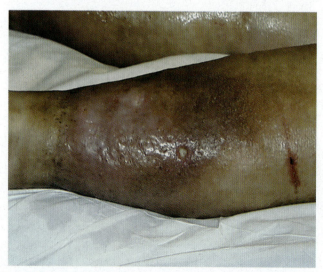

FIGURE 23-20. Hemosiderin staining associated with chronic stasis dermatitis. (Copyright Duke University, used with permission.)

b. Recurrence rate approaches 70%

c. Women affected three times more often than men but this decreases as both groups age

7. Assessment

a. History and physical examination

b. Complete review of medical history

(1) Previous pregnancies

(2) Leg trauma

(3) Cardiac disease

(4) Nutritional status

(5) History of DVT and/or pulmonary embolus

(6) Previous lower extremity surgery

c. Physical exam

(1) Varicose veins

(2) Lipodermatosclerosis and edema of the lower extremity usually present

(3) Stasis dermatitis: induration, erythematous hyperpigmentation, hemosiderin deposition, scaling, and weeping; may be pruritic

(4) Ankle flare sign: a collection of small venular channels inferior to the medial malleolus extending onto the medial foot

(5) Growth of hair: may indicate adequacy of arterial flow

(6) Atrophie blanche: atrophic plaques of white skin with telangiectasias

(7) Palpate dorsalis pedis and posterior tibial pulses

8. Diagnostic tests

a. Doppler ultrasonography: noninvasive assessment of deep venous system

b. Transcutaneous oxygen tension: greater than or equal to 30 mm Hg would indicate healing potential.

c. Duplex scanning with color-flow imaging: locates venous reflux in the superficial, deep, and perforator systems

d. Ankle–brachial index (ABI): noninvasive measure of arterial blood flow—greater than 80 mm Hg indicates healing potential. May not be reliable in patients with diabetes.

e. Contrast venography: invasive procedure utilizing radiopaque dye

f. Laboratory

(1) Visceral protein: of minimal value in patients with underlying conditions

(2) Glucose and HgbA1C

(3) CBC

9. Treatment

a. Treat underlying cause of venous dysfunction.

b. Compression and elevation to enhance venous return

c. Appropriate dressing for the wound based on assessment

d. Avoid restrictive garments.

e. Refer to vascular surgery for treatment of venous hypertension with ablation versus subfascial endoscopic perforating vein surgery versus open ligation vein surgery.

10. Nursing considerations (Table 23-3)

B. Arterial ulcers (Figure 23-21).
  1. Definition: ischemic ulcerations secondary to arterial insufficiency (PVD) with acute (e.g., thrombosis) or chronic (e.g., arteriosclerosis obliterans) presentation
  2. Etiology/pathophysiology
    a. Peripheral vascular disease
    b. Arteriosclerosis: thickening and decreased elasticity of arterial walls due to deposition of plaque, lipids, fibrin, platelets, and other cellular debris
    c. May involve bilateral lower extremities
    d. Contributing factors
      (1) Smoking
      (2) Diabetes mellitus
      (3) Hyperlipidemia
      (4) Hypertension
    e. Signs and symptoms of ischemic disease
      (1) Progressive pain; usually increases with leg elevation
        (a) Pain with exercise; relieved with rest (intermittent claudication)
        (b) Nocturnal pain; usually precedes rest pain (ischemic neuritis)
        (c) Pain at rest; demonstrates very advanced disease
      (2) Impaired circulation: seen prior to ulceration
        (a) Decreased pulses
        (b) Change in skin temperature
        (c) Delayed capillary and venous filling
        (d) Pallor on elevation
        (e) Dependent rubor
        (f) Development of gangrene
      (3) Ischemic skin changes
        (a) Smooth, shiny, thin epidermis
        (b) Absence of hair on lower extremities and feet
        (c) Slow nail growth

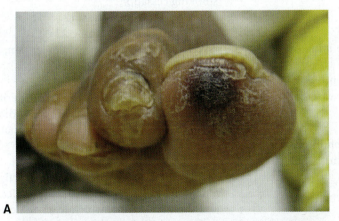

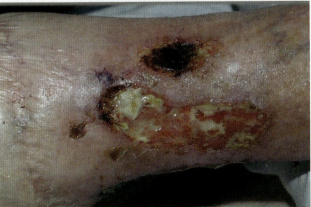
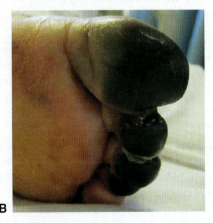

FIGURE 23-21. Arterial ulcers.
A: Arterial ulcer on the end of a toe, most likely due to an embolic event.
B: Arterial ulcers after use of vasoactive agents in a patient with preexisting compromised arterial blood flow.
C: Arterial leg ulcer. This ulcer has a more punched-out appearance than a venous ulcer. This patient has had arterial flood reestablished; granulation buds are visible in the wound base. (Copyright Duke University, used with permission.)

(4) Generally affects vessels below the knee (tibial and peroneal arteries) in diabetics

(5) Generally affects femoral, iliac, and aortic vessels in common population

3. Clinical presentation
   a. Punched-out appearance
   b. Well-demarcated borders
   c. Location: areas exposed to traumatic injury
      (1) Over toes
      (2) Interdigital spaces
      (3) Dorsum of the foot
      (4) Lateral malleolus
   d. May be deep, exposing tendon
   e. Base of ulcer generally necrotic and pale, lacking granulation tissue
   f. Gangrenous skin may be seen adjacent to or surrounding the ulcer

4. Incidence of PVD
   a. More common in diabetics
   b. More common at earlier age in diabetics
   c. Male/female ratio 2:1 in diabetics, 30:1 in nondiabetics
   d. Diabetics generally have bilateral lower extremity involvement.
   e. Nondiabetics generally have unilateral involvement.

5. Assessment
   a. History
      (1) Ask about events/symptoms specific to arterial insufficiency.
         (a) Pain
         (b) Impaired circulation
         (c) Ischemic skin changes
      (2) Evaluate history of the ulcer.
         (a) Length of time ulcer present
         (b) Any traumatic event that may have initiated the ulcer
         (c) Topical treatments used for treatment
         (d) History of diabetes, surgery, vascular problems
         (e) History of smoking
         (f) Presence of coexisting systemic conditions (anemia, sickle cell disease, arthritis, or venous insufficiency)

6. Physical examination
   a. Inspection
      (1) Ischemic skin changes
      (2) Evidence of gangrene
      (3) Pallor with delayed capillary filling
      (4) Wound bed: desiccated; dry leathery eschar or pale granulation
      (5) Drainage: scant to minimal
   b. Palpation
      (1) Decreased or absent pulses (femoral, popliteal, posterior tibial, and dorsalis pedis)
      (2) Mild (1+) to severe (3+) edema
      (3) Temperature of skin is cool in the presence of arterial disease

      (4) Wound bed
         (a) Palpate; probe wound bed to identify presence of tunnels and sinus tracts.
         (b) Palpate necrotic bed; if boggy/spongy, suspect liquefaction of necrotic tissue or infection.

7. Diagnostic tests
   a. Noninvasive
      (1) Doppler ultrasonography: assesses competency of deep arterial system; also measures ABI
      (2) Transcutaneous oxygen tension
   b. Invasive
      (1) Angiography
   c. Laboratory
      (1) Visceral protein: of minimal value in patients with underlying conditions
      (2) Glucose and HgbA1C
      (3) CBC
      (4) Culture (if infection suspected)

8. Treatment
   a. Avoid compression.
   b. Legs to be kept neutral or slightly dependent position (no elevation)
   c. Avoid restrictive garments.
   d. Eliminate causative factors: enhance arterial profusion either through surgery or pharmacotherapy.
   e. Optimize microenvironment: debridement; eradication of infection.
   f. Optimize the host: enhance nutritional status; control edema; control underlying medical conditions; smoking cessation.
   g. Appropriate wound dressing

9. Nursing considerations (Table 23-3)
   a. Five Ps of acute arterial ischemia: pain; paresthesia; paralysis; pallor; pulselessness

C. Neuropathic ulcers (Figure 23-22).
   1. Definition: skin ulcers secondary to peripheral neuropathy that commonly accompany diabetes mellitus; may also have peripheral neuropathy without diabetes.
   2. Etiology/pathophysiology
      a. Sensory neuropathy: decreased protective sensation places the patient at risk for mechanical, chemical, and thermal trauma, which leads to development of neuropathic ulcers.
      b. Motor neuropathy: muscular atrophy of the foot
         (1) Changes patient's gait
         (2) Causes claw toes
         (3) Repetitive stress on metatarsal head (callus buildup first sign of increased pressure): leads to ulceration
      c. Autonomic neuropathy—generally leads to infection/gangrene
         (1) Distal anhydrosis
         (2) Xerosis
         (3) Cracks/fissures (Figure 23-23)

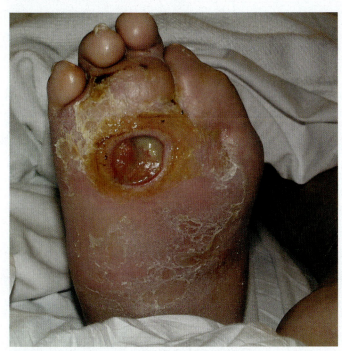

FIGURE 23-22. Neuropathic ulcer on the plantar aspect of foot, with surrounding hyperkeratosis. (Copyright Duke University, used with permission.)

3. Clinical presentation
   a. Usually isolated lesions on the plantar surface of the foot (correlate with areas of increased weight loading or friction)
   b. Round, dry, punched-out lesion (well-defined edges)
   c. Elevated hyperkeratotic rim
   d. Foot warm, pink, with pedal pulses present
   e. Xerosis and fissuring may be present.
   f. Eschar/necrotic debris possible
   g. Diminished or absence of normal protective skin sensation

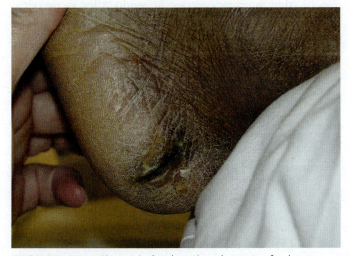

FIGURE 23-23. Fissure in heel setting the stage for bacterial entry and infection. (Copyright Duke University, used with permission.)

4. Incidence
   a. In patients with diabetes, the annual incidence rate for foot ulcers is 2.5% to 10.7%.
   b. A foot infection is most common reason for hospitalization of a patient with diabetes in the United States.
5. Assessment
   a. History
      (1) Complete medical history similar to that for ischemic ulcers
      (2) Previous trauma
      (3) Knowledge of and adherence with foot care (nail and skin care)
      (4) Types of shoes/orthotics being worn (examine for worn areas)
      (5) Pain relieved by walking
      (6) Paresthesias or insensate areas
   b. Physical examination: always distinguish between traumatic ulcers secondary to peripheral neuropathy and those secondary to arterial insufficiency
      (1) Diminished or absent sensation in feet as assessed with a Semmes–Weinstein monofilament
      (2) Deep, circular lesions
      (3) Indolent lesions
      (4) Pedal pulses generally present
      (5) Skin changes including in web spaces—xerosis, fissures
      (6) Foot and toe deformities
      (7) Foot may be warm.
   c. Diagnostic tests
      (1) Doppler ultrasonography and/or angiography to rule out macrovascular disease (PVD)
      (2) Toe pressures or transcutaneous oxygen measurements
      (3) ABI may be inaccurate due to microvascular calcification.
      (4) Screening tests for sensory loss:
          (a) Semmes–Weinstein monofilament: gold standard, quick and easy to perform in clinic setting
          (b) Vibratory sensation with a tuning fork: patient report of sensation when activated tuning fork held to the interphalangeal joint of the great toe.
          (c) Ipswich–Touch test: gentle touch of the distal end of the first, third, and fifth toe for 1 to 2 seconds. Two or more insensate areas equal a positive test.
   d. Laboratory
      (1) Visceral proteins: of minimal value with underlying conditions
      (2) CBC
      (3) Glucose and HgbA1C
      (4) Culture if infection suspected
      (5) C-reactive protein and erythrocyte sedimentation rate
6. Nursing considerations (Table 23-3)

D. Pressure ulcers.
1. Definition: a localized area of skin and/or tissue destruction as the result of pressure or pressure with shear. It is most commonly over a bony prominence but not always as they may be found associated with medical devices. Most common locations are the sacrum/buttocks in adults and posterior head in pediatrics. The heels are the second most common location for both populations.
2. Etiology: unrelieved pressure
3. Contributing factors
   a. Poor nutritional status
   b. Friction
   c. Excessive moisture and maceration (e.g., incontinence)
   d. Immobility
   e. Diminished sensation
4. Pathophysiology
   a. Pressure: amount of force exerted on a given area
      (1) Normal capillary filling pressure is approximately 32 mm Hg at arteriolar end, 12 mm Hg at venous end.
      (2) Pressure greater than 32 mm Hg restricts blood flow.
      (3) Increased pressure collapses capillaries leading to thrombosis, ischemia, and eventual cell death.
      (4) Decreased oxygen and nutrition reaches tissues and cellular waste products are not removed.
      (5) Muscle deformation causes damage on a microscopic scale leading to tissue death.
      (6) Skin, muscle, and adipose tissues respond differently to the amount and duration of pressure.
   b. Shear: a mechanical force that is parallel rather than perpendicular to a body area; combination of gravity and friction
      (1) Main effect is on deep tissue (sacral, coccygeal, trochanteric, ischial areas).
      (2) Blood vessels become angulated, obstructed, torn, and/or stretched.
      (3) Shearing decreases the time that tissues can tolerate pressure forces.
      (4) Undermining or tunneling commonly occurs as a result of shear.
   c. Friction: created by the forces of two surfaces moving across one another
      (1) Wound resembles an abrasion—not considered a pressure ulcer
      (2) Alters skin integrity, increasing potential for deeper tissue damage
   d. Excessive moisture: usually due to incontinence
      (1) Macerates epidermis
      (2) Causes epidermal sloughing
      (3) Predisposes to secondary yeast infection
5. Point prevalence
   a. Percentage of patients with a pressure ulcer at a specific point in time
   b. 6.3% to 14.9% of patients in acute care are estimated to have pressure ulcers.

   c. 4.1% to 32.2% of patients in long-term care are estimated to have pressure ulcers.
   d. 13.1% in US intensive care units and 45.5% in Chinese teaching hospital intensive care units
6. Cumulative incidence
   a. Percentage of patient who develop a pressure ulcer over a specified period of time—usually weeks to months
   b. 2.8% to 9% in acute care settings
   c. 3.6% to 59% in long-term care settings
   d. 3.3% to 53.4% in intensive care settings with rates varying with the type of ICU
7. Facility-acquired pressure ulcers: also known as nosocomial, hospital-acquired, or health care–acquired pressure ulcers
8. Prevention
   a. Not all pressure ulcers are preventable. Unavoidable pressure ulcers are those where all possible preventative measures have been employed and tissue damage occurs. This may been seen when patients refuse preventative care or where preventative care cannot be provided (hemodynamically unstable with offloading; unable to off-load a medical device).
   b. Risk factors for development of pressure ulcers: activity and mobility limitations, nutritional deficits, general skin status (including moisture), perfusion and oxygenation, sensory perception deficits, general health status, advanced age, and hematologic measures
   c. Risk assessment tool: use a structured risk assessment tool (e.g., Braden Scale, Norton Scale, Waterlow Scale) on admission and when the patient's condition changes. A routine reassessment with a tool may be the easiest way to ensure the patient risk for pressure ulcer development is reevaluated. Use the risk assessment to target appropriate prevention interventions (see Appendix A for an overview, sample protocol, and Braden Risk Assessment with Interventions).
   d. Skin assessment and care (e.g., see Appendix B protocol)
      (1) Assess the skin for intactness, generalized color, moisture, edema, localized erythema, and induration—pay close attention to bony prominences. May be difficult to see skin color changes in more darker pigmented skin.
      (2) Apply appropriate moisturizing creams and protective barriers (ointments and/or pastes) to protect the skin from moisture (urine and fecal incontinence the most concerning). Do not massage at-risk erythematous areas.
      (3) Keep the skin clean and dry. Use no-rinse cleansers when bed bathing is performed, avoiding detergents remaining on the skin after bath.
   e. Pressure redistribution: routine measures used to decrease the intensity and time of pressure on the soft tissues

(1) Provide the support surface based on the patient's needs (e.g., see Appendix C for sample protocol and algorithm).

(a) Level of activity and bed mobility

(b) Weight and size of patient

(c) Overall risk for development of pressure ulcer

(d) Need for microclimate control (moisture management)

(e) Status of any existing pressure ulcers

(2) Provide pressure redistribution seating cushion for patients with impaired mobility/sensation while in a chair. Provide routine repositioning while in the chair even with the chair cushion. Limit time in chair for patients with an existing pressure ulcer to no more than 60 minutes three times daily.

(3) Provide routine repositioning for all patient who are at risk for pressure ulcers who have impaired bed mobility unless it is contraindicated.

(4) Avoid positioning on an erythematous bony prominence or on an existing pressure ulcer.

(5) Consider placement of a prophylactic foam dressing to bony prominences and under medical devices at risk for damage from pressure, friction, and/or shear.

f. Nutrition: adequate intake of nutrients and fluids are important for the prevention of pressure ulcers and wounding healing in general. Refer patients who are at risk for malnutrition or who have an existing pressure ulcer to a registered dietician.

PATIENT EDUCATION
Pressure Ulcer Prevention

- Inspect skin at least daily and after any prolonged sitting/laying.
- Apply moisturizing cream to the skin after bathing daily and as needed to keep skin moist.
- Do not massage red areas over bony prominences.
- Eat a well-balanced diet. Ensure intake of adequate amounts of protein and fluids.
- Reposition every 15 minutes when in chair and regularly when recumbent.
- Seek care from health care provider for any red area than does not resolve and any open area.

9. Assessment (see Table 23-2 for parameters of targeted wound assessment)

a. Stages/categories: used only for pressure ulcer. Documents the tissue depth of the ulcer. Do not backstage as the ulcer heals.

(1) Stage/category I: nonblanchable erythema with intact skin

(2) Stage/category II: partial-thickness skin loss of the dermis. May be a serous filling blister/bulla. May often see hair follicles in the wound base

(3) Stage/category III: full-thickness skin loss to but not through the fascial layer of muscle. Adipose tissue may be visible but NOT muscle, tendon, or bone. Necrotic tissue may be visible but not obscuring the wound base.

(4) Stage/category IV: full-thickness skin loss with muscle, tendon, and/or bone visible in wound base. Necrotic tissue may be in the wound base.

(5) Unstageable: Full-thickness skin loss but full depth of the wound in unknown due to the covering of necrotic tissue

(6) Suspected deep tissue injury: purple or maroon intact skin or blood-filled blister/bulla. This may evolve despite interventions and eventually restaged to one of above stages/categories. Some SDTIs may resolve without further evolution.

(7) Mucosal: used to describe pressure ulcers on any mucosal surface

(8) Indeterminable: category established by the National Database for Nursing Quality Indicators (NDNQI). Includes mucosal category and any ulcer under a medical device or dressing that has not been assessed

b. Assess the pressure ulcer initially or upon admission and then at least weekly. Expect some sign of healing in 2 weeks.

10. Treatment

a. Pressure redistribution as noted in prevention

b. Clean the wound and surrounding skin with each dressing change.

c. Debride devitalized tissue from the wound if consistent with the overall goals. Consider close monitoring of dry intact eschar on heels.

d. Provide topical therapy based on wound characteristics, condition of surrounding skin, location of wound, goals of care, and costs of care and dressing provider level of expertise.

e. Surgical evaluation is appropriate for pressure ulcers with advancing cellulitis and/or stage III/IV for more rapid closure.

f. Interdisciplinary consultation may be appropriate for pressure ulcers that fail to show signs of healing.

11. Nursing considerations (Table 23-3)

E. Skin tear.

1. Definition: a separation of the skin layers due to friction, shear, and/or blunt trauma. It may be partial-thickness or full-thickness skin loss.

2. Etiology

a. Intrinsic factors

(1) Extreme of ages (>75 years and premature/neonate)

(2) Female

(3) Race (Caucasian)

(4) Long-term sun exposure

(5) Immobility

(6) Altered sensory perception (including neuropathy)

(7) Cognitive impairment

(8) Limb stiffness and/or spacity

TABLE 23-2 Characteristics of Common Problem Wounds

	Arterial Ulcer	Venous Ulcer	Neuropathic Ulcer	Pressure Ulcer	Skin Tear

Predisposing factors	Arteriosclerosis
	Peripheral vascular disease (PVD)
	Diabetes mellitus
	Advanced age
		History of:
		  Deep vein thrombosis
		  Thrombophlebitis
		  Pulmonary embolus
		  Incompetent valves in perforating veins
		  Calf pump failure
		  History of venous ulcers or family history of ulcers
		  Obesity
		  Pregnancy—multiparity
		  Advanced age
		  Sedentary lifestyle
			Diabetes
			Peripheral neuropathy
			Peripheral vascular disease
				Multiple medical diagnoses
				Advanced age
				Impaired mobility
				Loss of sensation
				Altered mental status
				Poor nutritional status
				Incontinence
				Impaired circulation
					Advance age or premature birth
					Solar-damaged skin
					Chronic steroid therapy
					Dependence in ADLs

Location	Usually distal to impaired arterial supply
	At sites subjected to trauma or rubbing of footwear:
	  Phalangeal heads
	  Lateral malleolus
	  Tips of toes
	  Interdigital spaces
		Can occur anywhere between the knee and ankle
		Medial malleolus is the most common site.
			Any sites on the foot and lower limb subjected to repetitive pressure, friction, shear, or trauma:
			Plantar surface over metatarsal heads (especially first and fifth)
			Great toe
			Calcaneus
				Can occur over any bony prominence subjected to pressure, friction, or shearing forces
				Sacrum, heels, elbows, and trochanter are the most common sites in bedridden patients.
				Occurs over ischial tuberosity with prolonged sitting
				Can occur anyplace medical devices are in use
					Forearms—for bedbound patients
					Pretibial surface—for ambulatory patients
					Skin areas subject to friction or shearing forces

Depth	Can be shallow but usually deep, crater-like wound Exposed tendons common	Usually shallow	Usually deep, but may be shallow depending on disease severity May have tracking and/or undermining Exposed tendons are common	Ranges in depth from circulatory compromise (stage 1) to deep tissue destruction involving underlying structures such as bone and tendon (stage 4)	Shallow (partial thickness to deep partial thickness) Full thickness
Wound appearance	Thick, dry, leathery eschar often present Digits may appear gangrenous. Pale, gray, or yellow wound base following debridement Absent or poor quality granulation tissue Cellulitis may be present and usually indicates advanced infection	Ruddy, "beefy" red granulation tissue Superficial fibrin deposits (looks like a gelatinous film) may occur suddenly on top of healthy-appearing granulation tissue	Often accompanied by thick, leathery eschar that requires sharp debridement Following debridement, base may appear dry and fibrotic. Wound granulates slowly, especially if PVD is present. Cellulitis or osteomyelitis is common	Stage 1—nonblanchable erythema over a pressure point Stage 2—superficial skin loss with exposure of pink, moist dermal tissue Stage 3—full-thickness crater with necrotic tissue possible. Stage 4—Extensive tissue necrosis down to and involving bone. Undermining, sinus tracts, or soft tissue tunneling may be present. Unstageable: full-thickness skin loss with base obscured by necrotic tissue Suspected deep tissue injury: maroon to dark purple skin discoloration	Superficial or deep partial-thickness skin flap (often partially attached at wound margin) Commonly occur over areas of purpura Pink to red moist dermal base Hematoma may be present

Exudate/ drainage	Minimal exudate Dry, fibrous wound base	Moderate-to-heavy exudate Exudate decreases with treatment of venous hypertension.	Small to moderate amounts of exudate Infected ulcers usually have purulent drainage. Excessive drainage may indicate underlying osteomyelitis.	Amount of drainage varies with stage of ulcer and whether or not the wound is infected.	Small to moderate amounts of exudate May have copious amount of drainage with underlying edema
Wound shape and margins	Sharp, well-defined margins that conform to the type of skin trauma "Punched-out" appearance	Irregular, poorly defined margins that make measurement difficult	Sharp, well-defined margins Wound may be small at the surface with a large subcutaneous abscess beneath. Callus around the ulcer in areas caused by ill-fitting shoes Edges often undermined	Usually shaped like the boney prominence below or the medical device causing the damage with well-defined margins Large ulcers caused by shearing forces may have irregular margins and extensive undermining	Shape of wound is consistent with a traumatic tear caused by skin friction or tissue shearing
Surrounding skin	Pale or cyanotic color Dependent rubor Skin is thin, shiny, and cool to the touch. Hair loss over skin surfaces Minimal to no edema	Brawny, hyperpigmented skin in gaiter (sock) area Moderate-to-severe edema Lipodermatosclerosis Localized areas of maceration from excessive drainage Dry, flaky skin (hyperkeratosis)	Dry, thin, frequently callused Periwound hyperkeratosis is common and indicates repeated pressure or trauma. Infection may be difficult to assess due to microcirculatory compromise	Skin may be macerated or have secondary yeast infection if patient is incontinent. Clinical infection is indicated by localized redness, warmth, and induration	Paper-thin, fragile skin Senile purpura (bruising)
Pain response	Often accompanied by severe pain at rest (claudication), numbness, and paresthesias Pain often increases with leg elevation. Pain may increase with ambulation (time of onset depends on severity of disease)	Pain varies unpredictably. Small, deep ulcers around malleoli are typically the most painful. May complain of a throbbing pain if leg edema is severe and not being adequately treated Pain often improves with leg elevation and edema control	Varies from no pain to constant or intermittent numbness or burning Neuropathic ulcers are almost always accompanied by numbness and paresthesias	Varies from mild to severe (pressure ulcers are less common in patients that have sensation and can communicate discomfort) Many patients experience pain but are unable to express it due to altered consciousness	Pain response varies Usually mild to moderate pain during cleansing, but subsides once wound is covered
Expected outcome	Rate of healing depends primarily on disease severity and adequacy of tissue perfusion. The presence of necrotic tissue will delay healing significantly. Open wounds will either not heal or recur if osteomyelitis is inadequately treated. If perfusion is poor and revascularization isn't an option, the outcome of a healed wound is very unlikely	Outcome depends on patient compliance with edema control measures. Average time to healing depends on: Disease severity Extent of lipodermatosclerosis Presence of cardiovascular disease Successful reversal of venous hypertension and edema control	Patient must comply with diet, glucose regulation, exercise, and foot care in order for healing to occur. Achieving a healed wound may require aggressive revascularization or appropriate antibiotic therapy. Open wounds will either not heal or recur if osteomyelitis is inadequately treated. Custom or specialized shoes will reduce pressure and help prevent ulcer recurrence	Must eliminate or significantly reduce pressure, shear, and friction in order to achieve a healed wound. Prevention measures and appropriate skin care are critical to maintaining intact skin once healing is achieved	Must prevent continued or recurrent skin trauma in order to achieve healing Adequate education of patient and caregivers should reduce recurrence rate

TABLE 23-3 Nursing Considerations for Wounds

Considerations	Outcomes	Interventions
Impaired skin integrity	Skin integrity will improve as evidenced by decrease in size of wound, decrease in drainage, and presence of granulation tissue.	Accurately assess the wound when first noted and then at least every week. Cleanse wound as indicated. Implement appropriate topical therapy using principles of wound care. Reevaluate wound and host factors if no healing in 2 weeks. Consider referral to wound specialist.
High risk for infection	Patient will be monitored closely for the development or progression of any infection; patient will be free of infection.	Assess wound and periwound skin for signs of infection. Use appropriate dressings to provide protection from infection (occlusive dressings in sacral area with incontinence noted).
Pain	Pain will be reduced or eradicated through appropriate interventions.	Use both topical and parenteral methods to reduce/relieve any pain associated with wounds. Consider use of progressive relaxation and/or therapeutic noncontact touch
Protein–calorie malnutrition leading to decrease healing	Nutritional status will be optimized leading to enhanced healing.	Assess patient's nutritional status, including serial weights. Provide dietary supplements as indicated to improve patient's nutritional status. Consider use of multivitamin. Refer to registered dietician.
Body image alteration secondary to the presence of wounds	Positive body image will be evident.	Assess patient's perceptions and feelings regarding the presence of open wounds. Allow patient to express feelings. Facilitate dressings that limit visibility of wound and decrease odor.
Immobility secondary to the presence of wounds	Maximum mobility is attained.	Assess limitations. Institute appropriate measures to enhance mobility (walker, cane). Refer to physical therapy.
Knowledge deficit	Patient will have knowledge regarding causative or exacerbating factors and comply with treatment regimen.	Assess knowledge or understanding of causative or exacerbating factors related to wound formation. Provide and document education to the patient and/or caregiver.
Ineffective coping mechanisms	Patient will develop healthier coping mechanisms.	Assess patient's psychosocial needs. Implement appropriate measures to assist patient in correcting problems. Refer to psychological services.

   (9) Underlying vascular, cardiac, and/or pulmonary issues
   (10) Inadequate nutritional intake
   (11) Long-term corticosteroid use
   (12) Incontinence
  b. Extrinsic factors
   (1) Assisted ADLs
   (2) Adhesive removal
   (3) Falls
   (4) Prosthetic devices
   (5) Use of mobility assistive devices (walkers, wheelchairs)
 3. Assessment
  a. ISTAP classification system (Figures 23-24 through 23-26)
   (1) Type 1: no skin loss—a linear or flap that can be completely reapproximated to cover the wound base
   (2) Type 2: partial flap loss—the skin flap cannot be repositioned such that it completely covers the wound bed.
   (3) Type 3: total flap loss—the entire wound bed is exposed with loss of the skin flap.
  b. Evaluate for modifiable intrinsic and extrinsic factors.

 4. Prevention
  a. Moisturizing skin after bathing with no-rinse product
  b. Avoid use of adhesive products on fragile skin.
  c. Protective clothing: long sleeves, long pants, skin/elbow guards
  d. Safe patient handling and fall prevention program
  e. Pad equipment and furniture
  f. Trim patient nails.

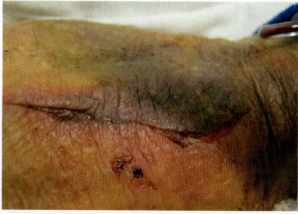

FIGURE 23-24. Skin tear, type 1. The skin flap is completely reapproximated to cover the wound base. (Copyright Duke University, used with permission.)

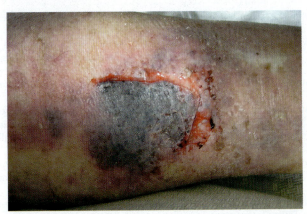

FIGURE 23-25. Skin tear, type 2. The skin flap cannot be completely reapproximated, and some wound base remains exposed. (Copyright Duke University, used with permission.)

PATIENT EDUCATION
Skin Tear Prevention

- Clean with mild soap (no-rinse cleanser if possible). Avoid detergents.
- Apply moisturizing cream to the skin after bathing daily and as needed to keep skin moist.
- Avoid any adhesive dressings on the skin, including dressing typically placed and a needlestick.
- Wear long sleeves and pants to protect skin from trauma.
- Wear sun block when in outdoors.

5. Treatment. (See Appendix D for sample protocol and algorithm.)
   a. Cleanse the skin tear at initial tear and with each dressing change.
   b. Using cotton-tipped swabs, reapproximate the skin flap as soon as possible and then secure in place with closure strips or liquid skin glue.
   c. Select a dressing that will:
      (1) Provide a moist wound environment.
      (2) Protect the surrounding skin from adhesive trauma.

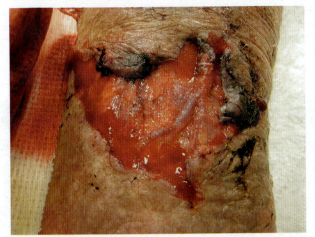

FIGURE 23-26. Skin tear, type 3. The skin flap is not salvageable, and the entire wound base is exposed. (Copyright Duke University, used with permission.)

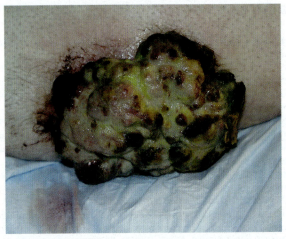

FIGURE 23-27. Fungating melanoma on the lateral calf. (Copyright Duke University, used with permission.)

   (3) Manage exudate.
   (4) Prevent infection.
   (5) Decrease caregiver time.
F. Palliative care for patients with wounds
   1. Determine the patient and/or family's understanding of and desire for preventative measures (pressure redistribution, nutrition interventions, and topical therapy).
   2. Select topical treatment that focuses on the following goals of care.
      a. Reduces pain associated with dressing changes
      b. Manages wound odor
         (1) Debridement of devitalized tissue
         (2) Topical metronidazole (crushed tablet or gel)
         (3) Charcoal or charcoal activated dressings
         (4) Environmental odor absorber
      c. Facilitates discharge to desired level of care
      d. Healing of wound may be secondary consideration for topical therapy.
   3. Wound commonly associated with palliative care
      a. Pressure ulcers
      b. Fungating malignant tumors (Figures 23-27 and 23-28)
      c. Marjolin ulcers: malignant transformation of a chronic wound

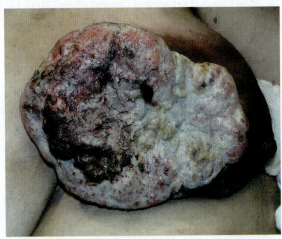

FIGURE 23-28. Fungating breast tumor. (Copyright Duke University, used with permission.)

BIBLIOGRAPHY

American Association for the Advancement of Wound Care. (2010) *Venous ulcer guideline*. Malvern, PA: AAWC

Angel, D., Lloyd, P., Carville, K., & Santamaria, N. (2011) The clinical efficacy of two semi-quantitative wound-swabbing techniques in identifying the causative organism(s) in infected cutaneous wounds. *International Wound Journal, 8*, 176–185.

Armstrong, D., & Meyr, A. (2013) Wound healing and risk factors for non-healing. In D. S. Basow (Ed.), *UpToDate*. Waltham, MA: UpToDate.

Ayello, E. A., & Braden, B. (2002). How and why to do pressure ulcer risk assessment. *Advances in Skin and Wound Care, 15*(3), 125–133.

Bien, P., Anda, C., & Prokocimer, P. (2014). Comparison of digital planimetry and ruler techniques to measure ABSSSI lesion sizes in the ESTABLISH-1 study. *Surgical Infections, 15*(2), 105–110.

Bilgin, M., & Güneş, Ü. (2013). A comparison of 3 wound measurement techniques: Effect of pressure ulcer size and shape. *Journal of Wound, Ostomy, and Continence Nursing, 40*(6), 590–593.

Black, J. M., Edsberg, L. E., Baharestani, M. M., Langemo, D., Goldberg, M., McNichols, L., Cuddingan, J., & National Pressure Ulcer Advisory Panel. (2011). Pressure ulcer: Avoidable or unavoidable? Results of the national pressure ulcer advisory panel consensus conference. *Ostomy/Wound Management, 57*(2), 24–37.

Bogie, K., & Ho, C. (2013). Pulsatile lavage for pressure ulcer management in spinal cord injury: A retrospective clinical safety review. *Ostomy/Wound Management, 59*(3), 35–38.

Cutting, K. (2008). Critical colonization. In K. Cutting (Ed.) *Advancing your practice: Understanding wound infection and the role of biofilm.* Malvern, PA: AAWC

Craig, A. H., Strauss, M. B., Daniller, A., & Miller, S. S. (2014). Foot sensation testing in the patient with diabetes: Introduction of the quick and easy assessment tool. *Wounds, 26*(8), 221–231.

Dorner, B., Posthauer, M., Thomas, D., & NPUAP. (2009). The role of nutrition in pressure ulcer prevention and treatment: National pressure ulcer advisory panel white paper. *Advances in Skin and Wound Care, 22*(5), 212–221.

Hunt, D. (2009). Diabetes: Foot ulcers and amputations. *American Family Physician, 80*(8), 789–790.

Krasner, D. L. (2014). *Chronic wound care: The essentials*. Malvern, PA: HMP Publications.

Lavery, L., Baranoski, E., & Ayello, E. (2004). Diabetic foot ulcers. In S. Baranoski, & E. Ayello (Eds.), *Wound care essentials: Practice principles.* Springhouse, PA: Lippincott Williams & Wilkins.

LeBlanc, K., & Baranoski, S. (2011). Skin tears: State of the science: Consensus statements for the prevention, prediction, assessment, and treatment of skin tears. *Advances in Skin and Wound Care, 24*(9), 2–15.

LeBlanc, K., & Baranoski, S. (2014). International skin tear advisory panel: Putting it all together, a tool kit to id in the prevention, assessment using a simplified classification system and treatment of skin tears. *World Council of Enterostomal Therapists Journal, 34*(1), 12–27.

Leung, L. (2013). Overview of hemostasis. In D. S. Basow (Ed.), *UpToDate*. Waltham, MA: UpToDate.

Levine, J., & Cioroiu, M. (2013). Wound healing in the geriatric patient. *Today's Wound Clinic, 7*(9).

Lewis, S., Raj, D. & Guzman, N. (2012). Renal failure: Implications of chronic kidney in the management of the diabetic foot. *Seminars in Vascular Surgery 28*, 82–88.

Milne, C. (2015, January 1) *Dressings*. Retrieved March 11, 2015, from http://www.woundsource.com/product-category/dressings

National Pressure Ulcer Advisory Panal, European Pressure Ulcer Advisory Panel and Pan Pacific Pressure Injury Alliance. (2014). *Prevention and treatment of pressure ulcers: Clinical practice guideline*. Perth, Australia: Cambridge Media.

Percival, S., Thomas, J., & Williams, D. (2010) Biofilms and bacterial imbalances in chronic wounds: Anti-Koch. *International Wound Journal 7*(3), 169–175.

Ramundo, J. & Gray, M. (2008). Enzymatic wound debridement, *Journal of Wound, Ostomy, and Continence Nursing, 35*(3), 273–280.

Rinker, B. (2013). The evils of nicotine: Evidenced-based guide to smoking and plastic surgery. *Annuals of Plastic Surgery, 70*(5):599-605.

Rondas, A., Schols, J., Halfens, R., & Stobberingh, E. (2013). Swab versus biopsy for the diagnosis of chronic infected wounds. *Advances in Skin and Wound Care, 26*(5), 211–219.

Scales, B., & Huffnagle, G. (2013) The microbiome in wound repair and tissue necrosis. *Journal of Pathology, 229*, 323–331.

Sherman, R. (2014) Mechanisms of maggot-induced wound healing: What do we know and where do we go from here? *Evidenced-Based Complementary and Alternative Medicine*. Art ID 592419.

Sinno, S., Lee, D., & Khachemoune, A. (2011) Vitamins and cutaneous wound healing. *Journal of Wound Care, 20*(6), 287–293.

Sorenson, L. (2012) Wound healing and infection in surgery: The pathophysiological impact of smoking, smoking cessation, and nicotine replacement therapy: A systematic review. *Annals of Surgery, 255*(6):1069–1079.

Stechmiller, J. (2010). Understanding the role of nutrition and wound healing. *Nutrition in Clinical Practice, 25*(1), 61–68.

Thomas, J. (2008) In K. Cutting (Eds) *Advancing Your Practice: Understanding Wound Infection and the Role of Biofilm*. AAWC: Malvern, PA.

Tobin, C., & Sanger, J. R. (2014). Marjolin's ulcers: A case series and literature review. *Wounds, 26*(9), 248–254.

White-Chu, E., & Conner-Kerr, T. (2014). Overview of guidelines for the prevention and treatment of venous leg ulcers: A US perspective. *Journal of Multidisciplinary Healthcare, 7*, 111–117.

Widegerou, A. (2012). Deconstructing the stalled wound. *Wounds, 24*(3), 58–66.

Wolcott, R., Cutting, K., & Ruiz, J. (2008). Biofilms and delayed wound healing. In K. F. Cutting (Ed.), *Advancing your practice understanding wound infection and the role of biofilms*. Malvern, PA: AAWC.

Wound Ostomy Continence Nurse Society (WOCN). (2010). *Guideline for prevention and management of pressure ulcers*. Mount Laurel, NJ: WOCN.

Wound Ostomy Continence Nurse Society (WOCN). (2011). *Guideline for management of wounds in patients with lower-extremity venous disease*. Mount Laurel, NJ: WOCN.

STUDY QUESTIONS

1. The proliferative phase of healing is characterized by all of the following *except*:
   a. Formation of new blood vessels
   b. Hemostasis
   c. Collagen deposition
   d. Collagen lysis
   e. Wound contraction

2. Which of the following is an example of a wound that heals by primary intention?
   a. Diabetic foot ulcer
   b. Venous leg ulcer
   c. Open abdominal wound
   d. Sutured laceration
   e. Skin tear

3. Intrinsic factors that can delay healing include all of the following *except*:
   a. Unrelieved pressure
   b. Protein malnutrition
   c. Increased capillary fragility
   d. Preexisting cardiac disease

4. Which of the following is the best example of a full-thickness wound?
   a. Skin tear
   b. Abrasion
   c. Stage IV pressure ulcer
   d. Callous
   e. Stage II pressure ulcer

5. Which of the following is the best clinical indicator of progress toward healing?
   a. Increase in slough tissue
   b. Decrease in wound volume
   c. Increase in percent of granulation tissue
   d. A and C
   e. B and C

6. An example of nonselective wound debridement is removal of necrotic tissue using:
   a. Dakin solution
   b. High-pressure saline irrigation
   c. Wet-to-dry dressings
   d. None of the above
   e. All of the above

7. Dressings that promote autolytic debridement include all of the following *except*:
   a. Hydrocolloid dressings
   b. Alginate packing
   c. Wet-to-dry saline dressings
   d. Semipermeable film dressings
   e. Absorption dressings

8. Clinical signs of inadequate wound perfusion include:
   a. Dry, fibrotic wound surface
   b. Nocturnal pain
   c. Pale granulation tissue
   d. Nonhealing for at least 2 weeks
   e. A and C
   f. All of the above

9. Appropriate prevention of neuropathic ulcers includes all of the following *except*:
   a. Liberal moisturization of feet and interdigit spaces
   b. Avoiding over-the-counter corn and callus removers
   c. Redistributing body weight to minimize pedal pressure points
   d. Avoiding the use of heating pads when feet are cold

10. A deep neuropathic foot ulcer with exposed tendon at the base should be classified as which of the following?
    a. Deep partial-thickness ulcer
    b. Stage IV ulcer
    c. Stage III ulcer
    d. Full-thickness ulcer

Answers to Study Questions: 1.b, 2.d, 3.a, 4.c, 5.e, 6.e, 7.c, 8.f, 9.a, 10.d

OVERVIEW

Pressure Ulcer Definition

A pressure ulcer is localized injury to the skin and/or underlying tissue usually over a bony prominence, as a result of pressure, or pressure in combination with shear and/or friction. A number of contributing or confounding factors are also associated with pressure ulcers; the significance of these factors is yet to be elucidated.

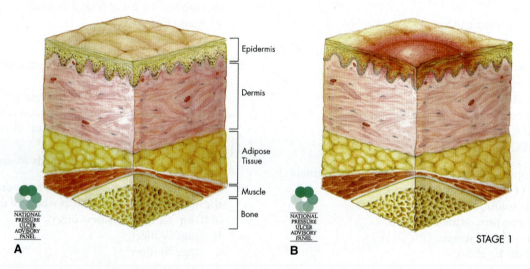

Stage I Pressure Ulcer

Intact skin with nonblanchable redness of a localized area usually over a bony prominence. Darkly pigmented skin may not have visible blanching; its color may differ from the surrounding area.

Stage I Further Description

The area may be painful, firm, soft, warmer, or cooler as compared to adjacent tissue. Stage I may be difficult to detect in individuals with dark skin tones. May indicate "at-risk" persons (a heralding sign of risk).

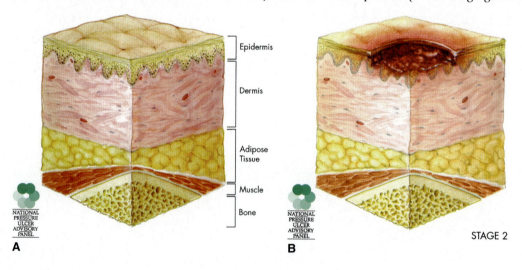

---

*Copyright and used with permission from Duke University Hospital.

Stage II Pressure Ulcer

Partial-thickness loss of dermis presenting as a shallow open ulcer with a red–pink wound bed, without slough. May also present as an intact or open/ruptured serum-filled blister.

Stage II Further Description

Presents as a shiny or dry shallow ulcer without slough or bruising.* This stage should not be used to describe skin tears, tape burns, perineal dermatitis, maceration, or excoriation.

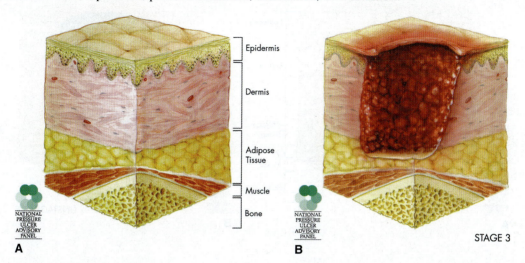

STAGE 3

A   B

Stage III Pressure Ulcer

Full-thickness tissue loss. Subcutaneous fat may be visible but bone, tendon, or muscle are not exposed. Slough may be present but does not obscure the depth of tissue loss. May include undermining and tunneling.

Stage III Further Description

The depth of a stage III pressure ulcer varies by anatomical location. The bridge of the nose, ear, occiput, and malleolus does not have subcutaneous tissue, and stage III ulcers can be shallow. In contrast, areas of significant adiposity can develop extremely deep stage III pressure ulcers. Bone/tendon is not visible or directly palpable.

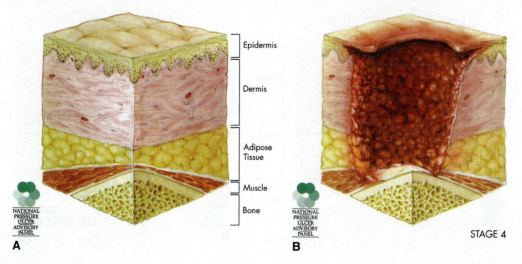

STAGE 4

A   B

Stage IV Pressure Ulcer

Full-thickness tissue loss with exposed bone, tendon, or muscle. Slough or eschar may be present on some parts of the wound bed. Often include undermining and tunneling.

*Bruising indicates suspected deep tissue injury.

Stage IV Further Description

The depth of a stage IV pressure ulcer varies by anatomical location. The bridge of the nose, ear, occiput, and malleolus does not have subcutaneous tissue and these ulcers can be shallow. Stage IV ulcers can extend into muscle and/or supporting structures (e.g., fascia, tendon, or joint capsule) making osteomyelitis possible. Exposed bone/tendon is visible or directly palpable.

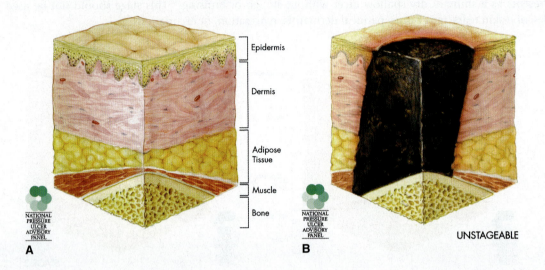

Unstageable Pressure Ulcer

Full-thickness tissue loss in which the base of the ulcer is covered by slough (yellow, tan, gray, green, or brown) and/or eschar (tan, brown, or black) in the wound bed.

Unstageable Further Description

Until enough slough and/or eschar is removed to expose the base of the wound, the true depth, and therefore stage, cannot be determined. Stable (dry, adherent, intact without erythema, or fluctuance) eschar on the heels serves as "the body's natural (biological) cover" and should not be removed.

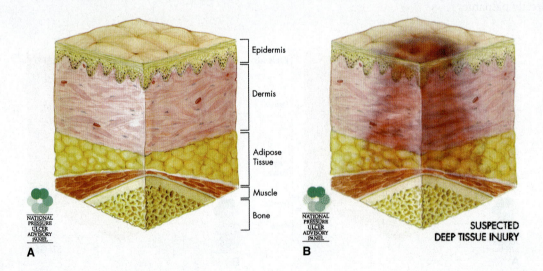

Suspected Deep Tissue Injury

Purple- or maroon-localized area of discolored intact skin or blood-filled blister due to damage of underlying soft tissue from pressure and/or shear. The area may be preceded by tissue that is painful, firm, mushy, boggy, warmer, or cooler as compared to adjacent tissue.

Suspected Deep Tissue Injury Further Description

Deep tissue injury may be difficult to detect in individuals with dark skin tones. Evolution may include a thin blister over a dark wound bed. The wound may further evolve and become covered by thin eschar. Evolution may be rapid exposing additional layers of tissue even with optimal treatment.

Indeterminant

The anatomic structure of mucous membranes is not compatible with the above staging system for pressure ulcers. Therefore, all pressure ulcers on any mucous membrane are defined as indeterminant per National Database of Nursing Quality Indicators.

Braden Scale for Predicting Pressure Sore Risk

Source: Barbara Braden and Nancy Bergstrom Copyright, 1988. Reprinted with permission.

Level: Interdependent—asterisked [*] items require an order from a health care practitioner licensed to prescribe medical therapy.

Policy Statement: To outline the care of the adult and pediatric patient at risk for the development of a pressure ulcer and/or with a pressure ulcer

A. Consult Wound Management Consult Service for:
  1. All pressure ulcers (stage II, III, and IV, unstageable, suspected deep tissue injury, or indeterminant) noted on admission
  2. All pressure ulcers that develop during admission
  3. Any skin deterioration after 48 to 72 hours of implementation of Advanced Skin Care Algorithm. Consider a consult for patients at risk for pressure ulcer development.
B. Assessment (refer to Braden Risk Assessment with Interventions, below).
  1. Document Braden score (8 years and older) or Braden Q score (7 years and younger) on admission and daily. Implement the pressure ulcer prevention and/or treatment plan of care for any subscale ≤ 3 and/or total Braden Scale Score ≤ 18 or Braden Q Scale score.
  2. Complete a head to toe skin assessment on admission and at least every shift.
      a. Be sure to look under any medical device (e.g., abdominal binder, TED hose, sequential compression sleeves).
      b. Reassess bony prominences with each dependent turn.
  3. Assess and document characteristics of pressure ulcer(s) on admission and with each dressing change:
      a. Location
      b. Dimensions: length, width, depth (recommend weekly)
      c. Characteristics of drainage
      d. Presence of granulation tissue or necrotic tissue (slough or eschar)
      e. Undermining/sinus tracts
      f. Surrounding skin
  4. Assess need for pain control during wound care procedures.
C. Self-concept.
  1. Encourage patient to express concerns/feelings regarding pressure ulcer.
  2. Reinforce and/or teach appropriate coping strategies to patient/caregiver.
  3. Collaborate with the health care team to provide stress management/coping skills.
D. Knowledge deficit.
  1. Institute teaching protocols as indicated.
      a. Prevention of pressure ulcers
      b. Treatment of pressure ulcers

Reportable Conditions

1. Temperature greater than 101.5°F
2. Increased size or stage of pressure ulcer
3. Less than 50%="" of="" po="" intake="" for="" 3="">
4. Increased pain associated with pressure ulcer
5. Change in characteristics of drainage indicating infection

Braden Pressure Ulcer Risk Assessment

Sensory Perception
Braden: Ability to respond meaningfully to pressure-related discomfort
Braden Q: The ability to respond in a developmentally appropriate way to pressure-related discomfort.

Braden/Braden Q Subscale	Patient Examples	Interventions

1. *Completely Limited*: Unresponsive (does not moan, flinch or grasp) to painful stimuli, due to diminished level of consciousness or sedation. OR limited ability to feel pain over most of body surface.	• Quadriplegia
	• Head injury
	• Anoxic brain injury
	• Sedated & paralyzed
	• Comatose
	• RASS Score of –5
		1. Turn and reposition trunk and limbs every 2 hours. Use microshifts only if patient unable to tolerate full repositioning
		2. Position extremities to avoid pressure on limb
		3. Avoid extreme hot or cold packs
		4. When needed, place hypothermia blankets over the patient
		5. Turn only slightly to side (not on trochanter) and brace with pillow
		6. Position top leg slightly posterior to bottom leg with a pillow between legs
		7. Reposition/Pad medical devices on/in the patient with above turning (e.g., rotate ear pulse oximeter with each turn)
		8. Retape nasoenteric tubes daily or use appropriate NG securement device. Tape such that the tube "floats" in the center of the nostril
		9. Implement the Tracheostomy Protocol for prevention of trach related pressure ulcers
		10. Remove TED hose at least once per shift for 1 hour
		11. Apply ear protectors (Ear Mates) for patients:
		  a. wearing a nasal cannula for > 24 hours;
		  b. wearing a nasal cannula who have an ear pressure ulcer;
		  c. wearing a nasal cannula who have fragile skin (e.g., skin tears)
		12. Provide the appropriate pressure distribution surface based on the Specialty Bed Algorithm (Insert Link)
		13. Provide pressure reduction device under head for patients at high risk for developing occipital ulcers, (i.e., patients that cannot be turned q 2 hours due to hemodynamic instability, unstable fractures, surgical flap instability, trauma, unstable gas exchange)
		14. Elevate heels off bed with pillow under calf or heel device.
		15. Apply heel protectors for patients with:
		  a. An existing heel pressure ulcer
		  b. Braden score <18
		  c. Immobility.
		  d. Do not turn orders regardless of bed surface

2. *Very Limited*: Responds only to painful stimuli. Cannot communicate discomfort except by moaning or restlessness. OR has a sensory impairment which limits the ability to feel pain or discomfort over half of body.	• Partially sedated • Moderate dementia • Epidural analgesia • Paraplegic • RASS score of –4	
3. *Slightly Limited*: Responds to verbal commands, but cannot always communicate discomfort or need to be turned. OR has some sensory impairment which limits ability to feel pain or discomfort in 1 or 2 extremities.	• Hemiplegia • Hemiparesis • Dementia	
4. *No Impairment*: Responds to verbal commands. Has no sensory deficit which would limit ability to	Alert and oriented RASS score of –1,0 or +1	No interventions may be required

MOISTURE: Degree to which skin is exposed to moisture

Braden/Braden Q Subscale	Patient Examples	Interventions
1. *Constantly Moist*: Skin is kept moist almost constantly by perspiration, urine, drainage, etc. Dampness is detected every time patient is moved or turned.	• Incontinent of urine/ stool with pad change every 2 hours when turned • Copious wound drainage • Anasarca • Weeping skin or tears	1. Implement the Skin Care Protocol (Insert link) 2. Avoid use of diapers for bedfast adult patients 3. Implement the Fecal Incontinence protocol (Insert link) 4. Assess for reversible causes of urinary or fecal incontinence 5. Consider consult with dietician for potential dietary cause and/or treatment interventions 6. Implement the Skin Tear Protocol (Insert link) 7. Consider applying an external urine containment device on adult males incontinent of urine 8. Consider consult with Ostomy team to contain copious amounts of wound drainage 9. Evaluate skin folds for fungal dermatitis or risk for skin breakdown 10 Collaborate with the physician team for antifungal treatment 10. Consider placing Interdry AG into anterior skin folds 11. Use only breathable underpads on low air loss and air fluidized surfaces 12. Secure the urinary catheter to the anterior thigh using a catheter securement device
2. *Very Moist*: Skin is often, but not always, moist. Linen must be changed at least once a shift *Braden Q: Skin is often, but not always, most. Linen must be changed at least every 8 hours.*	• Incontinent of urine or stools every 8h • Linen change every 8h • Moderate amount weeping	
3. *Occasionally Moist*: Skin is occasionally moist, requiring an extra linen change approximately once a day *Braden Q: Skin is occasionally moist, requiring linen change every 12 hours.*	• Foley but incontinent of stool • Rectal tube, but leaks periodically • Skin tears leaking small amount	
4. *Rarely Moist*: Skin is usually dry; linen requires changing only at routine intervals *Braden Q: Skin is usually dry, routine diaper changes; linen only requires changing every 24 hours.*	• Incontinent of formed stool once daily • Wound contained by pouch or dressing	No interventions may be required

MOBILITY: Ability to change and control body position

Braden/Braden Q Subscale	Patient Examples	Interventions
1. *Completely Immobile*: Does not make even slight changes in body or extremity position without assistance.	• Quadriplegia • Head injury • Sedated or paralyzed • Comatose • RASS Score –5	1. Provide appropriate interventions from Sensory Perception and Activity subscales 2. Instruct the patient/family regarding the importance of turning and repositioning every 2 hours 3. Keep HOB as low as tolerated unless medically contraindicated. 4. Document patient/family refusal to turn and reposition 5. Consider obtaining an overbed trapeze to facilitate bed mobility 6. Position carefully with any contractures (pillows between bony prominences)
2. *Very Limited*: Makes occasional slight changes in body or extremity position but unable to make frequent or significant changes independently. Unable to turn without assistance of at least one person. *Braden Q: Makes occasional slight changes in body or extremity position but unable to completely turn self independently.*	• Sedated, but not paralyzed	
3. *Slightly Limited*: Makes frequent though slight changes in body or extremity position independently.	• Can assist with turning • Unable to turn self completely	
4. *No Limitations*: Makes major or frequent changes in position without assistance.	• Paraplegic who can turn self in bed	No interventions may be required

ACTIVITY: Degree of physical activity

Braden/Braden Q Subscale	Patient Examples	Interventions

1. *Bedfast*: Confined to bed.	• Post procedure bedrest (cardiac cath or post op)
	• Quadriplegia or paraplegia that does not use wheelchair
	• Trauma related immobility
		1. Refer to Interventions for Sensory Perception for pressure redistribution interventions
		2. Facilitate Physical Therapy consult as indicated
		3. Consider ROM every 4 hours
		4. Maximize activity while in chair:
		  a. Reposition in chair every 1hr
		  b. Encourage position change every 15–20 min, if possible
		  c. limit time in chair if sacral, ischial or buttock pressure ulcer present (recommend chair time not to exceed 1 hour)
		  d. Provide pressure redistribution chair device
		5. Encourage to ambulate as much as possible

2. *Chairfast*: Ability to walk severely limited or nonexistent. Cannot bear own weight and/or must be assisted into chair or wheelchair.	• Receiving PT • Deconditioned re disease +/ or hospital stay • Up in wheelchair	
3. *Walks Occasionally*: Walks occasionally during day, but for very short distances, with or without assistance. Spends majority of each shift in bed or chair.	• Post-op recovery period • Ambulates with PT	
4. Walks Frequently: Walks outside the room at least twice a day and inside room at least once every 2 hours during waking hours. *Braden Q* 4. All patients too young to ambulate or walks frequently: Walks outside the room at least twice a day and inside room at least once every 2 hours during waking hours.	• Bathroom privileges • Ambulates with minimal or no assistance	No interventions may be required

NUTRITION: Usual food intake pattern

Braden/Braden Q Subscale	Patient Examples	Interventions

1. *Very Poor*: Never eats a complete meal. Rarely eats more than 1/3 of any food offered. Eats 2 servings or less of protein (meat or dairy products) per day. Takes fluids poorly. Does not take a liquid dietary supplement OR is NPO and/or maintained on clear liquids or IVs for more than 5 days.
Braden Q: NPO and/or maintained on clear liquids, or IVs for more than 5 days OR albumin <2.5 mg/dL OR never eats a complete meal. Rarely eats more than half of any food offered. Protein intake includes only 2 servings of meat or dairy products per day. Takes fluids poorly. Does not take a liquid dietary supplement.
	• Eats <30% meal
	• Refuses supplements
	• Albumin/Prealbumin decreased
		1. Obtain weight on admission and at least weekly
		2. Monitor food intake with each meal
		3. Recommend a consult with Dietician for patients with:
		  a. stage III/IV, unstageable and/or Suspected Deep Tissue Injury
		  b. subscale <2.
		4. Collaborate with physician team to obtain a appropriate labs to evaluate nutritional status.
		5. Collaborate with the Dietician/Provider to provide multivitamin and/or nutrition supplements
		6. Maximize the patient's ability to eat:
		  a. encourage patient to eat
		  b. assist into a sitting or chair position for meals
		  c. encourage family to visit during meal times
		  d. feed patients who are unable to feed themselves
		  e. provide hand washing prior to eating
		7. Encourage PO fluids (adults only) unless contraindicated

Braden/Braden Q Subscale	Patient Examples	Interventions
2. *Probably Inadequate*: Rarely eats a complete meal and generally eats only about 1/2 of any food offered. Protein intake includes only 3 servings of meat or dairy products per day. Occasionally will take a dietary supplement OR receives less than optimum amount of liquid diet or tube feeding. *Braden Q: 2. Inadequate: Is on a liquid diet or tube feedings/TPN, which provide inadequate calories and minerals for age OR albumin <3 mg/dL OR rarely eats a complete meal*	• Takes <50% meal • Not up to goal on tube feeding.	

FRICTION AND SHEAR

Braden Q: Friction occurs when skin moves against support surfaces. Shear occurs when skin and adjacent bony surface slide across one another.

Braden/Braden Q Subscale	Patient Examples	Interventions
Braden Q: 1. *Significant Problem: Spasticity, contractures, itching or agitation leads to almost constant thrashing and friction.* 1. *Problem*: Requires moderate to maximum assistance in moving. Complete lifting without sliding against sheets is impossible. Frequently slides down in bed or chair requiring frequent repositioning with maximum assistance. Spasticity, contractures or agitation lead to almost constant friction.		1. Keep HOB as low as tolerated unless medically contraindicated. 2. Slightly elevate knee gatch when HOB elevated 3. Use adequate personnel to turn, reposition patient 4. Use pull sheet/underpad to reposition patient 5. Use lift equipment per Minimal Manual Lift Environment Policy 6. Consider obtaining an overbed trapeze to facilitate bed mobility 7. Apply moisturizing cream to skin 8. Consider applying barrier products to bony prominences
Braden Q: 2. *Problem*: Requires moderate to maximum assistance in moving. Complete lifting without sliding against sheets is impossible. Frequently slides down in bed or chair, requiring frequent repositioning with maximum assistance. 2. *Potential Problem*: Moves freely or requires minimum assistance. During a move, skin probably slides to some extent against sheets, chair restraint or other devices. Maintains relative good position in chair or bed most of the time but occasionally		

Tissue Perfusion and Oxygenation (Braden Q Only)

Braden/Braden Q Subscale	Patient Examples	Interventions
1. *Extremely compromised*: Hypotensive (MAP < 50 mm Hg; <40 mm Hg in a newborn) or the patient does not physically tolerate position changes 2. *Compromised*: Normotensive, oxygen saturation may be <95%; hgb < 10 mg/dL; cap refill may be >2 seconds; serum pH is <7.40 3. *Adequate*: Normotensive; oxygen saturation may be <95%; hgb may be <10 mg/dL; cap refill may be >2 seconds; serum pH is normal		1. Refer to Interventions for Sensory Perception for pressure redistribution interventions
4. *Excellent*: Normotensive; O2 sats >95%; normal hgb; cap refill <2 seconds		No interventions required

BIBLIOGRAPHY

Baranoski, S., & Ayello, E. (2004). *Wound care essentials: Practice principles.* Philadelphia, PA: Lippincott Williams & Wilkins.

Bergstrom, N., Braden, B. J., Laguzza, A., & Holman, V. (1987). The Braden Scale for predicting pressure sore risk. *Nursing Research, 36,* 205–210.

Brem, H., & Lyder, C. (2004). Protocol for the successful treatment of pressure ulcers. *The American Journal of Surgery, 188*(Suppl), 9s–17s.

European Pressure Ulcer Advisory Panel and National Pressure Ulcer Advisory Panel. (2009). *Prevention and treatment of pressure ulcers: Clinical practice guideline.* Washington, DC: National Pressure Ulcer Advisory Panel.

Hess, C. (2005). *Clinical guide: Wound care* (5th ed.). Philadelphia, PA: Lippincott Williams & Wilkins.

Krasner, D., & Kane, D. (1997). *Chronic wound care: A clinical source book for health care professionals* (2nd ed.). Philadelphia, PA: Health Management Publications.

NDNQI. (2011). *Guidelines for data collection and submission on quarterly indicators.* Kansas City, KS: KU School of Nursing.

Pressure Ulcer Stages Revised by the NPUAP. (2007). http://npuap.org/pr2.htm

Wound, Ostomy and Continence Nurses Society. (2010). *Guideline for prevention and management of pressure ulcers.* Glenview, IL: WOCN.

APPENDIX B Advanced Skin Care Protocol*

Purpose: Promote and protect skin integrity across a high-risk population

Supportive Data: Patients with a Braden Score of less than 18 or Braden Q less than 16 are considered at risk for skin breakdown. Risk factors associated with altered skin integrity include moisture, dry cracked skin, and shear/friction forces. Promoting clean, dry, supple skin may deter more serious skin injuries such as pressure ulcers, skin tears, and incontinence-associated dermatitis. All patients identified at risk may benefit from the use of skin care products at the appropriate times.

Level: Independent

Equipment	No-rinse bath additive	No-rinse moisturizing cleanser
	Wash cloths	Moisturizing cream
	Extra protective cream	Protective ointment

Content

ASSESSMENT

1. Identify patients at risk for skin breakdown with Braden Scores of less than 18 or Braden Q less than 16 on admission and daily.
2. Assess skin integrity for excessive dryness, flaking, or callus every shift.
3. Assess skin exposed to moisture (urine, feces, and other body fluids) every shift:
   a. Color (pink, red, erythema)
   b. Erosions
   c. Wounds
   d. Maceration/denudation
   e. Fissure

CARE

4. Clean skin with no-rinse bath additive daily and PRN. Avoid use of soaps and detergents.
5. Follow the Incontinence Skin Care Algorithm for selection of skin protection and treatment (include link).

---

*Copyright and used with permission from Duke University Hospital.

6. Apply moisturizing cream to all at-risk patients based on their Braden/Braden Q score and patients with dry skin.
7. Avoid the use of diapers with patients that are confined to bed.
8. Avoid the use of plastic-lined, disposable underpads (blue chux).
9. Avoid use of powder in skin folds.
10. Use one underpad for all incontinent patients.
11. Use airflow pads on all low air loss and air-fluidized surfaces.
12. Consult wound management for patients with skin deterioration after implementation of Incontinence Skin Care Algorithm.
13. Utilize condom catheter containment device for incontinent adult males.
14. Implement the Fecal Incontinence Protocol (Adult) as indicated for fecal incontinence (add link).

Documentation
- Risk assessment (Braden/Braden Q) daily
- Implementation of Skin Care Protocol

Reportable Conditions
- Increased redness, progressing erosions, or wounds
- Increased pruritus and occurrence of a macular red rash with satellite lesions
- Temperature greater than 38.5°C

Resources

Patient Education
- Assess the patient and/or caregivers' readiness and ability to learn.
- Instruct patient and/or caregivers on appropriate skin care.

BIBLIOGRAPHY

Beckman, D., Schoonhoven, L., Verhaeghe, S., Heyneman, A., & Defloor, T. (2009). Prevention and treatment of incontinence-associated dermatitis: Literature review. *Journal of Advanced Nursing, 65*(6), 1141–1154.

Doughty, D., Junkin, J., Kurz, P., Selekof, J., Gray, M., Fader, M., …, Logan, S. (2012). Incontinence-associated dermatitis: Consensus statements, evidence-based guidelines for prevention and treatment, and current challenges. *Journal of Wound, Ostomy and Continence Nursing, 39*(3), 303–315.

European Pressure Ulcer Advisory Panel and National Pressure Ulcer Advisory Panel. (2009). *Prevention and treatment of pressure ulcers: Quick reference guide.* Washington, DC: National Pressure Ulcer Advisory Panel.

Gray, M., Ratliff, C., & Donovan, M. (2002). Perineal skin care for the incontinent patient. *Advances in Skin and Wound Care, 15*(4), 170–178.

Nix, D., & Ermer-Seltun, J. (2004). A review of perineal skin care protocol and skin barrier product use. *Ostomy/Wound Management, 50*(12), 59–67.

Wound, Ostomy and Continence Nurses Society. (2010). *Guideline for prevention and management of pressure ulcers.* Glenview, IL: WOCN.

APPENDIX C   Specialty Bed Selection Protocol and Algorithm*

Purpose: To describe the care of an adult or pediatric patient on a specialty bed

Level: Independent

Supportive Data
Specialty beds are primarily used.
a. In the prevention and treatment of pressure ulcers, including postsurgical treatment
b. For morbidly obese patients (refer to Bariatric Care Protocol)
c. Prevention of pneumonia (refer to Continuous Lateral Rotation Therapy Protocol)

They include:
a. Air-fluidized surfaces, for example, Clinitron Rite Height
b. Bariatric bed, for example, Sizewise Mighty Air, Sizewise Big Turn 2
c. Continuous lateral rotation therapy (CLRT) module, for example, Hill-Rom TotalCareSpO2RT Bed with rotation module and Stryker Intouch with XPRT surface
   A physician order is not required for placement and discontinuation of a specialty bed.

Content
A. Assessment.
   1. Assess for appropriate specialty bed selection (DUHS Specialty Bed Algorithm).
   2. Reassess the indication for specialty bed at minimum of every 7 days.
B. Interventions.
   1. Enter nursing order for specialty bed.
      a. In DHIS/CPOE at DUH
      b. Call WOCN and/or operations administrator at DRH.
      c. Call patient care equipment technician #5850 at DRAH. NOTE: Expect delivery within 2 hours. The technician will call to verify order of the bed.
   2. Use only airflow pads under patients on low air loss and air-fluidized surfaces. Do not use diapers, chux, or reusable underpads.
   3. Turn every 2 hours and more frequently as indicated for pulmonary toilet related to immobility.
   4. Confirm access of a call light. Call material services to obtain a handheld call light if not in the room.
   5. Assess temperature settings on air-fluidized surface. Adjust for patient comfort.
   6. Call specialty bed technician for any problems with the bed function, for example, deflation of surface and leaking "beads." If bed is not functional, obtain replacement bed.
   7. Obtain an overbed trapeze to assist with patient mobility as needed.
   8. Apply appropriate cream to patients on air-fluidized therapy. This therapy can result in excessive dry skin.

---

*Copyright and used with permission from Duke University Hospital.

Duke University Hospital Specialty Bed Algorithm

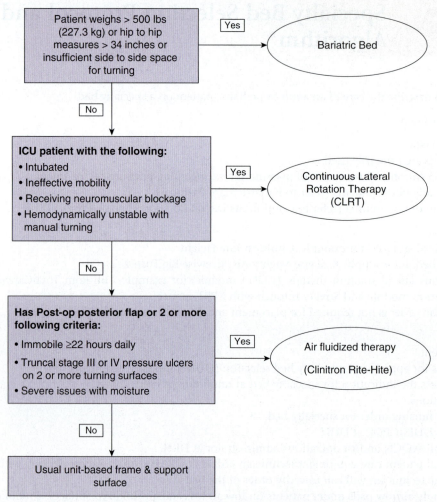

Copyright and used with permission of Duke University Hospital

BIBLIOGRAPHY

Baranoski, S., & Ayello, E. A. (2008). *Wound care essentials: Practice principles* (2nd ed.). Philadelphia, PA: Lippincott Williams & Wilkins.

European Pressure Ulcer Advisory Panel and National Pressure Ulcer Advisory Panel. (2009). *Prevention and treatment of pressure ulcers: Clinical practice guideline*. Washington, DC: National Pressure Ulcer Advisory Panel.

Hess, C. (2007). *Clinical guide: Skin and wound care* (6th ed.). Philadelphia, PA: Lippincott Williams & Wilkins.

Krasner, D., Sibbald, R., Woo, K., & Norton, L. (2012). Interprofessional perspectives on individualized wound device product selection. *Wound Source*, 3–16.

Krasner, D. (2007). *Chronic wound management: A clinical source book for healthcare professionals* (4th ed.). Pennsylvania, PA: Health Management Publications, Inc.

WOCN (Wound, Ostomy, and Continence Nurses Society). (2003). *Guideline for prevention and management of pressure ulcers #2WOCN clinical practice series*. Glenview, Ill.: WOCN Society.

Definitions

Skin tears occur most commonly on the arms and legs of older adults due to the weakening of the epidermal–dermal attachment and fragility of the capillaries resulting in senile purpura. Skin tears can result from trauma to the skin from minor friction or tape removal. Certain conditions also predispose patients to skin tears (long-term steroid use and sun exposure).

Level: Interdependent—asterisked [*] items require an order from a health care practitioner licensed to prescribe medical therapy.

Personnel: All RNs and LPNs

Competencies/Skills

Required Resources

Moisturizing cream (SAP# 313129 DUH, DRH, DRAH) and cotton-tipped applicator
Silicone foam dressing (4x4 SAP # 326961) and Xeroform gauze (SAP # 12804)
Rolled gauze
Self-adherent wrap (SAP # 318837)
Wound closure strips

Policy Statement

Purpose: Prevention and treatment of skin tears in adult and pediatric population

Content

A. Assessment.
  1. Identify patient's risk for skin tears daily.
  2. Assess wound on development and with each dressing change for:
      a. Color of wound base
      b. Size
      c. Location
      d. Presence/viability of epidermal skin flap
      e. Quality of surrounding skin—fragility of skin
      f. Characteristics of drainage
      g. Signs of infection
B. Care.
  1. Implement the Advanced Skin Care Protocol.
  2. Avoid use of tape and other adhesives on skin (transparent film, hydrocolloid).
  3. Spray skin with no-sting barrier film before applying all adhesives except silicone products.
  4. Use rolled gauze or self-adherent wrap to secure dressings to arms and legs.
  5. Provide topical dressing per the Skin Tear Algorithm.
  6. Consult wound management for skin tears greater than 3 cm in adults and greater than 2 cm in pediatrics 7 years and younger.
C. Patient education.
  1. Assess the patient and/or caregivers' readiness and ability to learn.
  2. Instruct patient and/or caregivers on appropriate preventive skin care.
  3. Instruct patient and/or caregivers on selected dressing change.

Reportable Conditions

  1. Increased size of wound
  2. Any sign of wound infection

---

*Copyright and used with permission from Duke University Hospital.

Duke University Health System Skin Tear Algorithm

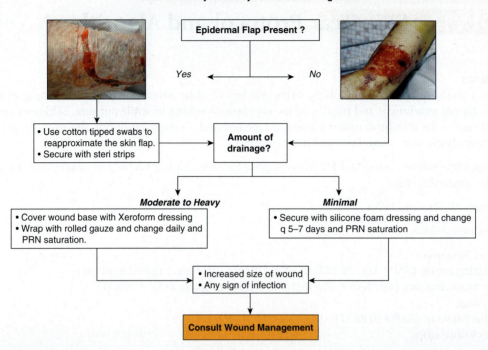

BIBLIOGRAPHY

Milne, C. T., & Corbett, L. Q. (2005). A new option in the treatment of skin tears for the institutionalized resident: Formulated 2-octylcyanoacrylate topical bandage. *Geriatric Nursing, 25*(5), 321–325.

Patient Safety Advisory. (2006). Skin Tears: The Clinical Challenge. *3*(3), 1–8.

Ratliff, C. R., & Fletcher, K. R. (2007). Skin tears: A review of the evidence to support prevention and treatment. *Ostomy/Wound Management, 53*(3), 32–42.

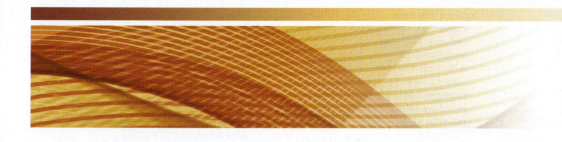

INDEX

Note: Page numbers followed by *f*, *t*, and *b* indicate figures, tables, and boxed text, respectively.